Laboratory Medicine

a LANGE medical book

Laboratory Medicine

The Diagnosis of Disease in the Clinical Laboratory

Edited by

Michael Laposata, MD, PhD

Edward and Nancy Fody Professor and
Executive Vice Chair of Pathology
Pathologist-in-Chief
Vanderbilt University Hospital
Professor of Medicine
Vanderbilt University School of Medicine
Nashville, Tennessee

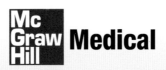

New York   Chicago   San Francisco   Lisbon   London   Madrid   Mexico City
Milan   New Delhi   San Juan   Seoul   Singapore   Sydney   Toronto

Laboratory Medicine: The Diagnosis of Disease in the Clinical Laboratory

Copyright © 2010 by The McGraw-Hill Companies, Inc. All rights reserved. Printed in China. Except as permitted under the United States Copyright Act of 1976, no part of this publication may be reproduced or distributed in any form or by any means, or stored in a data base or retrieval system, without the prior written permission of the publisher.

5 6 7 8 9 0 CTP/CTP 14

ISBN 978-0-07-162674-3
MHID 0-07-162674-3

This book was set in Minion Pro by Thomson Digital.
The editors were Michael Weitz and Robert Pancotti.
The production supervisor was Sherri Souffrance.
The illustration manager was Armen Ovsepyan.
Project management was provided by Aakriti Kathuria, Thomson Digital.
The cover art director was Margaret Webster-Shapiro.
The text designer was Elise Lansdon; the cover designer was Ty Nowicki.
Cover photos:
Small photo at top left: Color-enhanced transmission electron micrograph (TEM) of the Marburg virus. (Credit: Scott Camazine / Photo Researchers, Inc.)
Small photo at center: Umbilical cord blood stem cells. Technician holding blood stem cells harvested from a donated human placenta and umbilical cord. (Credit: Tek Image / Photo Researchers, Inc.)
Small photo at bottom: Red blood cells. (Credit: Steve Gschmeissner / Photo Researchers, Inc.)
Large background photo: Blood analysis. Part of a machine for automated analysis of donated blood. (Credit: Tek Image / Photo Researchers, Inc.)
China Translation & Printing Services, Ltd. was printer and binder.

Library of Congress Cataloging-in-Publication Data

Laboratory medicine : the diagnosis of disease in the clinical laboratory/editor, Michael Laposata.
    p. ; cm.
  Includes bibliographical references and index.
  ISBN-13: 978-0-07-162674-3 (pbk. : alk. paper)
  ISBN-10: 0-07-162674-3 (pbk. : alk. paper)
1. Diagnosis, Laboratory. I. Laposata, Michael.
  [DNLM: 1. Clinical Laboratory Techniques. 2. Diagnosis, Differential.
  3. Laboratory Techniques and Procedures. 4. Pathology, Clinical—methods.
  QY 25 L12355 2010]
  RB37.L27523 2010
  616.07'5—dc22
                    2009044316

McGraw-Hill books are available at special quantity discounts to use as premiums and sales promotions, or for use in corporate training programs. To contact a representative, please e-mail us at bulksales@mcgraw-hill.com.

My three wonderful children, Michael, Joe, and Maria, continue to inspire me to think about what I can do to make a difference for someone else. Without their love, this textbook would not have been created.

Key Features of
Laboratory Medicine

A complete full-color guide to selecting the correct laboratory test and accurately interpreting the results—covering the entire field of clinical pathology

- 36 clinical laboratory methods presented in easy-to-understand illustrations which include information on the expense and complexity of the assays

- More than 200 tables and full-color algorithms encapsulate important information and facilitate understanding

- Consistent presentation: chapters begin with a brief description of the disorder followed by a discussion of laboratory diagnosis that includes tables detailing the evaluation of the disorder

- Valuable learning aids in each chapter, including learning objectives, chapter outlines, and a general introduction

- Full-color blood-smear micrographs demonstrate common abnormal morphologies of red blood cells

- Logical systems-based organization parallels most textbooks

- 13-page table of Clinical Laboratory Reference Values showing the conversions between U.S. and SI units for each value

Blood-smear micrographs demonstrate common abnormal morphologies of red blood cells

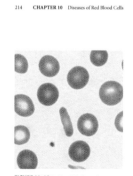

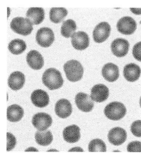

FIGURE 10–15 Peripheral blood smear from a patient with large numbers of elliptocytes.

FIGURE 10–16 A peripheral blood smear stained with Wright's stain showing a reticulocyte.

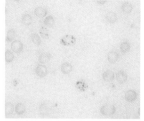

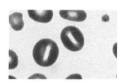

FIGURE 10–17 Two reticulocytes revealed by supravital staining.

FIGURE 10–18 A peripheral blood smear from a patient with stomatocytes.

Antimicrobial sensitivity tests

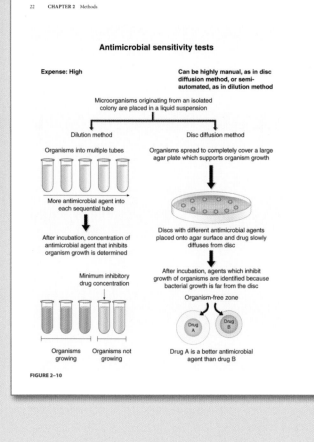

Expense: High

Can be highly manual, as in disc diffusion method, or semi-automated, as in dilution method

Microorganisms originating from an isolated colony are placed in a liquid suspension

Dilution method → Disc diffusion method

Organisms into multiple tubes

More antimicrobial agent into each sequential tube

After incubation, concentration of antimicrobial agent that inhibits organism growth is determined

Minimum inhibitory drug concentration

Organisms growing / Organisms not growing

Organisms spread to completely cover a large agar plate which supports organism growth

Discs with different antimicrobial agents placed onto agar surface and drug slowly diffuses from disc

After incubation, agents which inhibit growth of organisms are identified because bacterial growth is far from the disc

Organism-free zone

Drug A / Drug B

Drug A is a better antimicrobial agent than drug B

FIGURE 2–10

---

200 tables and full-color algorithms encapsulate important information

---

TABLE 5–23   Evaluation for Tuberculosis (TB)

	Pulmonary Tuberculosis	CNS Tuberculosis	Genitourinary Tuberculosis	Disseminated Tuberculosis
Clinical findings	Symptoms range from none to fever with productive cough and dyspnea; hemoptysis indicates presence of advanced disease	Fever, unremitting headache, nausea, and malaise; in the United States, elderly are frequently affected; where TB is common, it primarily affects children aged 1–5 years	Most common site for extrapulmonary TB is the kidney; dysuria, frequency, and hematuria are common; women may present with a chronic pelvic inflammatory process, menstrual irregularities, or sterility; men may present with an enlarging scrotal mass	More likely to occur in HIV-positive individuals; may be present without miliary pattern in chest radiographs; patient may present with fever, weight loss, and anorexia
Tests				
PPD	In the presence of compatible radiologic and clinical findings, a positive PPD in an unvaccinated patient suggests TB	In the presence of compatible radiologic and clinical findings, a positive PPD in an unvaccinated patient suggests TB	In the presence of compatible radiologic and clinical findings, a positive PPD in an unvaccinated patient suggests TB	In the presence of compatible radiologic and clinical findings, a positive PPD in an unvaccinated patient suggests TB
Microscopy	Acid-fast bacilli in sputum smears permit rapid diagnosis; sensitivity is variable, but increases with the number of specimens examined (up to 4)	Acid-fast bacilli in smears of CSF lead to identification of 20% or less of CNS TB cases; sputum samples also should be tested	Both urine and sputum samples should be examined, as a smear from a urine sample may not have detectable acid-fast bacilli	Urine, lymph node, liver, bone marrow, and sputum smears have low sensitivity for organism detection
Mycobacterial culture	Culture from sputum specimen on liquid and solid media is the most sensitive method in current use; for pediatric cases, multiple gastric lavage specimens can be used; liquid culture with DNA probe hybridization also enables TB confirmation	Culture of CSF may reveal organisms in CNS TB cases	Urine specimens for mycobacterial culture are positive in 60%–80% of cases, though it is more likely to be positive in men than in women	Culture may be performed using bone marrow, liver, urine, and sputum specimens
Nucleic acid amplification	May be useful for rapid diagnostic confirmation of specimens negative by direct examination	May provide a rapid diagnosis but cannot replace culture	Utility not well defined	Sputum specimens may be used for amplification
Other findings	Pleural fluid, if present, is an exudate (not a transudate) with mononuclear cells	With lumbar puncture, there may be an increased opening pressure and 100–1,000 cells/μL of CSF (mostly mononuclear cells) and elevated CSF protein	In the appropriate clinical setting, TB may be considered if negative routine urine cultures show WBCs in acid urine	Impaired function of infected organs may be noted in routine laboratory tests of those organ systems
Radiology	Chest radiograph may detect adenopathy, effusion, or nodule in HIV-infected patients, the chest radiograph is more likely to be normal	If TB is established in the brain, it may produce a mass, or "tuberculoma," visible by CT scan	40%–75% of cases have a positive chest radiograph; other radiologic studies are not very useful	Chest radiograph may be normal and repeat testing may prove useful; CT scan or MRI may be useful to detect TB in extrapulmonary sites such as the brain or vertebrae
Anatomic pathology	Caseating granulomas may be observed in biopsies of enlarged lymph nodes	Biopsy may be diagnostic	Renal biopsy may be helpful to identify genitourinary lesions	If bronchial washings do not provide diagnosis, granulomas in bone marrow or liver biopsy may be diagnostic

CNS, central nervous system; CSF, cerebrospinal fluid; CT, computed tomography; MRI, magnetic resonance imaging; PPD, purified protein derivative.

The Endocrine System

Michael Laposata, Samir L. Aleryani, and Alison Woodworth

C H A P T E R

22

LEARNING OBJECTIVES
1. Learn the physiology and biochemistry of the relevant hormones and other important mediators.
2. Understand the laboratory tests used in the diagnosis of the more commonly encountered disorders.
3. Identify the clinical disorders associated with each of the endocrine glands and the role of specific laboratory tests in their diagnosis.

CHAPTER OUTLINE

Valuable learning aids are included in each chapter

Contents

Authors

Yash Pal Agrawal, MD, PhD
Associate Professor of Clinical Pathology and Laboratory Medicine, Weill Cornell Medical College; Director, Central Laboratory; Director, Point of Care Testing Services, Department of Pathology and Laboratory Medicine, New York Presbyterian Hospital, New York, New York

Samir L. Aleryani, PhD
Instructor of Pathology, Medical Director, Laboratory Support Services, Department of Pathology, Vanderbilt University Medical Center, Nashville, Tennessee

Fred S. Apple, PhD
Medical Director, Clinical Laboratories, Hennepin County Medical Center; Professor, Laboratory Medicine and Pathology, University of Minnesota School of Medicine, Minneapolis, Minnesota

Sheila Dawling, PhD, CChem, FRSC
Associate Professor of Pathology, Vanderbilt University School of Medicine; Director, Toxicology/TDM Laboratory; Associate Director, Clinical Chemistry, Vanderbilt University Medical Center, Nashville, Tennessee

D. Robert Dufour, MD, FCAP, FACB
Consultant, Pathology and Hepatology, Veterans Affairs Medical Center; Emeritus Professor of Pathology, The George Washington University Medical Center, Washington, District of Columbia

Karin E. Finberg, MD, PhD
Medical Instructor in Pathology, Department of Pathology, Duke University Medical Center, Durham, North Carolina

Jacqueline J. Haas, MD
Staff Pathologist, Clinical Pathology Associates; Laboratory Medical Director, St. David's Medical Center, Austin, Texas

Michael Laposata, MD, PhD
Edward and Nancy Fody Professor and Executive Vice Chair of Pathology, Pathologist-in-Chief, Vanderbilt University Hospital; Professor of Medicine, Vanderbilt University School of Medicine, Nashville, Tennessee

Daniel D. Mais, MD
Medical Director for Hematopathology, St. Joseph Mercy Hospital and Warde Medical Laboratory, Ann Arbor, Michigan

Stacy E.F. Melanson, MD, PhD
Associate Medical Director, Clinical Chemistry, Brigham and Women's Hospital; Assistant Professor, Harvard Medical School, Boston, Massachusetts

Mandakolathur R. Murali, MD
Director, Clinical Immunology Laboratory, Massachusetts General Hospital; Assistant Professor, Harvard Medical School, Boston, Massachusetts

Fritz F. Parl, MD, PhD
Professor of Pathology, Director of Clinical Chemistry, Vanderbilt University Medical Center, Nashville, Tennessee

Daniel E. Sabath, MD, PhD
Associate Professor, Department of Laboratory Medicine; Adjunct Associate Professor, Department of Medicine (Medical Genetics), University of Washington School of Medicine; Head, Hematology Division, Department of Laboratory Medicine; Director, Clinical Laboratory Services, Seattle Cancer Care Alliance, Seattle, Washington

Susan L. Saidman, PhD
Director, Histocompatibility Laboratory, Massachusetts General Hospital; Associate Professor, Harvard Medical School, Boston, Massachusetts

Eric D. Spitzer, MD, PhD
Associate Professor of Pathology and Molecular Genetics and Microbiology, Chief of Clinical Microbiology, Stony Brook University Medical Center, Stony Brook, New York

Paul Steele, MD
Medical Director, Clinical Laboratories, Cincinnati Children's Hospital Medical Center; Clinical Associate Professor, Department of Pathology and Laboratory Medicine, University of Cincinnati, Cincinnati, Ohio

Christopher P. Stowell, MD, PhD
Director, Blood Transfusion Service, Massachusetts General Hospital; Assistant Professor, Harvard Medical School, Boston, Massachusetts

Elizabeth M. Van Cott, MD
Director, Coagulation Laboratory; Medical Director, Core Laboratory, Massachusetts General Hospital; Associate Professor, Harvard Medical School, Boston, Massachusetts

William E. Winter, MD
Professor, Department of Pathology, Immunology, and Laboratory Medicine, University of Florida College of Medicine, Gainesville, Florida

Alison Woodworth, PhD
Assistant Professor of Pathology, Director, Esoteric Chemistry, Vanderbilt University Medical Center, Nashville, Tennessee

Preface

Everyone accepts that a physician caring for a patient cannot accurately interpret biopsy specimens and complex imaging studies. The roles of the anatomic pathologist and the radiologist as diagnostic physicians are well accepted and regarded as necessary for patient safety. Currently, most hospitals in the United States do not have a pathologist capable of interpreting the wide array of laboratory test results and guiding a clinical laboratory assessment to completion.

This means that, to care effectively for patients, the practicing physician today must have a working knowledge of his or her own about appropriate test selection and result interpretation, in an era when new tests are appearing every week. The tests appearing now are increasingly expensive and scientifically complex, particularly because so much of the new diagnostic testing relates to genetic variations. Before the 1980s, the number of clinical laboratory tests was so small that most physicians had no difficulty selecting the correct tests and interpreting the test results. However, the last 3 decades, and especially the last 10 years, have witnessed a dramatic increase in the number of clinical laboratory tests. Many physicians caring for patients today openly admit that they do not know which clinical laboratory tests to select or how to interpret the test results in a growing percentage of their cases.

The health care system has presumed that the ordering physician knows precisely which coagulation factor test to order when the PTT is prolonged or which serologic tests should be ordered when the antinuclear antibody test is strongly positive and speckled. Unfortunately, this assumption is incorrect. These 2 simple examples are extremely common occurrences in clinical practice. Because there is so much to know and because there is so little teaching of laboratory medicine and clinical pathology in medical school, most physicians today are forced to make guesses about appropriate diagnostic tests and their clinical significance. To consider the impact of molecular testing on the complexity of test selection, a diagnosis of cystic fibrosis not long ago was associated with a single test for sweat chloride. Now there are more than 1,300 mutations described for the cystic fibrosis gene, many of which can be identified by genetic testing in the clinical laboratory, and the information has clinical importance because there are differences in prognosis and treatment among the mutations. A single test with a single clinical meaning has changed into something of enormous size and complexity. A physician whose knowledge about testing for cystic fibrosis goes beyond the sweat chloride test is more clinically successful, to the great benefit of the patient.

There is now increased recognition of a major patient safety problem related to physicians selecting incorrect tests and misinterpreting test results. As a physician with a specialty practice in coagulation disorders (in addition to being a clinical pathologist), who has been receiving referrals for more than a decade, I have seen cases in which fathers were charged with child abuse because a well-intentioned physician misinterpreted the test results for bleeding in a child; a case in which a pregnancy was unhappily terminated as a result of a misinterpretation of a test result for protein S; inappropriate decisions about anticoagulation therapy because of a poor understanding of the laboratory tests that predict thrombotic risk; and many more cases involving severe harm to the patient.

Consider what is taught to medical students in the preclinical years about myocardial infarction. Given the current sensitivity regarding patient safety, it is surprising that virtually every medical school pathology course teaches the cardiac histopathology associated with a myocardial infarction, while instruction about the appropriate use and result interpretation for circulating markers of cardiac ischemia, such as troponin, varies widely in quantity and quality among medical schools. In some medical schools, there is only passing attention in the preclinical years to most of the diagnostic tests in the clinical laboratory. From the perspective of the patient with chest pain, a physician is most valuable if he or she has knowledge about the troponin level and can confidently use this test result to identify cardiac ischemia and separate it from other causes of chest pain. Nevertheless, in many medical schools, probably in most medical schools, much more attention is directed toward instruction on the histopathology of the infarct.

I believe that a major reason why laboratory medicine and clinical pathology have been overlooked in the teaching of medical students in the preclinical years is the absence of a single comprehensive textbook, written at the medical student level, that approximately parallels the topics in anatomic pathology. Such a textbook is also greatly needed in medical school because there are areas of diagnostic pathology, such as toxicology and coagulation, where there is little anatomic pathology and much clinical pathology. Commonly encountered topics such as drug testing may or may not be taught in a pathology course if there is little emphasis on clinical pathology. It is my greatest hope that this textbook will spur the development of systematic teaching of laboratory medicine and clinical pathology in the preclinical years of medical school and will lead to a better balance of teaching time between clinical pathology and anatomic pathology. It is empowering to the practicing physician, and protective of the patient, for medical students in the preclinical years, and beyond, to learn appropriate test selection and test result interpretation.

Michael Laposata
Nashville, Tennessee

Acknowledgments

I would first like to acknowledge all of the expert chapter authors associated with this textbook. It has been a pleasure to work with each of you, and I am honored to be your colleague. I would also like to recognize the professionalism of the McGraw-Hill publishing company, particularly my editors, Michael Weitz and Robert Pancotti, who have moved this textbook forward and included it among the books in the Lange series, which has such a proud tradition in medical education.

Clinical Laboratory Reference Values

The conventional units in this table are the ones most commonly used in the United States. Outside the United States, SI units are the predominant nomenclature for laboratory test results. The base units in the SI system related to laboratory testing that are found in this table include the mole (amount of substance), meter (length), kilogram (mass), second (time), and Celsius (temperature).

Reference ranges vary depending on the instrument and the reagents used to perform the test. Therefore, the reference ranges shown in this table are only close approximations to the reference ranges found in an individual clinical laboratory. It is also important to understand that reference ranges can be significantly affected by age and sex.

Conversion factors are provided in the table to allow the reader to convert conventional units to SI units and vice versa. The conversion of the conventional unit to SI unit requires a multiplication with the conversion factor, and conversion of the SI unit to the conventional unit requires division by the conversion factor.

The sample fluid is sometimes highly restrictive. For example, coagulation tests must be performed using plasma samples and serum samples are unacceptable. For other compounds, plasma samples and serum samples may both be acceptable. However, there may be differences, often minor, in the results obtained using plasma versus serum. Potassium is 1 such compound in which reference ranges may be different for plasma and serum. There is a significant movement away from the use of serum in favor of plasma. The principal reason for this is that extra time is required for samples to clot so that serum may be generated. A sample collected into a tube with anticoagulant results in the generation of plasma rather than serum after the tube is centrifuged. The clotting step is omitted when plasma samples are prepared, and therefore the turnaround time for the performance of the test is shortened. In some circumstances, whole blood is used for analysis, but the number of tests performed using whole blood is very limited. Urine and other body fluids, such as pleural fluid and cerebrospinal fluid, are also used for testing. Some of the entries in the table are associated with a fluid other than plasma, serum, or whole blood.

	Specimen	Traditional Reference Interval	Traditional Units	Conversion Factor, Multiply →, ← Divide	SI Reference Interval	SI Units
Acetaminophen (therapeutic)	Serum, plasma	10–30	µg/mL	6.62	70–200	µmol/L
Acetoacetic acid	Serum, plasma	<1	mg/dL	0.098	<0.1	mmol/L
Acetone	Serum, plasma	<2.0	mg/dL	0.172	<0.34	mmol/L
Acetylcholinesterase	Red blood cells	30–40	U/g of Hb	0.0645	2.13–2.63	MU/mol of Hb
Activated partial thromboplastin time (APTT)	Whole blood	25–40	seconds	1	25–40	Seconds
Adenosine deaminase[a]	Serum	11.5–25.0	U/L	0.017	0.20–0.43	µKat/L
Adrenocorticotropic hormone (ACTH) (see corticotropin)						
Alanine[b]	Serum	1.87–5.89	mg/dL	112.2	210–661	µmol/L
Alanine amino-transferase (ALT, SGPT)[b]	Serum	10–40	U/L	1	10–40	U/L
Albumin[b]	Serum	3.5–5.0	g/dL	10	35–50	g/L
Alcohol (see ethanol, isopropanol, methanol)						
Alcohol dehydrogenase[a]	Serum	<2.8	U/L	0.017	<0.05	µKat/L
Aldolase[a, b]	Serum	1.0–7.5	U/L	0.017	0.02–0.13	µKat/L
Aldosterone[b]	Serum, plasma	7–30	ng/dL	0.0277	0.19–0.83	nmol/L
Aldosterone	Urine	3–20	µg/24 hours	2.77	8–55	nmol/day
Alkaline phosphatase[b]	Serum	50–120	U/L	1	50–120	U/L
Alprazolam (therapeutic)	Serum, plasma	10–50	ng/mL	3.24	32–162	nmol/L
Aluminum	Serum	0–6	ng/mL	37.06	0.0–222.4	nmol/L
Amikacin (therapeutic, peak)	Serum, plasma	20–30	µg/mL	1.71	34–52	µmol/L
Amino acid fractionation						
Alanine[b]	Serum	1.87–5.89	mg/dL	112.2	210–661	µmol/L
α-Aminobutyric acid[b]	Plasma	0.08–0.36	mg/dL	97	8–35	µmol/L
Arginine[b]	Plasma	0.37–2.40	mg/dL	57.4	21–138	µmol/L
Asparagine[b]	Plasma	0.40–0.91	mg/dL	75.7	30–69	µmol/L
Aspartic acid[b]	Plasma	<0.3	mg/dL	75.1	<25	µmol/L
Citrulline[b]	Plasma	0.2–1.0	mg/dL	57.1	12–55	µmol/L
Cystine[b]	Plasma	0.40–1.40	mg/dL	83.3	33–117	µmol/L
Glutamic acid[b]	Plasma	0.2–2.8	mg/dL	67.97	15–190	µmol/L
Glutamine[b]	Plasma	6.1–10.2	mg/dL	68.42	420–700	µmol/L
Glycine[b]	Plasma	0.9–4.2	mg/dL	133.3	120–560	µmol/L
Histidine[b]	Plasma	0.5–1.7	mg/dL	64.5	32–110	µmol/L
Hydroxyproline[b]	Plasma	<0.55	mg/dL	76.3	<42	µmol/L
Isoleucine[b]	Plasma	0.5–1.3	mg/dL	76.24	40–100	µmol/L
Leucine[b]	Plasma	1.0–2.3	mg/dL	76.3	75–175	µmol/L
Lysine[b]	Plasma	1.2–3.5	mg/dL	68.5	80–240	µmol/L
Methionine[b]	Plasma	0.1–0.6	mg/dL	67.1	6–40	µmol/L
Ornithine[b]	Plasma	0.4–1.4	mg/dL	75.8	30–106	µmol/L
Phenylalanine[b]	Plasma	0.6–1.5	mg/dL	60.5	35–90	µmol/L
Proline[b]	Plasma	1.2–3.9	mg/dL	86.9	104–340	µmol/L
Serine[b]	Plasma	0.7–2.0	mg/dL	95.2	65–193	µmol/L
Taurine[b]	Plasma	0.3–2.1	mg/dL	80	24–168	µmol/L
Threonine[b]	Plasma	0.9–2.5	mg/dL	84	75–210	µmol/L
Tryptophan[b]	Plasma	0.5–1.5	mg/dL	48.97	25–73	µmol/L
Tyrosine[b]	Plasma	0.4–1.6	mg/dL	55.19	20–90	µmol/L
Valine[b]	Plasma	1.7–3.7	mg/dL	85.5	145–315	µmol/L
α-Aminobutyric acid[b]	Plasma	0.08–0.36	mg/dL	97	8–35	µmol/L
Amiodarone (therapeutic)	Serum, plasma	0.5–2.5	µg/mL	1.55	0.8–3.9	µmol/L

The sample type listed under Specimen in this table shows the reference interval for that specimen type. Thus, if the specimen for a test is listed as serum, the reference interval shown is for serum specimens. For many tests listed with serum as the specimen type, plasma is also acceptable, often with a similar reference interval.

Continued next page—

	Specimen	Traditional Reference Interval	Traditional Units	Conversion Factor, Multiply →, ← Divide	SI Reference Interval	SI Units
δ-Aminolevulinic acid	Urine	1.0–7.0	mg/24 hours	7.626	8–53	µmol/day
Amitriptyline (therapeutic)	Serum, plasma	80–250	ng/mL	3.61	289–903	nmol/L
Ammonia (as NH_3)[b]	Plasma	19–60	µg/dL	0.587	11–35	µmol/L
Amobarbital (therapeutic)	Serum	1–5	µg/mL	4.42	4–22	µmol/L
Amoxapine (therapeutic)	Plasma	200–600	ng/mL	1	200–600	µg/L
Amylase[a,b]	Serum	27–130	U/L	0.017	0.46–2.21	µKat/L
Androstenedione,[b] male	Serum	75–205	ng/dL	0.0349	2.6–7.2	nmol/L
Androstenedione,[b] female	Serum	85–275	ng/dL	0.0349	3.0–9.6	nmol/L
Angiotensin I	Plasma	<25	pg/mL	1	<25	ng/L
Angiotensin II	Plasma	10–60	pg/mL	1	10–60	ng/L
Angiotensin-converting enzyme (ACE)[a,b]	Serum	8–52	U/L	0.017	0.14–0.88	µKat/L
Anion gap (Na^+)–(Cl^- + HCO_3^-)	Serum, plasma	8–16	mEq/L	1	8–16	nmol/L
Antidiuretic hormone (ADH, vasopressin) (varies with osmolality: 285–290 mOsm/kg)	Plasma	1–5	pg/mL	0.926	0.9–4.6	pmol/L
α2-Antiplasmin	Plasma	80–130	%	0.01	0.8–1.3	Fraction of 1.0
Antithrombin III	Plasma	21–30	mg/dL	10	210–300	mg/L
Antithrombin III activity	Plasma	80–130	%	0.01	0.8–1.3	Fraction of 1.0
α1-Antitrypsin	Serum	126–226	mg/dL	0.01	1.26–2.26	g/L
Apolipoprotein A[b] Male Female	Serum Serum	80–151 80–170	mg/dL mg/dL	0.01 0.01	0.8–1.5 0.8–1.7	g/L g/L
Apolipoprotein B[b] Male Female	Serum, plasma Serum, plasma	50–123 25–120	mg/dL mg/dL	0.01 0.01	0.5–1.2 0.25–1.20	g/L g/L
Arginine[b]	Plasma	0.37–2.40	mg/dL	57.4	21–138	µmol/L
Arsenic (As)	Whole blood	<23	µg/L	0.0133	<0.31	µmol/L
Arsenic (As), acute poisoning	Whole blood	600–9300	µg/L	0.0133	7.9–123.7	µmol/L
Ascorbate, ascorbic acid (see vitamin C)						
Asparagine[b]	Plasma	0.40–0.91	mg/dL	75.7	30–69	µmol/L
Aspartate amino transferase (AST, SGOT)[a,b]	Serum	20–48	U/L	0.017	0.34–0.82	µKat/L
Aspartic acid[b]	Plasma	<0.3	mg/dL	75.1	<25	µmol/L
Atrial natriuretic hormone	Plasma	20–77	pg/mL	1	20–77	ng/L
Barbiturates (see individual drugs; pentobarbital, phenobarbital, thiopental)						
Basophils (see complete blood count, white blood cell count)						
Benzodiazepines (see individual drugs; alprazolam, chlordiazepoxide, diazepam, lorazepam)						
Bicarbonate	Plasma	21–28	mEq/L	1	21–28	mmol/L
Bile acids (total)	Serum	0.3–2.3	µg/mL	2.448	0.73–5.63	µmol/L
Bilirubin Total[b] Direct (conjugated)	Serum Serum	0.3–1.2 <0.2	mg/dL mg/dL	17.1 17.1	2–18 <3.4	µmol/L µmol/L

Continued next page—

	Specimen	Traditional Reference Interval	Traditional Units	Conversion Factor, Multiply →, ← Divide	SI Reference Interval	SI Units
Biotin	Whole blood, serum	200–500	pg/mL	0.0041	0.82–2.05	nmol/L
Bismuth	Whole blood	1–12	µg/L	4.785	4.8–57.4	nmol/L
Blood gases						
P_{CO_2}	Arterial blood	35–45	mmHg	1	35–45	mmHg
pH	Arterial blood	7.35–7.45	—	1	7.35–7.45	—
P_{O_2}	Arterial blood	80–100	mmHg	1	80–100	mmHg
Blood urea nitrogen (BUN, see urea nitrogen)						
C1 esterase inhibitor	Serum	12–30	mg/dL	0.01	0.12–0.30	g/L
C3 complement[b]	Serum	1200–1500	µg/mL	0.001	1.2–1.5	g/L
C4 complement[b]	Serum	350–600	µg/mL	0.001	0.35–0.60	g/L
Cadmium (nonsmoker)	Whole blood	0.3–1.2	µg/L	8.897	2.7–10.7	nmol/L
Caffeine (therapeutic, infants)	Serum, plasma	8–20	µg/mL	5.15	41–103	µmol/L
Calciferol (see vitamin D)						
Calcitonin	Serum, plasma	<19	pg/mL	1	<19	ng/L
Calcium, ionized	Serum	4.60–5.08	mg/dL	0.25	1.15–1.27	mmol/L
Calcium, total	Serum	8.2–10.2	mg/dL	0.25	2.05–2.55	mmol/L
Calcium, normal diet	Urine	<250	mg/24 hours	0.025	<6.2	mmol/day
Carbamazepine (therapeutic)	Serum, plasma	8–12	µg/mL	4.23	34–51	µmol/L
Carbon dioxide	Serum, plasma, venous blood	22–28	mEq/L	1	22–28	mmol/L
Carboxyhemoglobin (carbon monoxide), as fraction of hemoglobin saturation						
Nonsmoker	Whole blood	<2.0	%	0.01	<0.02	Fraction of 1.0
Toxic	Whole blood	>20	%	0.01	>0.2	Fraction of 1.0
β-Carotene	Serum	10–85	µg/dL	0.0186	0.2–1.6	µmol/L
Catecholamines, total (see norepinephrine)						
Ceruloplasmin[b]	Serum	20–40	mg/dL	10	200–400	mg/L
Chloramphenicol (therapeutic)	Serum	10–25	µg/mL	3.1	31–77	µmol/L
Chlordiazepoxide (therapeutic)	Serum, plasma	0.7–1.0	µg/mL	3.34	2.3–3.3	µmol/L
Chloride	Serum, plasma	96–106	mEq/L	1	96–106	mmol/L
Chloride	CSF	118–132	mEq/L	1	118–132	mmol/L
Chlorpromazine (therapeutic, adult)	Plasma	50–300	ng/mL	3.14	157–942	nmol/L
Chlorpromazine (therapeutic, child)	Plasma	40–80	ng/mL	3.14	126–251	nmol/L
Chlorpropamide (therapeutic)	Plasma	75–250	mg/L	3.61	270–900	µmol/L
Cholesterol, high-density lipoproteins (HDL)						
Male	Plasma	35–65	mg/dL	0.02586	0.91–1.68	mmol/L
Female	Plasma	35–80	mg/dL	0.02586	0.91–2.07	mmol/L
Cholesterol, low-density lipoproteins (LDL)[b]	Plasma	60–130	mg/dL	0.02586	1.55–3.37	mmol/L
Cholesterol (total), adult						
Desirable	Serum	<200	mg/dL	0.02586	<5.17	mmol/L
Borderline high	Serum	200–239	mg/dL	0.02586	5.17–6.18	mmol/L
High	Serum	>240	mg/dL	0.02586	>6.21	mmol/L

Continued next page—

	Specimen	Traditional Reference Interval	Traditional Units	Conversion Factor, Multiply →, ← Divide	SI Reference Interval	SI Units
Cholesterol (total), children						
Desirable	Serum	<170	mg/dL	0.02586	4.40	mmol/L
Borderline high	Serum	170–199	mg/dL	0.02586	4.40–5.15	mmol/L
High	Serum	>200	mg/dL	0.02586	>5.18	mmol/L
Cholesterol esters (as percent of total cholesterol)	Plasma	60–75	%	0.01	0.60–0.75	Fraction of 1.0
Chromium	Whole blood	0.7–28.0	µg/L	19.2	13.4–538.6	nmol/L
Citrate	Serum	1.2–3.0	mg/dL	52.05	60–160	µmol/L
Citrulline[b]	Plasma	0.2–1.0	mg/dL	57.1	12–55	µmol/L
Clonazepam (therapeutic)	Serum	15–60	ng/mL	3.17	48–190	nmol/L
Coagulation factor I (fibrinogen)	Plasma	150–400	mg/dL	0.01	1.5–4.0	g/L
Coagulation factor II (prothrombin)	Plasma	60–140	%	0.01	0.60–1.40	Fraction of 1.0
Coagulation factor V	Plasma	60–140	%	0.01	0.60–1.40	Fraction of 1.0
Coagulation factor VII	Plasma	60–140	%	0.01	0.60–1.40	Fraction of 1.0
Coagulation factor VIII	Plasma	50–200	%	0.01	0.50–2.00	Fraction of 1.0
Coagulation factor IX	Plasma	60–140	%	0.01	0.60–1.40	Fraction of 1.0
Coagulation factor X	Plasma	60–140	%	0.01	0.60–1.40	Fraction of 1.0
Coagulation factor XI	Plasma	60–140	%	0.01	0.60–1.40	Fraction of 1.0
Coagulation factor XII	Plasma	60–140	%	0.01	0.60–1.40	Fraction of 1.0
Cobalt	Serum	4.0–10.0	µg/L	16.97	67.9–169.7	nmol/L
Codeine (therapeutic)	Serum	10–100	ng/mL	3.34	33–334	nmol/L
Complete blood count (CBC)						
Hematocrit[b]						
Male	Whole blood	41–50	%	0.01	0.41–0.50	Fraction of 1.0
Female	Whole blood	35–45	%	0.01	0.35–0.45	Fraction of 1.0
Hemoglobin (mass concentration)[b]						
Male	Whole blood	13.5–17.5	g/dL	10	135–175	g/L
Female	Whole blood	12.0–15.5	g/dL	10	120–155	g/L
Hemoglobin (substance concentration, Hb [Fe])						
Male	Whole blood	13.6–17.2	g/dL	0.6206	8.44–10.65	mmol/L
Female	Whole blood	12.0–15.0	g/dL	0.6206	7.45–9.30	mmol/L
Mean corpuscular hemoglobin (MCH), mass concentration[b]	Whole blood	27–33	pg/cell	1	27–33	pg/cell
Mean corpuscular hemoglobin (MCH), substance concentration, Hb [Fe]	Whole blood	27–33	pg/cell	0.06206	1.70–2.05	fmol
Mean corpuscular hemoglobin concentration (MCHC), mass concentration	Whole Blood	33–37	g Hb/dL	10	330–370	g Hb/L
Mean corpuscular hemoglobin concentration (MCHC), substance concentration, Hb [Fe]	Whole Blood	33–37	g Hb/dL	0.6206	20–23	mmol/L
Mean cell volume (MCV)[b]	Whole Blood	80–100	µm³	1	80–100	fl
Platelet count	Whole blood	150–450	10^3 µL^{-1}	1	150–450	10^9 L^{-1}
Red blood cell count						
Female	Whole blood	3.9–5.5	10^6 µL^{-1}	1	3.9–5.5	10^{12} L^{-1}
Male	Whole blood	4.6–6.0	10^6 µL^{-1}	1	4.6–6.0	10^{12} L^{-1}
Reticulocyte count[b]	Whole blood	25–75	10^3 µL^{-1}	1	25–75	10^9 L^{-1}
Reticulocyte count[b] (fraction)	Whole blood	0.5–1.5	% of RBCs	0.01	0.005–0.015	Fraction of RBCs
White blood cell count[b]	Whole blood	4.5–11.0	10^3 µL^{-1}	1	4.5–11.0	10^9 L^{-1}

Continued next page—

	Specimen	Traditional Reference Interval	Traditional Units	Conversion Factor, Multiply →, ← Divide	SI Reference Interval	SI Units
(Continue complete blood count, white blood cell count)						
Differential count[b] (absolute)						
Neutrophils	Whole blood	1800–7800	µL^{-1}	1	1.8–7.8	10^9 L^{-1}
Bands	Whole blood	0–700	µL^{-1}	1	0.00–0.70	10^9 L^{-1}
Lymphocytes	Whole blood	1000–4800	µL^{-1}	1	1.0–4.8	10^9 L^{-1}
Monocytes	Whole blood	0–800	µL^{-1}	1	0.00–0.80	10^9 L^{-1}
Eosinophils	Whole blood	0–450	µL^{-1}	1	0.00–0.45	10^9 L^{-1}
Basophils	Whole blood	0–200	µL^{-1}	1	0.00–0.20	10^9 L^{-1}
Differential count[b] (number fraction)						
Neutrophils	Whole blood	56	%	0.01	0.56	Fraction of 1.0
Bands	Whole blood	3	%	0.01	0.03	Fraction of 1.0
Lymphocytes	Whole blood	34	%	0.01	0.34	Fraction of 1.0
Monocytes	Whole blood	4	%	0.01	0.04	Fraction of 1.0
Eosinophils	Whole blood	2.7	%	0.01	0.027	Fraction of 1.0
Basophils	Whole blood	0.3	%	0.01	0.003	Fraction of 1.0
Copper[b]	Serum	70–140	µg/dL	0.1574	11.0–22.0	µmol/L
Coproporphyrin	Urine	<200	µg/24 hours	1.527	<300	nmol/day
Corticotropin[b]	Plasma	<120	pg/mL	0.22	<26	pmol/L
Cortisol, total[b]						
Fasting, 8 a.m. to noon	Plasma	5–25	µg/dL	27.6	138–690	nmol/L
Noon to 8 p.m.	Plasma	5–15	µg/dL	27.6	138–414	nmol/L
8 p.m. to 8 a.m.	Plasma	0–10	µg/dL	27.6	0–276	nmol/L
Cortisol, free[b]	Urine	30–100	µg/24 hours	2.759	80–280	nmol/day
Cotinine (smoker)	Plasma	16–145	ng/mL	5.68	91–823	nmol/L
C peptide	Serum	0.5–2.5	ng/mL	0.333	0.17–0.83	nmol/L
Creatine, male	Serum	0.2–0.7	mg/dL	76.3	15.3–53.3	µmol/L
Creatine, female	Serum	0.3–0.9	mg/dL	76.3	22.9–68.6	µmol/L
Creatine kinase (CK)[a]	Serum	50–200	U/L	0.017	0.85–3.40	µKat/L
Creatine kinase-MB fraction	Serum	<6	%	0.01	<0.06	Fraction of 1.0
Creatinine[b]	Serum, plasma	0.6–1.2	mg/dL	88.4	53–106	µmol/L
Creatinine	Urine	1–2	g/24 hours	8.84	8.8–17.7	mmol/day
Creatinine clearance	Serum, urine	75–125	mL/min	0.01667	1.24–2.08	mL/second
Cyanide (toxic)	Whole blood	>1.0	µg/mL	38.4	>38.4	µmol/L
Cyanocobalamin (see vitamin B$_{12}$)						
Cyclic adenosine monophosphate (cAMP)	Plasma	4.6–8.6	ng/mL	3.04	14–26	nmol/L
Cyclosporine (toxic)	Whole blood	>400	ng/mL	0.832	>333	nmol/L
Cystine[b]	Plasma	0.40–1.40	mg/dL	83.3	33–117	µmol/L
D-dimer	Plasma	Negative (<500)	ng/mL	1	Negative (<500)	ng/mL
Dehydroepiandrosterone (DHEA) (unconjugated, male)[b]	Plasma, serum	180–1250	ng/dL	0.0347	6.2–43.3	nmol/L
Dehydroepiandrosterone sulfate (DHEA-S) (male)[b]	Plasma, serum	10–619	µg/dL	0.027	0.3–16.7	µmol/L
Desipramine (therapeutic)	Plasma, serum	50–200	ng/mL	3.75	170–700	nmol/L
Diazepam (therapeutic)	Plasma, serum	100–1000	ng/mL	0.00351	0.35–3.51	µmol/L
Digoxin (therapeutic)	Plasma	0.5–2.0	ng/mL	1.281	0.6–2.6	nmol/L

Continued next page—

	Specimen	Traditional Reference Interval	Traditional Units	Conversion Factor, Multiply →, ← Divide	SI Reference Interval	SI Units
Disopyramide (therapeutic)	Plasma, serum	2.8–7.0	mg/L	2.95	8–21	µmol/L
Doxepin (therapeutic)	Plasma, serum	150–250	ng/mL	3.58	540–890	nmol/L
Electrolytes						
Chloride	Serum, plasma	96–106	mEq/L	1	96–106	mmol/L
Carbon dioxide (CO_2)	Serum, plasma, venous blood	22–28	mEq/L	1	22–28	mmol/L
Potassium	Plasma	3.5–5.0	mEq/L	1	3.5–5.0	mmol/L
Sodium[b]	Plasma	136–142	mEq/L	1	136–142	mmol/L
Eosinophils (see complete blood count, white blood cell count)						
Epinephrine	Plasma	<60	pg/mL	5.46	<330	pmol/L
Epinephrine[b]	Urine	<20	µg/24 hours	5.46	<109	nmol/day
Erythrocyte count (see complete blood count, red blood cell count)						
Erythrocyte sedimentation rate (ESR)[b]	Whole blood	0–20	mm/hour	1	0–20	mm/hour
Erythropoietin	Serum	5–36	mU/mL	1	5–36	IU/L
Estradiol (E2, unconjugated),[b] female						
Follicular phase	Serum	20–350	pg/mL	3.67	73–1285	pmol/L
Mid-cycle peak	Serum	150–750	pg/mL	3.67	551–2753	pmol/L
Luteal phase	Serum	30–450	pg/mL	3.67	110–1652	pmol/L
Post-menopausal	Serum	<59	pg/mL	3.67	<218	pmol/L
Estradiol (unconjugated),[b] male	Serum	<20	pg/mL	3.67	<184	pmol/L
Estriol (E3, unconjugated), varies with length of gestation	Serum	5–40	ng/mL	3.47	17.4–138.8	nmol/L
Estrogens (total),[b] female						
Follicular phase	Serum	60–200	pg/mL	1	60–200	ng/L
Luteal phase	Serum	160–400	pg/mL	1	160–400	ng/L
Post-menopausal	Serum	<130	pg/mL	1	<130	ng/L
Estrogens (total),[b] male	Serum	20–80	pg/mL	1	20–80	ng/L
Estrone (E1),[b] female						
Follicular phase	Plasma, serum	1.5–25	pg/mL	37	55–925	pmol/L
Luteal phase	Plasma, serum	1.5–20	pg/mL	37	55–740	pmol/L
Post-menopausal	Plasma, serum	1.5–5.5	pg/mL	37	55–204	pmol/L
Estrone (E1),[b] male	Plasma, serum	1.5–6.5	pg/mL	37	55–240	pmol/L
Ethanol (ethyl alcohol), toxic	Serum, whole blood	>100	mg/dL	0.2171	>21.7	mmol/L
Ethosuximide	Plasma, serum	40–100	µg/mL	7.08	283–708	µmol/L
Ethylene glycol (toxic)	Plasma, serum	>30	mg/dL	0.1611	>5	mmol/L
Fatty acids (nonesterified)	Plasma	8–25	mg/dL	0.0354	0.28–0.89	mmol/L
Fecal fat (as stearic acid)	Stool	2.0–6.0	g/day	1	2–6	g/day
Ferritin[b]	Plasma	15–200	ng/mL	1	15–200	µg/L
α1-Fetoprotein[b]	Serum	<10	ng/mL	1	<10	µg/L
Fibrinogen	Plasma	150–400	mg/dL	0.01	1.5–4.0	g/L
Fibrin breakdown products (fibrin split products)	Serum	<10	µg/mL	1	<10	mg/L
Folate (folic acid)	Red blood cells	166–640	ng/mL	2.266	376–1450	nmol/L
Folate (folic acid)	Serum	5–25	ng/mL	2.266	11–57	nmol/L

Continued next page—

	Specimen	Traditional Reference Interval	Traditional Units	Conversion Factor, Multiply →, ← Divide	SI Reference Interval	SI Units
Follicle-stimulating hormone (FSH, follitropin),[b] female						
Follicular phase	Serum	1.37–9.9	mIU/mL	1	1.3–9.9	IU/L
Ovulatory phase	Serum	6.17–17.2	mIU/mL	1	6.1–17.2	IU/L
Luteal phase	Serum	1.09–9.2	mIU/mL	1	1.0–9.2	IU/L
Post-menopausal	Serum	19.3–100.6	mIU/mL	1	19.3–100.6	IU/L
Follicle-stimulating hormone (FSH, follitropin),[b] male	Serum	1.42–15.4	mIU/mL	1	1.4–15.4	IU/L
Follicle-stimulating hormone (FSH, follitropin),[b] female	Urine	2–15	IU/24 hours	1	2–15	IU/day
Follicle-stimulating hormone (FSH, follitropin),[b] Male	Urine	3–12	IU/24 hours	1	3–11	IU/day
Fructosamine[b]	Serum	1.5–2.7	mmol/L	1	1.5–2.7	mmol/L
Fructose	Serum	1–6	mg/dL	55.5	55–333	µmol/L
Galactose	Plasma, serum	<20	mg/dL	0.0555	<1.10	mmol/L
Gastrin (fasting)	Serum	<100	pg/mL	1	<100	ng/L
Gentamicin (therapeutic, peak)	Serum	6–10	µg/mL	2.1	12–21	µmol/L
Glucagon[b]	Plasma	20–100	pg/mL	1	20–100	ng/L
Glucose[b]	Serum, plasma	70–110	mg/dL	0.05551	3.9–6.1	mmol/L
Glucose	CSF	50–80	mg/dL	0.05551	2.8–4.4	mmol/L
Glucose-6-phosphate dehydrogenase	Red blood cells	10–14	U/g of Hb	0.0645	0.65–0.90	MU/mol of Hb
Glutamic acid[b]	Plasma	0.2–2.8	mg/dL	67.97	15–190	µmol/L
Glutamine	Plasma	6.1–10.2	mg/dL	68.42	420–700	µmol/L
γ-Glutamyltransferase (GGT; γ-glutamyl transpeptidase)[b]	Serum	0–30	U/L	0.017	0–0.51	µKat/L
Glycerol (free)[b]	Serum	<1.5	mg/dL	0.1086	<0.16	mmol/L
Glycine[b]	Plasma	0.9–4.2	mg/dL	133.3	120–560	µmol/L
Glycosylated hemoglobin (glycated hemoglobin; hemoglobin A1, A1c)	Whole blood	4–7	% of total Hb	0.01	0.04–0.07	Fraction of total Hb
Gold (therapeutic)	Serum	100–200	µg/dL	0.05077	5.1–10.2	µmol/L
Growth hormone, adult (GH, somatotropin)[b]	Plasma, serum	<20	ng/mL	1	<20	µg/L
Haloperidol (therapeutic)	Serum, plasma	5–20	ng/mL	2.6	13–52	nmol/L
Haptoglobin[b]	Serum	40–180	mg/dL	0.01	0.4–1.8	g/L
Hematocrit (see complete blood count)						
Hemoglobin (see complete blood count)						
Hemoglobin A1c (see glycosylated hemoglobin)						
Hemoglobin A2[b]	Whole blood	2.0–3.0	%	0.01	0.02–0.03	Fraction of 1.0
Hemoglobin F[b] (fetal hemoglobin in adult)	Whole blood	<2	%	0.01	<0.02	Fraction of 1.0
High-density lipoprotein cholesterol (HDL)						
Male	Plasma	35–65	mg/dL	0.02586	0.91–1.68	mmol/L
Female	Plasma	35–80	mg/dL	0.02586	0.91–2.07	mmol/L
Histidine[b]	Plasma	0.5–1.7	mg/dL	64.5	32–110	µmol/L
Homocysteine (total)	Plasma, serum	4–12	µmol/L	1	4–12	µmol/L

Continued next page—

	Specimen	Traditional Reference Interval	Traditional Units	Conversion Factor, Multiply →, ← Divide	SI Reference Interval	SI Units
Homovanillic acid[b]	Urine	<8	mg/24 hours	5.489	<45	µmol/day
Human chorionic gonadotropin (HCG) (nonpregnant adult female)	Serum	<3	mIU/mL	1	<3	IU/L
β-Hydroxybutyric acid	Serum	0.21–2.81	mg/dL	96.05	20–270	µmol/L
5-Hydroxyindoleacetic acid (5-HIAA)	Urine	<25	mg/24 hours	5.23	<131	µmol/day
17α-Hydroxyprogesterone,[b] female						
Follicular phase	Serum	15–70	ng/dL	0.03	0.4–2.1	nmol/L
Luteal phase	Serum	35–290	ng/dL	0.03	1.0–8.7	nmol/L
Post-menopausal	Serum	<70	ng/dL	0.03	<2.1	nmol/L
17α-Hydroxyprogesterone,[b] male	Serum	27–199	ng/dL	0.03	0.8–6.0	nmol/L
Hydroxyproline	Plasma	<0.55	mg/dL	76.3	<42	µmol/L
5-Hydroxytryptamine (see serotonin)						
Ibuprofen (therapeutic)	Plasma, serum	10–50	µg/mL	4.85	49–243	µmol/L
Imipramine (therapeutic)	Plasma	150–250	ng/mL	3.57	536–893	nmol/L
Immunoglobin A (IgA)[b]	Serum	50–350	mg/dL	0.01	0.5–3.5	g/L
Immunoglobin D (IgD)	Serum	0.5–3.0	mg/dL	10	5–30	mg/L
Immunoglobin E (IgE)	Serum	10–179	IU/mL	2.4	24–430	µg/L
Immunoglobin G (IgG)[b]	Serum	650–1600	mg/dL	0.01	6.5–16.0	g/L
Immunoglobin M (IgM)[b]	Serum	54–222	mg/dL	0.01	0.5–2.2	g/L
Insulin	Plasma	5–20	µU/mL	6.945	34.7–138.9	pmol/L
Insulin C peptide (see C peptide)						
Insulin-like growth factor[b]	Plasma	130–450	ng/mL	1	130–450	µg/L
Ionized calcium (see calcium)						
Iron (total)[b]	Serum	60–150	µg/dL	0.179	10.7–26.9	µmol/L
Iron binding capacity	Serum	250–400	µg/dL	0.179	44.8–71.6	µmol/L
Isoleucine[b]	Plasma	0.5–1.3	mg/dL	76.24	40–100	µmol/L
Isoniazid (therapeutic)	Plasma	1–7	µg/mL	7.29	7–51	µmol/L
Isopropanol (toxic)	Plasma, serum	>400	mg/L	0.0166	>6.64	mmol/L
Lactate (lactic acid)	Arterial blood	3–11.3	mg/dL	0.111	0.3–1.3	mmol/L
Lactate (lactic acid)	Venous blood	4.5–19.8	mg/dL	0.111	0.5–2.2	mmol/L
Lactate dehydrogenase (LDH)	Serum	50–200	U/L	1	50–200	U/L
Lactate dehydrogenase isoenzymes						
LD1	Serum	17–27	%	0.01	0.17–0.27	Fraction of 1.0
LD2	Serum	27–37	%	0.01	0.27–0.37	Fraction of 1.0
LD3	Serum	18–25	%	0.01	0.18–0.25	Fraction of 1.0
LD4	Serum	8–16	%	0.01	0.08–0.16	Fraction of 1.0
LD5	Serum	6–16	%	0.01	0.06–0.16	Fraction of 1.0
Lead	Whole blood	<25	µg/dL	0.0483	<1.21	µmol/L
Leucine[b]	Plasma	1.0–2.3	mg/dL	76.3	75–175	µmol/L
Leukocyte count (see complete blood count, white blood cell count)						
Lidocaine (therapeutic)	Serum, plasma	1.5–6.0	µg/mL	4.27	6.4–25.6	µmol/L
Lipase[a]	Serum	0–160	U/L	0.017	0–2.72	µKat/L

Continued next page—

	Specimen	Traditional Reference Interval	Traditional Units	Conversion Factor, Multiply →, ← Divide	SI Reference Interval	SI Units
Lipoprotein(a) [Lp(a)]	Serum, plasma	10–30	mg/dL	0.01	0.1–0.3	g/L
Lithium (therapeutic)	Serum	0.6–1.2	mEq/L	1	0.6–1.2	mmol/L
Lorazepam (therapeutic)	Serum, plasma	50–240	ng/mL	3.11	156–746	nmol/L
Low-density lipoprotein cholesterol (LDL)[b]	Plasma	60–130	mg/dL	0.02586	1.55–3.37	mmol/L
Luteinizing hormone (LH)[b], female						
Follicular phase	Serum	2.0–15.0	mIU/L	1	2.0–15.0	IU/L
Ovulatory peak	Serum	22.0–105.0	mIU/L	1	22.0–105.0	IU/L
Luteal phase	Serum	0.6–19.0	mIU/L	1	0.6–19.0	IU/L
Post-menopausal	Serum	16.0–64.0	mIU/L	1	16.0–64.0	IU/L
Luteinizing hormone (LH),[b] male	Serum	2.0–12.0	mIU/L	1	2.0–12.0	IU/L
Lymphocytes (see complete blood count, white blood cell count)						
Lysine[b]	Plasma	1.2–3.5	mg/dL	68.5	80–240	µmol/L
Lysozyme (muramidase)	Serum	4–13	mg/L	1	4–13	mg/L
Magnesium[b]	Serum	1.5–2.5	mg/dL	0.4114	0.62–1.03	mmol/L
Magnesium[b]	Serum	1.3–2.1	mEq/L	0.5	0.65–1.05	mmol/L
Manganese	Whole blood	10–12	µg/L	18.2	182–218	nmol/L
Maprotiline (therapeutic)	Plasma	200–600	ng/mL	1	200–600	µg/L
Mean corpuscular hemoglobin (see complete blood count)						
Mean corpuscular hemoglobin concentration (see complete blood count)						
Meperidine (therapeutic)	Serum, plasma	0.4–0.7	µg/mL	4.04	1.6–2.8	µmol/L
Mercury	Whole blood	0.6–59.0	µg/L	4.99	3.0–294.4	nmol/L
Metanephrines (total)[b]	Urine	<1.0	mg/24 hours	5.07	<5	µmol/day
Methadone (therapeutic)	Serum, plasma	100–400	ng/mL	0.00323	0.32–1.29	µmol/L
Methanol	Whole blood, serum	<1.5	mg/L	0.0312	<0.05	mmol/L
Methemoglobin	Whole blood	<0.24	g/dL	155	<37.2	µmol/L
Methemoglobin	Whole blood	<1.0	% of total Hb	0.01	<0.01	Fraction of total Hb
Methionine[b]	Plasma	0.1–0.6	mg/dL	67.1	6–40	µmol/L
Methsuximide (therapeutic)	Serum	10–40	µg/mL	5.29	53–212	µmol/L
Methyldopa (therapeutic)	Serum, plasma	1–5	µg/mL	4.73	5–24	µmol/L
Metoprolol (therapeutic)	Serum, plasma	75–200	ng/mL	3.74	281–748	nmol/L
β2-Microglobulin	Serum	<2	µg/mL	85	<170	nmol/L
Monocytes (see complete blood count, white blood cell count)						
Morphine (therapeutic)	Serum, plasma	10–80	ng/mL	3.5	35–280	nmol/L
Muramidase (see lysozyme)						
Myoglobin	Serum	19–92	µg/L	1	19–92	µg/L
Naproxen (therapeutic trough)	Plasma, serum	>50	µg/mL	4.34	>217	µmol/L
Neutrophils (see complete blood count, white blood cell count)						
Niacin (nicotinic acid)	Urine	2.4–6.4	mg/24 hours	7.3	17.5–46.7	µmol/day
Nickel	Whole blood	1.0–28.0	µg/L	17	17–476	nmol/L

Continued next page—

	Specimen	Traditional Reference Interval	Traditional Units	Conversion Factor, Multiply →, ← Divide	SI Reference Interval	SI Units
Nicotine (smoker)	Plasma	0.01–0.05	mg/L	6.16	0.062–0.308	µmol/L
Nitrogen (nonprotein)	Serum	20–35	mg/dL	0.714	14.3–25.0	mmol/L
Norepinephrine[b]	Plasma	110–410	pg/mL	5.91	650–2423	nmol/L
Norepinephrine[b]	Urine	15–80	µg/24 hours	5.91	89–473	nmol/day
Nortriptyline (therapeutic)	Serum, plasma	50–150	ng/mL	3.8	190–570	nmol/L
Ornithine[b]	Plasma	0.4–1.4	mg/dL	75.8	30–106	µmol/L
Osmolality[b]	Serum	275–295	mOsm/kg H_2O	1	275–295	mmol/kg H_2O
Osmolality	Urine	250–900	mOsm/kg H_2O	1	250–900	mmol/kg H_2O
Osteocalcin[b]	Serum	3.0–13.0	ng/mL	1	3.0–13.0	µg/L
Oxalate	Serum	1.0–2.4	mg/L	11.4	11–27	µmol/L
Oxazepam (therapeutic)	Serum, plasma	0.2–1.4	µg/mL	3.49	0.7–4.9	µmol/L
Oxycodone (therapeutic)	Plasma, serum	10–100	ng/mL	3.17	32–317	nmol/L
Oxygen, partial pressure (P_{O_2})	Arterial blood	80–100	mmHg	1	80–100	mmHg
Pantothenic acid (see vitamin B_5)						

Parathyroid hormone
  Intact[b]
  N-terminal specific[b]
  C-terminal (mid-molecule)
	
	Serum
	Serum
	Serum
		
		10–50
		8–24
		0–340
			
			pg/mL
			pg/mL
			pg/mL
				
				1
				1
				1
					
					10–50
					8–24
					0–340
						
						ng/L
						ng/L
						ng/L

Pentobarbital (therapeutic)	Serum, plasma	1–5	µg/mL	4.42	4.0–22	µmol/L
Pepsinogen I[b]	Serum	28–100	ng/mL	1	28–100	µg/L
pH (see blood gases)						
Phenobarbital (therapeutic)	Serum, plasma	15–40	µg/mL	4.31	65–172	µmol/L
Phenylalanine[b]	Plasma	0.6–1.5	mg/dL	60.5	35–90	µmol/L
Phenytoin (therapeutic)	Serum, plasma	10–20	µg/mL	3.96	40–79	µmol/L
Phosphorus (inorganic)[b]	Serum	2.3–4.7	mg/dL	0.3229	0.74–1.52	mmol/L
Phosphorus (inorganic)[b]	Urine	0.4–1.3	g/24 hours	32.29	12.9–42.0	mmol/day
Phospholipid phosphorus (total)	Serum	8.0–11.0	mg/dL	0.3229	2.58–3.55	mmol/L
Placental lactogen (5–38-week gestation)	Serum	0.5–11	µg/mL	46.3	23–509	nmol/L
Plasminogen	Plasma	8.4–14.0	mg/dL	10	84–140	mg/L
Plasminogen	Plasma	80–120	%	0.01	0.80–1.20	Fraction of 1.0
Plasminogen activator inhibitor	Plasma	<15	IU/mL	1	<15	kIU/L
Platelet count (see complete blood count, platelet count)						
Porphobilinogen deaminase	Red blood cells	>7.0	nmol/second/L	1	>7.0	nmol/(second·L)
Porphyrins (total)	Urine	<320	nmol/L	1	<320	nmol/L
Potassium	Plasma	3.5–5.0	mEq/L	1	3.5–5.0	mmol/L

Pregnanediol,[b] female
  Follicular phase
  Luteal phase
	
	Urine
	Urine
		
		<2.6
		2.3–10.6
			
			mg/24 hours
			mg/24 hours
				
				3.12
				3.12
					
					<8
					8–33
						
						µmol/day
						µmol/day

Pregnanediol,[b] male	Urine	0–1.9	mg/24 hours	3.12	0–5.9	µmol/day
Pregnanetriol[b]	Urine	<2.5	mg/24 hours	2.97	<7.5	µmol/day

Continued next page—

	Specimen	Traditional Reference Interval	Traditional Units	Conversion Factor, Multiply →, ← Divide	SI Reference Interval	SI Units
Primidone (therapeutic)	Plasma	5–12	µg/mL	4.58	23–55	µmol/L
Procainamide (therapeutic)	Serum, plasma	4–10	µg/mL	4.23	17–42	µmol/L
Progesterone,[b] female						
Follicular phase	Serum	0.1–0.7	ng/mL	3.18	0.5–2.2	nmol/L
Luteal phase	Serum	2.0–25.0	ng/mL	3.18	6.4–79.5	nmol/L
Progesterone,[b] male	Serum	0.13–0.97	ng/mL	3.18	0.4–3.1	nmol/L
Prolactin (nonlactating subject)	Serum	1–25	ng/mL	1	1–25	µg/L
Proline[b]	Plasma	1.2–3.9	mg/dL	86.9	104–340	µmol/L
Propoxyphene (therapeutic)	Serum	0.1–0.4	µg/mL	2.946	0.3–1.2	µmol/L
Propanolol (therapeutic)	Serum	50–100	ng/mL	3.86	190–386	nmol/L
Protein (total)[b]	Serum	6.0–8.0	g/dL	10	60–80	g/L
Protein C	Plasma	70–140	%	0.01	0.70–1.40	Fraction of 1.0
Protein electrophoresis (SPEP), fraction of total protein						
Albumin	Serum	52–65	%	0.01	0.52–0.65	Fraction of 1.0
α1-Globulin	Serum	2.5–5.0	%	0.01	0.025–0.05	Fraction of 1.0
α2-Globulin	Serum	7.0–13.0	%	0.01	0.07–0.13	Fraction of 1.0
β-Globulin	Serum	8.0–14.0	%	0.01	0.08–0.14	Fraction of 1.0
γ-Globulin	Serum	12.0–22.0	%	0.01	0.12–0.22	Fraction of 1.0
Protein electrophoresis (SPEP), concentration						
Albumin	Serum	3.2–5.6	g/dL	10	32–56	g/L
α1-Globulin	Serum	0.1–0.4	g/dL	10	1–10	g/L
α2-Globulin	Serum	0.4–1.2	g/dL	10	4–12	g/L
β-Globulin	Serum	0.5–1.1	g/dL	10	5–11	g/L
γ-Globulin	Serum	0.5–1.6	g/dL	10	5–16	g/L
Protein S (activity)	Plasma	70–140	%	0.01	0.70–1.40	Fraction of 1.0
Prothrombin time (PT)	Plasma	10–13	seconds	1	10–13	Seconds
Protoporphyrin	Red blood cells	15–50	µg/dL	0.0177	0.27–0.89	µmol/L
Pyridoxine (see vitamin B$_6$)						
Pyruvate (as pyruvic acid)	Whole blood	0.3–0.9	mg/dL	113.6	34–102	µmol/L
Quinidine (therapeutic)	Serum	2.0–5.0	µg/mL	3.08	6.2–15.4	µmol/L
Red blood cell count (see complete blood count)						
Red cell folate (see folate)						
Renin (normal sodium diet)[b]	Plasma	1.1–4.1	ng/mL/hour	1	1.1–4.1	ng/(mL hour)
Reticulocyte count[b]	Whole blood	25–75	$10^3 \, \mu L^{-1}$	1	25–75	$10^9 \, L^{-1}$
Reticulocyte count[b] (fraction)	Whole blood	0.5–1.5	% of RBCs	0.01	0.005–0.015	Fraction of RBCs
Retinol (see vitamin A)						
Rheumatoid factor	Serum	<30	IU/mL	1	<30	kIU/L
Riboflavin (see vitamin B$_2$)						
Salicylates (therapeutic)	Serum, plasma	15–30	mg/dL	0.0724	1.08–2.17	mmol/L
Sedimentation rate (see erythrocyte sedimentation rate)						
Selenium	Whole blood	58–234	µg/L	0.0127	0.74–2.97	µmol/L
Serine[b]	Plasma	0.7–2.0	mg/dL	95.2	65–193	µmol/L
Serotonin (5-hydroxytryptamine)	Whole blood	50–200	ng/mL	0.00568	0.28–1.14	µmol/L

Continued next page—

	Specimen	Traditional Reference Interval	Traditional Units	Conversion Factor, Multiply →, ← Divide	SI Reference Interval	SI Units
Serum protein electrophoresis (SPEP, see protein electrophoresis)						
Sex hormone binding globulin[b]	Serum	0.5–1.5	µg/dL	34.7	17.4–52.1	nmol/L
Sodium[b]	Plasma	136–142	mEq/L	1	136–142	mmol/L
Somatostatin	Plasma	<25	pg/mL	1	<25	ng/L
Somatomedin C (see insulin-like growth factor)						
Strychnine (toxic)	Whole blood	>0.5	mg/L	2.99	>1.5	µmol/L
Substance P	Plasma	<240	pg/mL	1	<240	ng/L
Sulfhemoglobin	Whole blood	<1.0	% of total Hb	0.01	<0.010	Fraction of total Hb
Taurine[b]	Plasma	0.3–2.1	mg/dL	80	24–168	µmol/L
Testosterone,[b] male	Plasma, serum	300–1200	ng/dL	0.0347	10.4–41.6	nmol/L
Testosterone,[b] female	Plasma, serum	<85	ng/dL	0.0347	2.95	nmol/L
Theophylline (therapeutic)	Plasma, serum	10–20	µg/mL	5.55	56–111	µmol/L
Thiamine (see vitamin B₁)						
Thiocyanate (nonsmoker)	Plasma, serum	1–4	mg/L	17.2	17–69	µmol/L
Thiopental (therapeutic)	Plasma, serum	1–5	µg/mL	4.13	4–21	µmol/L
Thioridazine (therapeutic)	Plasma, serum	1.0–1.5	µg/mL	2.7	2.7–4.1	µmol/L
Thrombin time	Plasma	16–24	seconds	1.0	16–24	seconds
Threonine[b]	Plasma	0.9–2.5	mg/dL	84	75–210	µmol/L
Thyroglobulin[b]	Serum	3–42	ng/mL	1	3–42	µg/L
Thyrotropin (thyroid-stimulating hormone, TSH)[b]	Serum	0.5–5.0	µIU/mL	1	0.5–5.0	mU/L
Thyroxine, free (FT4)[b]	Serum	0.9–2.3	ng/dL	12.87	12–30	pmol/L
Thyroxine, total (T4)[b]	Serum	5.5–12.5	µg/dL	12.87	71–160	nmol/L
Thyroxine-binding globulin (TBG),[b] as T4 binding capacity	Serum	10–26	µg/dL	12.9	129–335	nmol/L
Tissue plasminogen activator	Plasma	<0.04	IU/mL	1000	<40	IU/L
Tobramycin (therapeutic, peak)	Plasma, serum	5–10	µg/mL	2.14	10–21	µmol/L
Tocainide (therapeutic)	Plasma, serum	4–10	µg/mL	5.2	21–52	µmol/L
α-Tocopherol (see vitamin E)						
Transferrin (siderophilin)[b]	Serum	200–380	mg/dL	0.01	2.0–3.8	g/L
Triglycerides[b]	Plasma, serum	10–190	mg/dL	0.01129	0.11–2.15	mmol/L
Triiodothyronine, free (FT3)[b]	Serum	260–480	pg/dL	0.0154	4.0–7.4	pmol/L
Triiodothyronine, resin uptake[b]	Serum	25–35	%	0.01	0.25–0.35	Fraction of 1.0
Triiodothyronine, total (T3)[b]	Serum	70–200	ng/dL	0.0154	1.08–3.14	nmol/L
Troponin I (cardiac)	Serum	0–0.4	ng/mL	1	0–0.4	µg/L
Troponin T (cardiac)	Serum	0–0.1	ng/mL	1	0–0.1	µg/L
Tryptophan[b]	Plasma	0.5–1.5	mg/dL	48.97	25–73	µmol/L
Tyrosine[b]	Plasma	0.4–1.6	mg/dL	55.19	20–90	µmol/L
Urea nitrogen (BUN)[b]	Serum	8–23	mg/dL	0.357	2.9–8.2	mmol/L

Continued next page—

	Specimen	Traditional Reference Interval	Traditional Units	Conversion Factor, Multiply →, ← Divide	SI Reference Interval	SI Units
Uric acid[b]	Serum	4.0–8.5	mg/dL	0.0595	0.24–0.51	mmol/L
Urobilinogen[b]	Urine	0.05–2.5	mg/24 hours	1.693	0.1–4.2	µmol/day
Valine[b]	Plasma	1.7–3.7	mg/dL	85.5	145–315	µmol/L
Valproic acid (therapeutic)	Plasma, serum	50–150	µg/mL	6.93	346–1040	µmol/L
Vancomycin (therapeutic, peak)	Plasma, serum	18–26	µg/mL	0.69	12–18	µmol/L
Vanillylmandelic acid (VMA)[b]	Urine	2.1–7.6	mg/24 hours	5.046	11–38	µmol/day
Vasoactive intestinal polypeptide	Plasma	<50	pg/mL	1	<50	ng/L
Verapamil (therapeutic)	Plasma, serum	100–500	ng/mL	2.2	220–1100	nmol/L
Vitamin A (retinol)[b]	Serum	30–80	µg/dL	0.0349	1.05–2.80	µmol/L
Vitamin B$_1$ (thiamine)	Whole blood	2.5–7.5	µg/dL	29.6	74–222	nmol/L
Vitamin B$_2$ (riboflavin)	Plasma, serum	4–24	µg/dL	26.6	106–638	nmol/L
Vitamin B$_5$ (pantothenic acid)	Whole blood	0.2–1.8	µg/mL	4.56	0.9–8.2	µmol/L
Vitamin B$_6$ (pyridoxine)	Plasma	5–30	ng/mL	4.046	20–121	nmol/L
Vitamin B$_{12}$ (cyanocobalamin)[b]	Serum	160–950	pg/mL	0.7378	118–701	pmol/L
Vitamin C (ascorbic acid)	Plasma, serum	0.4–1.5	mg/dL	56.78	23–85	µmol/L
Vitamin D, 1,25-dihydroxyvitamin D	Plasma, serum	16–65	pg/mL	2.6	42–169	pmol/L
Vitamin D, 25-hydroxyvitamin D	Plasma, serum	14–60	ng/mL	2.496	35–150	nmol/L
Vitamin E (α-tocopherol)[b]	Plasma, serum	0.5–1.8	mg/dL	23.22	12–42	µmol/L
Vitamin K	Plasma, serum	0.13–1.19	ng/mL	2.22	0.29–2.64	nmol/L
von Willebrand's factor (ranges vary according to blood type)	Plasma	70–140	%	0.01	0.70–1.40	Fraction of 1.0
Warfarin (therapeutic)	Plasma, serum	1.0–10	µg/mL	3.24	3.2–32.4	µmol/L
White blood cell count[b]	Whole blood	4.5–11.0	$10^3\ \mu L^{-1}$	1	4.5–11.0	$10^9\ L^{-1}$
White blood cell, differential count (see complete blood count)						
Xylose absorption test (25-g dose)[b]	Whole blood	>25 mg/dL	mg/dL	0.06661	>1.7	mmol/L
Zidovudine (therapeutic)	Plasma, serum	0.15–0.27	µg/mL	3.74	0.56–1.01	µmol/L
Zinc	Serum	50–150	µg/dL	0.153	7.7–23.0	µmol/L

The normal ranges listed here are included as a helpful guide and are by no means comprehensive. The listed reference, unless noted, pertains to adults. Laboratory results are method dependent and can have intra-laboratory variation. Conversion factors are not affected by age-related differences. This table is compiled from data in the following sources: 1) Tietz NW, ed. *Clinical Guide to Laboratory Tests*. 3rd ed. Philadelphia: WB Saunders Co; 1995; 2) Laposata M. *SI Unit Conversion Guide*. Boston: NEJM Books; 1992; 3) *American Medical Association Manual of Style: A Guide for Authors and Editors*. 9th ed. Chicago: AMA; 1998:486–503. Copyright 1998, American Medical Association; 4) Jacobs DS, DeMott WR, Oxley DK, eds. *Jacobs & DeMott Laboratory Test Handbook with Key Word Index*. 5th ed. Hudson, OH: Lexi-Comp Inc; 2001; 5) Henry JB, ed. *Clinical Diagnosis and Management by Laboratory Methods*. 20th ed. Philadelphia: WB Saunders Co; 2001; 6) Kratz A, et al. Laboratory reference values. *N Engl J Med*. 2006;351:1548–1563.

[a]The SI unit katal is the amount of enzyme generating 1 mol of product per second. Although provisionally recommended as the SI unit for enzymatic activity, it has not been universally accepted. It is suitable to maintain use of U/L in these circumstances (conversion factor 1.0).

[b]For this analyte, there is age dependence for the reference range. There may be several different normal ranges for different pediatric age ranges. Consult your clinical laboratory for the local institution age-specific reference range. Pediatric reference values may also be found in Soldin SJ, Brugnara C, Wong, EC, eds.; Hicks JM, editor emeritus. *Pediatric References Intervals*. 5th ed. (formerly *Pediatric Reference Ranges*). Washington, DC: AACC Press; 2005.

Concepts in Laboratory Medicine

Michael Laposata

LEARNING OBJECTIVES

1. To understand the concepts of sensitivity, specificity, predictive value, prevalence, and incidence.
2. To learn the frequently encountered preanalytical variables that influence laboratory test results.
3. To identify the well-known interferences in many of the laboratory tests.
4. To understand the individual steps in specimen processing and handling.
5. To understand the guidelines for appropriate selection of laboratory tests.
6. To understand how cell injury and inflammation result in the generation of plasma markers of these processes.

CHAPTER OUTLINE

An understanding of the principles set forth in this chapter is essential for the appropriate selection of laboratory tests and the accurate interpretation of the test results.

ANALYTICAL AND STATISTICAL CONCEPTS IN DATA ANALYSIS

Ranges Used in the Interpretation of Test Results

In clinical practice, the laboratory test result is typically placed alongside a range of values for that test. In most cases, this is the reference range, which is often considered to be the normal range. It is important to understand that individuals with values inside the reference range may have subclinical disease, despite the presence of an apparently normal value. The reference range is dependent on the instrument and reagent used to perform the test. The reference ranges are ideally established inside the laboratory where the test is being performed. Reference ranges supplied by instrument and reagent manufacturers are not likely to correspond perfectly to ranges generated within an individual laboratory. This is because the population used to establish the range by the manufacturer and/or the instruments and reagents used by the manufacturer are likely to be different from those in an individual clinical laboratory.

The Reference Range

To obtain a reference range, individuals without disease and on no medications donate samples for testing. A distribution of these values, which should be numerous enough to be statistically reliable, is plotted. The data are not always distributed in a Gaussian pattern. Therefore, statistical methods that are nonparametric are used to identify the central 95% of values. This range, representing the middle 95% of results, is the reference range. As an indication that being outside the reference range does not always reflect the disease, 5% of normal healthy, nonmedicated individuals who donated samples for the reference range determination now fall outside of what has become the reference range for the test.

> To obtain a reference range, individuals without disease and on no medications donate samples for testing. The middle 95% of results is the reference range.

The Desirable Range

Several decades ago, the results for cholesterol testing demonstrated that individuals eating a high-fat diet showed high cholesterol levels that were associated with atherosclerotic vascular disease. When these apparently healthy, nonmedicated individuals provided samples for reference range determinations, the central 95% of values from this population provided an inappropriately high reference range. Therefore, the use of the classical reference range for selected laboratory tests in certain populations was not recommended. For that reason, desirable or prognosis-related ranges were developed. These are commonly established by groups of experts associating laboratory test results with clinical outcome.

Therapeutic Range

For certain medications, a therapeutic window exists to provide a target for a blood, plasma, or serum level for the medication. Values below the therapeutic range typically reflect an inadequate amount of medication, and values above the therapeutic range may be associated with a particular toxic effect. In some cases, the therapeutic range does not reflect the amount of medication in the blood, but instead reflects a therapeutic effect produced by the drug. For example, patients taking the drug warfarin are not monitored with warfarin levels in the blood. Instead, the warfarin decreases the level of coagulation factors, which results in a prolonged prothrombin time (PT), and a calculated value known as the international normalized ratio or INR. The therapeutic range of warfarin, therefore, is determined by its effect rather than its concentration in the blood.

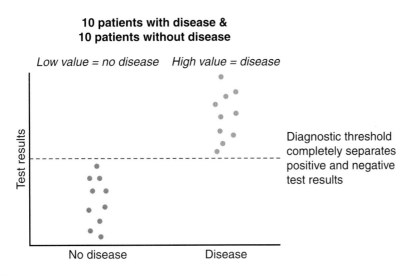

**10 patients with disease &
10 patients without disease**

Low value = no disease   *High value = disease*

Test results

Diagnostic threshold
completely separates
positive and negative
test results

No disease   Disease

FIGURE 1–1 A clinical situation in which the diagnostic threshold completely separates those with disease from those without disease.

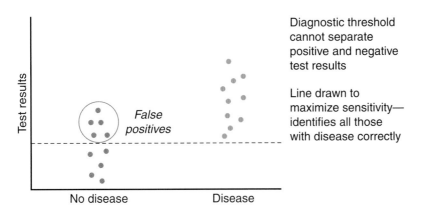

Test results

Diagnostic threshold
cannot separate
positive and negative
test results

Line drawn to
maximize sensitivity—
identifies all those
with disease correctly

*False
positives*

No disease   Disease

FIGURE 1–2 A clinical situation in which a diagnostic threshold is selected to maximize sensitivity.

For certain laboratory
tests, the presence of
disease is associated
with a value that is
above a threshold.

Interpretations of Clinical Laboratory Test Results that Do Not Involve the Use of a Range

For certain laboratory tests, the presence of disease is associated with a value that is above a threshold. The use of troponin as a marker for myocardial infarction involves a threshold value, such that a level above the threshold is consistent with cardiac ischemia. Another prominent example is related to the detection of drugs of abuse. Any level above zero, as a threshold value, provides evidence for the ingestion of an illicit drug.

For laboratory tests that show too much variability to permit the use of a range or a threshold, an individual laboratory result for a specific patient can be compared to a result for that same patient that was generated previously. The longitudinal analysis of results over time can indicate the progression or regression of the disease.

The Need for a Diagnostic Cutoff

Figure 1–1 shows 2 populations of individuals and their results for a particular test. All of the individuals who do not have disease have a low value for the test, and all of the individuals with disease have a high value for the test. There is no overlap between groups in **Figure 1–1**. In **Figure 1–2**, a more commonly encountered situation is shown. There is overlap in laboratory values between individuals with disease and those without disease. This means that the diagnostic threshold will necessarily misclassify some patients to create false-positives, false-negatives, or both.

The Definition of Sensitivity of a Laboratory Test

The population of individuals who have disease is the focus of sensitivity. The sensitivity of a laboratory test is its capacity to identify all individuals with disease. The threshold used in **Figure 1–2** maximizes sensitivity by placing all those with disease above the line. This placement of the diagnostic threshold would decrease the number of false-negatives (those with disease who fall below the line), because everybody with the disease would have a positive test result. However, there is a significant misclassification of individuals without disease. As the diagnostic threshold is lowered, an increasing number of patients without disease would be told they have a positive test result, and by implication, the disease in question. The formula for sensitivity is:

$$\frac{\text{true-positives}}{\text{true-positives} + \text{false-negatives}} \times 100$$

True-positives and false-negatives are groups with disease; as noted above, sensitivity focuses on those with disease.

The Definition of Specificity of a Laboratory Test

The population of individuals without disease is the focus of specificity. Specificity is a statistical term that indicates the effectiveness of a test to correctly identify those without disease. When used to describe a laboratory test, it does not refer to its ability to diagnose a "specific" disease among a group of related disorders. One could maximize specificity by raising the threshold shown in **Figure 1–3** to place all those without disease below the line. This would decrease the number of false-positives because everyone without disease would have a negative test result. However, there would be a significant misclassification of the individuals with disease. As the diagnostic threshold is raised, an increasing number of patients with disease would be told they have a negative test result and, by implication, no disease. The formula for specificity is:

$$\frac{\text{true-negatives}}{\text{true-negatives} + \text{false-positives}} \times 100$$

True-negatives and false-positives are the groups without disease; as noted above, specificity focuses on those without disease.

The Identification of the Appropriate Value for the Diagnostic Threshold

For diseases that are serious and treatable, and for which a second confirmatory laboratory test exists, it is important to maximize sensitivity as in **Figure 1–2**. For example, for diagnosis of

> The sensitivity of a laboratory test is its capacity to identify all individuals with disease. Specificity is a statistical term that indicates the effectiveness of a test to correctly identify those without disease.

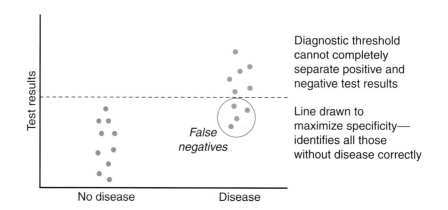

FIGURE 1–3 A clinical situation in which a diagnostic threshold is selected to maximize specificity.

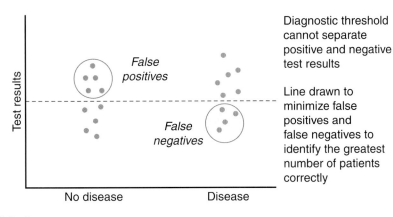

FIGURE 1–4 A clinical situation in which a diagnostic threshold is selected to minimize the number of false-positives and false-negatives.

AIDS, it is better to have a few false-positives that can be subsequently correctly identified with a confirmatory test than to fail to identify individuals with HIV infection who might unknowingly infect others. However, for diseases that are serious and not curable, a false-positive result is catastrophic for the patient. For such diseases, such as pancreatic cancer, it is better to use the threshold shown in **Figure 1–3** for diagnosis because if individuals with disease are missed, it will have no effect on the treatment or outcome. When there are no compelling reasons to maximize either sensitivity or specificity, the threshold value should be established to minimize the total number of false-positives and false-negatives, as shown in **Figure 1–4**.

The Definition of Predictive Value of a Positive Test

The population of individuals with a positive test result is the focus of positive predictive value. The positive predictive value for a laboratory test indicates the likelihood that a positive test result identifies someone with disease. It should be noted that the predictive value of a positive test is greatly influenced by the prevalence of the disease in the area where testing is performed. As an example, a screening test for HIV infection is more likely to be confirmed as positive in an area where many individuals are infected with HIV, as opposed to a location where there is only a rare case of HIV infection. In the latter situation, most of the positive HIV tests in the initial evaluation of a patient are found to be false-positives by confirmatory tests. A high percentage of false-positives from a low prevalence disease, as shown in the following formula, decreases the predictive value of the positive test:

$$\frac{\text{true-positives}}{\text{true-positives} + \text{false-positives}} \times 100$$

> The positive predictive value for a laboratory test indicates the likelihood that a positive test result identifies someone with disease. The negative predictive value for a laboratory test indicates the likelihood that a negative test result identifies someone without disease.

True-positives and false-positives are the groups with a positive test result; as noted above, positive predictive value focuses on those with a positive test.

The Definition of Predictive Value of a Negative Test

The population of individuals with a negative test result is the focus of the negative predictive value. The negative predictive value for a laboratory test indicates the likelihood that a negative test result identifies someone without disease. It is not greatly influenced by the prevalence of disease because false-positives are not included in the formula for negative predictive value. The formula for predictive value of a negative test result is:

$$\frac{\text{true-negatives}}{\text{true-negatives} + \text{false-negatives}} \times 100$$

True-negatives and false-negatives are the groups with a negative test result; as noted above, negative predictive value focuses on those with a negative test result.

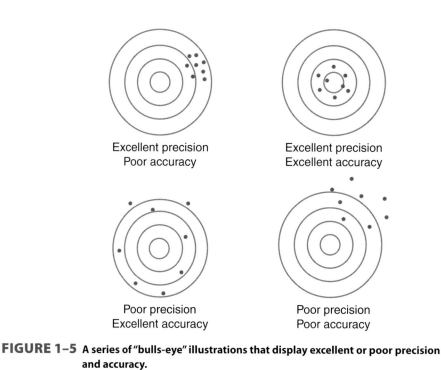

FIGURE 1–5 **A series of "bulls-eye" illustrations that display excellent or poor precision and accuracy.**

The Difference Between Prevalence and Incidence

The prevalence of a disease reflects the number of existing cases in a population. It is usually expressed as a percentage of a certain population. Incidence refers to the number of new cases occurring within a period of time, usually 1 year. For example, in the United States, sore throat has a low prevalence because considering the size of the population there is a low percentage of individuals at a given time afflicted with sore throat. However, it has a high incidence because many new cases of sore throat appear each year.

Precision versus Accuracy

Precision refers to the ability to test 1 sample and repeatedly obtain results that are close to each other. This does not infer that the mean of these very similar numbers is the correct number (see **Figure 1–5**). Some analyses, which have great precision, are very inaccurate. The accuracy reflects the relationship between the number obtained and the true result. Thus, a sample could have high accuracy but low precision if it provides the correct answer but has substantial variability as the sample is repeatedly tested.

Analyzing Errors in Laboratory Performance

There are 3 phases of laboratory analysis. The first of these is the preanalytical phase. This time frame is from patient preparation for the laboratory test, through the time of sample collection, until the sample arrives in the laboratory. Most of the errors in laboratory test performance occur in this phase. Examples of preanalytical errors are: inappropriate preparation of the patient, such as not fasting for a particular test in which fasting is required; ingesting drugs that will interfere with the laboratory tests; collection of the specimen in the wrong tube; delayed transport of the specimen to the laboratory; storage of the sample at an incorrect temperature; and collection of an inadequate amount of blood in vacuum tubes containing a fixed amount of anticoagulants. All these errors occur before the sample arrives for analysis and make it impossible, no matter how great the analytical precision within the laboratory, to provide a test result that truly reflects the patient's condition. The second phase is the analytical phase, which is the time that the sample is being analyzed in the laboratory. Errors can occur during this process, but they are much less common now because of

Precision refers to the ability to test 1 sample and repeatedly obtain results that are close to each other. This does not infer that the mean of these very similar numbers is the correct number.

the high level of automation of many laboratory instruments. Examples of analytical errors are: incorrect use of the instrumentation and the use of expired reagents. The third phase of laboratory test performance is the postanalytical phase, which begins when the result is generated and ends when the result is reported to the physician. Example of errors in this phase, which are more common than analytical errors, but less common than preanalytical errors are: delay in time to enter a completed result into the laboratory information system and reporting results for the wrong patient.

PREANALYTICAL VARIABLES THAT AFFECT LABORATORY TEST RESULTS

The Effect of Age on Laboratory Tests

There are a number of laboratory tests that have different normal ranges for patients of different ages. This is particularly important in pediatrics. Newborns especially have many different normal ranges than adults or older children for substances in blood and other bodily fluids. For example, several of the coagulation factors do not reach adult levels for many months after birth. As a second well-known example, the cholesterol level rises with age.

The Effect of Gender on Laboratory Tests

Gender has a significant bearing on many laboratory tests. Testosterone and estradiol are obvious examples. In addition, among women there are variations in the serum concentration of various hormones throughout the menstrual cycle.

The Effect of Body Mass on Laboratory Tests

Muscle mass can affect the level of certain compounds, such as creatine kinase, in the blood. It is also known that there is an increase in the serum cholesterol level with obesity, because the cholesterol level is related to the amount of body fat.

Preparation of the Patient for Laboratory Testing

For certain laboratory tests, there are a number of special preparations of the patient that are necessary to provide the most clinically useful, accurate, and precise result. One of the most commonly encountered patient preparations is fasting, usually for 8 to 12 hours, depending on the test. The serum triglyceride level can be significantly affected by eating, and fasting is absolutely required. Another test for which fasting is required is the fasting blood glucose used in the evaluation of a patient for diabetes.

One of the most commonly encountered patient preparations is fasting, usually for 8 to 12 hours, depending on the test. The serum triglyceride level can be significantly affected by eating, and fasting is absolutely required. Another test for which fasting is required is the fasting blood glucose.

Patient Posture for Blood Collection

Patient posture may affect the result for certain tests. There is a lower plasma volume when the patient is upright because there is pooling of fluid in the dependent parts of the body when standing. When the patient is supine, there is a movement of fluid back into the circulation from the tissues. The extra volume in the circulation can dilute certain compounds in the blood. It is best to monitor the patient in the same postural position if the test result is affected by posture and if the values need to be compared with one another over time.

Differences in Test Results Between Samples of Venous, Arterial, and Capillary Blood

Venous blood may have a different concentration of a compound than arterial blood. The best examples are the blood gases that show marked differences between arterial and venous blood because of the exchange of gases in the lungs. There may also be a difference between capillary blood and arterial and venous blood. Blood glucose values may differ significantly in capillary (fingerstick) samples from venous or arterial blood.

INTERFERENCES IN LABORATORY TESTS

Analytical Interferences in Laboratory Testing

Interferences may result in falsely high or falsely low values, depending on the interfering substance and the particular test. Although there are many compounds that can interfere with the accurate and precise quantitation of a compound, there are 3 major interferences that must be considered when selecting and interpreting results of laboratory tests. These are hemolysis that makes plasma and serum red; elevated bilirubin that makes plasma and serum shades of orange, green, or brown; and lipemia that makes plasma and serum milky white. There are many drugs, particularly those that color the plasma and serum, which can produce significant analytical interference. Many automated laboratory tests are spectrophotometric, and therefore depend on measurable changes in the color of plasma or serum after a chemical reaction. This is why alterations in the color of the serum or plasma often interfere with laboratory test performance.

Impact of Drugs on Laboratory Test Results

Drugs can affect laboratory tests in 2 ways—as an interfering substance in the laboratory test only and by producing an effect in the body that alters a laboratory test result. For example, there are many drugs that will increase the PT in patients receiving warfarin (coumadin) by an in vivo potentiation or diminution of warfarin-induced anticoagulation. There are a number of drug effects, however, that alter the result of a particular test strictly in vitro, and do not change anything in vivo.

TEST SELECTION GUIDELINES

The Use of Screening Tests Before Esoteric Tests

Screening laboratory tests are typically inexpensive, easy-to-perform assays that indicate whether additional tests need to be performed to reach a diagnosis. Whenever possible, if a screening test is available, it should be used before the more expensive or time-consuming tests are performed. An example of the use of a screening test is the partial thromboplastin time (result within minutes/hours and at low cost) to assess a major portion of the coagulation cascade. Only if this value is elevated should tests be performed for PTT-related coagulation factor deficiencies (results within several hours and at high cost).

The Danger of Ordering Too Many Laboratory Tests

As noted in the discussion of the normal range, 5% of individuals who have no disease can fall outside of the reference range established by the central 95% of healthy individuals. Thus, if an individual without disease has 20 different tests, it is likely on a statistical basis that he/she will have 1 abnormal value (5% = 1 of 20). In medical practice, the abnormal test result for the normal patient often leads to further evaluation and raises suspicion for a disease that does not exist. Thus, by limiting the number of tests ordered for a patient to those relevant to the clinical presentation of the patient, one is less likely to encounter false-positive or false-negative results.

SPECIMEN PROCESSING AND HANDLING

The Importance of Turnaround Time

An accurate and precise laboratory test result provided after a decision has been made regarding patient management is of no value. Since results for all laboratory tests cannot be provided immediately, the physicians and laboratory personnel must decide on clinically relevant turnaround times for each laboratory test. In addition, if a patient is not discharged from the hospital because of a delay in laboratory testing, this may have a significant financial impact from unnecessary

TABLE 1–1 Cap Color and Contents of Tubes for Blood Collection

Cap Color	Contents
Red	Nothing—the sample clots and the product is serum
Light blue	Citrate anticoagulant
Purple (lavender)	EDTA anticoagulant
Green	Heparin anticoagulant
Red/green with gel	No anticoagulant, but a gel is present that separates the serum or plasma and the cells after centrifugation
Gray	Fluoride (glycolysis inhibitor for optimum glucose measurements) with oxalate anticoagulant
Yellow	Acid-citrate-dextrose solution (ACD) that anticoagulates the blood and helps preserve the blood cells during processing
Dark blue	Nothing—but the tube is specially treated to permit accurate measurement of trace heavy materials

length of stay. All steps related to turnaround time, from ordering of the test to the reporting of the result, must be carefully analyzed and shortened as much as possible.

Tubes for Blood Collection

There are a number of different tubes into which blood may be collected. The tubes used for the vast majority of collections contain a vacuum to help draw the blood into the tube. The tops of the tubes have a different color depending on the contents of the tube prior to blood collection (**Table 1–1**). Several of the tubes contain anticoagulants to prevent the clotting of the blood in the tube. Clotted blood that is centrifuged to remove the clot and any cells is known as serum. Blood that has not been clotted and is then centrifuged to remove any cells is known as plasma. For many laboratory tests, the same result is obtained in an assay if serum or plasma is used. However, this is often not the case. The clotting of the blood, for example, makes blood cell counts and coagulation tests impossible because the clotting factors are consumed in the clot and the blood cells become trapped in it. If the clotting of the blood to form serum is not absolutely necessary, tests can be performed with a shorter turnaround time using plasma because there is no requisite time to wait for the blood clot to form. The amount of anticoagulant in the light blue-top tube must be in a specific proportion to the blood volume in the tube, usually 9 parts blood to 1 part citrate solution. When an inadequate amount of blood is collected into a blue-top tube, the ratio of blood to anticoagulant is less than 9:1. This can result in spuriously high values for the PT and PTT tests. Thus, light blue-top tubes must be filled appropriately to obtain accurate results for clotting tests.

> Clotted blood that is centrifuged to remove the clot and any cells is known as serum. Blood that has not been clotted and is then centrifuged to remove any cells is known as plasma.

Timing of Blood Collection

Patients may have a need to present for phlebotomy at a certain time of the day if the parameter being measured has a diurnal variation in its concentration.

Dynamic tests involve the measurement of a patient response to a treatment or stimulus, and timing of collection is important in these studies. The oral glucose tolerance test, in which plasma glucose levels are measured after the oral ingestion of a glucose solution, is an example of such a test.

A third situation in which timing of sample collection is important is in therapeutic drug monitoring. The serum level of certain drugs is measured to determine if the concentration is within the therapeutic window. The serum level of a drug varies greatly as the drug is absorbed, distributed, and metabolized, so the timing of collection must be consistent. For the monitoring of many drugs, a "trough" level is obtained just before the next dose of the drug is administered.

EFFECTS OF CELL INJURY AND INFLAMMATION ON SELECTED LABORATORY TESTS

The Release of Plasma Markers of Organ Damage from Injured Cells

When cells are injured, components of the cells can leak out of the damaged or dead cells and make their way into the systemic circulation. This permits the measurement of these "marker" compounds in the serum or plasma as a test for injury to the organ. The most important features of plasma markers of cell injury are that: 1) they are not rapidly removed from the circulation; 2) they are relatively organ specific so that the damaged organ is identified; and 3) the compound is precisely and accurately measured in the clinical laboratory. A well-known example includes the release of the creatine kinase-MB fraction and troponin from myocardial cells injured by ischemia in myocardial infarction.

Markers of Inflammation and the Acute Phase Response

The concentration of many plasma proteins changes significantly in patients with inflammation. Infections (even minor viral illnesses), autoimmune disorders, and many other conditions result in an increased concentration of proteins known as acute-phase reactants. Commonly used tests to assess the severity of inflammation, from whatever cause, are the erythrocyte sedimentation rate (ESR) and C-reactive protein (CRP). Examples of acute-phase reactant proteins include fibrinogen, which can rise as much as 10-fold over baseline, and von Willebrand factor, which can rise 2- to 3-fold over baseline. The rise in von Willebrand factor with inflammation can mask a deficiency of von Willebrand factor in patients with von Willebrand disease, and this highlights the need to obtain baseline values after an acute-phase response subsides for accurate diagnosis.

The Serologic Diagnosis of Infectious Disease

It is not uncommon to suffer an infection with an organism that is not identifiable by Gram staining or other microscopic analysis and is not readily cultured. For these infections, the diagnosis is often made by identifying and measuring the amount of antibody produced in response to an antigen derived from the infectious agent. The antibody response typically takes several days to a week or 2 (dependent on past exposure) to emerge, and the appearance of IgM antibody before IgG occurs in most infections. This is why the presence of IgM antibody in a serologic test is likely to reflect an acute infection rather than past exposure. Serologic tests may also be designed to detect and measure an antigen associated with the infectious agent. This obviates the inherent delay in diagnosis of the infection of up to approximately 2 weeks while waiting for the antibody response to occur.

REFERENCES

Gornall AG. Basic concepts in laboratory investigation [Chapter 1]. In: Gornall AG, ed. *Applied Biochemistry of Clinical Disorders*. Philadelphia, PA: Harper and Row; 1980.

McPherson RA. Laboratory statistics [Chapter 9]. In: McPherson RA, Pincus MR, eds. *Henry's Clinical Diagnosis and Management by Laboratory Methods*. 21st ed. Philadelphia, PA: WB Saunders; 2006.

When cells are injured, components of the cells can leak out of the damaged or dead cells and make their way into the systemic circulation. This permits the measurement of these "marker" compounds in the serum or plasma as a test for injury to the organ.

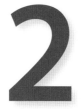

Methods

Michael Laposata

CHAPTER OUTLINE

No textbook in laboratory medicine would be complete without a description of methods used in the clinical laboratory. The methods described in this chapter are predominantly the common ones found in clinical laboratories. Each method description provides an overview of the basic concept of the assay, minimizing the details, while including clinically important information and a comment on the expense of the test and the complexity of the assay in the laboratory.

Some methods describe specific assays used almost exclusively in the clinical laboratory. For example, the PT and PTT are tests used for clinical assessment, with the goal to identify factor deficiencies in the coagulation cascade. Other methods are standard techniques used inside and outside the clinical laboratory. As an example, flow cytometry is a standard technique used in a variety of settings, and in this chapter it is shown how it is used in clinical laboratory testing.

The expense assessment attached to each assay described in this chapter is an approximation, listed as low, moderate, or high. It should be understood that the charge for the test set by the institution operating the laboratory is usually proportional to the expense of the reagents, supplies, and labor required to perform the test. On occasion, however, there is a great disparity between the actual expense to perform the test and the amount charged by the institution for the assay. With this in mind, the expense estimation provided for each method in this chapter is more closely related to the actual cost of reagents, supplies, and labor in the laboratory, with the understanding that the amount charged for the test should be in the same range of low, moderate, or high—but it is not always the case.

Each method also has a descriptor to reflect whether it is manual, semi-automated, or highly automated. A comment has been added if microscopy is involved, as this makes any technique highly manual. It should be noted that for some methods, there is an option for manual performance or for using some level of automation. Manual methods are often less expensive. There is usually greater automation in the larger clinical laboratories because larger laboratories are more likely to have the test volume and the financial resources to justify the automated option. The term semi-automated indicates that there is a manual component associated with the use of an instrument that performs some steps of the analysis.

The turnaround time for an assay is not provided because it is impossible to know all of the elements associated with the turnaround time for a test within an individual institution. Broadly speaking, the turnaround time is shorter for assays that are highly automated and less expensive, and longer for assays that are manual and highly expensive. It is important to understand that the turnaround time for an assay can be calculated using different starting points. For example, 1 starting point is the time a sample is collected. Another starting point is the time that a sample enters the laboratory. However, the most relevant starting time clinically, which predates the previous 2 starting times, is the time at which the physician orders the test. Similarly, there are different endpoints in the assessment of turnaround time. Most commonly, the endpoint is the time at which the result is reported by the laboratory into the laboratory information system. However, it is most important to know when the physician becomes aware of the result. This endpoint is extremely difficult to ascertain, and, therefore, virtually always the endpoint is considered to be the time at which the result is reported by the laboratory.

Finally, it should be noted what methods are not presented in this chapter. There are a number of methods that have been used progressively less over time, and in many institutions these assays are no longer performed at all in the clinical laboratory. These are numerous and include the radioimmunoassay (RIA), immunoelectrophoresis, lipoprotein electrophoresis, and the bleeding time. Also less frequently performed assays are not described in this chapter. Though this number of methods may be large, the number of tests performed using these methods account for a small percentage of the total tests performed in a typical hospital clinical laboratory.

Broadly speaking, the turnaround time is shorter for assays that are highly automated and less expensive, and longer for assays that are manual and highly expensive.

Antinuclear antibody (ANA) testing

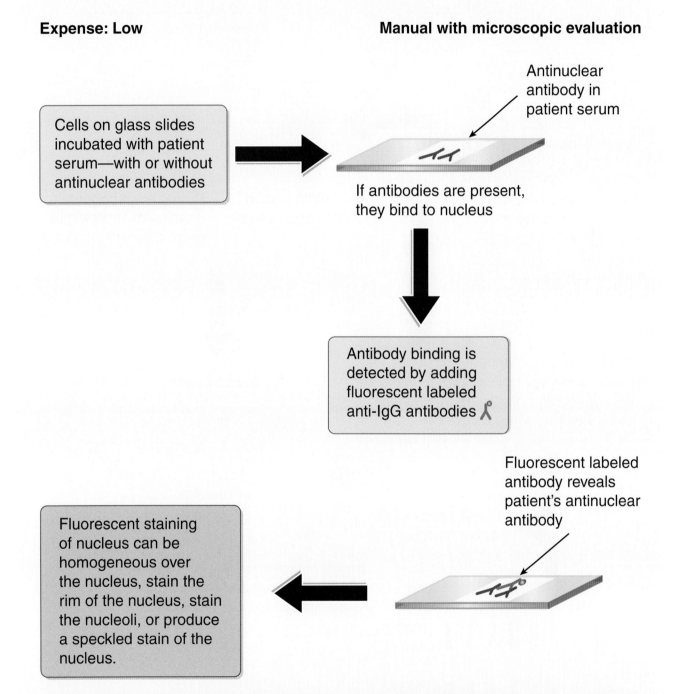

Expense: Low

Manual with microscopic evaluation

Cells on glass slides incubated with patient serum—with or without antinuclear antibodies

Antinuclear antibody in patient serum

If antibodies are present, they bind to nucleus

Antibody binding is detected by adding fluorescent labeled anti-IgG antibodies

Fluorescent labeled antibody reveals patient's antinuclear antibody

Fluorescent staining of nucleus can be homogeneous over the nucleus, stain the rim of the nucleus, stain the nucleoli, or produce a speckled stain of the nucleus.

If an antibody is detected, the patient's serum is progressively diluted until the staining is no longer detected. The final result includes the highest serum dilution producing a detectable response and the pattern of nuclear staining.

FIGURE 2–1

Protein electrophoresis (PEP)

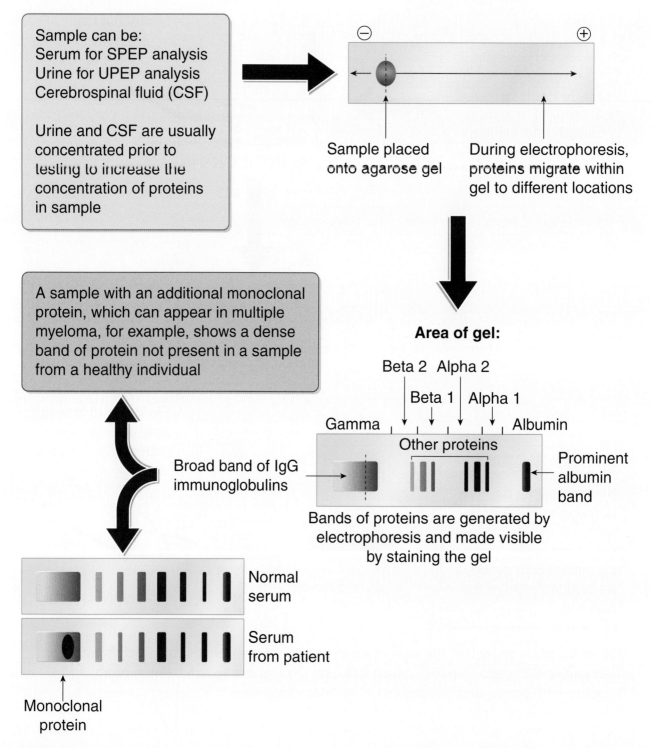

Expense: Moderate

Sample can be:
Serum for SPEP analysis
Urine for UPEP analysis
Cerebrospinal fluid (CSF)

Urine and CSF are usually concentrated prior to testing to increase the concentration of proteins in sample

Semi-automated

Sample placed onto agarose gel

During electrophoresis, proteins migrate within gel to different locations

A sample with an additional monoclonal protein, which can appear in multiple myeloma, for example, shows a dense band of protein not present in a sample from a healthy individual

Area of gel:

Beta 2   Alpha 2
Beta 1 | Alpha 1
Gamma   Albumin
Other proteins

Broad band of IgG immunoglobulins

Prominent albumin band

Bands of proteins are generated by electrophoresis and made visible by staining the gel

Normal serum

Serum from patient

Monoclonal protein

FIGURE 2–2

Immunofixation to identify monoclonal immunoglobulins

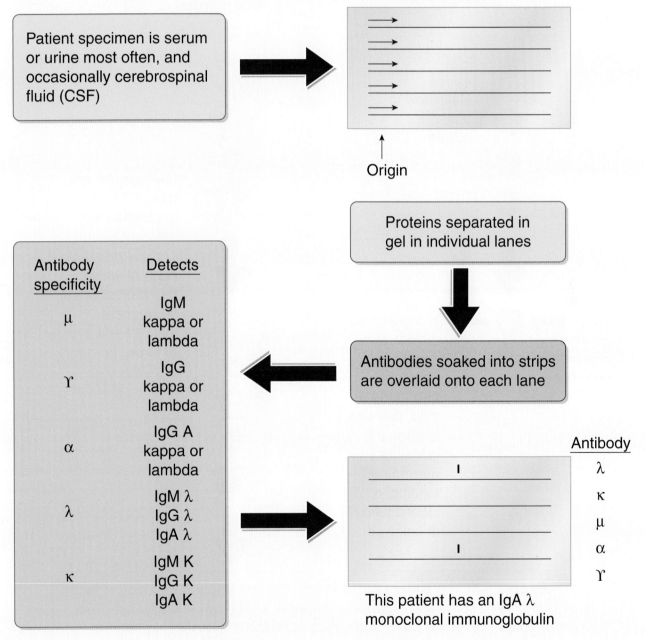

Expense: Moderate

Patient specimen is serum or urine most often, and occasionally cerebrospinal fluid (CSF)

Semi-automated

Multiple aliquots of same sample onto an agarose gel

Origin

Proteins separated in gel in individual lanes

Antibodies soaked into strips are overlaid onto each lane

Antibody specificity	Detects
μ	IgM kappa or lambda
ϒ	IgG kappa or lambda
α	IgG A kappa or lambda
λ	IgM λ IgG λ IgA λ
κ	IgM K IgG K IgA K

Antibody

λ
κ
μ
α
ϒ

This patient has an IgA λ monoclonal immunoglobulin

FIGURE 2–3

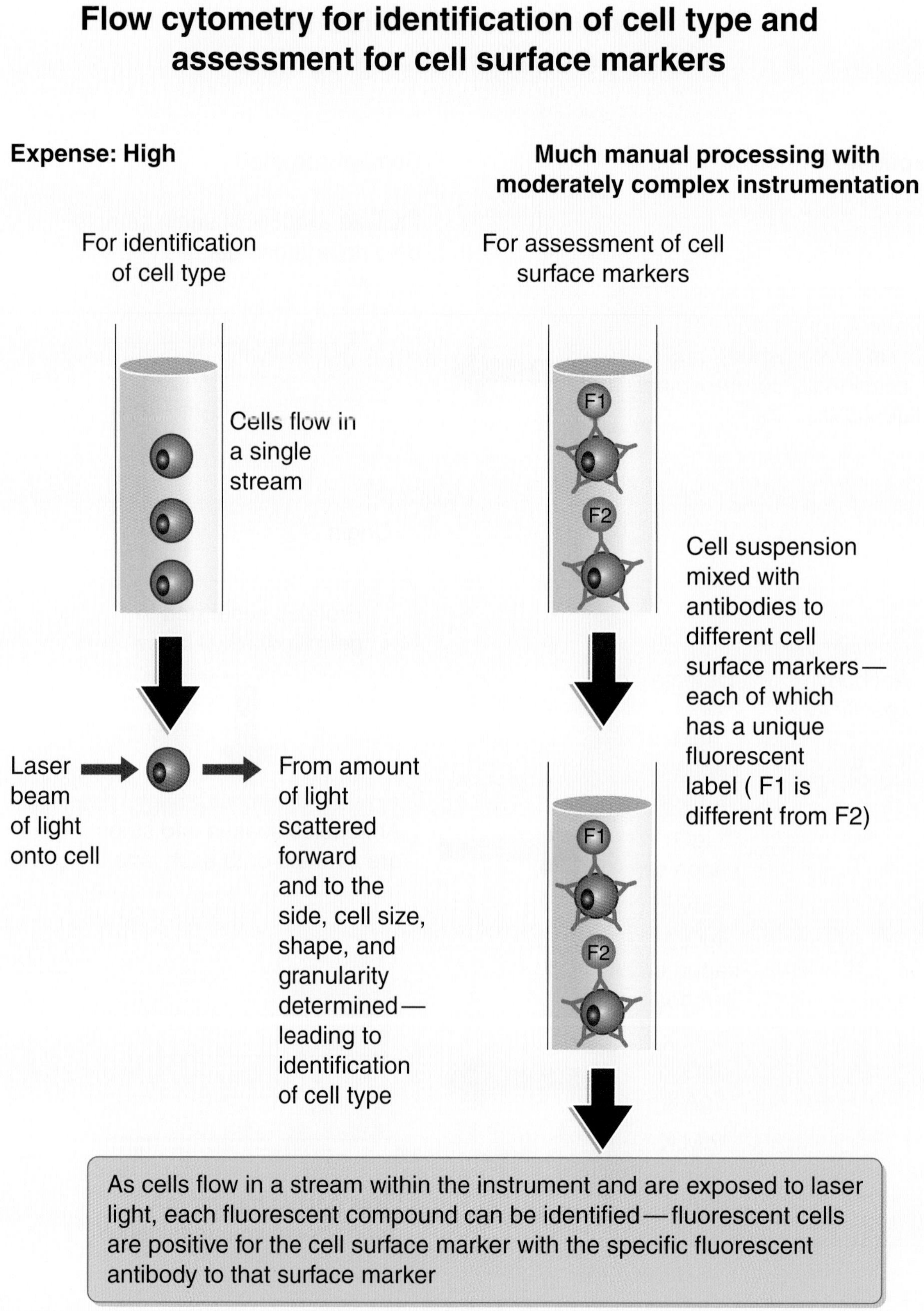

Flow cytometry for identification of cell type and assessment for cell surface markers

Expense: High

Much manual processing with moderately complex instrumentation

For identification of cell type

For assessment of cell surface markers

Cells flow in a single stream

Laser beam of light onto cell

From amount of light scattered forward and to the side, cell size, shape, and granularity determined— leading to identification of cell type

Cell suspension mixed with antibodies to different cell surface markers— each of which has a unique fluorescent label (F1 is different from F2)

As cells flow in a stream within the instrument and are exposed to laser light, each fluorescent compound can be identified—fluorescent cells are positive for the cell surface marker with the specific fluorescent antibody to that surface marker

FIGURE 2–4

Nephelometry for quantitation of selected proteins and other compounds

Expense: Moderate   **Semi-automated**

Sample of any body fluid is incubated with an antibody to the compound being measured	When the compound is present, antigen–antibody complexes form

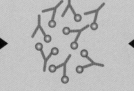

Antibody to the compound is the reagent added to the sample		Antigen is compound being measured

The amount of scattered light is proportional to the amount of compound being measured	Antigen–antibody complexes scatter light from a beam of light shown through the sample

FIGURE 2–5

Cryoglobulin analysis

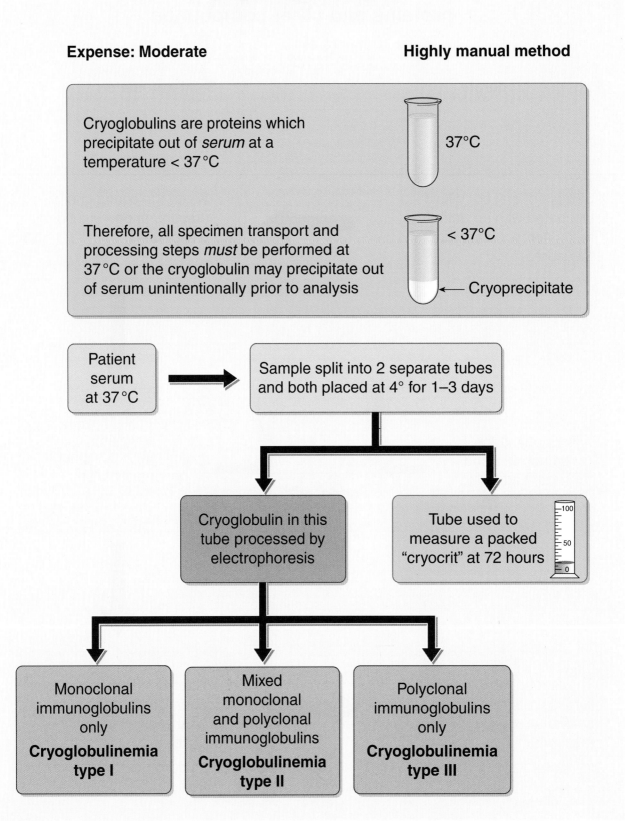

Expense: Moderate

Highly manual method

Cryoglobulins are proteins which precipitate out of *serum* at a temperature < 37°C

37°C

Therefore, all specimen transport and processing steps *must* be performed at 37°C or the cryoglobulin may precipitate out of serum unintentionally prior to analysis

< 37°C

Cryoprecipitate

Patient serum at 37°C

Sample split into 2 separate tubes and both placed at 4° for 1–3 days

Cryoglobulin in this tube processed by electrophoresis

Tube used to measure a packed "cryocrit" at 72 hours

Monoclonal immunoglobulins only
Cryoglobulinemia type I

Mixed monoclonal and polyclonal immunoglobulins
Cryoglobulinemia type II

Polyclonal immunoglobulins only
Cryoglobulinemia type III

FIGURE 2–6

Gram stain

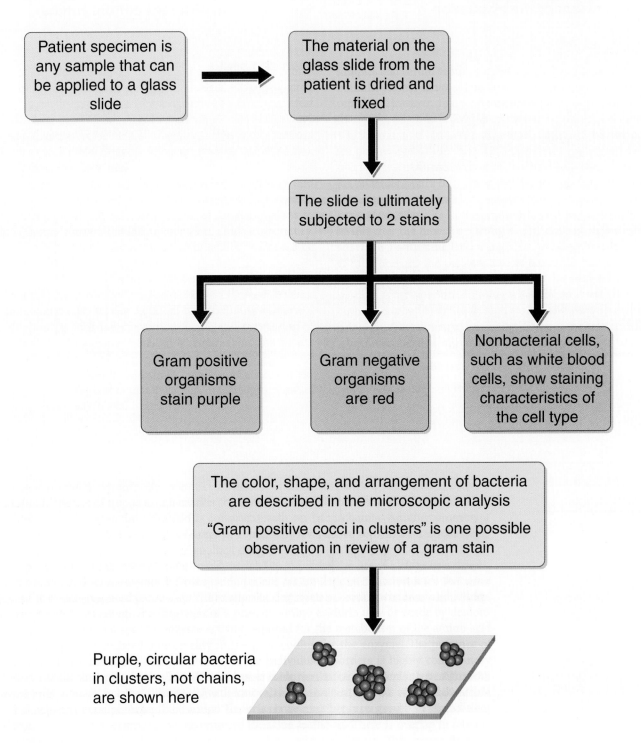

FIGURE 2–7

Microbiologic culture and organism identification

Expense: Moderate to high, depending on the extent of the evaluation

Mostly manual with much visual inspection of colonies in different culture media

Sample collection	The sample to be processed can be:		
	Liquid—such as body fluids other than blood, which is processed differently	Solid or semisolid— such as sputum, stool, or tissue	On a swab from an infected site— such as a wound

Growth of organisms— in aerobic or anaerobic environments	The sample can be:		
	Plated onto ≥1 agar plate to permit organisms to grow into colonies	Inoculated into a broth which promotes growth of microorganisms	Inoculated onto agar within a tube which promotes the growth of certain bacteria

Isolation of organisms	Colonies growing on agar surfaces are first characterized by colony morphology which provides an early clue to organism identification—and then colonies of interest can be subcultured for species identification

Identification of organisms	Microorganisms originating from an isolated colony can be tested in a panel of biochemical tests—the results of which identify the microorganism with a percent likelihood

FIGURE 2–8

Blood cultures

Expense: High

**In most laboratories it
is now highly automated**

| Sample collection | The surface of the arm overlying the venipuncture site must be meticulously cleaned with agents that eliminate skin microorganisms before venipuncture– if not, non-pathogenic skin bacteria can contaminate the blood culture |
| | Blood with or without microorganisms is collected into bottles for growth in aerobic or anaerobic environments |

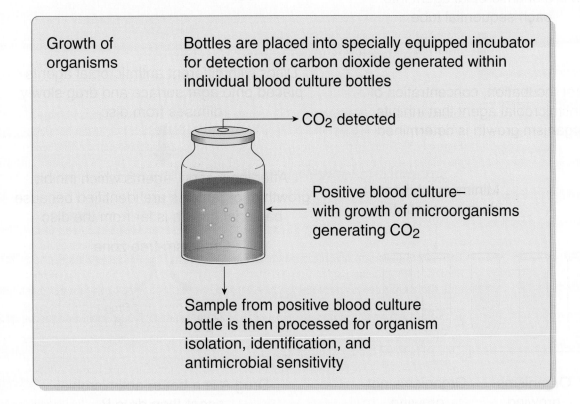

| Growth of organisms | Bottles are placed into specially equipped incubator for detection of carbon dioxide generated within individual blood culture bottles |

CO_2 detected

Positive blood culture– with growth of microorganisms generating CO_2

Sample from positive blood culture bottle is then processed for organism isolation, identification, and antimicrobial sensitivity

FIGURE 2–9

Antimicrobial sensitivity tests

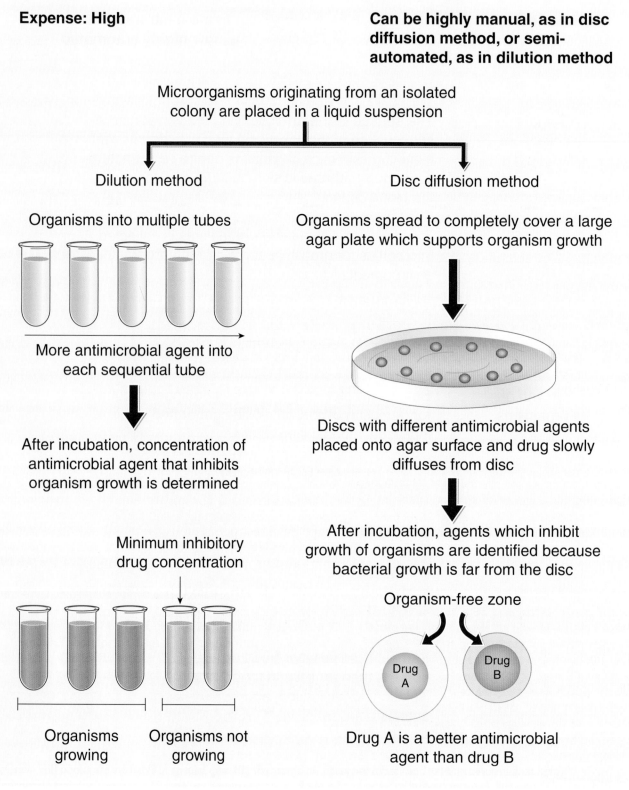

Expense: High

Can be highly manual, as in disc diffusion method, or semi-automated, as in dilution method

Microorganisms originating from an isolated colony are placed in a liquid suspension

Dilution method

Disc diffusion method

Organisms into multiple tubes

Organisms spread to completely cover a large agar plate which supports organism growth

More antimicrobial agent into each sequential tube

After incubation, concentration of antimicrobial agent that inhibits organism growth is determined

Discs with different antimicrobial agents placed onto agar surface and drug slowly diffuses from disc

Minimum inhibitory drug concentration

After incubation, agents which inhibit growth of organisms are identified because bacterial growth is far from the disc

Organism-free zone

Drug A

Drug B

Organisms growing

Organisms not growing

Drug A is a better antimicrobial agent than drug B

FIGURE 2–10

Direct and indirect immunofluorescence for antigen detection

Expense: Moderate   **Manual with microscopic evaluation**

Direct immunofluorescence   Indirect immunofluorescence

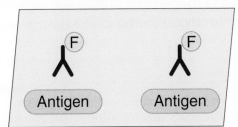

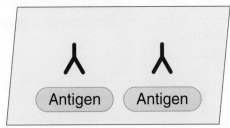

Fluorescent Ⓕ labeled antibody
binds to antigen of interest on
a glass slide or other surface

Antibody which is *not*
fluorescent-labeled binds
to antigen of interest on a
glass slide or other surface

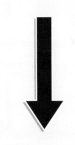

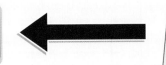
Slides read using a
fluorescent microscope

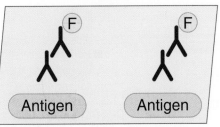

Fluorescent Ⓕ labeled antibody
to IgG is added and binds to
antibody previously bound to
antigen

FIGURE 2–11

Counting of blood cells with automated white blood cell differential count

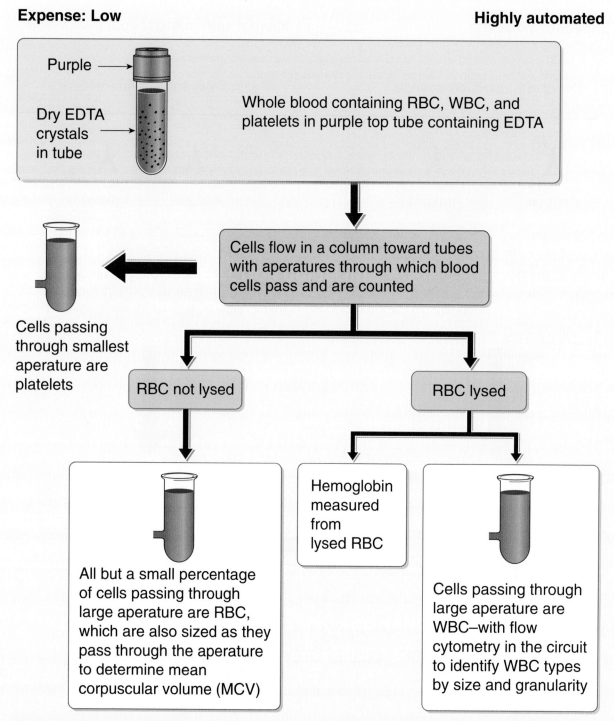

Hematocrit or packed RBC volume is calculated from number and size of RBC

FIGURE 2–12

Peripheral blood smear analysis

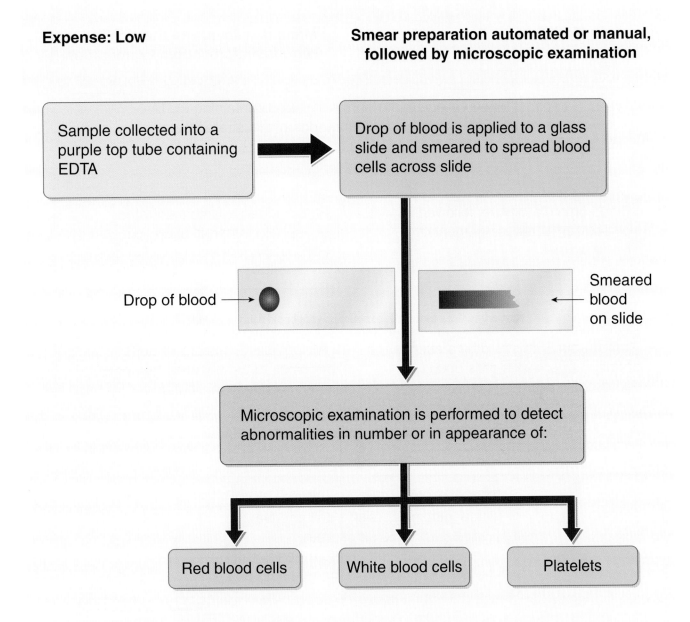

Expense: Low

Smear preparation automated or manual, followed by microscopic examination

Sample collected into a purple top tube containing EDTA

Drop of blood is applied to a glass slide and smeared to spread blood cells across slide

Drop of blood →

Smeared blood on slide ←

Microscopic examination is performed to detect abnormalities in number or in appearance of:

Red blood cells

White blood cells

Platelets

The peripheral blood smear is commonly used early in the diagnostic process to assess a patient for an abnormality involving circulating blood cells

FIGURE 2–13

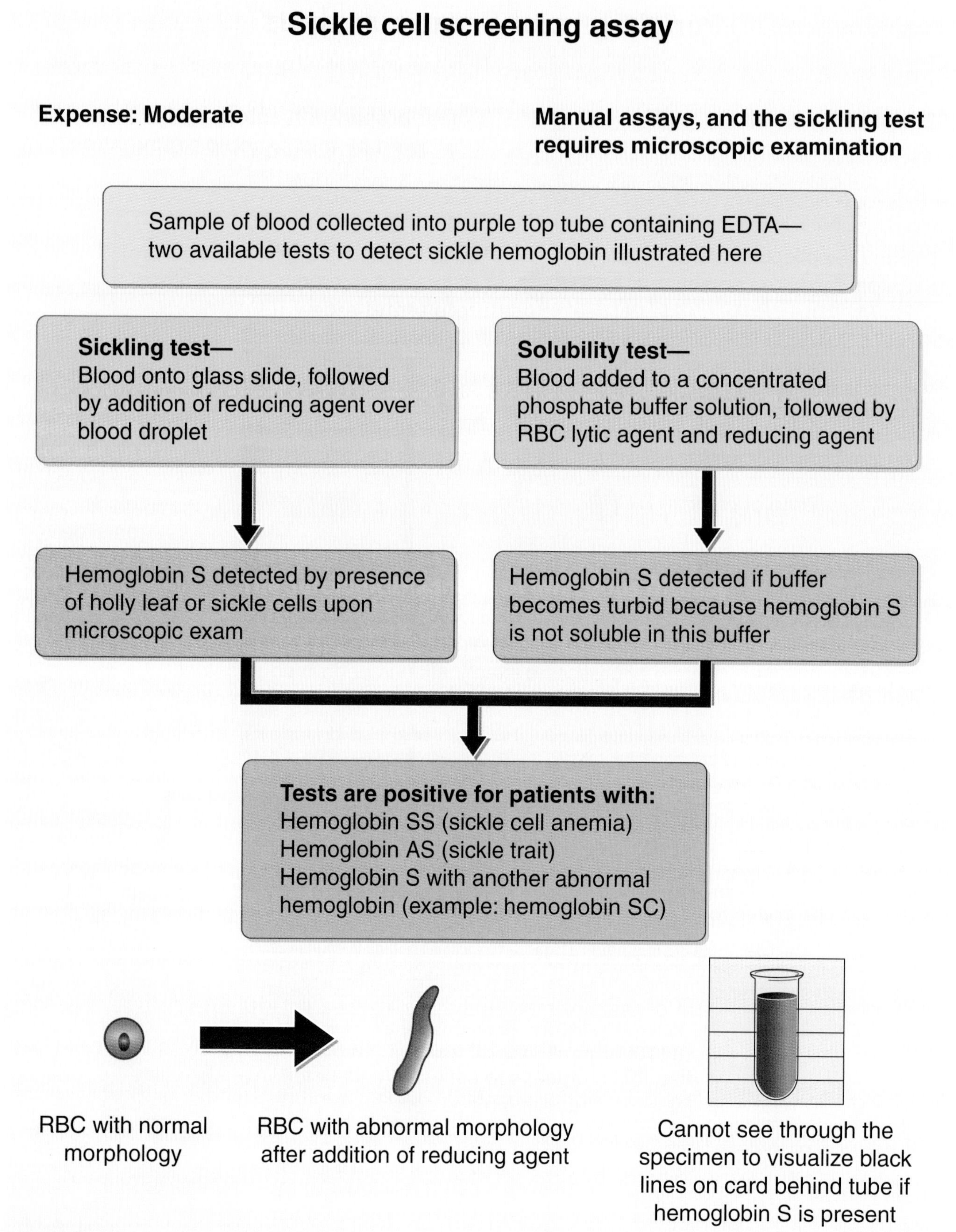

Sickle cell screening assay

Expense: Moderate

Manual assays, and the sickling test requires microscopic examination

Sample of blood collected into purple top tube containing EDTA—two available tests to detect sickle hemoglobin illustrated here

Sickling test—
Blood onto glass slide, followed by addition of reducing agent over blood droplet

Solubility test—
Blood added to a concentrated phosphate buffer solution, followed by RBC lytic agent and reducing agent

Hemoglobin S detected by presence of holly leaf or sickle cells upon microscopic exam

Hemoglobin S detected if buffer becomes turbid because hemoglobin S is not soluble in this buffer

Tests are positive for patients with:
Hemoglobin SS (sickle cell anemia)
Hemoglobin AS (sickle trait)
Hemoglobin S with another abnormal hemoglobin (example: hemoglobin SC)

RBC with normal morphology

RBC with abnormal morphology after addition of reducing agent

Cannot see through the specimen to visualize black lines on card behind tube if hemoglobin S is present

FIGURE 2–14

Hemoglobin electrophoresis

Expense: Moderate   **Semi-automated**

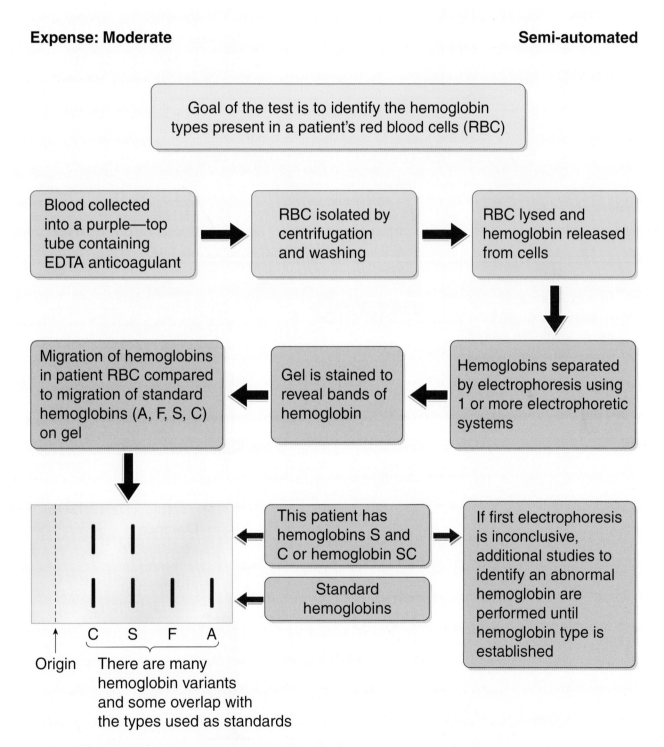

Goal of the test is to identify the hemoglobin types present in a patient's red blood cells (RBC)

Blood collected into a purple—top tube containing EDTA anticoagulant

RBC isolated by centrifugation and washing

RBC lysed and hemoglobin released from cells

Hemoglobins separated by electrophoresis using 1 or more electrophoretic systems

Gel is stained to reveal bands of hemoglobin

Migration of hemoglobins in patient RBC compared to migration of standard hemoglobins (A, F, S, C) on gel

This patient has hemoglobins S and C or hemoglobin SC

Standard hemoglobins

If first electrophoresis is inconclusive, additional studies to identify an abnormal hemoglobin are performed until hemoglobin type is established

C   S   F   A

Origin

There are many hemoglobin variants and some overlap with the types used as standards

Hemoglobin types can also be separated by isoelectric focusing and by high performance liquid chromatography (HPLC)

FIGURE 2–15

Erythrocyte sedimentation rate

Expense: Low   **Manual or semi-automated**

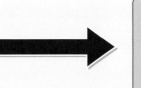

Goal of the test is to measure the height of
sedimented RBC after an incubation, often 1 hour

Whole blood placed
in a cylindrical vessel
with markings to
assess column height

→

RBC allowed to sediment
undisturbed within
cylindrical vessel

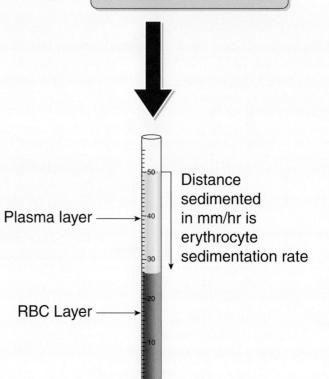

Plasma layer →

RBC Layer →

Distance
sedimented
in mm/hr is
erythrocyte
sedimentation rate

FIGURE 2–16

The PT and PTT assays

Expense: Low   **Highly automated**

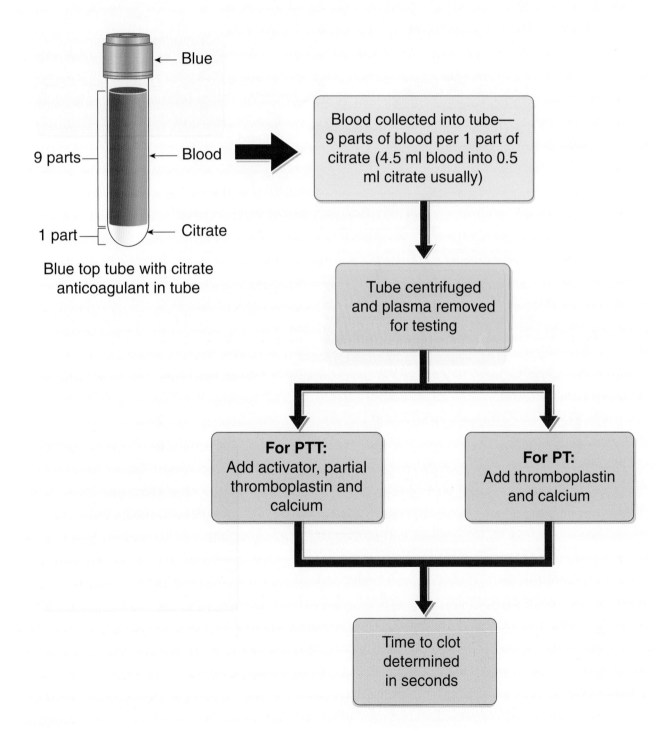

FIGURE 2–17

PT and PTT mixing studies

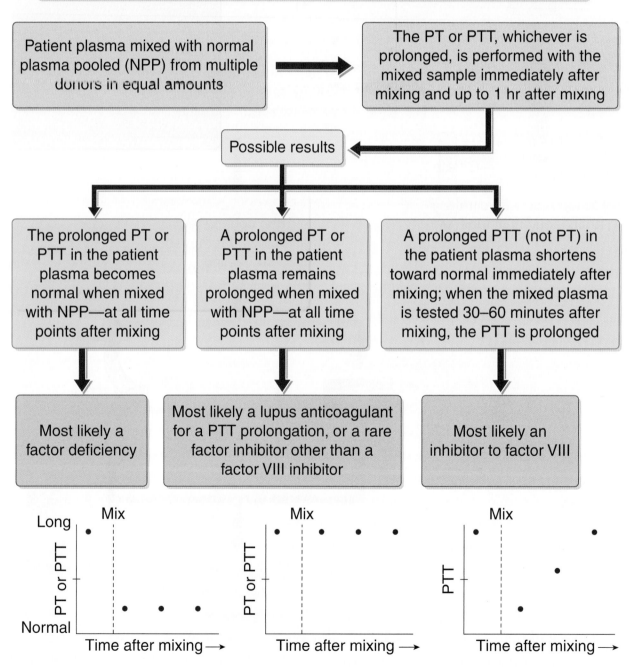

Expense: Low   **After samples are mixed, the testing is highly automated**

The goal of the test is to determine if a prolonged PT or prolonged PTT is a result of ≥1 factor defiencies or an inhibitor of the PT or PTT clotting reaction

Patient plasma mixed with normal plasma pooled (NPP) from multiple donors in equal amounts

The PT or PTT, whichever is prolonged, is performed with the mixed sample immediately after mixing and up to 1 hr after mixing

Possible results

The prolonged PT or PTT in the patient plasma becomes normal when mixed with NPP—at all time points after mixing

A prolonged PT or PTT in the patient plasma remains prolonged when mixed with NPP—at all time points after mixing

A prolonged PTT (not PT) in the patient plasma shortens toward normal immediately after mixing; when the mixed plasma is tested 30–60 minutes after mixing, the PTT is prolonged

Most likely a factor deficiency

Most likely a lupus anticoagulant for a PTT prolongation, or a rare factor inhibitor other than a factor VIII inhibitor

Most likely an inhibitor to factor VIII

FIGURE 2–18

Coagulation factor assays

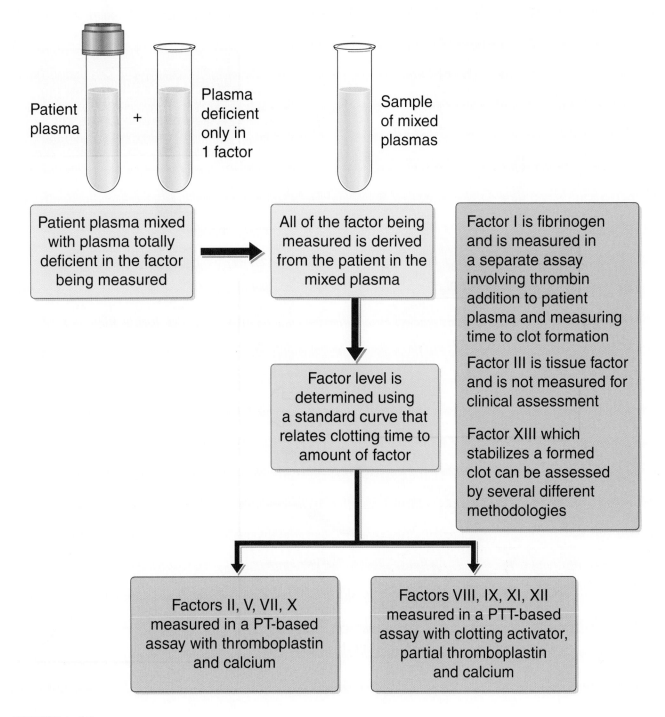

Expense: Moderate, due to reagents used

Highly automated after dilution and mixing steps

Patient plasma + Plasma deficient only in 1 factor

Sample of mixed plasmas

Patient plasma mixed with plasma totally deficient in the factor being measured

All of the factor being measured is derived from the patient in the mixed plasma

Factor level is determined using a standard curve that relates clotting time to amount of factor

Factor I is fibrinogen and is measured in a separate assay involving thrombin addition to patient plasma and measuring time to clot formation

Factor III is tissue factor and is not measured for clinical assessment

Factor XIII which stabilizes a formed clot can be assessed by several different methodologies

Factors II, V, VII, X measured in a PT-based assay with thromboplastin and calcium

Factors VIII, IX, XI, XII measured in a PTT-based assay with clotting activator, partial thromboplastin and calcium

FIGURE 2–19

von Willebrand factor assays

Expense: High

Test for ristocetin cofactor is largely manual, and tests for von Willebrand factor antigen can be semi-automated

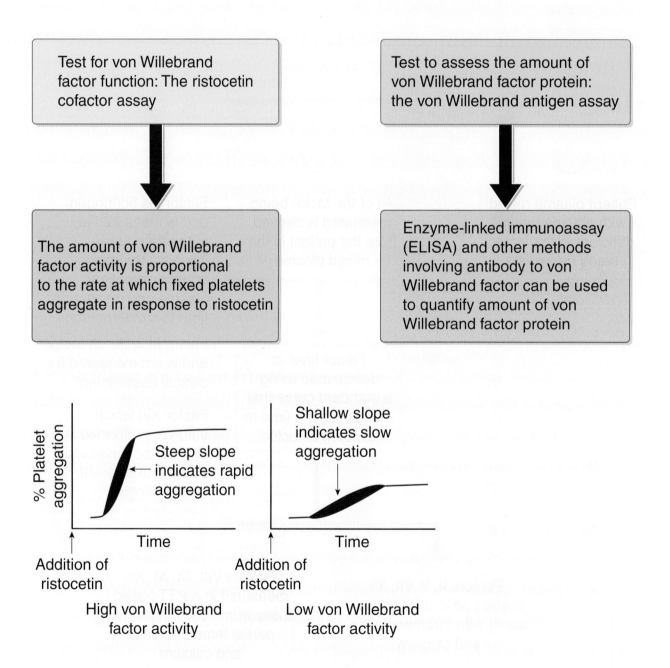

Test for von Willebrand factor function: The ristocetin cofactor assay

The amount of von Willebrand factor activity is proportional to the rate at which fixed platelets aggregate in response to ristocetin

Test to assess the amount of von Willebrand factor protein: the von Willebrand antigen assay

Enzyme-linked immunoassay (ELISA) and other methods involving antibody to von Willebrand factor can be used to quantify amount of von Willebrand factor protein

% Platelet aggregation

Steep slope indicates rapid aggregation

Shallow slope indicates slow aggregation

Time

Time

Addition of ristocetin

Addition of ristocetin

High von Willebrand factor activity

Low von Willebrand factor activity

FIGURE 2–20

Platelet aggregation

Expense: High

Manual test requiring careful performance to generate accurate result

Goal of the test is to assess the function of circulating platelets

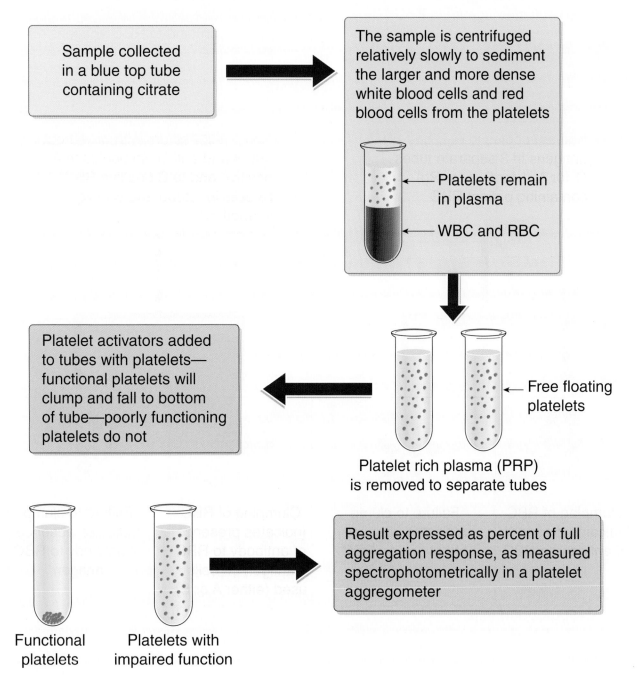

Sample collected in a blue top tube containing citrate

The sample is centrifuged relatively slowly to sediment the larger and more dense white blood cells and red blood cells from the platelets

Platelets remain in plasma

WBC and RBC

Platelet activators added to tubes with platelets— functional platelets will clump and fall to bottom of tube—poorly functioning platelets do not

Free floating platelets

Platelet rich plasma (PRP) is removed to separate tubes

Functional platelets

Platelets with impaired function

Result expressed as percent of full aggregation response, as measured spectrophotometrically in a platelet aggregometer

FIGURE 2–21

ABO/Rh typing

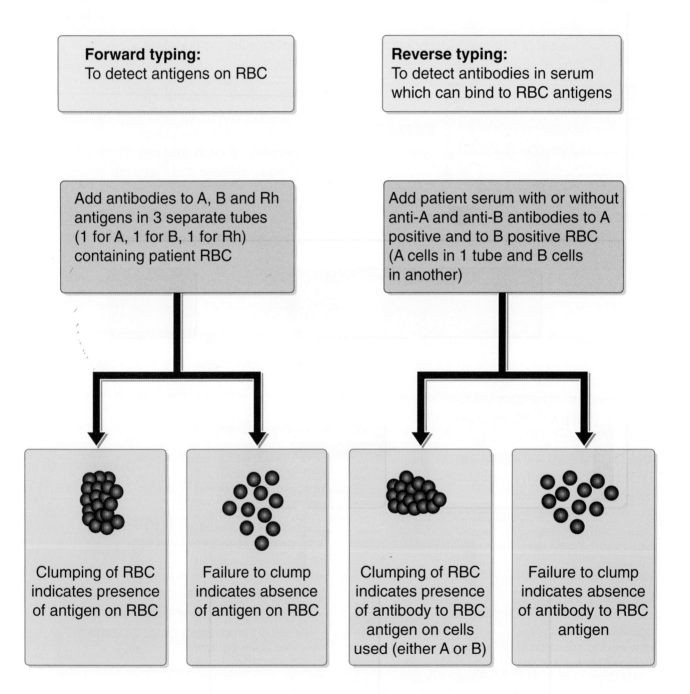

Expense: Low

Automated or manual

Forward typing:
To detect antigens on RBC

Reverse typing:
To detect antibodies in serum which can bind to RBC antigens

Add antibodies to A, B and Rh antigens in 3 separate tubes (1 for A, 1 for B, 1 for Rh) containing patient RBC

Add patient serum with or without anti-A and anti-B antibodies to A positive and to B positive RBC (A cells in 1 tube and B cells in another)

Clumping of RBC indicates presence of antigen on RBC

Failure to clump indicates absence of antigen on RBC

Clumping of RBC indicates presence of antibody to RBC antigen on cells used (either A or B)

Failure to clump indicates absence of antibody to RBC antigen

FIGURE 2–22

Blood component preparation

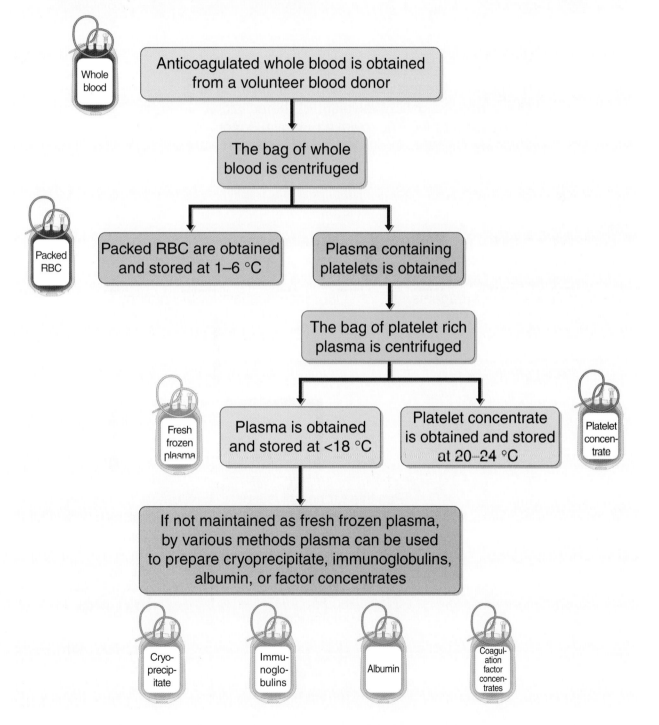

Expense: Blood products are expensive; separation of whole blood into blood components is moderately expensive

The process of component preparation is manual

Whole blood

Anticoagulated whole blood is obtained from a volunteer blood donor

The bag of whole blood is centrifuged

Packed RBC

Packed RBC are obtained and stored at 1–6 °C

Plasma containing platelets is obtained

The bag of platelet rich plasma is centrifuged

Fresh frozen plasma

Plasma is obtained and stored at <18 °C

Platelet concentrate is obtained and stored at 20–24 °C

Platelet concentrate

If not maintained as fresh frozen plasma, by various methods plasma can be used to prepare cryoprecipitate, immunoglobulins, albumin, or factor concentrates

Cryo-precipitate

Immuno-globulins

Albumin

Coagulation factor concentrates

FIGURE 2–23

Blood crossmatch

Expense: Low   **Process described below is manual**

The goal of the test is to determine if anything in the blood of a patient recipient will hemolyze or agglutinate the RBC from a potential donor

Patient serum mixed with RBC from a potential donor, followed by centrifugation, incubation, and addition of other reagents

Sample checked for hemolysis or agglutination—either of which makes the potential donor blood incompatible for the patient

Positive for hemolysis or agglutination—incompatible unit—do not transfuse

Agglutination

Hemolysis

Negative for hemolysis or agglutination—compatible unit suitable for transfusion

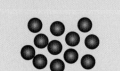

Intact RBC with no agglutination

FIGURE 2–24

Direct antiglobulin test (DAT)

Expense: Moderate   **Largely manual method**

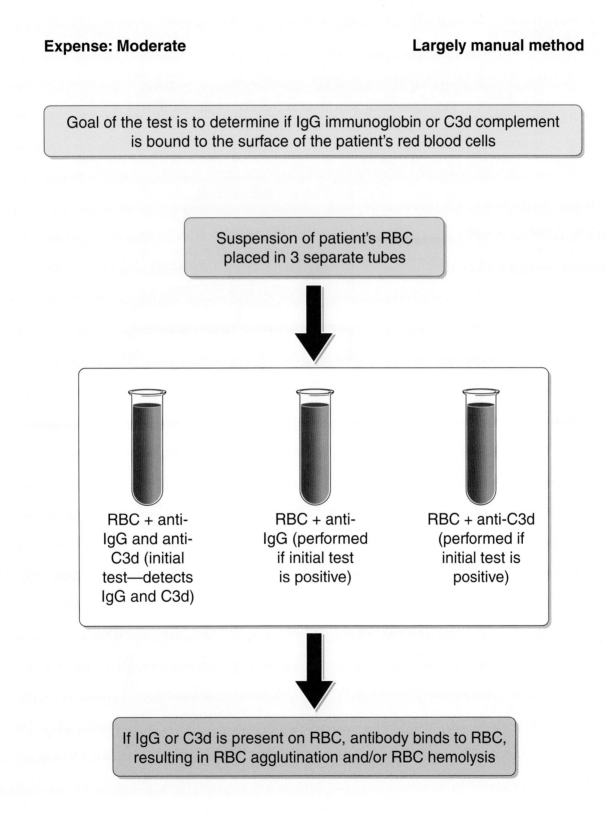

Goal of the test is to determine if IgG immunoglobin or C3d complement is bound to the surface of the patient's red blood cells

Suspension of patient's RBC placed in 3 separate tubes

RBC + anti-IgG and anti-C3d (initial test—detects IgG and C3d)

RBC + anti-IgG (performed if initial test is positive)

RBC + anti-C3d (performed if initial test is positive)

If IgG or C3d is present on RBC, antibody binds to RBC, resulting in RBC agglutination and/or RBC hemolysis

FIGURE 2–25

Indirect antiglobulin test (IAT)

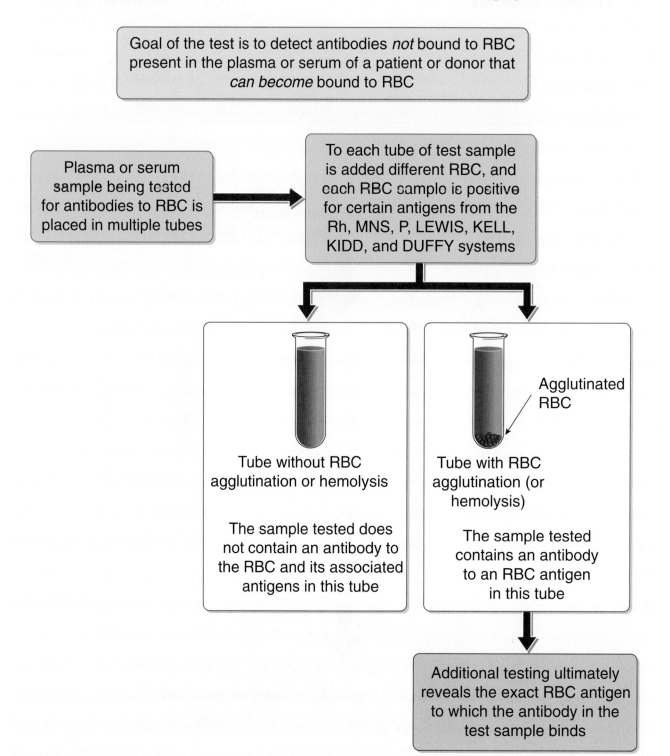

Expense: Moderate   **Largely manual method**

Goal of the test is to detect antibodies *not* bound to RBC present in the plasma or serum of a patient or donor that *can become* bound to RBC

Plasma or serum sample being tested for antibodies to RBC is placed in multiple tubes

To each tube of test sample is added different RBC, and each RBC sample is positive for certain antigens from the Rh, MNS, P, LEWIS, KELL, KIDD, and DUFFY systems

Tube without RBC agglutination or hemolysis

The sample tested does not contain an antibody to the RBC and its associated antigens in this tube

Agglutinated RBC

Tube with RBC agglutination (or hemolysis)

The sample tested contains an antibody to an RBC antigen in this tube

Additional testing ultimately reveals the exact RBC antigen to which the antibody in the test sample binds

FIGURE 2–26

Apheresis

Expense: Very high

**Moderately invasive
clinical procedure**

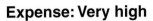

Intravenous line takes blood
out of patient

Intravenous line returns
non-collected components
and replacement fluids
and/or cells

Plasma and cells separated
by centrifugation in
apheresis device within a
sterile circuit

Collection could be for:
Plasma (plasmapheresis)
Platelets (plateletpheresis)
WBC (leukapheresis)
RBC (red blood cell exchange)

Goal of the procedure is to selectively remove
from the patient's circulation either plasma, platelets,
white blood cells or red blood cells—replacement of
plasma or red blood cells can occur depending
upon the clinical indication for the procedure

FIGURE 2–27

Western blot

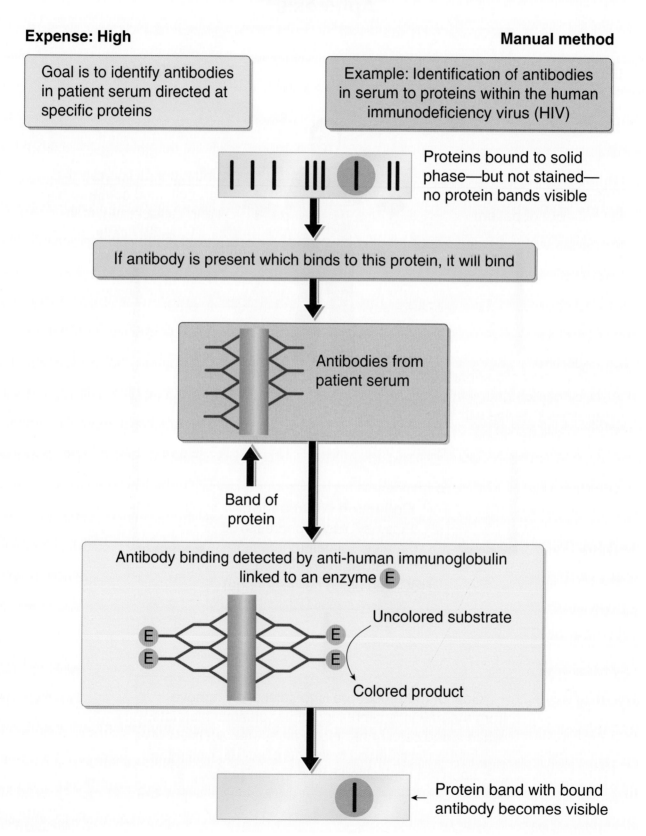

Expense: High

Goal is to identify antibodies in patient serum directed at specific proteins

Manual method

Example: Identification of antibodies in serum to proteins within the human immunodeficiency virus (HIV)

Proteins bound to solid phase—but not stained—no protein bands visible

If antibody is present which binds to this protein, it will bind

Antibodies from patient serum

Band of protein

Antibody binding detected by anti-human immunoglobulin linked to an enzyme E

Uncolored substrate

Colored product

Protein band with bound antibody becomes visible

FIGURE 2–28

Electrolyte measurements: Sodium–Na, Potassium–K, Chloride–Cl

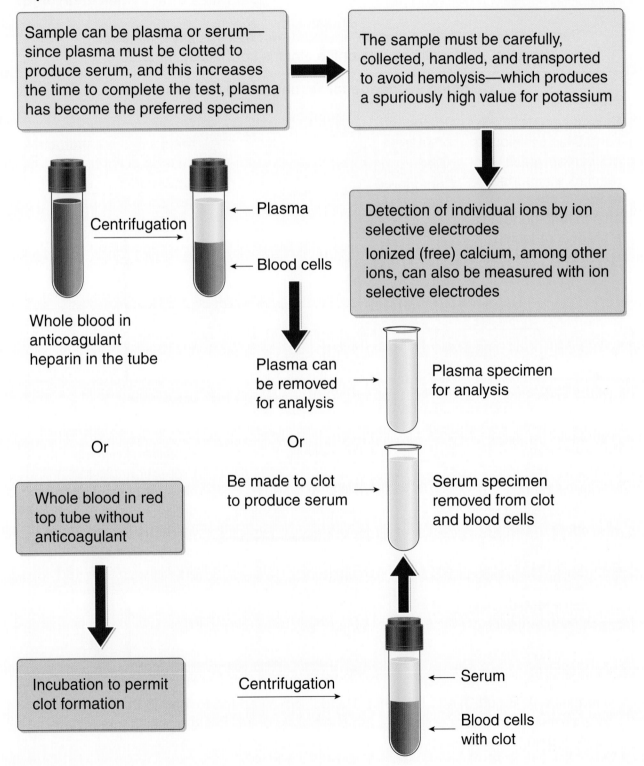

Expense: Low

Sample can be plasma or serum—since plasma must be clotted to produce serum, and this increases the time to complete the test, plasma has become the preferred specimen

Highly automated

The sample must be carefully, collected, handled, and transported to avoid hemolysis—which produces a spuriously high value for potassium

Centrifugation

← Plasma

← Blood cells

Whole blood in anticoagulant heparin in the tube

Detection of individual ions by ion selective electrodes

Ionized (free) calcium, among other ions, can also be measured with ion selective electrodes

Plasma can be removed for analysis

Plasma specimen for analysis

Or

Or

Whole blood in red top tube without anticoagulant

Be made to clot to produce serum

Serum specimen removed from clot and blood cells

Incubation to permit clot formation

Centrifugation

← Serum

Blood cells with clot

FIGURE 2–29

Assays measuring concentration by spectrophotometry

Expense: Low

Highly automated assays for most substances or activities measured

Sample is usually patient plasma or serum—for many assays, either can be used and for others, one or the other is specifically required

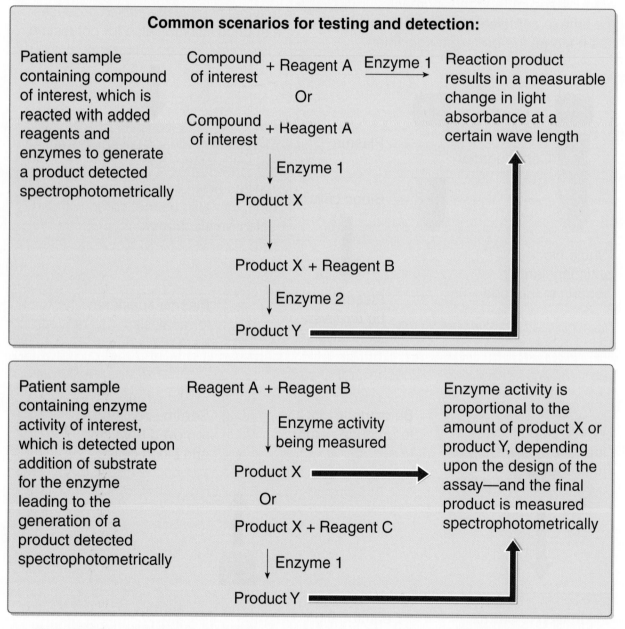

Common scenarios for testing and detection:

Patient sample containing compound of interest, which is reacted with added reagents and enzymes to generate a product detected spectrophotometrically

Compound of interest + Reagent A → Enzyme 1 →

Or

Compound of interest + Reagent A
↓ Enzyme 1
Product X
↓
Product X + Reagent B
↓ Enzyme 2
Product Y

Reaction product results in a measurable change in light absorbance at a certain wave length

Patient sample containing enzyme activity of interest, which is detected upon addition of substrate for the enzyme leading to the generation of a product detected spectrophotometrically

Reagent A + Reagent B
↓ Enzyme activity being measured
Product X →

Or

Product X + Reagent C
↓ Enzyme 1
Product Y

Enzyme activity is proportional to the amount of product X or product Y, depending upon the design of the assay—and the final product is measured spectrophotometrically

Reagents A, B and C, and enzymes 1 and 2 are all added to lead to the generation of a product that is proportional to the compound of interest or reflects the enzyme activity being measured

FIGURE 2–30

Blood gas measurements

Expense: Low

Requires injection of whole blood sample into instrument with no additional manipulation

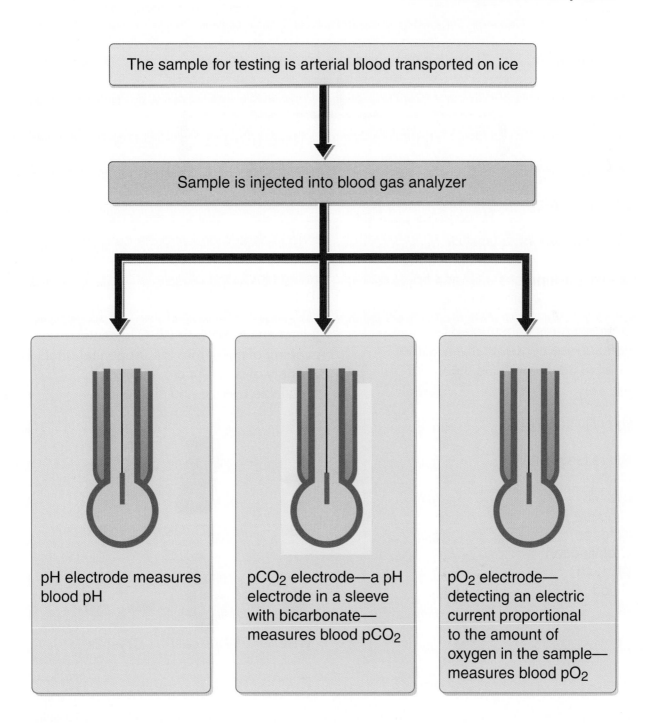

The sample for testing is arterial blood transported on ice

Sample is injected into blood gas analyzer

pH electrode measures blood pH

pCO_2 electrode—a pH electrode in a sleeve with bicarbonate— measures blood pCO_2

pO_2 electrode— detecting an electric current proportional to the amount of oxygen in the sample— measures blood pO_2

FIGURE 2–31

Urinalysis

Expense: Low

Can be completely manual or highly automated—sediment is examined microscopically which can be aided by automation in some instruments

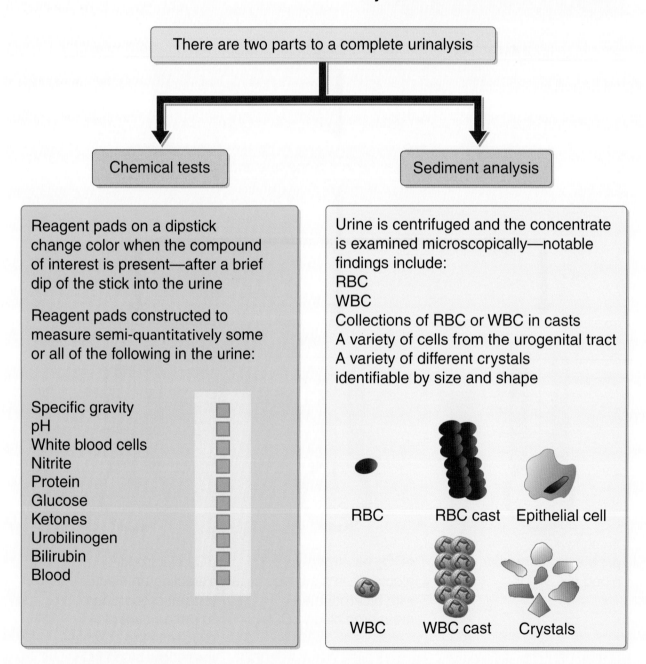

There are two parts to a complete urinalysis

Chemical tests

Sediment analysis

Reagent pads on a dipstick change color when the compound of interest is present—after a brief dip of the stick into the urine

Reagent pads constructed to measure semi-quantitatively some or all of the following in the urine:

Specific gravity
pH
White blood cells
Nitrite
Protein
Glucose
Ketones
Urobilinogen
Bilirubin
Blood

Urine is centrifuged and the concentrate is examined microscopically—notable findings include:
RBC
WBC
Collections of RBC or WBC in casts
A variety of cells from the urogenital tract
A variety of different crystals identifiable by size and shape

RBC   RBC cast   Epithelial cell

WBC   WBC cast   Crystals

FIGURE 2–32

Enzyme-linked immunosorbent assay (ELISA)

Expense: Moderate

Semi-automated to almost fully automated

To detect antibodies in the patient's serum

To detect an antigen in the patient's serum

Antibodies are detected by binding to a corresponding antigen fixed to a surface

Antigens are detected by binding to corresponding antibodies fixed to a surface

Antibody in patient serum

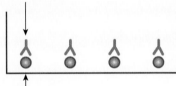

Antigen fixed to surface

Antigen in patient serum

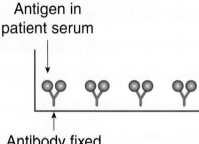

Antibody fixed to surface

Detection with anti-human antibody linked to an enzyme Ⓔ

Detection with antibody to antigen that has an enzyme Ⓔ linked to the antibody

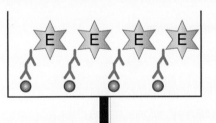

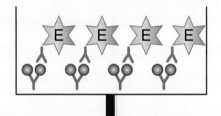

Add uncolored substrate for enzyme and enzyme converts it to a colored product—the darker the color, the more antibody or antigen in the patient serum

Uncolored substrate → Colored product

FIGURE 2–33

Latex agglutination

Expense: Low   **Automated or manual**

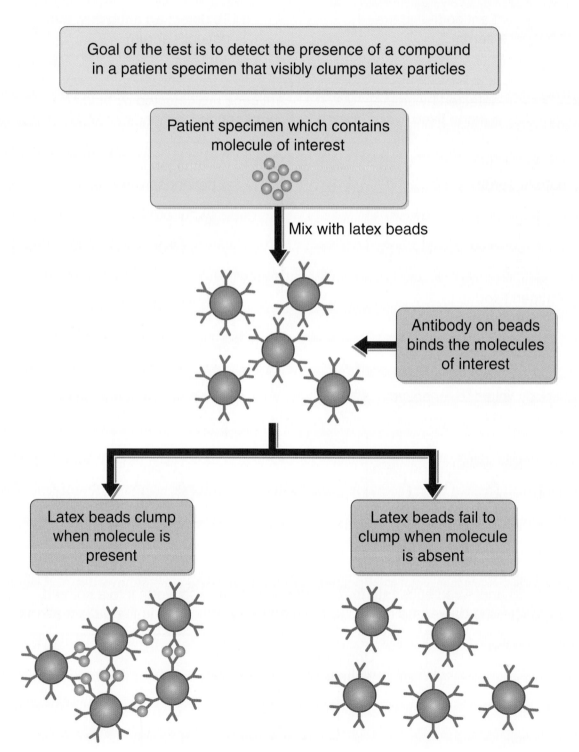

Goal of the test is to detect the presence of a compound in a patient specimen that visibly clumps latex particles

Patient specimen which contains molecule of interest

Mix with latex beads

Antibody on beads binds the molecules of interest

Latex beads clump when molecule is present

Latex beads fail to clump when molecule is absent

FIGURE 2–34

Mass spectrometry for molecular identification

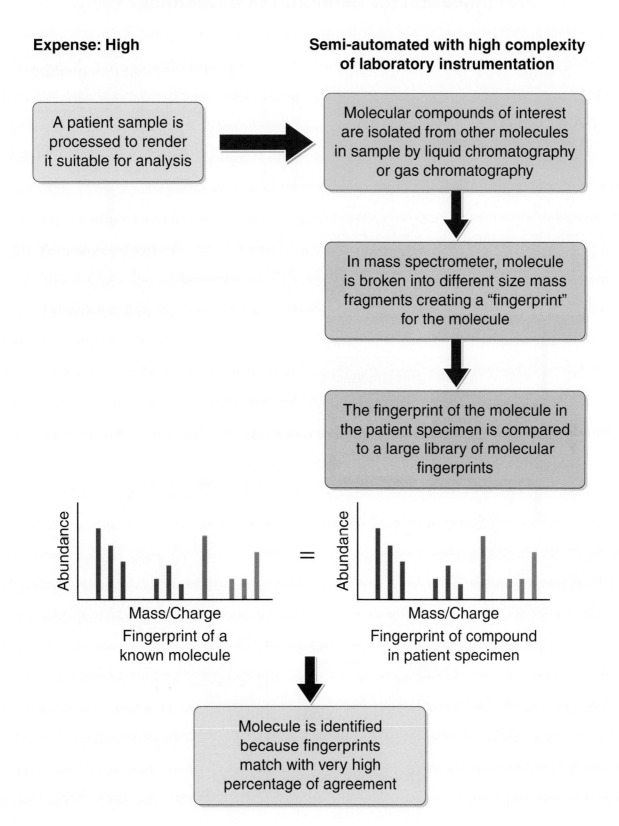

FIGURE 2–35

Polymerase chain reaction with restriction enzyme digestion for detection of mutations

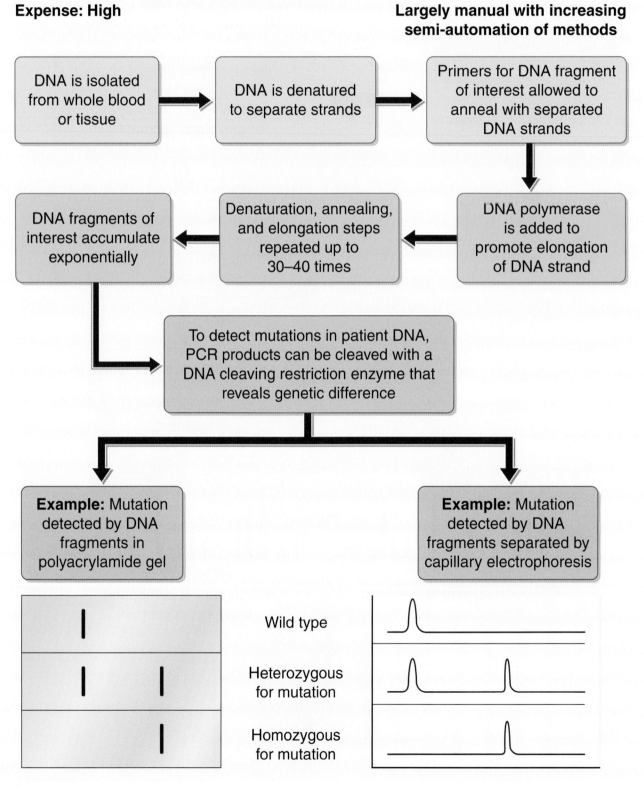

FIGURE 2–36

Autoimmune Disorders Involving the Connective Tissue and Immunodeficiency Diseases

CHAPTER

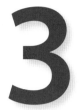

Mandakolathur R. Murali

LEARNING OBJECTIVES

1. Learn the common autoimmune diseases involving primarily the connective tissue.

2. Understand the disorders associated with immune deficiencies and their underlying pathophysiology.

3. Learn the diagnostic tests required to establish a diagnosis for autoimmune disorders and for immunodeficiency disorders.

CHAPTER OUTLINE

The immune system is a tightly regulated network that is both innate and adaptive. The genes regulating the innate system are coded in the germ line. The innate immune system is not antigen specific. The cells and soluble factors of the innate system have **p**attern **r**ecognition **r**eceptors (PRRs, such as toll-like receptors) to common motifs on pathogens and altered self-motifs. The motifs on pathogens are called **p**athogen-**a**ssociated **m**olecular **p**atterns (PAMPs). Altered self-antigens include **d**anger-**a**ssociated **m**olecular **p**atterns (DAMPs) as found in heat shock protein, and **a**poptosis-**a**ssociated **m**olecular **p**atterns (AAMPs) as found in ds DNA, RNP, and histones. This response is rapid and there is no memory of the encounter.

The receptors on the T and B cells of the adaptive immune system are antigen or epitope specific and clonally variable, and their diversity is derived from gene recombination. The cells retain memory of the encounter and on subsequent engagement with that antigen, the cells exhibit more rapid and robust responses.

TABLE 3-1   Systemic Autoimmune Diseases: Diseases Associated with Positive Test Results for Antinuclear Antibodies (ANA)

Disease	% ANA Positive	Titer	Common Patterns
Systemic lupus erythematosus—active	95–98	High	H > S > R
Systemic lupus erythematosus—remission	90	Moderate-high	H > S
Mixed connective tissue disease	93	High	S > N
Scleroderma/CREST	85	High	S > C > N
Sjogren syndrome	48	Moderate-high	S > H
Polymyositis/dermatomyositis	61	Low-moderate	S > N
Rheumatoid arthritis	41	Low-moderate	S
Drug-induced lupus	100	Low-moderate	S
Pauciarticular juvenile chronic arthritis	71	Low-moderate	S

Note: ANA patterns on Hep 2 cells by indirect immunofluorescent technique (IFA). Patterns: H, homogeneous; S, speckled; R, rim; C, centromere; N, nucleolar. Titers: high = 1:1280 to 1:5120; moderate = 1:160 to 1:640; low = 1:40 to 1:80.

TABLE 3-2   Specific Organ Autoimmune Diseases: Diseases Associated with Positive Test Results for Antinuclear Antibodies (ANA)

Disease	% ANA Positive	Titer	Common Patterns
Graves disease	50	Low-moderate	S
Hashimoto thyroiditis	46	Low-moderate	S
Autoimmune hepatitis	63–91	Low-moderate	S
Primary biliary cirrhosis	10–40	Low-moderate	S

Patterns: H, homogeneous; S, speckled; R, rim; C, centromere; N, nucleolar. Miscellaneous causes: low titer positive ANA patterns (mostly speckled) have been described in chronic infectious diseases such as infectious mononucleosis, hepatitis C infection, HIV, subacute bacterial endocarditis, and certain lymphoproliferative diseases.

The following 2 groups of disorders are the focus of this chapter: the autoimmune diseases involving the connective tissue and the immunodeficiency diseases.

The immune network is tightly regulated by cells and cytokines, and a derangement in this immune homeostasis can result in immune response to self-antigens as in autoimmunity (failure of self-tolerance), or failure to recognize pathogens and eliminate them as occurs in immunodeficiency syndromes (failure of immunity). The following 2 groups of disorders are the focus of this chapter: the autoimmune diseases involving the connective tissue and the immunodeficiency diseases.

Diseases in which immune responses to self-antigens occur in the context of a genetic predisposition to disease expression are called autoimmune diseases. Some involve organ-specific pathologic autoimmunity such as Hashimoto's thyroiditis and celiac disease, and these are discussed in chapters on those organ systems. The autoimmune disorders discussed in this chapter are systemic diseases with predominant involvement of the connective tissue, manifesting clinical features including inflammation of the joints, skin, muscles, and other soft tissues (see **Tables 3–1** and **3–2** and **Figure 3–1**).

The immunodeficiency diseases are subdivided into the relatively rare primary and the more common secondary immunodeficiency diseases. Primary immunodeficiency diseases are a direct consequence of either structural or functional derangement in the immune network. Secondary immune deficiency is the manifestation of a primary infectious disease, such as HIV infection; a malignancy as seen in lymphoma and multiple myeloma; or exposure to a therapeutic regimen such as immunosuppression or radiation.

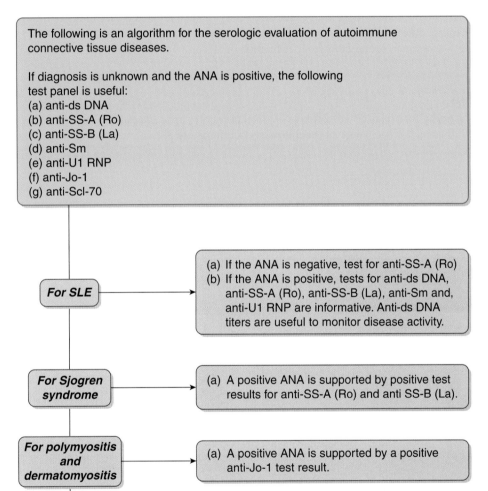

The clinical features of the disease, the morphologic pattern of the ANA test, and the serum titer of the positive ANA test are established.

If the ANA is positive, the pattern of staining suggests the differential diagnosis. The results of specific antinuclear antibody tests often establish the diagnosis.
A negative ANA test can occur in rheumatoid arthritis, inflammatory muscle diseases, and when there are connective tissue manifestations in patients with selected chronic infectious diseases.

The following is an algorithm for the serologic evaluation of autoimmune connective tissue diseases.

If diagnosis is unknown and the ANA is positive, the following test panel is useful:
(a) anti-ds DNA
(b) anti-SS-A (Ro)
(c) anti-SS-B (La)
(d) anti-Sm
(e) anti-U1 RNP
(f) anti-Jo-1
(g) anti-Scl-70

For SLE
(a) If the ANA is negative, test for anti-SS-A (Ro)
(b) If the ANA is positive, tests for anti-ds DNA, anti-SS-A (Ro), anti-SS-B (La), anti-Sm and, anti-U1 RNP are informative. Anti-ds DNA titers are useful to monitor disease activity.

For Sjogren syndrome
(a) A positive ANA is supported by positive test results for anti-SS-A (Ro) and anti SS-B (La).

For polymyositis and dermatomyositis
(a) A positive ANA is supported by a positive anti-Jo-1 test result.

For mixed connective tissue disease
(a) A positive ANA is supported by a positive result for anti-U1RNP.

For Scleroderma
(a) If the ANA pattern is the speckled or centromeric, anti-Scl-70 (anti-topoisomerase 1) provides additional diagnostic confirmation.

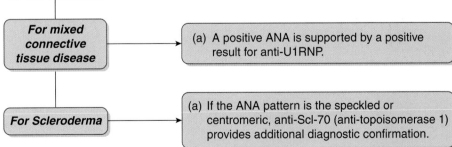

FIGURE 3–1 An approach to the diagnosis of autoimmune disorders involving connective tissue.

SYSTEMIC AUTOIMMUNE DISEASES INVOLVING THE CONNECTIVE TISSUE

Systemic Lupus Erythematosus

Description

Systemic lupus erythematosus (SLE) is a multisystem autoimmune disease, associated with the production of antibodies to a variety of nuclear and cytoplasmic antigens. The hallmark characteristic is the generation of antibodies to ds DNA. These antibodies complex to these self-antigens, and the ensuing immune complexes contribute to the inflammation in many organs, particularly the skin, joints, kidney, and, to a lesser extent, the nervous system, lung, and hemopoietic cells.

The disease is more common in women than men and usually appears in early adulthood, though it is seen in children as well. It is not only more common in African Americans than in Caucasians, but it also has a more severe clinical phenotype with renal and vasculitic manifestations in African Americans.

Table 3–3 summarizes the laboratory evaluation of SLE and **Table 3–4** lists the autoantibodies associated with SLE.

> Systemic lupus erythematosus (SLE) is a multisystem autoimmune disease, associated with the production of antibodies to a variety of nuclear and cytoplasmic antigens. The hallmark characteristic is the generation of antibodies to ds DNA.

Diagnosis

According to the American Rheumatologic Association criteria for diagnosis of SLE, the diagnosis of SLE is made if 4 or more of the following 11 criteria are present at any time during the course of the disease:

Malar rash	Flat or raised fixed erythema over the malar eminences and sparing the nasolabial folds
Discoid rash	Erythematous raised patches with adherent keratotic scaling and follicular plugging; scarring may occur in older lesions
Photosensitivity	Skin rash resulting from reaction to light
Arthritis	Nonerosive arthritis involving 2 or more peripheral joints that are swollen or tender and evidence of effusion
Oral ulcers	Mostly painless ulcers in the oral cavity and pharynx
Serositis	Pleuritis with pleural rub or effusion; pericarditis documented by rub, EKG change, or pericardial effusion
Renal diseases	Persistent proteinuria greater than 0.5 g/day or 3+ on dipstick
Neurologic	Seizures or psychosis in the absence of metabolic or drug-induced causes
Hematologic	Any immune cytopenia—RBC, WBC, or platelets
Immunologic	Positive anti-ds DNA antibody, positive antiphospholipid antibody, positive anti-Sm antibody, and false-positive serologic test for syphilis
Antinuclear antibody	An abnormal ANA titer by immunofluorescence or an equivalent assay in the absence of drugs known to be associated with "drug-induced lupus"

Tests utilized in the initial evaluation and subsequent monitoring of patients with SLE are shown in **Tables 3–3** and **3–4** and **Figure 3–1**.

Sjogren Syndrome

Description

Sjogren syndrome (SS) is a systemic connective tissue disease, more common in women than men. Pathologically, it is an autoimmune exocrinopathy involving the lacrimal glands, salivary glands, and less often the pancreas. The immune inflammation of these glands contributes to

TABLE 3–3 Laboratory Evaluation of Systemic Lupus Erythematosus (SLE): General Laboratory Tests

Laboratory Tests	Results/significance
Complete blood count and erythrocyte sedimentation rate (ESR)	Decrease in RBC, WBC, and platelets either singly or in combination suggests the presence of autoimmune cytopenias; serial CBC is useful to monitor bone marrow response to immunosuppressive therapy; ESR if elevated is a useful parameter to follow with therapy
Urinalysis and BUN/creatinine	Urinalysis is useful to evaluate proteinuria and any cellular sediments and casts; 24-hour protein excretion and BUN/creatinine are useful to monitor renal function
Liver function tests and lipid profile	For evaluation of possible autoimmune hepatitis; alterations in plasma lipids either due to disease or as a sequelae of therapy are to be appropriately managed to prevent cardiovascular complications
VDRL/RPR test for syphilis	False-positive VDRL test is noted in SLE; a positive VDRL in the absence of syphilis (negative RPR) is a diagnostic criterion for SLE
Antinuclear antibody	95%–98% of patients with active SLE have a positive ANA
Complement assay	C3, C4, and factor B are useful to evaluate complement activation; CH50 to detect congenital complement deficiency especially in familial SLE; low complement values may reflect disease activity

TABLE 3–4 Autoantibodies and Clinical Associations in Systemic Lupus Erythematosus (SLE)

Antigen Specificity	Prevalence Percent (%)	Pattern on Hep-2 Cells	Clinical Associations
ds DNA	40–60	Homogeneous	Marker of active disease; titers fluctuate with disease activity; correlates best with renal disease
SSA/Ro	40	Speckled, fine	Subacute cutaneous lupus (75%), neonatal lupus with heart block, complements deficiencies and photosensitivity
SSB/La	10–15	Speckled, fine	Neonatal lupus
Sm	20–30	Speckled, coarse	Specific marker for SLE; may be associated with CNS disease; not useful in monitoring disease activity
RNP (U1-RNP)	30–40	Speckled, coarse	Generally co-exists with Sm; a marker for MCTD
Histones	50–95	Homogeneous	50%–70% in SLE and >95% in drug-induced SLE
Phospholipids (beta-2 glycoprotein I antibodies)	30	None specific	Associated with thrombocytopenia, later trimester abortions, and hypercoagulable states
Proliferating cell nuclear antigen (PCNA)	3	Finely granular nuclear staining in rapidly dividing cells	Not sensitive but specific (>95); not seen in RA, other connective tissue disease; antibody rapidly diminished by steroids and immunosuppressive drugs; correlates with arthritis

the sicca syndrome, with dry eyes (keratoconjunctivitis) and dry mouth (xerostomia) as characteristic clinical features. The disease can be primary or secondary. The primary syndrome is characterized by dry eyes, dry mouth, decreased production of tears as tested by the Schirmer's test, and a lip biopsy that demonstrates inflammation of the minor salivary glands. Serologically, patients with primary Sjogren show a positive ANA, positive SS-A (Ro), positive SS-B (La), and positive rheumatoid factor (RF) in the absence of another connective tissue disease. A prospective study of 80 patients with primary SS followed for a median of 7.5 years reported the following frequencies of clinical manifestations: a) keratoconjunctivitis sicca and/or xerostomia

TABLE 3–5   Laboratory Evaluation for Sjogren Syndrome

	Findings in Sjogren Syndrome
Diagnostic tests for dry eyes	
Schirmer test	<8 mm wet zone on filter paper
Rose Bengal dye test	Visualization of devitalized areas in cornea
Tear break-up time	Measuring break-up time and tear osmolality after installation of fluorescein; identifies those who respond to anti-inflammatory therapy
Diagnostic tests for dry mouth	
Salivary gland scintigraphy	Low uptake of radionuclide is specific for SS, but 33% of patients have a positive test; not a sensitive test
Lower lip biopsy	Presence of lymphoid infiltrate around salivary glands is consistent with disease
Magnetic resonance imaging (MRI)	MRI is superior to ultrasonography and CT studies and is equivalent to sialography; correlates well with salivary gland biopsy
Laboratory tests for autoimmunity	
Antinuclear antibody (ANA) titer	Commonest pattern is speckled; titer greater than 1:160; in 75% of patients
Antibodies to SS-A (Ro)	With ELISA >90% have a positive test
Antibodies to SS-B (La)	With ELISA >90% have a positive test
Rheumatoid factor	70% have positive RF
Cryoglobulins, C3, and C4	Presence of cryoglobulins and low C3 and C4 are found with multisystem DISEASE
Anti-ds DNA antibody	In 25%–30% of patients with primary SS

occurred in all patients and were the only disease manifestations in 31%; b) extraglandular involvement occurred in 25%; and c) non-Hodgkin lymphoma developed in 2.5%. Secondary SS is clinically similar to the primary disorder, but it is additionally associated with clinical and serologic features of another connective tissue disease, such as rheumatoid arthritis (RA) or scleroderma.

Diagnosis

The diagnostic features are revealed by tests that document the sicca features. The dry eyes are evaluated by the Schirmer test. This test is a measurement of tear flow over a 5-minute period. Filter paper is allowed to hang from the lower eyelid, and the length of the paper that becomes wet is measured. This test is not reliable, as early in the disease there is excessive lacrimation giving a false-negative test. Demonstration of devitalized corneal epithelium due to keratoconjunctivitis is evaluated by rose Bengal or fluorescein stain. The most accurate test is the slit lamp examination of the cornea and conjunctiva. Tests for quantitating salivary secretion are not standardized and also are not specific to SS. Biopsy of the minor salivary gland in the lower lip demonstrating focal lymphocytic infiltration is a useful confirmatory test.

Table 3–5 summarizes the laboratory tests useful in diagnosis of both primary and secondary SS.

Systemic Sclerosis/Scleroderma

Description

Systemic sclerosis is characterized by excessive and widespread deposition of collagen in many organ systems of the body. Pathologically, the hallmark is the deposition of altered collagen in the extracellular matrix.

Systemic sclerosis is characterized by excessive and widespread deposition of collagen in many organ systems of the body. Pathologically, the hallmark is the deposition of altered collagen in the extracellular matrix.

TABLE 3-6   Laboratory Evaluation for Systemic Sclerosis/Scleroderma

Laboratory Test	Scleroderma	CREST Syndrome
Pattern of ANA (Hep-2)	Speckled	Centromeric
Commonly found autoantibody	Anti-Scl 70 (greater in diffuse disease than localized disease)	Mostly anticentomeric with a distinctive pattern on Hep-2 cells

The immunologic basis is not well understood, but an aberration in TGF-B-mediated deposition of collagen has been observed. Antibodies to platelet-derived growth factor receptors have been incriminated in the development of fibrosis. Both the triggering event and genetic predisposition are not well defined. Though the common organ involved is the skin, the gastrointestinal tract, kidney, lung, and muscles are also affected as the disease progresses. Renal ischemia leading to hypertension escalates the complications of this disease. Preponderance in females is common.

Clinically there are 4 major subtypes described:

1. Diffuse cutaneous scleroderma with widespread involvement of skin and visceral organs.
2. Limited cutaneous scleroderma, in which the disease is limited to the digital extremities and face. CREST syndrome is a variant of this entity. The name is derived from its features— **C**alcinosis, **R**aynauds syndrome, **E**sophageal dysmotility, **S**clerodactyly, and **T**elangiectasia.
3. Localized scleroderma that affects primarily the skin of the forearms, the fingers, and later the systemic organs.
4. Overlap syndromes with features of RA or muscle involvement.

Diagnosis

Ninety percent to 95% of all patients with scleroderma have a positive ANA test. The most common pattern is finely speckled, followed by centomeric and nucleolar patterns. The ANA activity is directed against DNA topoisomerase (also known as Scl-70). A definitive diagnosis is achieved when the characteristic clinical findings are accompanied by a positive ANA test, and often confirmed by an antibody directed to Scl-70 by ELISA. Table 3-6 summarizes the laboratory evaluation for systemic sclerosis/scleroderma.

Inflammatory Muscle Diseases

Description

Inflammation of the muscle leading to injury and weakness is the basis of the 3 most common but distinct diseases in this category. They are dermatomyositis (DM), polymyositis (PM), and inclusion body myositis. These diseases are more common in women, and their etiology remains unknown, though immune mechanisms have been incriminated. DM may occur as a specific entity or be associated with scleroderma or mixed connective tissue disease. Rarely, it is a manifestation of a malignancy. Skin manifestations such as a heliotrope rash, the shawl sign, and Gottron's papules are common in DM. Like DM, PM may also be associated with another connective tissue disease. In addition, it may be associated with viral, parasitic, or bacterial infections. DM is characterized by immune complex deposition in the vessels and is considered to be in part a complement-mediated vasculopathy. In contrast, PM appears to reflect direct T-cell-mediated muscle injury. Inclusion body myositis is a disease of older individuals and is not associated with malignancy. It is occasionally associated with another connective tissue disease.

Antisynthetase syndrome, characterized by antisynthetase antibodies that are highly specific for DM and PM, is seen in about 30% of patients with DM or PM. These patients typically experience a relatively acute onset of disease, constitutional symptoms such as fever, Raynaud's phenomenon, arthritis, and interstitial lung diseases. The antisynthetase antibodies include antibodies to aminoacyl-tRNA synthetase; antihistidyl-tRNA synthetase, also known as Jo-1; anti-signal recognition particle (SRP) antibodies directed against SRP; and anti-Mi-2 antibodies directed against a helicase involved in transcriptional activation.

Inflammation of the muscle leading to injury and weakness is the basis of the 3 most common but distinct diseases in this category. They are dermatomyositis (DM), polymyositis (PM), and inclusion body myositis.

TABLE 3–7   Laboratory Evaluation for Inflammatory Muscle Diseases

Test	Polymyositis	Dermatomyositis	Inclusion Body Myositis (IBM)
Creatine kinase (CK)	The CK concentration is elevated >50 times and levels reflect disease activity	The CK concentration is elevated >50 times and levels reflect disease activity	CK concentrations may be normal or elevated no more than 10 times the upper limit of normal
Muscle biopsy	The inflammatory infiltrates are usually within the fascicles surrounding the healthy muscle fibers; no perifascicular atrophy; increased CD8+ cells and enhanced expression of major histocompatibility antigens by muscle fibers	The inflammatory infiltrate is usually around the fascicles. The presence of perifascicular atrophy is diagnostic; complement-mediated vasculopathy is present	The pattern of inflammation is similar to that seen in polymyositis, with the addition of basophilic-rimmed vacuoles within the muscle fiber sarcoplasm that are characteristic of IBM; the presence of all 3 of the following on muscle biopsy confirms IBM and effectively excludes other idiopathic inflammatory myopathies: 1) vacuolated muscle fibers, 2) muscle fiber inclusions with staining characteristics of beta-amyloid deposits, and 3) demonstration of paired helical fibers by electron microscopy or immunohistologic staining
Anti Jo-1 antibodies	Present in about 40% of patients	Present in about 40% of patients	Present in about 40% of patients

Diagnosis

Although there are several common features between DM and PM, a characteristic feature of DM itself is the heliotrope hue around the eyes. Pulmonary interstitial fibrosis is seen in about 10% of cases in both diseases, occurring in the context of antisynthetase syndromes. There are 5 distinctive features described for both of these diseases. At least 3 of the following features are essential to fulfill the clinical diagnostic criteria for each:

1. proximal and symmetrical muscle weakness
2. history of muscle pain and tenderness on palpation
3. electromyographic evidence of spontaneous muscle activity and myopathic changes
4. elevated serum or plasma concentrations of muscle enzymes such as aldolase, creatinine kinase (CK), and AST
5. muscle biopsy demonstrating cellular inflammation

The laboratory diagnosis begins with documentation of muscle inflammation and injury as shown by elevation of serum or plasma concentrations of muscle enzymes such as aldolase, CK, and AST, together with the expected inflammatory histological features on muscle biopsy. The detection of autoantibodies is found in about one-third of the patients, and supports a diagnosis of inflammatory muscle disease. The antibodies are directed at tRNA-synthetases. Jo-1 is such an antibody, with specificity to histidyl-tRNA synthetase. It is found in about 40% of patients with PM, and generally indicates a worse prognosis. It is also more commonly found in patients with pulmonary fibrosis. Jo-1 is more commonly detected in cases of autoimmune myositis than those with other causes of muscle inflammation. As with many autoimmune diseases, the integration of clinical features with laboratory findings forms the basis of definitive diagnosis. **Table 3–7** presents the laboratory evaluation for inflammatory muscle disorders.

Mixed Connective Tissue Disease
Description

The entity known as mixed connective tissue disorder (MCTD) has some of the features of SLE, some of systemic sclerosis, and some of PM. The patients have variable clinical presentations with arthralgias, myalgias, fatigue, and Raynaud phenomenon. These features are superimposed on other findings that can add in over time, including malar rash, sclerodactyly,

> The entity known as mixed connective tissue disorder (MCTD) has some of the features of SLE, some of systemic sclerosis, and some of polymyositis.

TABLE 3–8   Laboratory Evaluation for Mixed Connective Tissue Disorders

Laboratory Tests	Results
Antinuclear antibody	Speckled pattern on Hep-2 cells
Autoantibody to extractable nuclear antigens (ENA)	Predominantly anti-U1 RNP
Autoantibodies for SLE, SS, and polymyositis	Often positive, except for anti-Sm which is negative

arthritis of the hands, and Raynaud phenomenon. Pulmonary manifestations occur in over 85% of these patients and include interstitial pneumonitis, pulmonary hypertension, progressive interstitial fibrosis, and, rarely, dysfunction of diaphragm and esophagus. On rare occasion, patients with MCTD develop diffuse proliferative glomerulonephritis, psychosis, or seizures. The appropriate constellation of clinical findings suggests the need for laboratory testing, described in **Table 3–8**.

Diagnosis

The diagnosis of MCTD is largely made on the basis of the clinical features consistent with multiple autoimmune diseases. It is supported by a high titer of anti-U1 RNP in the serum.

Rheumatoid Arthritis

Description

RA is a systemic autoimmune connective tissue disorder that primarily affects the synovial joints, often starting as a synovitis. It affects 1% to 2% of the adult population worldwide, and is predominantly a disease of young women. Susceptibility and resistance to RA is associated with HLA genotypes. The criteria for diagnosis of RA were revised in 1987 to include clinical features, laboratory values, and radiographic findings. To establish a definitive diagnosis, at least 3 of the following 7 criteria must be present along with morning stiffness for a period of at least 6 weeks:

1. arthritis in 3 or more small joints
2. morning stiffness lasting >30 minutes
3. arthritis of the small joints of the hand
4. rheumatoid nodules
5. symmetrical arthritis, often with synovitis
6. a positive test for RF
7. radiographic changes of the affected joints

> RA is a systemic autoimmune connective tissue disorder that primarily affects the synovial joints, often starting as a synovitis. It affects 1% to 2% of the adult population worldwide, and is predominantly a disease of young women.

Diagnosis

An increased serum titer of RF has been a longstanding marker of RA, until the validation of anti-cyclic citrullinated peptide antibody (anti-CCP). This antibody is not only highly associated with RA, but it is also a marker for progressive and erosive joint disease. Anti-CCP is approximately 98% specific and 85% sensitive as a serum marker for RA. RF is an IgM autoantibody directed against the Fc region of IgG. While high titers of RF are associated with severe RA, it is not specific for diagnosis of RA, as it is also found in chronic infections and other connective tissue diseases. **Table 3–9** summarizes the laboratory tests useful in the evaluation of RA.

Amyloidosis

Description

Amyloidosis and cryoglobulinemia (which follows) are systemic diseases resulting from the deposition in the tissues of insoluble proteins from a soluble circulating precursor. Both represent the consequences of immune dysregulation, and their diagnosis depends on laboratory evaluation and confirmation.

TABLE 3–9   Laboratory Evaluation for Rheumatoid Arthritis

Laboratory Test	Results and Significance
Complete blood count (CBC)	Patients with RA may have a normochromic, normocytic anemia (Hbg of about 10 g/dL), and elevated platelet count with neutrophilia; in Felty's syndrome there is neutropenia; patients on immunosuppressive therapy have decreased counts of all lineages
ESR	An index of inflammation and often elevated; in RA patients, its level often parallels disease activity
C-reactive protein	This acute phase reactant is increased in RA and is an index of inflammation; useful in monitoring disease activity over time and in response to therapy
Rheumatoid factor (RF) titer	RF is detectable in 70%–80% of patients with RA; diagnostic utility is limited by its lack of specificity as it is found in almost all patients with cryoglobulinemia, in 70% of patients with Sjogren's syndrome, 20%–30% of those with SLE, and 5%–10% of healthy individuals; its prevalence increases with age
Anti-CCP antibodies	Most useful as its specificity is 90%–96% and sensitivity is around 85%; predicts erosive disease in RA; valuable in diagnosis of early RA; positive titers to CCP have better predictive value in diagnosis of RA in the IgM-RF negative subgroup; negative RF in combination with negative anti-CCP is better in excluding RA than either alone in patients with polyarthritis
Serum cryoglobulins	Presence correlates with extra-articular disease
Radiological studies	Periarticular osteoporosis, soft tissue swelling, joint space reduction and erosions should be determined at baseline and monitored with use of disease-modifying antirheumatic drugs; MRI is sensitive but expensive
Joint fluid analysis	If a single joint exhibits heightened inflammation in a patient with polyarticular disease, need to exclude septic arthritis or crystal-induced arthritis by cell count and differential, culture, and crystal identification

Amyloidosis is a heterogeneous group of diseases resulting from the extracellular deposition of low molecular weight fibrils from a soluble circulating precursor giving a "waxy" or "lardaceous" appearance to the infiltrated organs. Ultrastructurally, amyloid deposits are composed of unbranching fibrils 8 to 10 nm in width and with a molecular weight of 5 to 25 kD. At least 25 biochemically distinct forms of human amyloid protein have been identified. The 2 most common forms are primary, with amyloid light chain (AL) derived from light chains of plasma cells, and secondary, with amyloid-associated protein (AA), a nonimmunoglobulin protein. Congo red staining of amyloid deposits demonstrates a characteristic apple-green birefringence on polarized microscopy, while staining with thioflavine T produces yellow-green fluorescence.

The classification of amyloidosis is based on whether the amyloidosis is associated with a plasma cell dyscrasia such as multiple myeloma or light chain myeloma (primary amyloidosis), or the sequelae of an infectious or inflammatory disease (secondary or reactive amyloidosis). Amyloidosis may also be classified as hereditary or acquired, localized or systemic, or by the type of fibril deposited in tissues, such as transthyretin (TTR) and Alzheimer amyloid precursor protein (APP).

The most common form of the disease, representing 75% to 80% of the cases, is primary amyloidosis, as an acquired disorder, with multiorgan systemic involvement. Primary amyloidosis has a male to female preponderance of 2:1. Its incidence increases with age, often starting at age 40 years.

> The diagnosis of amyloidosis is based on the histological and immunochemical demonstration of amyloid deposits in affected organs and tissues. The preferred tissue for biopsy is obtained by fine needle aspiration of the abdominal fat pad.

Diagnosis

The diagnosis of amyloidosis is based on the histological and immunochemical demonstration of amyloid deposits in affected organs and tissues. The preferred tissue for biopsy is obtained by fine needle aspiration of the abdominal fat pad. Its advantages over rectal biopsy are that multiple samples can be obtained for study, and it is less painful and invasive. Since a plasma cell dyscrasia is commonly found in patients with amyloidosis, a serum protein electrophoresis together with a determination of serum free kappa and lambda light chains by nephelometry and a calculation of the kappa/lambda ratio are necessary to exclude a monoclonal gammopathy as the cause of the

TABLE 3-10   Laboratory Evaluation for Amyloidosis

Laboratory Tests	Results/Comments
Abdominal fat pad biopsy	Preferred site due to ease of obtaining multiple samples, better yield than rectal biopsy, and less invasive; has replaced rectal biopsy
Serum and urine protein electrophoresis	Primary amyloidosis is often associated with a monoclonal gammopathy; serum and urine electrophoresis followed by immunofixation studies to identify the specific monoclonal protein; assays for free serum light chains and their ratio in serum are essential to detect light chain disease
Bone marrow biopsy	Indicated when serum electrophoresis, serum-free light chain assays, and urine electrophoresis indicate a monoclonal gammopathy; flow cytometry and special stains for amyloid facilitate diagnosis
Coagulation factor X level	About 10% of patients with primary amyloidosis have factor X deficiency; about half of the patients with isolated and acquired factor X deficiency have primary amyloidosis; detection of this deficiency prior to biopsy with prothrombin time and factor X assay is essential
Protein sequencing	Useful in identifying genetic abnormalities in hereditary amyloidosis and identifying rare forms of amyloidosis
Serum amyloid P (SAP) component scanning	Scintigraphy with radiolabeled SAP used to identify and estimate total body burden of amyloid; its value is limited because SAP is obtained from blood donors and carries potential infectious risk

amyloidosis. Amyloid fibrils may bind to coagulation factor X causing a coagulopathy. Determination of the factor X level is important to explain bleeding tendencies in amyloidosis patients and is useful prior to biopsy of organs and tissues to identify a coagulopathy that would permit excess bleeding at the biopsy site.

To define the extent of the disease and the type of amyloidosis, the patient should be evaluated for renal, cardiac, pulmonary, neurologic, cutaneous, articular, liver, and spleen involvement. Cardiac involvement is extremely common in primary amyloidosis and much less in secondary amyloidosis. Virtually all of the familial amyloidosis manifests with nephropathic, neuropathic, or cardiopathic features. Laboratory evaluation for amyloidosis is summarized in **Table 3-10**.

Cryoglobulinemia

Description

Cryoglobulinemia refers to the presence in the serum of 1 or more immunoglobulins that precipitate at a temperature below 37°C. This precipitation is reversible, as it redissolves on warming to 37°C. The cause of cryoprecipitation remains to be determined.

Cryoglobulins are classified into 3 types. Type I consists of a single monoclonal immunoglobulin that does not have RF activity. It is typically IgM or IgG and less often IgA. Type I, also called simple cryoglobulinemia, is often associated with lymphoproliferative malignancies such as Waldenstrom macroglobulinemia or multiple myeloma. Patients with this disorder may present with features of vasculopathy involving the digits, resulting in gangrene. Type II consists of monoclonal IgM RF mixed with polyclonal IgG or IgA. The most common association for this form of cryoglobulinemia is hepatitis C infection. Type II may rarely be associated with lymphoma. Type III is also a mixed cryoglobulinemia, with polyclonal IgM RF associated with polyclonal IgG or IgA. Type III is found in patients with connective tissue disease and chronic infections. Both type II and III cryoglobulinemia patients may show fixation of complement and be associated with hypocomplementemia. Immune complex vasculitis, arthritis, neuropathy, and renal involvement may be the presenting features in patients with type II or III cryoglobulinemia.

Diagnosis

When present, the cryoglobulins are quantitated using a Wintrobe tube, and the amount of cryoglobulin present is reported as a cryocrit. When a cryoglobulin is identified, the components

TABLE 3–11   Laboratory Evaluation for Cryoglobulinemia

Laboratory Test	Comment
Cryocrit	This is the (volume of the cryoprecipitate/volume of serum) × 100; necessary to keep the sample at 37°C until it reaches the laboratory and serum is separated; serum is then refrigerated at 4°C for 72 hours; the cryocrit is then measured after centrifugation at 4°C; increased fibrinogen and lipids may lead to falsely elevated values
Immunofixation and immunodiffusion	Used to evaluate the constituents of the cryoglobulin, their clonality and allow classification as type I, II, or III
Urinalysis, BUN, creatinine	To evaluate renal function
C3, C4, and RF	To assess for complement fixation by RF in the cryoglobulin
Liver enzymes	To evaluate liver function
Hepatitis serology	To evaluate hepatitis B or C infections
Renal biopsy and immunofluorescence studies	Proteinuria, abnormal urinalysis, and altered renal function are an indication for renal biopsy with immunofluorescence for renal pathology
Lymph node and bone marrow biopsy	Indicated when a lymphoproliferative disease is suspected from the type of cryoglobulin, usually type I or II

comprising the cryoprotein are tested by immunodiffusion and immunofixation, using specific antisera directed at the immunoglobulin isotypes and against C3 and C4. Based on the clonality and the constituent isotypes, the cryoglobulin is then categorized as type I, II, or III. **Table 3–11** summarizes the laboratory evaluation for cryoglobulinemia.

DISEASES OF THE IMMUNE SYSTEM

X-linked Agammaglobulinemia

Description

X-linked agammaglobulinemia (XLA), also known as Bruton's agammaglobulinemia, is the pro-type humoral immune deficiency. It is a disease restricted to males, and is characterized by a near total absence of B lymphocytes from an arrest in B lymphocyte development. The deficiency of B cells results in pan hypogammaglobulinemia. Patients with XLA are asymptomatic for the first several months of life. Recurrent infections manifest between 4 and 12 months after birth as the maternal antibodies wane. Lack of the opsonic antibodies results in recurrent bacterial infections due to pyogenic, encapsulated bacteria such as *Streptococcus pneumonia*, *Haemophilus influenza*, *Staphylococcus aureus*, and *Pseudomonas species*. Upper and lower respiratory tract infections are most common, including otitis media, sinusitis, bronchitis, and pneumonia. Skin infections and urinary tract infections also occur. The cause of XLA is due to loss of function mutations of a tyrosine kinase protein known as *btk* that is essential for B-cell development.

Diagnosis

Early diagnosis is essential to prevent infections and complications of infections, such as bronchiectasis, meningitis, bacterial sepsis, septic arthritis, and even osteomyelitis. Recognizing that B cells are CD19 and CD20 positive, a definitive diagnosis can be made at birth by enumerating B cells in cord blood by flow cytometry using monoclonal antibodies to CD19 and CD20. In children less than 6 months of age, measuring serum immunoglobulin concentration is not diagnostically useful due to the presence of transplacentally acquired maternal antibody in the blood. Thus, to establish a diagnosis in the first 6 months, it is necessary to enumerate B cells by flow cytometry. The molecular diagnosis is made by mutational analysis of the *btk* gene. This is seldom needed in clinical practice as clinical features of the lack of tonsils and CD19 or CD20 cells can establish the diagnosis. Deficient expression of *btk* protein can be detected by flow cytometry, a

X-linked agammaglobulinemia (XLA) is the protype humoral immune deficiency. It is a disease restricted to males, and is characterized by a near total absence of B lymphocytes from an arrest in B lymphocyte development.

TABLE 3–12   Laboratory Evaluation for X-linked Agammaglobulinemia (XLA)

Laboratory Test	Result for XLA	Result for Carriers
Serum IgG	<200 mg/dL in patients greater than 6 months of age	Normal
Serum IgM and IgA	Low to absent if greater than 6 months of age	Normal
B-cell markers—CD19 and CD20	Low at birth and is diagnostic even at <6 months of age	Normal
btk gene mutation	Though not clinically needed, it is the definitive diagnostic test	Definitive test for carrier state
Antibody response to childhood vaccines	Markedly decreased to absent	Normal

TABLE 3–13   Laboratory Evaluation for Common Variable Immunodeficiency (CVID)

Laboratory Test	Result/Comments
Serum protein electrophoresis	Marked decrease in the gamma globulin fraction; rarely it may be normal in the dysfunctional variant
Serum IgM, IgG, and IgA levels	Usually low, but may be normal in dysfunctional variant
CD19 and CD20 cells	Usually normal, may be increased; rarely, low normal but never absent
Response to polysaccharide and protein antigens	There is a failure to respond to these antigens; the expected 4-fold rise in titer following vaccination is not observed; defines the functional defect

technique that can also be used for carrier detection. **Table 3–12** summarizes the laboratory approach to the diagnosis of this disorder.

Common Variable Immunodeficiency

Description

Common variable immunodeficiency (CVID) affects both males and females equally. The phenotypic expression of this disease is characterized by hypogammaglobulinemia, and there are many genetic defects in the B-cell maturation pathway that apparently cause this disorder. The disease usually manifests in adult life. Unlike agammaglobulinemia, in which B cells and tonsils are absent, patients with CVID have tonsils and normal numbers of B cells in blood and lymphoid tissues. Some patients even have mediastinal and abdominal lymphadenopathy. The primary defect in CVID is that the B cells are dysfunctional, and do not differentiate into plasma cells and secrete antibody. The clinical presentation is the consequence of the hypogammaglobulinemia, namely, recurrent pyogenic infections, often of the upper and lower respiratory tracts. Lack of mucosal immunity also results in enteroviral infections and giardiasis. Autoimmune diseases such as immune hemolytic anemia, neutropenia, and pernicious anemia occur. B-cell lymphomas may manifest with time. Studies of B-cell function in CVID have revealed a subset of CVID patients who have normal or low normal IgM, IgG, and IgA but fail to make functional antibody to polysaccharide and protein antigens. Therapy with intravenous gamma globulin has improved the clinical outcome for CVID patients.

Diagnosis

Table 3–13 describes the laboratory tests useful to establish the clinical diagnosis. **Figure 3–2** shows the molecular tests available to define the genetic defects.

Common variable immunodeficiency (CVID) affects both males and females equally. The phenotypic expression of this disease is characterized by hypogammaglobulinemia, and there are many genetic defects in the B-cell maturation pathway that apparently cause this disorder.

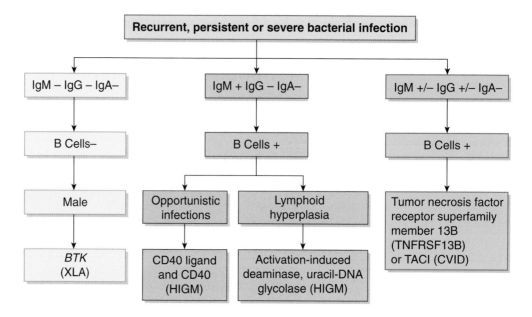

FIGURE 3–2 Molecular defects in B-cell immunodeficiencies—X-linked agammaglobulinemia (XLA), hyper-IgM syndrome (HIGM), and common variable immunodeficiency (CVID).

Hyper-IgM Syndrome

Description

Hyper-IgM syndrome (HIGM) is characterized by markedly reduced IgG and IgA, with normal to elevated IgM and normal numbers of circulating B cells. The low IgG and IgA is due to an inability of IgM-positive B cells to switch to other isotypes. The increased IgM reflects polyclonal expansion of IgM synthesis in response to infections from encapsulated bacteria. Both X-linked and autosomal recessive forms exist. The molecular causes include the X-linked loss of function mutation of the CD40 ligand (CD154) found on activated T cells, which is needed to engage with CD40 on B cells to promote the isotype switch. Other causes include loss of functional mutations of activation-induced deaminase (AID) and of uracil-DNA glycolase (UNG). These enzymes are involved in class switch recombination and in mending error-prone repair.

Selective IgA deficiency is the most common primary immunodeficiency syndrome. The defect is due to a B-cell differentiation arrest in the IgG to IgA isotype switch.

Diagnosis

The diagnosis is established by measuring serum IgM, IgG, and IgA along with enumerating CD19 and CD20 cells by flow cytometry. Normal or elevated IgM, with low IgG and IgA, with normal B cells, suggests the diagnosis, which can be confirmed by molecular studies, as shown in **Figure 3–2**.

Selective IgA Deficiency

Description

Selective IgA deficiency is the most common primary immunodeficiency syndrome. Its prevalence varies from 1 in 500 in Caucasians to 1 in 10,000 to 15,000 in Asians. The clinical picture is variable, and includes asymptomatic individuals and those with allergies, autoimmune disorders, recurrent infections, and gastrointestinal diseases. The defect is due to a B-cell differentiation arrest in the IgG to IgA isotype switch. There are low numbers of IgA bearing B cells. Anti-IgA antibodies are found in the serum of some patients, and these individuals can experience an anaphylactoid reaction to any blood or blood product containing IgA. These patients are to be given IgA-deficient blood and blood products and washed red blood cells.

Diagnosis

The diagnosis is made by documenting an IgA level of <5 mg/dL in the presence of normal IgG and IgM. It is important to evaluate for IgG subclasses, as subjects with IgA deficiency and a low IgG2 subclass are prone to recurrent infections.

DiGeorge Syndrome

Description

DiGeorge syndrome is due to deletion of chromosome 22q11.2 and is part of the spectrum described as "CATCH 22" (**C**ardiac anomalies, **A**bnormal facies, **T**hymic hypoplasia, **C**left palate, and **H**ypocalcemia). This deletion leads to failure of the development of third and fourth pharyngeal pouches and consequent abnormalities in the development of the thymus and parathyroid glands. Thymic dysfunction leads to T-cell abnormalities, and also B-cell dysfunction, while parathyroid abnormalities cause hypocalcaemia and tetany. Defects in the third and fourth pharyngeal pouches also result in congenital heart diseases, anomalies of the great vessels and abnormal facies with low set ears, fish-like mouth, and cleft palate. Patients with complete DiGeorge syndrome manifest marked defects in T-cell function and are prone to viral infections. Those with partial DiGeorge syndrome have fewer infections but have cardiac and facial abnormalities.

Diagnosis

A child with neonatal tetany and abnormal facies should be evaluated for DiGeorge syndrome by enumerating T and B cells, along with measurement of serum calcium and parathyroid hormone (PTH). Chromosome 22q11.2 deletion is documented by fluorescence in situ hybridization (FISH).

Severe Combined Immunodeficiency (SCID) Syndrome

Description and Diagnosis

As the name implies, SCID syndrome is characterized by profound defects of both cellular and humoral immunity. Affected neonates manifest severe and widespread viral, fungal, and bacterial infections soon after birth. The protection from maternal antibody is minimal, and the child fails to thrive. Respiratory failure often supervenes and is a cause of death. Patients with this disorder were the "bubble babies" decades earlier. Haploidentical, allogeneic bone marrow transplantation has altered the natural history of the disease. The path to recovery is often accompanied by graft-versus-host disease, and restitution of B-cell function is often incomplete. As a result, SCID patients may need intravenous gamma globulin to increase their antibody repertoire.

Based on T-cell, B-cell, and NK-cell enumeration, the SCID syndrome is classified as shown in **Figure 3–3**. This classification permits an insight to the molecular mechanisms of the disease and provides a framework for evaluating patients for SCID.

SCID syndrome is characterized by profound defects of both cellular and humoral immunity. Affected neonates manifest severe and widespread viral, fungal, and bacterial infections soon after birth.

Deficiencies of Complement Proteins

Description

The complement system of proteins and their receptors protect the host against pathogens or non-self-antigens and also abrogate the emergence of autoimmune diseases by scavenging self-antigens such as DNA so that they do not become immunogenic. Deficiencies of the complement system, therefore, result in susceptibility to infections and predispose to autoimmune diseases such as SLE. Deficiency of C3 results in increased susceptibility to infections by encapsulated, pyogenic bacteria. Deficiencies of C5, C6, C7, and C8 result in recurrent or disseminated Neisseria infections. Deficiencies of C1q (which scavenges DNA released from apoptotic cells), C2, and C4 predispose to SLE and other autoimmune diseases. Deficiency of C1 inhibitor causes hereditary angioedema (HAE). In type 1 HAE, there is a deficiency of both the antigenic and functional C1 inhibitor protein. In type 2, the protein is antigenically normal and hence normal serum levels are noted when it is measured by an antigenic assay. However, in type 2 HAE, the protein is functionally abnormal and hence cannot inhibit the kinin, complement, kallikrein, and

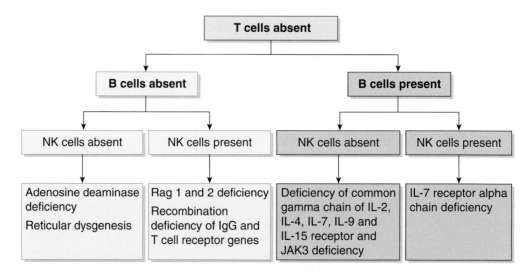

FIGURE 3–3 Classification of severe combined immunodeficiency (SCID).

plasminogen pathways. This results in generation of bradykinin that causes angioedema. Lack of C1 inhibitor causes C4 consumption even in the basal state so that C4 is always low. In HAE patients with angioedema, C2 is also decreased. C3 is normal as this activation occurs in the fluid phase. Factor I deficiency is associated with recurrent infections, and factor H deficiency with hemolytic uremic syndrome and age-related macular degeneration. Deficiency of membrane inhibitors such as decay accelerating factor (DAF or CD55) and homologous restriction factor (HRF or CD 59) causes paroxysmal nocturnal hemoglobinuria.

Diagnosis

The traditional method to measure the functional integrity of the complement cascade was to measure the ability of this system to hemolyze antibody-coated sheep red cells in a hemolytic assay. In this test, the result is reported as titer or the concentration of serum that supports 50% hemolysis in the S-shaped titration curve. Serum depleted of complement due to consumption by immune complexes and serum that is congenitally deficient in complement proteins yield low

TABLE 3–14   Patterns of Complement Activation

Pattern of Activation	CH50	C4	C3	Factor B	Conditions with Activation Pattern
Classic	Decreased	Decreased	Decreased	No change	SLE, SS, RA, and cryoglobulinemia
Alternative	Decreased	No change	Decreased	Decreased	Endotoxemia; type II MPGN
Classical and alternative	Decreased	Decreased	Decreased	Decreased	SLE, shock, and immune complex diseases
Fluid phase activation—classical	Decreased	Decreased	No change	No change	Hereditary angioedema; malarial infection (P. vivax)
Acute phase pattern	Significantly increased	Significantly increased	Significantly increased	Significantly increase	Acute and chronic inflammation; pregnancy

SLE, systemic lupus erythematosus; SS, Sjogren syndrome; RA, rheumatoid arthritis; MPGN, membranoproliferative glomerularnephritis.

CH50 values. This assay has been replaced by enzyme assays that detect neoantigens exposed during the activation of terminal complement components. In inherited deficiencies of the complement system, specific assays for the individual complement component must be performed. Further, it must be shown that addition of that component alone will restore the full hemolytic activity. **Table 3–14** provides a profile of complement activation that is useful in clinical diagnosis.

REFERENCES

Alarcon Segovia D, Villareal M. Classification and diagnostic criteria for mixed connective tissue disease. In: Kasukawa R, Sharp G, eds. *Mixed Connective Tissue Disease and Anti-nuclear Antibodies.* Amsterdam: Elsevier; 1987:33.

Alspaugh MA, Tan EM. Antibodies to cellular antigens in Sjogren's syndrome. *J Clin Invest.* 1975:55:1067.

Arbuckle MR, et al. Development of autoantibodies before the clinical onset of systemic lupus erythematosus. *N Engl J Med.* 2003:349:1526.

Betteridge Z, et al. Anti-synthetase syndrome: a new auto antibody to phenylalanyl transfer RNA synthetase (anti-Zo) associated with polymyositis and interstitial pneumonia. *Rheumatology.* 2007:46:1005.

Bhat A, et al. Current concepts on the immunopathology of amyloidosis [published online: July 21, 2009]. *Clin Rev Allergy Immunol.*

Buckley RH, et al. Human severe combined immunodeficiency: genetic, phenotypic, functional diversity in one hundred eight infants. *J Pediatr.* 1997:130:378.

Castigli E, Geha RS. Molecular basis of common variable immunodeficiency. *J Allergy Clin Immunol.* 2006:117:740.

Cavazzana-Calvo M, et al. Gene therapy of human severe combined immunodeficiency (SCID)—X1 disease. *Science.* 2000:288:669.

Conley ME, et al. Genetic analysis of patients with defect in early B-cell development. *Immunol Rev.* 2005:203:216.

Cunningham-Rundles C, Ponda PP. Molecular defects in T- and B-cell primary immunodeficiency diseases. *Nat Rev Immunol.* 2005:11:880.

Dalakas MC, Hohlfeld R. Polymyositis and dermatomyositis. *Lancet.* 2003:362:971.

Davis AE 3rd. The pathophysiology of hereditary angioedema. *Clin Immunol.* 2005:114:3.

Dispenzieri A, et al. International Myeloma Working Group guidelines for serum-free light analysis in multiple myeloma and related disorders. *Leukemia.* 2009:23:215.

Durand A, et al. Hyper-immunoglobulin M syndromes caused by intrinsic B-lymphocyte defects. *Immunol Rev.* 2005:203:67.

Ferri C, et al. Cryoglobulin. *J Clin Pathol.* 2002:55:4.

Glovsky MM, et al. Complement determinations in human disease. *Ann Allergy Asthma Immunol.* 2004:93:513.

Griggs RC, et al. Inclusion body myositis and myopathies. *Ann Neurol.* 1995:705:13.

Harley JB. Autoantibodies are central to the diagnosis and clinical manifestations of lupus. *J Rheumatol.* 1994:21:1183.

Heinlen LD, et al. Clinical criteria for systemic lupus erythematosus precede diagnosis, and associated autoantibodies are present before clinical symptoms. *Arthritis Rheum.* 2007:56:2344.

Hochberg MC. Updating the American College of Rheumatology Revised criteria for the classification of systemic lupus erythematosus. *Arthritis Rheum.* 1997:40:1725.

Hu PQ, et al. Correlation of serum anti-DNA topoisomerase I antibody levels with disease severity and activity in systemic sclerosis. *Arthritis Rheum.* 2003:48:1363.

Kawai T, Akira S. Pathogen recognition with Toll-like receptors. *Curr Opin Immunol.* 2005:17:338.

Kissel JT, et al. Microvascular deposition of complement membrane attack complex in dermatomyositis. *N Engl J Med.* 1986:329:34.

Nakamura RM, Bylund DJ. Contemporary concepts for the clinical and laboratory evaluation of systemic lupus erythematosus and "lupus-like" syndromes. *J Clin Lab Anal.* 1994:8:347.

Phan TG, et al. Autoantibodies to extractable nuclear antigens: making detection and interpretation more meaningful. *Clin Diagn Lab Immunol.* 2002:9:1.

Pratt G. The evolving use of serum free light chain assays in hematology. *Br J Haematol.* 2008:141:413.

Ramos-Casals M, et al. Primary Sjogren's syndrome: new clinical and therapeutic concepts. *Ann Rheum Dis.* 2005:64:347.

Reveille JD, Solomon DH. Evidence-based guidelines for the use of immunologic tests: anticentromere, Sci-70, and nucleolar antibodies. *Arthritis Rheum.* 2003:49:399.

Rider LG, Miller FW. Laboratory evaluation of the inflammatory myopathies. *Clin Diagn Lab Immunol.* 1995:2:1.

Rojas-Serrano J, et al. Very recent arthritis: the value of initial rheumatological evaluation and anti-cyclic citrullinated peptide antibodies in the diagnosis of rheumatoid arthritis. *Clin Rheumatol*. 2009:28:1135.

Rothfield NF. Autoantibodies in scleroderma. *Rheum Dis Clin North Am*. 1992:18:483.

Sanchez-Guerrero J, et al. Utility of Sm, anti-RNP, anti-Ro/SS-A and anti-La/SS-B (extractable nuclear antigens) detected by enzyme-linked immunosorbent assay for the diagnosis of systemic lupus erythematosus. *Arthritis Rheum*. 1996:39:1055.

Schroeder HW Jr, et al. The complex genetics of common variable immunodeficiency. *J Invest Med*. 2004:52:90.

Smeenk R, et al. Antibodies to DNA in patients with systemic lupus erythematosus. Their role in diagnosis, the follow-up and the pathogenesis of the disease. *Clin Rheumatol*. 1990:9:100.

Solomon DH, et al. Evidence-based guidelines for the use of immunologic tests: antinuclear antibody testing. *Arthritis Rheum*. 2002:47:434.

Talal N. Sjogren's syndrome: historical overview and clinical spectrum of disease. *Rheum Dis Clin North Am*. 1992:18:507.

Tedeschi A, et al. Cryoglobulinemia. Blood Rev. 2007:21:183.

Von Muhlen CA, Tan EM. Autoantibodies in the diagnosis of systemic rheumatic diseases. *Semin Arthritis Rheum*. 1995:24:323.

Walport MJ. Complement. First of two parts. *N Engl J Med*. 2001:344:1058.

Walport MJ. Complement. Second of two parts. *N Engl J Med*. 2001:344:1140.

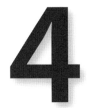

Histocompatibility Testing and Transplantation

Yash Pal Agrawal and Susan L. Saidman

LEARNING OBJECTIVES

1. Learn the organization of human leukocyte antigen (HLA) genes and the molecular details of their gene products.

2. Understand the clinical laboratory tests used to assess histocompatibility.

3. Learn the histocompatibility requirements for the solid organ and stem cell transplants in clinical use.

CHAPTER OUTLINE

INTRODUCTION

An animal will generally accept an organ transplant from itself, but will reject a transplant from other animals, even if the donor animal is of the same species. Organ rejection is a consequence of the interactions between the immune system of the transplant recipient and the histocompatibility antigens present on the transplanted cells. Clinical laboratories play an important role in the histocompatibility testing for solid organ and bone marrow transplantation (BMT). This chapter provides a brief background to some of the issues and techniques involved in histocompatibility testing.

The histocompatibility antigens that are the primary stimulus in graft rejection are encoded by a complex of closely linked genes called the major histocompatibility complex (MHC). In mice, these genes are located on the H2 region of chromosome 17. In humans, the analogous MHC region is located in a 4,000-kb region on the short arm of chromosome 6 and encodes for the HLA system (**Figure 4–1**).

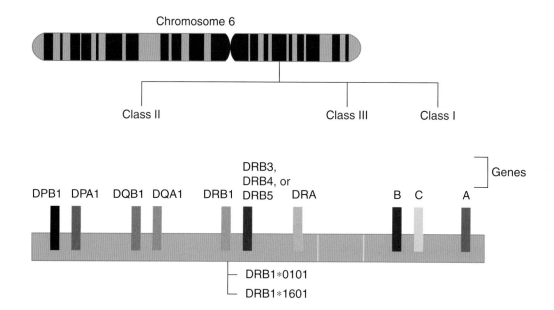

FIGURE 4–1 Genes of the human MHC system. The human major histocompatibility complex (MHC) is located on the short arm of chromosome 6. It contains over 200 genes that can be divided into different regions (class I–III). Only the major genes encoding the HLA molecules important in transplantation are shown. The class I region contains genes that encode the α chains of the classic transplantation antigens, HLA-A, -B, and -C. The class II region has genes that encode both the α and β chains of HLA-DP, -DQ, and -DR molecules. Genes encoding the α and β chains are designated as "A" or "B," and are followed by a number if there is more than 1 gene encoding a particular chain. For example, DRB1 is 1 of the genes that encodes the β chain of DR molecules. Different alleles at each gene location are indicated by an asterisk (*) and then a number. Thus, HLA-DRB1*0101 and HLA-DRB1*1601 are different alleles of the DRB1 gene. The class III region is located between regions I and II and does not encode for HLA molecules (adapted with permission from: Clinical Laboratory Reviews [a newsletter publication of the Massachusetts General Hospital] 2000;8:3).

HLA GENES AND GENE PRODUCTS

The HLA class I region encodes for certain glycoprotein molecules that are present on all nucleated cells. The main function of the HLA class I molecules is to bind to fragments resulting from the breakdown of intracellular pathogens, such as viruses. The HLA molecule and the bound peptide are then presented on the cell surface so that an immune response can be initiated against the pathogen. Class I molecules consist of 2 noncovalently linked chains. A gene in the MHC encodes the heavy chain, and a gene outside the MHC on chromosome 15 encodes the β2-microglobulin light chain. In humans there are 3 important class I genes known as HLA-A, -B, and -C. These genes are highly polymorphic. Polymorphism refers to multiple variations of a single genetic locus and its gene product. Each variation of the gene is called an *allele*. The HLA-A, -B, and -C genes encode for over 80 gene products that can be defined by serology—that is, by matching antibodies against the different HLA antigens (**Table 4–1**). However, the antigens identified by serotyping are far outnumbered by the alleles that are recognized by sequencing the gene. This is because not all gene polymorphisms result in distinct antibody specificities.

The class II region encodes for the α and β chains that make up the HLA-DR, -DQ, and -DP molecules (**Figure 4–1**). These HLA class II molecules have a more restricted expression than the class I molecules. They are found mainly on B lymphocytes, dendritic cells, monocytes, activated T cells, and some endothelial cells. Antigen-presenting cells such as macrophages can phagocytose and engulf bacteria and other parasites via endocytosis. Once these pathogens gain entry to the cell, they can be broken down by proteases into peptides that are able to bind to the class II molecules. These peptides are then presented on the cell surface and an immune response is initiated. The class III region contains approximately 40 genes that do not encode HLA molecules, but

In humans there are 3 important class I genes known as HLA-A, -B, and -C. The class II region encodes for the α and β chains that make up the HLA-DR, -DQ, and -DP molecules.

TABLE 4–1 Number of HLA Alleles and Serologic Specificities

HLA Gene	Number of Alleles Determined by Gene Sequencing[a]	Number of Serologic Specificities
HLA-A	>450	28
HLA-B	>850	70
HLA-C	>250	10
HLA-DRB1	>450	21
HLA-DQB1	>75	9

[a]This number increases continually as new sequences are identified.

encode certain complement components and numerous other proteins not involved in transplantation or the immune response.

The HLA genes are linked together—in what is called a *haplotype*—on the chromosome and inherited en bloc. Each individual inherits 1 haplotype from each parent, and the 2 haplotypes represent the HLA genotype. The alleles from both of these haplotypes are expressed on an individual's cells. This is referred to as a codominant expression of the gene. Therefore, even though there are multiple HLA genes, usually only 4 genotypes are possible in the offspring. There is a 25% chance of any 2 siblings being HLA identical and a 50% chance of the siblings sharing a haplotype.

SEROLOGIC HISTOCOMPATIBILITY TESTING ASSAYS

HLA Typing

The HLA type of a potential graft recipient or donor can be determined using a microlymphocytotoxicity assay. T lymphocytes are used for typing class I antigens, and B lymphocytes for typing class II antigens. The assay involves mixing known HLA typing sera with the separated lymphocytes, followed by the addition of complement. Complement-mediated lysis of lymphocytes follows when the antibody in the serum binds to the appropriate HLA antigen. The extent of cell lysis is visualized under a fluorescence microscope after exposing the cells to DNA binding dyes such as ethidium bromide. The dye stains the nuclear DNA of lysed cells but does not permeate the cell membranes of viable cells. HLA typing for class I and II antigens typically involves mixing the cells with over 200 different HLA typing sera, each in a different well of a microtiter tray.

HLA Antibody Screening

The patient's serum can be screened for the presence of antibodies that may have resulted from prior transfusions, pregnancies, or transplants. Serum from patients awaiting renal transplantation is usually collected at monthly intervals and screened for reactivity against a panel of lymphocytes or purified HLA molecules from individuals (panel cells) with known HLA types. Screening can be done using either cell-based or solid-phase assays. In the cell-based assays, patient serum is mixed with different panel cells. If the cells are lysed (in a cytotoxicity assay) or if antibody binds to them (detected using a flow cytometry assay), then it is evident that the patient's serum contains HLA antibody against the antigens expressed on that panel cell. In the solid-phase assays, HLA antigens are extracted from the panel cells. The antigens are purified and bound to a solid support, either to the wells of an ELISA plate or to colored beads that can be detected using flow cytometry or Luminex technology. Antibody binding to the molecules on the well or bead is detected using an enzyme or fluorescence conjugated anti-immunoglobulin reagent.

The number of panel cells showing lysis or antibody binding is noted, and the results are expressed as percent panel reactive antibody (PRA). Patients with a high PRA are referred to as "sensitized." If the patient's serum reacts with 90% of the panel cells, it is likely that the patient will have to wait longer for a compatible donor than someone who shows a PRA of 0% (i.e., no HLA

The HLA genes are linked together—in what is called a *haplotype*—on the chromosome and inherited en bloc. Each individual inherits 1 haplotype from each parent, and the 2 haplotypes represent the HLA genotype.

antibody). Identification of the HLA antigen specificity of the antibody is an important feature of the antibody screening assays, and may reduce unnecessary crossmatches between patients who have antibodies against specific HLA antigens and donors who are positive for those antigens. Knowledge of antibody specificity can also increase opportunities for identifying compatible donors for these difficult-to-match patients. Highly sensitized (high PRA) patients may also be managed differently posttransplant since they have a higher risk of rejection. Pretransplant screening for HLA antibodies is also indicated in patients undergoing autologous stem cell transplants, since posttransplant patients with a high PRA are more likely to become refractory to platelet transfusions and may require careful observation regarding their need for HLA-matched platelets.

Crossmatching

The lymphocyte crossmatch is a critical step, especially before renal transplantation. It is also important in sensitized patients who are undergoing a heart or lung transplant. In this assay, the graft recipient's serum is mixed with donor lymphocytes (similar to that shown for red blood cells in Chapter 2 under Blood Crossmatch). If the recipient has preformed HLA antibodies against donor antigens, the cells will be lysed, the crossmatch is considered positive, and the transplant will likely not be done. The test may be performed using a variation of the microlymphocytotoxicity assay that is used for HLA typing. In this test, antihuman globulin (AHG) is added to the microtiter wells after mixing the serum with the lymphocytes, which greatly increases the sensitivity of the assay. The crossmatch may also be performed by measuring antibody binding to cells by flow cytometry.

MOLECULAR TECHNIQUES FOR HLA TYPING

Molecular methods allow high-resolution HLA typing at the allele level, so different alleles that cannot be distinguished by serologic assays can be identified. Such techniques also have applications in typing nonlymphocytes (e.g., blasts) and in patients with cytopenias. One technique involves amplification of genomic DNA by polymerase chain reaction (PCR) (see Chapter 2) using primers that are *locus specific* (e.g., all DQB1 alleles) or *group specific* (e.g., all DR4 alleles). The amplified DNA is then hybridized with a panel of labeled, sequence-specific oligonucleotide probes (PCR-SSOP) specific for each allele or group of alleles. Even a single nucleotide mismatch will prevent the annealing of the probe. The bound probe is visualized using various methods, including autoradiography and color development, by blotting the DNA onto multiple membranes (dot blot hybridization). Alternatively, the probes may be bound to a single membrane or to groups of different colored beads (reverse hybridization).

In a related technique, *sequence-specific* primers for an allele are used in a PCR amplification reaction (PCR-SSP). The presence or absence of PCR amplification is detected by gel electrophoresis and ethidium bromide visualization. In this technique, a positive amplification reaction signifies the presence of that specific allele.

HISTOCOMPATIBILITY REQUIREMENTS FOR SOLID ORGAN AND STEM CELL TRANSPLANTS

In general, HLA matching is not an absolute requirement with respect to solid organ transplants (**Table 4–2**). It is usually a requirement for BMT. The application of HLA typing, crossmatching, and antibody screening in histocompatibility testing prior to transplantation of specific organs or tissues is described hereafter.

In general, HLA matching is not an absolute requirement with respect to solid organ transplants. It is usually a requirement for bone marrow transplantation.

Kidney

Renal transplantation from living donors, whether HLA matched or unmatched, is preferable to kidney transplantation from deceased donors. The half-life of a transplanted deceased donor kidney is about 8 years, as compared to 12 and 26 years for kidneys matched at 1 or 2 haplotypes

TABLE 4-2 General Requirements for HLA and ABO Blood Group Matching in Transplants

Organ	HLA	ABO
Kidney	No[a]	Yes
Cornea	No	No
Liver	No	Yes
Heart	No	Yes
Lung	No	Yes
Pancreas	No[a]	Yes
Stem cell/bone marrow	Yes	No

[a]HLA matching preferable but not required.

from living donors. In the United States, nearly 50% of the kidney transplants are from living donors, including genetically unrelated donors such as spouses or friends. In a large multicenter study involving primary cadaveric renal transplants, multiple factors were shown to influence the outcome. These included the age of donor and recipient, presence of diabetes in the recipient, the cause of the donor's death, cold ischemic time of the donated kidney prior to transplant, the transplant center, and matching for HLA antigens. The advantages of HLA-matched transplants include a reduced need for antirejection treatment and posttransplant dialysis, as well as significantly improved long-term survival. Other important predictors of outcome are ABO-blood group compatibility, PRA, and crossmatch between donor lymphocytes and recipient serum. A positive crossmatch is usually a contraindication to transplant. However, techniques to remove recipient circulating HLA and/or ABO antibody have been recently developed, allowing successful transplantation with previously incompatible kidneys.

> In the United States, nearly 50% of the kidney transplants are from living donors, including genetically unrelated donors such as spouses or friends.

Liver

HLA matching does not appear to correlate with better outcomes in liver transplantation and, in some cases, even appears to have a deleterious effect. There are conflicting reports regarding the importance of a negative crossmatch in the pretransplant setting. In general, high-titer IgG antibodies against HLA antigens are likely to be significant, but are not an absolute contraindication to transplantation. ABO matching, in contrast, is associated with better outcomes in both adult and pediatric populations.

Heart

The benefits of HLA matching in heart transplantation are difficult to evaluate because there are few studies that utilize prospective HLA matching. The usual priorities in cardiac transplantation are short ischemia time for the donated heart prior to transplant (<4 hours), heart size, and blood group matching. Most centers screen for HLA antibodies prior to transplant surgery and perform, when possible, a prospective crossmatch using donor cells only on sensitized patients. The presence of HLA-specific antibodies and a positive crossmatch against donor cells are generally accepted to be associated with an adverse outcome.

Lung

While there may be a small survival advantage with HLA-matched lung transplants, there is no consensus on the hierarchical importance of the various HLA loci. Lungs are allocated on the basis of ABO compatibility and size. Similar to heart transplant patients, crossmatches are usually done only on patients known to have HLA antibody.

Pancreas

Pancreata are transplanted based on ABO compatibility. HLA antibody screening is performed on transplant candidates, and a positive crossmatch is usually a contraindication to transplantation with that donor. Patients with pancreas-only transplantation have a lower survival rate than those undergoing combined pancreas and kidney transplantation. Most pancreata are transplanted in patients undergoing kidney transplants for diabetic renal failure. Evidence suggests that the kidney–pancreas transplant combination is associated with a long-term reduction in mortality, as compared to renal transplant only, in end-stage diabetic renal disease.

Cornea

The cornea is the most commonly transplanted tissue. There is no convincing evidence for the utility of HLA and ABO group matching for corneal transplants. However, the long-term graft survival is approximately 50% and rejection remains the most common cause of graft loss. Because corneal rejection is not life threatening, the routine use of systemic immunosuppression for prevention of rejection is not a consideration.

HEMATOPOIETIC STEM CELL TRANSPLANTATION

Hematopoietic bone marrow/stem cell transplantation is a therapeutic option in which normal hematopoietic stem cells are used to replace abnormal hematopoietic stem cells or to reconstitute the bone marrow of patients undergoing high-dose cytotoxic therapy for malignancy. The hematopoietic stem and progenitor cells can be harvested from the bone marrow under general anesthesia or from the peripheral blood after giving the donor multiple doses of growth factors/cytokines such as granulocyte colony stimulating factor (G-CSF) or granulocyte–monocyte colony stimulating factor (GM-CSF).

HLA matching is usually a requirement for allogeneic stem cell transplantation. A positive crossmatch between donor and recipient is a strong predictor of graft failure, but because most patients and donors are HLA matched, this is rarely a concern. Some success has been obtained in cases involving partially mismatched BMT. This is based on animal studies that show that an MHC-mismatched BMT can mediate a potent antitumor effect in excess of that achieved by an MHC-matched BMT and without significant graft-versus-host disease (GVHD) when special conditioning regimens are used.

In the past, serologic techniques were used extensively for HLA typing in BMT. As noted earlier, it is now known that the number of identifiable serologic specificities at any locus is far less than the number of true alleles at that locus (**Table 4–1**). Individuals who appear to be HLA matched after serologic typing may in fact have some mismatched alleles. Patients transplanted with genotypically HLA-matched marrow from siblings or unrelated individuals have a graft failure rate of approximately 2%. The risk of graft failure is much higher in the presence of a mismatch of 2 or more class I alleles.

The widespread availability of high-resolution allelic typing methods that allow better matching of donors with recipients has resulted in improved outcomes.

A substantial portion of this chapter also appeared previously in Clinical Laboratory Reviews (a newsletter publication of the Massachusetts General Hospital, 2000;8:3).

REFERENCES

Agrawal YP, Saidman SL. Histocompatibility testing for solid organ and bone marrow transplantation. *Clin Lab Rev,* A publication of the Massachusetts General Hospital. 2000;8:3.

Donaldson PT, Williams R. Cross-matching in liver transplantation [Review]. *Transplantation.* 1997;63:789.

Dyer PA, et al. HLA and clinical solid organ transplantation: recent publications and novel approaches. In: Gjertson DW, Terasaki PI, eds. *HLA 1998.* American Society for Histocompatibility and Immunogenetics; 1998:13.

Futagawa Y, Terasaki PI. An analysis of the OPTN/UNOS Liver Transplant Registry. *Clin Transplants.* 2004;315.

Gebel HM, et al. Pre-transplant assessment of donor-reactive, HLA-specific antibodies in renal transplantation: contraindication vs. risk. *Am J Transplantation.* 2003;3:1488.

Magee CC. Transplantation across previously incompatible immunological barriers [Review]. *Transplant Int.* 2006;19:87.

Marsh SGE. Nomenclature of factors of the HLA system. http://www.anthonynolan.org.uk/HIG/lists/nomenc.html. Accessed October 17, 2006.

McCluskey J, Peh CA. The human leucocyte antigens and clinical medicine: an overview. *Rev Immunogenet.* 1999;1:3.

Morris PJ, et al. Analysis of factors that affect outcome of primary cadaveric renal transplantation in the UK. *Lancet.* 1999;354:1147.

Petersdorf EW, et al. Human leukocyte antigen matching in unrelated donor hematopoietic cell transplantation [Review]. *Semin Hematol.* 2005;42:76.

Reinsmoen NL, et al. Anti-HLA antibody analysis and crossmatching in heart and lung transplantation [Review]. *Transplant Immunol.* 2004;13:63.

Smets YFC, et al. Effect of simultaneous pancreas-kidney transplantation on mortality of patients with type-1 diabetes mellitus and end-stage renal failure. *Lancet.* 1999;353:1915.

Sykes M, et al. Mixed lymphohaemopoietic chimerism and graft-versus-lymphoma effects after non-myeloablative therapy and HLA-mismatched bone-marrow transplantation. *Lancet.* 1999;353:1755.

Wolfe RA, et al. Comparison of mortality in all patients on dialysis, patients on dialysis awaiting transplantation, and recipients of a first cadaveric transplant. *N Engl J Med.* 1999;341:1725.

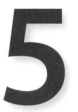

Infectious Diseases

Eric D. Spitzer

CHAPTER OUTLINE

INTRODUCTION

Humans live in a world of microbes. Many types of microbes are part of the normal human flora and rarely cause disease. Other organisms have a greater potential for virulence and can cause disease depending on complex interactions between the host and the microbe. A small group of organisms is highly virulent and usually causes disease whenever it infects humans. This chapter on infectious diseases and clinical microbiology focuses on common pathogens and frequently encountered clinical syndromes. Infectious agents include a daunting array of viruses, bacteria, fungi, protozoans, and helminths. **Table 5–1** provides information on the basic microbiology and clinical significance of common pathogens. The organisms are grouped based on shared properties because this is often relevant to the diagnostic process.

TABLE 5–1   Selected Clinically Significant Microorganisms

Aerobic Gram-Positive Cocci

Occur singly or in pairs, tetrads, chains, or clusters

Catalase Positive
Micrococcus
Staphylococcus

Catalase Negative
Aerococcus
Enterococcus avium (group D enterococcus)
Enterococcus durans (group D enterococcus)
Enterococcus faecalis (group D enterococcus)
Enterococcus faecium (group D enterococcus)
Gemella
Helcococcus
Lactococcus
Leuconostoc
Streptococcus agalactiae (group B streptococci)
Streptococcus bovis (group D nonenterococcus)
Streptococcus dysgalactiae (multiple species within group C or group G streptococci are classified as *Streptococcus dysgalactiae*)
Streptococcus milleri group (viridans streptococci)
Streptococcus mitis (viridans streptococci)
Streptococcus mutans group (viridans streptococci)
Streptococcus pneumoniae (pneumococcus)
Streptococcus pyogenes (group A streptococci)
Streptococcus salivarius group (viridans streptococci)
Streptococcus sanguis group (viridans streptococci)
Streptococcus zooepidemicus (group C streptococci)
Vagococcus

Aerobic Gram-Negative Cocci

Occur singly or in pairs or clumps; catalase positive, oxidase positive

Moraxella catarrhalis (*Branhamella catarrhalis*)
Neisseria gonorrhoeae
Neisseria meningitidis

Aerobic Gram-Positive Bacilli

Rod-like organisms; only *Bacillus* species produce spores, some organisms in category are partially acid-fast

Actinomyces (some species are aerobic/anaerobic)
Bacillus
Corynebacterium
Erysipelothrix
Gardnerella vaginalis (*Haemophilus vaginalis*)
Lactobacillus
Listeria
Nocardia

Mycobacteria

Rod-like organisms; acid-fast stain positive; some stains are gram-positive; most are slow growing

Mycobacterium tuberculosis
Mycobacterium avium complex
Mycobacterium kansasii
Mycobacterium marinum
Mycobacterium fortuitum complex (rapid grower)
Mycobacterium abscessus (rapid grower)
Mycobacterium chelonae (rapid grower)

Aerobic Gram-Negative Bacilli

Enterobacteriaceae; rod-like organisms; oxidase negative; ferment sugars

Citrobacter
Edwardsiella
Enterobacter
Escherichia
Ewingella
Hafnia
Klebsiella
Morganella morganii (*Proteus morganii*)
Proteus
Providencia
Salmonella
Serratia
Shigella
Yersinia enterocolitica
Yersinia pestis
Yersinia pseudotuberculosis

Aerobic Gram-Negative Bacilli

Nonenterobacteriaceae, fermentative; rod-like organisms; oxidase positive; ferment sugars

Aeromonas
Chromobacterium

Pasteurella
Plesiomonas
Vibrio

Aerobic Gram-Negative Bacilli

Nonenterobacteriaceae; rod-like organisms; catalase positive; do not ferment sugars; oxidase variable

Acinetobacter
Alcaligenes
Burkholderia
Chryseobacterium (*Flavobacterium*)
Empedobacter (*Flavobacterium*)
Flaviomonas
Flavobacterium
Pseudomonas

Aerobic Gram-Negative Coccobacilli

Small, straight or curved gram-negative bacilli or coccobacilli; may require special conditions for adequate growth

Actinobacillus
Afipia
Bartonella henselae
Bartonella quintana
Bordetella
Brucella
Campylobacter (microaerophilic)
Chlamydia (obligate intracellular pathogen)
Coxiella (obligate intracellular pathogen)
Ehrlichia (obligate intracellular pathogen)
Eikenella (obligate intracellular pathogen)
Francisella tularensis
Haemophilus
Helicobacter pylori
Legionella
Rickettsia
Streptobacillus

***Mycoplasma* (also known as Pleuropneumonia-like Organisms or PPLO)**

Small highly pleomorphic organisms; difficult to observe with routine stains and require complex medium for growth

Mycoplasma
Ureaplasma

Continued next page—

TABLE 5-1   Selected Clinically Significant Microorganisms (continued)

Treponemes

Spiral organisms that may or may not stain with routine stains and require complex medium or animal host for growth

Borrelia
Leptospira
Spirillum
Treponema

Anaerobic Gram-Negative Bacilli

Bacteroides
Bilophila
Fusobacterium
Leptotrichia

Anaerobic Gram-Negative Cocci

Acidaminococcus
Veillonella

Anaerobic Gram-Positive Bacilli: Nonspore Forming

Actinomyces (all anaerobic species are aerobic/anaerobic)

Lactobacillus (all anaerobic species are aerobic/anaerobic)
Propionibacterium

Anaerobic Gram-Positive Bacilli: Spore Forming

Clostridium
Filifactor

Anaerobic Gram-Positive Cocci

Gemella (aerobic/anaerobic)
Peptococcus
Peptostreptococcus
Staphylococcus saccharolyticus (aerobic/anaerobic)
Other *Staphylococcus* species are aerobic
Streptococcus intermedius (aerobic/anaerobic)

Fungi of Medical Significance[a]

Acremonium
Aspergillus
Blastomyces
Candida
Coccidioides
Cryptococcus
Epidermophyton
Fonsecaea
Fusarium
Geotrichum
Histoplasma
Malassezia
Microsporum
Mucor
Pseudallescheria (Scedosporium)
Rhizomucor
Rhizopus
Sporothrix
Trichophyton
Trichosporon
Wangiella

Viruses[b]

Family	Representative Species Pathogenic for Humans	Family	Representative Species Pathogenic for Humans
DNA Viruses			Hantaviruses (rodent-associated)
Poxviridae	Vaccinia virus		Hantaan virus (hemorrhagic fever with renal syndrome), Sin Nombre virus (hantavirus pulmonary syndrome)
	Variola virus (smallpox)	Arenaviridae	Lymphocytic choriomeningitis virus
	Molluscum contagiosum virus		Lassa fever virus
Herpesviridae	Herpes simplex virus, type 1		Junin (Argentine hemorrhagic fever virus)
	Herpes simplex virus, type 2		Machupo (Bolivian hemorrhagic fever virus)
	Varicella zoster virus	Picornaviridae	Enteroviruses
	Epstein–Barr virus		Poliovirus (3 types)
	Cytomegalovirus		Coxsackie A virus (23 types)
	Human herpesvirus 6 (HHV 6)		Coxsackie B virus (6 types)
	Human herpesvirus 8 (HHV 8, Kaposi's sarcoma-associated herpesvirus)		Echovirus (30 types)
			Enteroviruses 68–71 (4)
Adenoviridae	Human adenoviruses (51 serotypes)		Rhinovirus (common cold virus) (>115 types)
Papillomaviridae	Human papilloma viruses (>96 types)		Hepatitis A virus (enterovirus 72)
Polyomaviridae	BK virus	Caliciviridae	Noroviruses
	JC virus		Norwalk and Norwalk-like gastroenteritis viruses
Parvoviridae	B19 virus (human parvovirus)	Hepeviridae	Hepatitis E virus (enterically transmitted)
Hepadnaviridae	Hepatitis B virus	Astroviridae	Human astroviruses
RNA Viruses		Coronaviridae	Human coronaviruses
Reoviridae	Orthoreoviruses		SARS-CoV
	Colorado tick fever virus	Flaviviridae	Flaviviruses (mosquito-borne)
	Rotaviruses A–C		St. Louis and Japanese encephalitis viruses, West Nile virus, yellow fever virus, dengue virus
Paramyxoviridae	Respiroviruses		Flaviviruses (tick-borne)
	Parainfluenza virus, types 1 and 3		Omsk hemorrhagic fever, European and Far Eastern tick-borne encephalitis viruses
	Morbilliviruses		Hepatitis C virus (parenterally transmitted)
	Measles virus	Togaviridae	Alphaviruses
	Rubulaviruses		Western, Eastern, and Venezuelan equine encephalitis viruses; Ross River and Semliki Forest viruses (mosquito-borne)
	Mumps virus, parainfluenza virus, types 2 and 4		
	Pneumoviruses		Rubivirus
	Respiratory syncytial virus		Rubella virus
	Metapneumovirus	Retroviridae	Human T-cell lymphotropic virus (HTLV) 1 and 2
Rhabdoviridae	Rabies virus		
Filoviridae	Marburg and Ebola viruses		Human immunodeficiency virus (HIV) 1 and 2
Orthomyxoviridae	Influenza A virus		
	Influenza B virus		
Bunyaviridae	Orthobunyaviruses (mosquito-transmitted)		
	California serogroup (e.g., *California encephalitis* and *La Crosse* viruses)		

Continued next page—

TABLE 5–1   Selected Clinically Significant Microorganisms (continued)

Subviral Agents

Satellites
  Hepatitis delta (D) virus
Prions
  Kuru, Creutzfeldt–Jakob disease (CJD),
  Gerstmann–Straussler–Scheinker
  syndrome (GSS), fatal familial
  insomnia (FFI)

Parasites of Clinical Significance[c]

Protozoa

Amebae (intestinal)
Entamoeba
Endolimax
Iodamoeba
Blastocystis

Amebae (other body sites)
Naegleria
Acanthamoeba
Balamuthia

Flagellates (intestinal)
Giardia
Dientamoeba
Trichomonas hominis

Flagellates (blood, tissue)
Leishmania
Trypanosoma

Flagellates (other body sites)
Trichomonas vaginalis

Ciliates (intestinal)
Balantidium

Coccidia (intestinal)
Cryptosporidium
Cyclospora
Isospora

Coccidia (other body sites)
Toxoplasma

Microsporidia (intestinal)
Enterocytozoon
Encephalitozoon

Microsporidia (other body sites)
Encephalitozoon
Enterocytozoon (not a true genus—for species
unidentified by genus and/or species)

Sporozoa (blood, tissue)
Plasmodium
Babesia

**Fungal-like organism (formerly classified
as a protozoan)**
Pneumocystis

Nematodes (Roundworms)

(Intestinal)
Ascaris
Enterobius
Ancylostoma
Necator
Strongyloides
Trichostrongylus
Trichuris

(Tissue)
Trichinella
Visceral larva migrans (*Toxocara canis* or
  Toxocara cati)
Ocular larva migrans (*Toxocara canis* or
  Toxocara cati)
Cutaneous larva migrans (*Ancylostoma
  braziliense* or *Ancylostoma caninum*)
Dracunculus
Angiostrongylus
Gnathostoma

Anisakis
Capillaria
Thelazia

(Blood and Tissues)
Wuchereria
Brugia
Loa
Onchocerca

Cestodes (Tapeworms)

(Intestinal)
Diphyllobothrium
Hymenolepis
Taenia solium
Taenia saginata

(Tissue—larval forms)
Taenia solium
Echinococcus
Diphyllobothrium

Trematodes (Flukes)

(Intestinal)
Fasciolopsis
Echinostoma
Metagonimus

(Liver/Lung)
Clonorchis
Opisthorchis
Fasciola
Paragonimus

(Blood and Tissue)
Schistosoma mansoni (intestine)
Schistosoma japonicum (intestine)
Schistosoma haematobium (bladder)

[a]The fungi are listed by genus. As with the bacteria, certain species within a genus are more commonly associated with infections than other species. The list includes the fungi associated with the majority of human fungal infections. There are many more fungi in nature than are listed here. Compiled from data in McGinnis MR, Rinaldi MG. *Clin Infect Dis.* 1997; 25:15.

[b]The viruses are grouped by family. Listed within each family are representative viral species that are pathogenic for humans. Compiled from data in Miller MJ. *Clin Infect Dis.* 1997; 25:18–20 and updated based on Knipe DM, Howley PM, eds. *Fields' Virology*, 5th ed. Wolters Kluwer; 2007.

[c]These organisms are listed by type of organism and most common site of infection. They are listed by genus only unless an individual species within a genus is located in 1 category and another species within the same genus is in a different category. Compiled from data in Garcia LS. *Clin Infect Dis.* 1997; 25:21.

Because of the large number of potential pathogens, it is not technically possible, practical, or cost effective to attempt to rule out all of them in each patient who may have an infection. It is therefore important for the clinician to know what organisms are most likely in a particular patient and whether routine diagnostic tests will detect them or whether specialized tests are needed. **Table 5–2** lists organisms that are often associated with infections at specific sites.

Identification of the causative agent is usually important for determining the most appropriate therapy. It can also have infection control or public health implications. The clinical findings are the first major clues in determining the site of infection and identifying a pathogenic organism. For example, a cough is usually indicative of a process in the respiratory tract while pain on urination is a clue to a urinary tract infection (UTI). Radiographic studies can further clarify the type of process and may point to specific categories of organisms.

TABLE 5-2   Bacteria, Fungi and Viruses most likely to cause Acute Infections[a]

Blood (Septicemia)

Newborn infants

Escherichia coli (or other gram-negative
   bacilli)
Streptococcus (group B)
Listeria monocytogenes
Staphylococcus aureus
Streptococcus pyogenes (group A)
Enterococcus
Streptococcus pneumoniae

Children

Streptococcus pneumoniae
Neisseria meningitides
Haemophilus influenzae
Streptococcus pyogenes (group A)
Escherichia coli (or other gram-negative
   bacilli)

Adults

Escherichia coli (or other enteric gram-
   negative bacilli)
Staphylococcus aureus
Streptococcus pneumoniae
Nonenteric gram-negative bacilli
   (*Pseudomonas, Acinetobacter, Aeromonas*)
Bacteroides
Streptococcus pyogenes (group A)
Other streptococci (nongroup A and
   not Lancefield groupable)
Staphylococcus epidermidis
Enterococcus
Neisseria meningitides
Candida spp. and other fungi
Neisseria gonorrhoeae
Fusobacterium
Mycobacteria
Rickettsia
Ehrlichia spp.
Brucella spp.
Leptospira

Meninges

Viruses (enterovirus, mumps, herpes simplex,
   HIV, and others)
Neisseria meningitidis
Streptococcus pneumoniae
Haemophilus influenzae (in children)
Streptococcus group B; infants less than
   2 months old)
Escherichia coli (or other gram-negative
   bacilli)
Streptococcus pyogenes (group A)
Staphylococcus aureus (with endocarditis or
   after neurosurgery, brain abscess)
Mycobacterium tuberculosis
Cryptococcus neoformans and other fungi
Listeria monocytogenes
Enterococcus (neonatal period)
Treponema pallidum
Leptospira
Borrelia burgdorferi
Toxoplasma gondii

Paranasal Sinuses

Streptococcus pneumoniae
Haemophilus influenzae
Moraxella catarrhalis
Streptococcus pyogenes (group A)
Anaerobic streptococci (chronic sinusitis)
Staphylococcus aureus (chronic sinusitis)
Klebsiella (or other gram-negative bacilli)
Mucor, Aspergillus (especially in
   diabetics

Mouth, periodontal, submandibular

Herpes simplex viruses
Candida albicans
Bacteroides
Mixed anaerobes
Actinomyces

Throat

Respiratory viruses
Streptococcus pyogenes (group A)
Neisseria meningitidis or *gonorrhoeae*
Leptotrichia buccalis
Candida albicans
Corynebacterium diphtheriae
Bordetella pertussis
Haemophilus influenzae
Fusobacterium necrophorum

Larynx, Trachea, and Bronchi

Respiratory viruses
Streptococcus pneumoniae
Haemophilus influenzae
Streptococcus pyogenes (group A)
Corynebacterium diphtheriae
Staphylococcus aureus
Gram-negative bacilli
Fusobacterium necrophorum

Pleura

Streptococcus pneumoniae
Staphylococcus aureus
Haemophilus influenzae
Gram-negative bacilli
Anaerobic streptococci
Bacteroides
Streptococcus pyogenes (group A)
Mycobacterium tuberculosis
Actinomyces, Nocardia
Fungi
Fusobacterium necrophorum

Brain and Perimeningeal Spaces

Herpes simplex (encephalitis)
Anaerobic streptococci and/or *Bacteroides*
   (cerebritis, brain abscess, and subdural
   empyema)
Staphylococcus aureus (cerebritis, brain
   abscess, epidural abscess)
Haemophilus influenzae (subdural
   empyema)
Arbovirus (encephalitis)

Mumps (encephalitis)
Toxoplasma gondii (encephalitis)
HIV
Mycobacterium tuberculosis
Nocardia (brain abscess)
Listeria monocytogenes (encephalitis)
Treponema pallidum
Cryptococcus neoformans
   and other fungi
Borrelia burgdorferi

Endocardium

Streptococci viridans
Enterococcus
Staphylococcus aureus
Streptococcus bovis
Staphylococcus epidermidis
Candida albicans and other fungi
Gram-negative bacilli
Streptococcus pneumoniae
Streptococcus pyogenes (group A)
Corynebacterium (especially with prosthetic
   valves)
Haemophilus, Actinobacillus,
   Cardiobacterium, Eikenella, or *Kingella*

Bones (Osteomyelitis)

Staphylococcus aureus
Salmonella (or other gram-negative
   bacilli)
Streptococcus pyogenes (group A)
Mycobacterium tuberculosis
Anaerobic streptococci (chronic)
Bacteroides (chronic)

Joints

Staphylococcus aureus
Streptococcus pyogenes (group A)
Neisseria gonorrhoeae
Gram-negative bacilli
Streptococcus pneumoniae
Neisseria meningitides
Haemophilus influenzae (in children)
Mycobacterium tuberculosis and
   other mycobacteria
Fungi
Borrelia burgdorferi

Skin and Subcutaneous Tissues

Burns
Staphylococcus aureus
Streptococcus pyogenes (group A)
Pseudomonas aeruginosa (or other
   gram-negative bacilli)

Skin infections
Staphylococcus aureus
Streptococcus pyogenes (group A)
Dermatophytes
Candida albicans
Herpes simplex or zoster
Gram-negative bacilli
Treponema pallidum
Bartonella henselae or *quintana*

Continued next page—

TABLE 5–2   Bacteria, Fungi and Viruses most likely to cause Acute Infections (continued)

Decubitus wound infections
Staphylococcus aureus
Escherichia coli (or other
   gram-negative bacilli)
Streptococcus pyogenes (group A)
Anaerobic streptococci
Clostridia
Enterococcus
Bacteroides

Traumatic and surgical wounds
Staphylococcus aureus
Anaerobic streptococci
Gram-negative bacilli
Clostridia
Streptococcus pyogenes (group A)
Enterococcus

Lungs

Pneumonia
Respiratory viruses
Mycoplasma pneumoniae
Streptococcus pneumoniae
Haemophilus influenzae
Anaerobic streptococci, fusospirochetes
Bacteroides
Staphylococcus aureus
Klebsiella (or other gram-negative bacilli)
Legionella pneumophila
Chlamydia pneumoniae
Streptococcus pyogenes (group A)
Rickettsia
Mycobacterium tuberculosis
Pneumocystis carinii
Fungi
Moraxella catarrhalis
Legionella micdadei (L. pittsburgensis)
Chlamydia psittaci
Fusobacterium necrophorum

Abscess
Anaerobic streptococci
Bacteroides
Staphylococcus aureus
Klebsiella (or other gram-negative bacilli)
Streptococcus pneumoniae
Fungi
Actinomyces, Nocardia

Gastrointestinal Tract

Gastrointestinal viruses
Campylobacter jejuni
Salmonella
Escherichia coli
Shigella
Yersinia enterocolitica
Entamoeba histolytica
Giardia lamblia
Staphylococcus aureus
Vibrio cholerae

Vibrio parahaemolyticus
Herpes simplex viruses (anus)
Treponema pallidum (anus)
Neisseria gonorrhoeae (anus)
Candida albicans
Clostridium difficile
Cryptosporidium parvum
Cytomegalovirus
HIV
Mycobacterium avium complex
Helicobacter pylor

Urinary Tract

Escherichia coli (or other gram-negative
   bacilli)
Staphylococcus aureus and epidermidis
Neisseria gonorrhoeae (urethra)
Enterococcus
Candida albicans
Chlamydia (urethra)
Treponema pallidum (urethra)
Trichomonas vaginalis (urethra)
Ureaplasma urealyticum

Eyes (Cornea and Conjunctiva)

Herpes and other viruses
Neisseria gonorrhoeae (in newborn)
Staphylococcus aureus
Streptococcus pneumoniae
Haemophilus influenzae (in children),
   including biotype aegyptius
   (Koch–Weeks bacillus)
Moraxella lacunata
Pseudomonas aeruginosa
Other gram-negative bacilli
Chlamydia trachomatis (trachoma and
   inclusion conjunctivitis)
Fungi

Ears

Auditory canal
Pseudomonas aeruginosa (or other
   gram-negative bacilli)
Staphylococcus aureus
Streptococcus pyogenes (group A)
Streptococcus pneumoniae
Haemophilus influenzae (in children)
Fungi

Middle ear
Streptococcus pneumoniae
Haemophilus influenzae (in children)
Moraxella catarrhalis
Streptococcus pyogenes (group A)
Staphylococcus aureus
Anaerobic streptococci (chronic)
Bacteroides (chronic)
Other gram-negative bacilli (chronic)
Mycobacterium tuberculosis

Female Genital Tract

Vagina
Trichomonas vaginalis
Candida albicans
Neisseria gonorrhoeae
Streptococcus pyogenes (group A)
Gardnerella vaginalis and associated
   anaerobes
Treponema pallidum

Uterus
Anaerobic streptococci
Bacteroides
Neisseria gonorrhoeae (cervix)
Clostridia
Escherichia coli (or other gram-negative
   bacilli)
Herpes simplex virus, type 2 (cervix)
Streptococcus pyogenes (group A)
Streptococcus, groups B and C
Treponema pallidum
Actinomyces spp. (most common infection
   associated with intrauterine devices)
Staphylococcus aureus
Enterococcus
Chlamydia trachomatis
Mycoplasma hominis

Fallopian tubes
Neisseria gonorrhoeae
Escherichia coli (or other gram-negative bacilli)
Anaerobic streptococci
Bacteroides
Chlamydia trachomatis

Male Genital Tract

Seminal vesicles
Gram-negative bacilli
Neisseria gonorrhoeae

Epididymis
Chlamydia
Gram-negative bacilli
Neisseria gonorrhoeae
Mycobacterium tuberculosis

Prostate gland
Gram-negative bacilli
Neisseria gonorrhoeae

Peritoneum

Gram-negative bacilli
Enterococcus
Bacteroides
Anaerobic streptococci
Clostridia
Streptococcus pneumoniae
Streptococcus (group B)

aReproduced with permission from: *The Medical Letter on Drugs & Therapeutics Handbook of Antimicrobial Therapy,* Revised Edition, 1998.

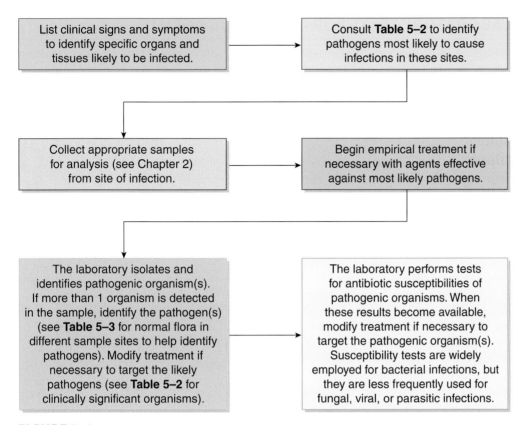

FIGURE 5-1 A general clinical approach to the patient with an infectious disease.

Often, a single species of microbe can cause multiple syndromes. Similarly, a single syndrome may be caused by multiple organisms. This can lead to a potentially vast array of diagnostic possibilities. In order to determine the diagnosis in a timely and cost-efficient manner, it is essential to take into consideration the clinical setting. For example, the organisms responsible for a community-acquired infection such as pneumonia are usually different from those that cause corresponding nosocomial infections. If the patient is immunosuppressed, this further enlarges the list of potential organisms. It also matters whether the immunosuppression is due to decreased cell-mediated immunity, for example, due to HIV infection or inhibitors of tumor necrosis factor (TNF), versus neutropenia secondary to chemotherapy because each has its own associated group of opportunistic infections. Other underlying conditions such as diabetes or sickle cell disease, or the presence of prosthetic devices, are associated with specific infections. A history of travel or exposure to arthropod vectors may raise the possibility of additional organisms.

The organization of this chapter reflects the common associations between selected organisms and the site of infection. The discussion of a particular organism in a specific anatomic site in this chapter does not imply that infection by that organism is restricted to that location. Several infectious diseases, such as viral hepatitis (see Chapter 16) and *Helicobacter pylori* infections (see Chapter 15), are presented elsewhere in this book because these infections are intimately associated with a specific organ or tissue. The organisms and diseases selected for presentation in this chapter were chosen primarily by their incidence, with a preference for common infections. Many lower incidence infections also have been included because they are often within a differential diagnosis, new information on their diagnosis and treatment is emerging, or they can be overlooked if appropriate tests are not requested. The chapter focuses on infections commonly encountered in the United States, although several travel-associated infections are discussed.

A general clinical approach to the patient with an infectious disease is diagrammed in **Figure 5-1**.

The organization of this chapter reflects the common associations between selected organisms and the site of infection.

LABORATORY TESTS FOR INFECTIOUS AGENTS

The laboratory diagnosis of infectious disease utilizes 5 distinct types of tests: direct examination, culture, antigen detection, nucleic acid detection, and serology. Each of these tests has strengths and weaknesses. The types of test(s) that are used in a specific case depend in large part on the organisms that are in the differential diagnosis as well as the type of specimens that are available. See Chapter 2 for illustrations of these laboratory methods.

Direct Stains

Direct examination involves preparing a smear of the specimen and then using an appropriate staining technique to detect the relevant microorganisms. The Gram stain is rapid and detects most types of bacterial pathogens if they are present in sufficient numbers. The Gram stain provides a preliminary characterization in terms of the Gram reaction, that is, positive or negative, as well as the morphology (cocci, coccobacilli, or bacilli) and arrangement of the cells (individual cells, pairs, chains, or clusters). It also provides information on the host response, for example, the presence or absence of neutrophils. This stain is routinely performed on most specimen types including respiratory specimens, sterile fluids, tissue biopsies, wounds, and abscesses. It is not routinely performed on stool because of the large numbers of normal flora, urine because similar information is available from the urinalysis, and blood because of the small number of organisms typically found in cases of bacteremia. The analytic sensitivity of the Gram stain is relatively low because the observation of an average of 1 organism per oil immersion field corresponds to a concentration of 10^5 organisms per milliliter in the specimen. The sensitivity can be increased by concentration of the specimen through centrifugation. Other direct stains include acid-fast stains for mycobacteria and calcofluor white for fungi. Wright stains of peripheral blood are used to detect *Plasmodium* and *Babesia* infections. Routine hematoxylin and eosin stains as well as Gram, acid-fast bacteria (AFB), and Gomori-methenamine-silver (GMS) stains can reveal the presence of microorganisms in paraffin-embedded tissue in the surgical pathology laboratory.

> The laboratory diagnosis of infectious disease utilizes 5 distinct types of tests: direct examination, culture, antigen detection, nucleic acid detection, and serology.

Culture

Isolation of organisms in pure culture continues to be the mainstay of microbiologic diagnosis. In general, culture is very sensitive and specific and remains the "gold standard" for diagnosing many types of infection. Culture provides relatively rapid detection (within usually 1 to 3 days) of a wide array of organisms that are then available for definitive identification and antimicrobial susceptibility testing. One of the great advantages of culture assays is that microbiology laboratories routinely inoculate a combination of nonselective and selective media that will support the growth of many types of pathogenic bacteria. The person ordering the test does not need to specify which organism or organisms are suspected of causing the infection. A clinician who submits a blood culture bottle does not have to order a *Staphylococcus* culture, a *Streptococcus* culture, a gram-negative rod culture, etc. Nonetheless, it is essential to remember that routine cultures only detect typical bacteria. If other classes of agents, such as mycobacteria, fungi, parasites, or viruses, are in the differential diagnosis, then the clinician must request the appropriate tests. For example, mycobacteria and fungal cultures utilize media designed to inhibit the growth of routine bacteria and they also require prolonged incubation.

Antigen Detection

Antigen detection tests do not require the growth of microorganisms. Therefore, they have the potential to provide rapid detection of infectious agents. Immunoassays that detect soluble antigens vary in speed, complexity, sensitivity, and specificity. Usually there is a tradeoff between simplicity and sensitivity. Immunochromatographic assays require very few procedural steps and are the basis of many rapid point-of-care tests. These assays are less sensitive than traditional solid-phase enzyme immunoassays (EIAs) that are used for batch testing in the laboratory. Unlike culture-based assays, an immunoassay can only detect the organism that binds to the reagent antibodies; a separate assay must be performed for each organism. Immunoassays generally exhibit good but not perfect specificity. Furthermore, they cannot distinguish viable from nonviable organisms. Direct or indirect fluorescent immunoassays utilize microscopy to identify organisms that bind the reagent antibody. These assays often have high sensitivity and specificity compared to other types of immunoassays but they require extensive training to insure proper interpretation.

Nucleic Acid Amplification

The introduction of nucleic acid amplification techniques (NAAT) has revolutionized several areas of infectious disease testing including HIV viral load testing, diagnosis of Herpes simplex virus (HSV) encephalitis, and rapid detection of MRSA. They are particularly valuable for detecting difficult-to-grow or slow-growing organisms that may be present in small numbers. NAAT tests have the potential for very high sensitivity and specificity. However, as with antigen tests, they can only be used to diagnose infections caused by organisms that the assay detects. Current technology is not at the stage where it can replace traditional culture methods. Nonetheless, this is a rapidly changing field and there are already commercially available multiplexed NAAT assays that can detect a battery of common respiratory viruses.

Serology

Serologic tests detect host antibodies that are produced in response to infection with a particular infectious agent. The most important limitation of these assays is that antibody is usually not detectable early in the course of infection. Even if antibody is detected, it may represent a past infection. Serologic diagnosis usually requires demonstration of seroconversion, a fourfold rise in IgG titer between sequential specimens, or a positive IgM assay. While the latter is usually thought of as a marker of acute infection, IgM can persist for 6 to 12 months. For the reasons outlined above, serologic assays are mainly used to diagnose infections that cannot be detected using more direct methods.

SEPSIS AND BLOODSTREAM INFECTIONS

Bacteremia

Description

Normally the blood is sterile. Infection in any of the organs or tissues can result in entry of bacteria into the circulation. Replication of bacteria in the blood can contribute to the signs and symptoms of sepsis (e.g., fever, tachycardia, leukocytosis, and hypotension) and may lead to dissemination of the organism to other tissues and organs; however, patients can be septic without having demonstrable bacteria in their blood. Bacteremia is often described as transient, intermittent, or continuous based on the number of positive specimens. Transient bacteremia occurs when small numbers of a commensal organism present on a mucosal surface gain access to the bloodstream. These infections are usually not clinically significant when they occur in an otherwise healthy host. Intermittent bacteremias are usually associated with a sequestered infection somewhere in the organs or tissues (e.g., an abscess). Continuous bacteremias are associated with an intravascular focus of infection. Examples include endocarditis or an infected vascular catheter.

> Normally the blood is sterile. Infection in any of the organs or tissues can result in entry of bacteria into the circulation. Blood cultures are routinely collected as part of the diagnostic evaluation of patients who present with signs and symptoms of sepsis or disseminated infection.

Diagnosis

Blood cultures are routinely collected as part of the diagnostic evaluation of patients who present with signs and symptoms of sepsis or disseminated infection. To maximize sensitivity and specificity, it is recommended that 2 to 3 sets of blood cultures be collected per septic episode.

To identify intermittent bacteremias, the timing of the blood collection is important to maximize the likelihood of finding organisms while they are in the blood (see the section on sample collection in microbiology in Chapter 2). Ideally, blood from patients with intermittent bacteremias is collected during the hour before a temperature spike, but this is not practical because the febrile episodes are often not predictable. It is common practice for blood to be collected at 30- to 60-minute intervals (if possible) when a febrile patient is suspected of having an intermittent bacteremia. As one might expect, one is much more likely to detect a continuous bacteremia in the first blood culture than to detect an intermittent bacteremia.

TABLE 5-3   Normal Body Flora[a]

Mouth	Vagina	Sputum
More common	*More common*	Often contaminated from upper respiratory tract, most commonly *Staphylococcus aureus*, *Staphylococcus epidermidis*, *Haemophilus* spp., *Corynebacterium*, *Streptococcus viridans*, Enterobacteriaceae, *Candida* spp., *Neisseria* spp.
Anaerobic streptococci	*Bacteroides*	
Aerobic streptococci (not group A)	*Veillonella*	
Staphylococcus epidermidis	Anaerobic streptococci	
Lactobacillus	Aerobic streptococci (groups B and D)	
Streptococcus pneumoniae	*Lactobacillus*	
Moraxella catarrhalis	*Staphylococcus epidermidis*	**Jejunum**
Bacteroides	*Staphylococcus aureus*	
Veillonella	*Corynebacterium*	*Lactobacillus*
Nonpathogenic *Neisseria*	*Gardnerella vaginalis*	*Enterococcus*
Candida	*Candida*	
Less common	*Less common*	**Terminal Ileum and Colon (95% are Anaerobes)**
Streptococcus pyogenes (group A)	*Listeria monocytogenes*	
Neisseria meningitides	*Ureaplasma*	
Staphylococcus aureus	*Neisseria*	*More common*
Haemophilus influenzae	*Clostridium perfringens*	*Peptococcus*
Enterobacteriaceae	*Actinomyces*	*Peptostreptococcus*
Actinomyces		*Clostridium*
Throat (Nasopharynx and Oropharynx)	**Skin**	*Bacteroides*
		Fusobacterium
		Enterobacteriaceae
More common	*More common*	*Lactobacillus*
Streptococcus	*Staphylococcus epidermidis* and other coagulase-negative *staphylococci*	*Enterococcus* spp.
Nonpathogenic *Neisseria*	*Staphylococcus aureus*	*Less common*
Staphylococcus aureus	*Corynebacterium*	*Pseudomonas*
Corynebacterium	*Malassezia*	*Staphylococcus aureus*
Haemophilus influenzae	*Less common*	*Staphylococcus epidermidis*
Less common	*Streptococcus* (group A)	*Actinomyces*
Streptococcus pyogenes (group A)	*Bacillus*	Nontuberculous mycobacteria
Neisseria meningitidis	*Peptostreptococcus*	*Treponema*
Enterobacteriaceae	Nontuberculous mycobacteria	*Candida*
Bacteroides	*Candida*	*Clostridium difficile*
Candida		*Bacillus subtilis*
Nose	**Eye**	**Sterile Areas (Selected)**
More common	*More common*	Bronchi
Corynebacterium	*Staphylococcus epidermidis*	Blood
Staphylococcus epidermidis	*Haemophilus*	Cerebrospinal fluid
Aerobic *Streptococcus* (nongroup A)	*Corynebacterium*	Joint fluid
Streptococcus aureus	*Uncommon*	Pleural fluid
Haemophilus spp.	*Streptococcus pyogenes*	Pericardial fluid
Less common	*Moraxella*	Peritoneal fluid
Streptococcus pneumoniae	*Neisseria*	
Haemophilus influenzae	*Streptococcus pneumoniae*	
Neisseria meningitidis	Enterobacteriaceae	
Streptococcus pyogenes		

[a]Listed by genus only if species is not specified (e.g., *Bacteroides*) or by genus and species (e.g., *Haemophilus influenzae*) if specific organism is known. Modified from: Ravel R. *Clinical Laboratory Medicine*, 6th ed. St. Louis, MO: Mosby-Year Book; 1995:666–667.

A major problem in the interpretation of the blood culture results is incidental contamination of the specimen with the normal bacterial flora from the skin.

A major problem in the interpretation of the blood culture results is incidental contamination of the specimen with the normal bacterial flora from the skin (**Table 5–3**). The clinical significance of a positive blood culture is dependent on both the number of positive specimens and the type of organism. The isolation of recognized pathogens such as *Staphylococcus aureus*, *Streptococcus pneumoniae*, beta-hemolytic streptococci (*Streptococcus pyogenes* and *Streptococcus agalactiae*), enterococci, gram-negative rods (aerobic and anaerobic), or yeast from 1 or more blood cultures is almost always clinically significant. In contrast, if only 1 of the multiple blood culture specimens is positive for an organism found on the skin (e.g., coagulase-negative staphylococci or *Corynebacterium* spp.), the result is likely to reflect contamination during specimen collection rather than true septicemia. This frequently encountered problem is 1 reason why at least 2 blood samples should be collected for blood cultures. Although skin-derived bacteria are often thought of as nonpathogenic, it is important to remember that they can cause clinically significant infections, particularly in immunosuppressed patients and in patients with intravascular catheters or

TABLE 5–4   Evaluation for Rickettsial Diseases and Selected Disorders Caused by Related Organisms

Disease	Etiologic Agent	Mechanism of Transmission to Humans	Clinical Features	Laboratory Tests
Rocky Mountain spotted fever	*Rickettsia rickettsii*	Tick vector	Higher rate seasonally and in specific geographic areas; rash from a vasculitis, fever, and headache	Serology: increase in antibody titer after exposure; immunohistochemical tests give rapid result but sensitivity is low at about 70%
Boutonneuse fever	*Rickettsia conorii*	Tick vector	Seasonal: distribution in Europe, Asia, and Africa; rash, fever, headache, and black spot at the site of tick attachment	Same as for Rocky Mountain spotted fever
Rickettsial pox	*Rickettsia akari*	Bite of mouse mite	Similar to but milder than Rocky Mountain spotted fever and Boutonneuse fever; rare in United States	Serology: increase in antibody titer after exposure
Murine typhus	*Rickettsia typhi*	Flea feces inoculated into flea bite wound on human	Seasonal and geographic; rash, fever, and headache	Serology: increase in antibody titer after exposure
Epidemic typhus	*Rickettsia prowazekii*	Infected louse feces inoculated into human skin wounds	In areas of poor sanitation; clinically similar to Rocky Mountain spotted fever	Serology: increase in antibody titer after exposure
Scrub tuphus	*Orientia tsutsugamushi*	Bite of a larval mite	Rash, fever, and headache	Serology: increase in antibody titer after exposure
Q fever	*Coxiella burnetii*	Inhalation of infected aerosols, ingestion of contaminated dairy products, or, rarely, by tick vector	Acutely, it is usually an asymptomatic or self-limited febrile pneumonia; can become chronic with damage to heart valves and bone	Serology: increase in antibody titer after exposure
Erhlichiosis	*Ehrlichia chaffeensis*	Tick vector	From asymptomatic to a severe Rocky Mountain spotted fever-like illness	Serology: increase in antibody titer after exposure; PCR
Anaplasmosis	*Anaplasma phagocytophilium*	Tick vector	Fever, headache, myalgia	Serology, PCR

prosthetic devices. The isolation of the same skin flora organism in 2 separately collected specimens increases the probability that it represents a clinically significant bacteremia.

To avoid the problem of contamination of the blood culture bottles with skin organisms, meticulous preparation of the skin with a bactericidal agent is necessary. The number of blood cultures required for detection of a pathogenic organism is determined by the volume of blood collected per bottle, the timing of the blood collection, the type of organism producing the infection, and previous antibiotic exposure. Three or more blood culture collections may be required to document the presence of certain organisms.

To avoid the problem of contamination of the blood culture bottles with skin organisms, meticulous preparation of the skin with a bactericidal agent is necessary.

Infections Caused by *Rickettsia*, *Ehrlichia*, and Related Organisms
Description

Rickettsia, *Ehrlichia*, and *Anaplasma* are obligate intracellular bacteria that cannot be detected in routine bacterial cultures. These organisms are transmitted to humans by ticks; therefore, the risk of acquiring these infections depends on geography and the time of year (see **Table 5–4**).

Rickettsia rickettsii, the agent of Rocky Mountain spotted fever (RMSF), is transmitted by dog ticks and infects endothelial cells. The resulting vascular injury elicits a widespread vasculitis, consisting of vasodilation with perivascular edema, and at times complicated by thrombosis and hemorrhage. Erythrocytes extravasating into the dermis form nonblanching petechial or purpuric lesions. The characteristic rash is often absent during the early stages of infection, and the infection can progress to a life-threatening encephalitis if not promptly treated.

Ehrlichia chafeensis and other species are transmitted by the lone star tick and dog tick and infect monocytes. Patients present with nonspecific findings including fever, leukopenia, thrombocytopenia, and/or elevations of hepatic enzymes. Similar clinical manifestations are seen with *Anaplasma* (*formerly Ehrlichia*) *phagocytophilum* that is transmitted by deer ticks and infects granulocytes.

Diagnosis

None of these agents can be cultured on artificial media. RMSF is usually diagnosed retrospectively with serologic tests; however, this should not delay treatment that should be initiated based on clinical findings and potential history of exposure. If the rash is present, organisms can be demonstrated by immunohistochemical staining of a skin biopsy in 70% of cases. Examination of peripheral blood smears in patients with *Anaplasma* can reveal the presence of organisms within inclusions in neutrophils but many cases are negative. *Ehrlichia* is rarely observed in monocytes. Polymerase chain reaction (PCR) of blood and/or serologic tests are the best methods for diagnosing *Anaplasma* and *Ehrlichia* infections.

Fungemia
Description

Yeast belonging to the genus *Candida* are a major cause of hospital-acquired bloodstream infections. These organisms are frequently part of the oral and gastrointestinal flora. Treatment with broad-spectrum antibiotics that disrupt the normal bacterial flora, the presence of intravenous catheters, and neutropenia all predispose to the development of candidemia.

Cryptococcus neoformans and *Histoplasma capsulatum* are important causes of fungemia in patients with markedly depressed cell-mediated immunity (*Cryptococcus* is further discussed in the section "Chronic Meningitis" and *Histoplasma* is further discussed in the section "Infections of the Lung and Pleurae"). Although molds such as *Aspergillus* spp. can cause disseminated infections in immunosuppressed patients, they are rarely detected in the bloodstream.

Diagnosis

Candidemia can usually be detected with routine blood cultures. Specialized techniques (e.g., lysis–centrifugation cultures) are required to detect *H. capsulatum* and may enhance the detection of *C. neoformans*. Immunoassays that detect antigens produced by *H. capsulatum* and *C. neoformans* are also used to diagnose disseminated infections caused by these organisms.

Parasitic Infections of the Blood
Overview

Several vector-borne parasites can infect the blood. These include protozoans such as *Plasmodium* spp. (malaria), *Babesia* spp., and *Trypanosoma* spp., and nematodes such as the agents of lymphatic filariasis. *Plasmodium* infections are an important cause of nonspecific febrile illnesses in returning travelers, and *Babesia* infections are endemic in the United States; these infections are discussed below. Other blood parasites are uncommon in the United States.

Malaria
Description

> Malaria is one of the largest causes of mortality and morbidity in the world. Individuals who travel to areas where malaria is endemic and develop fever within weeks of return should be suspected of suffering from malaria.

Malaria is one of the largest causes of mortality and morbidity in the world. Individuals who travel to areas where malaria is endemic and develop fever within weeks of return should be suspected of suffering from malaria.

There are 4 species of *Plasmodium* that produce malaria in humans. These parasites are transmitted by *Anopheles* mosquitoes that are widely distributed throughout Africa, Asia, and Latin America. The most dangerous of the 4 species is *Plasmodium falciparum*. This organism can achieve very high levels of parasitemia and adheres to capillary endothelium that can lead

TABLE 5–5   Laboratory Evaluation for Malaria

Laboratory Test	Results/Comments
Identification of organisms within RBC in blood smears	The first line test in the diagnosis of malaria; for best results, blood should be collected from the patient during or after a febrile episode and before the administration of anti-parasitic medications; to rule out malaria, it is recommended that negative results be demonstrated in blood samples collected every 6–8 hours for 24 hours
	Preparation of smears: thick and thin blood smears should be prepared; thick smears allow for a rapid examination of a relatively large volume of blood and have approximately a 10-fold increase in sensitivity over thin smears; thin smears allow for superior preservation of morphology and are needed for species determination; the best stain is the aqueous Giemsa stain buffered with phosphate to pH 7.2
	Reading of smears: no single criterion except for the crescentiform (banana-shaped) gametocyte of *Plasmodium falciparum* is pathognomonic; multiple morphologic criteria are used to make the diagnosis of malaria and determine speciation of the *Plasmodium*; it is very difficult to speciate when mixed *Plasmodium* infections occur
Quantitation of parasitemia	Reported as percent of RBC parasitized or as number of parasites per 100 WBC; quantitation should be repeated after treatment to monitor effectiveness

to severe organ damage. *P. falciparum* infection may be fatal within days. *P. vivax* and *P. ovale* are morphologically similar and generally cause less severe infection but unlike *P. falciparum*, they can establish persistent infection and cause relapses several months after the initial infection. *P. malariae* is the least virulent species and can cause low-level infection that may cause few symptoms, but it can persist for years.

Diagnosis

Currently, the diagnosis of malaria and the identification of each of the 4 species of *Plasmodium* responsible for malaria is based on the microscopic examination of stained erythrocytes in thick and thin blood films. These organisms have maturation cycles involving a variety of specific structures in the RBC, including ring trophozoites, growing trophozoites, mature schizonts, and gametocytes. The stippling of the RBCs with different dot patterns is also important in differentiating between the 4 species. Thus, the size and shape of the various malarial forms, their alteration of RBC morphology, and the stippling pattern in the RBCs provide the identification of the particular type of malaria. Quantitation of the level of parasitemia is also important. Marked parasitemia is a poor prognostic sign for *P. falciparum* infection. However, ill patients may have relatively low levels of parasitemia due to trapping of organisms in capillaries. PCR is starting to be used for the diagnosis of malaria and is particularly useful when low levels of parasitemia make it difficult to identify individual species. **Table 5–5** summarizes the relevant laboratory information for the diagnosis of malaria.

Babesiosis
Description

Babesia are protozoa that, like *Plasmodium* species, infect erythrocytes. They are delivered to the infected host by the same tick (*Ixodes*) that transmits the agent of Lyme disease. Babesiosis mimics malaria in that it causes hemolysis, fever, anorexia, and hemoglobinuria. In the United States, *B. microti* is responsible for most cases of human babesiosis. In Europe, *B. bovis* and *B. bigemina* have been implicated as agents of human disease. Babesiosis occurs mainly in the Northeast and upper Midwest in the United States. It affects patients of all ages, but most cases occur during the sixth and seventh decades of life. The infection from *Babesia* tends to be self-limited. In most cases, it lasts from weeks to months, following an incubation period of 1 to 6 weeks. Mild symptoms, including malaise, fever, and headache, characterize the disease in normal hosts, but asplenic patients often develop severe infections with high levels of parasitemia.

Diagnosis

The laboratory diagnosis rests upon the identification of the *Babesia* organisms inside erythrocytes in stained thick and thin peripheral blood smears. There are a number of morphological features that differentiate *Babesia* from *Plasmodium*. Despite its relative shortcomings, serologic

Babesia are protozoa that, like *Plasmodium* species, infect erythrocytes. They are delivered to the infected host by the same tick (*Ixodes*) that transmits the agent of Lyme disease.

TABLE 5–6   **Laboratory Evaluation for *Babesia***

Laboratory Test	Results/Comments
Identification of organism in RBC on blood film	Differentiating features in infected RBC suggesting *Babesia* rather than *Plasmodium* include 1) a tetrad of structures that resembles a "Maltese cross" and 2) the absence of pigment granules
Indirect immunofluorescent testing for antibodies to *B. microti*	A titer of >1:64 is considered indicative of exposure to the organisms, and a titer of >1:256 is diagnostic for an acute *Babesia* infection; at titers <1:256, the result does not clearly differentiate between patients who were exposed in the past and those who are actively infected

testing for *B. microti* can be performed as noted in **Table 5–6**. The level of parasitemia with *Babesia* does not always correlate with the severity of symptoms.

Viral Infections of the Blood
Overview
Many viruses such as varicella zoster virus (VZV), measles, Enteroviruses, and Arboviruses (such as West Nile virus) exhibit a viremic phase. These viruses also exhibit organ-specific manifestations and are discussed in other sections of this chapter. Cytomegalovirus (CMV), Epstein–Barr virus (EBV), and parvovirus B19 are discussed below because they are common viruses that can have a direct effect on the blood.

Infectious Mononucleosis/Epstein–Barr Virus
Description
Most cases of mononucleosis are caused by EBV, a member of the herpesvirus family that infects B lymphocytes and causes them to proliferate. This in turn stimulates the proliferation of cytotoxic T cells that control the active infection but do not eradicate the latent state. Infection with EBV is extremely common, and most individuals have asymptomatic infections. Patients with infectious mononucleosis typically present with fever, sore throat, and enlarged cervical lymph nodes.

In addition to mononucleosis, EBV is associated with 2 types of human tumor (Burkitt's lymphoma and nasopharyngeal carcinoma) and is responsible for lymphoproliferative disorders in patients with severe immunosuppression following organ transplantation or AIDS. It also causes oral hairy leukoplakia in HIV-infected patients.

Diagnosis
Large atypical lymphocytes (cytotoxic T cells) are usually present in peripheral blood smears of patients with infectious mononucleosis, but they are also found in many other disease states as well. The diagnosis of EBV-associated infectious mononucleosis is usually confirmed by a positive serum heterophile antibody test that detects the presence of antibodies that agglutinate horse or cow erythrocytes. The heterophile test is often negative in young children or in patients with atypical presentations; EBV-specific serologic tests are especially important in establishing the diagnosis in these situations.

The use of laboratory tests in the diagnosis of infectious mononucleosis is shown in **Table 5–7**.

Cytomegalovirus
Description
CMV infections produce significant morbidity and mortality in immunocompromised patients. CMV infects leukocytes, where it remains latent in immunocompetent individuals but readily reactivates in immunosuppressed individuals. CMV is a leading cause of opportunistic infections in transplant recipients and AIDS patients. In transplant recipients, it often presents as a nonspecific febrile illness but it can also cause more invasive infections including esophagitis,

The diagnosis of EBV-associated infectious mononucleosis is usually confirmed by a positive serum heterophile antibody test that detects the presence of antibodies that agglutinate horse or cow erythrocytes.

TABLE 5-7   Evaluation for Infectious Mononucleosis

Laboratory Tests	Comments
Heterophile antibody tests	Heterophile antibodies are IgM antibodies reactive with antigens on the cells from multiple species, and on this basis are termed heterophilic; they are detected in agglutination assays with horse or sheep RBCs or by their capacity to induce an agglutination response on antigen-coated latex particles; in infectious mononucleosis, the heterophile antibody test result is positive approximately 1 week after the symptoms first appear; the highest titers appear in the second to third week of the illness; relatively high titers persist for up to 8 weeks
Antibodies to EBV-specific antigens	Although heterophile-negative infectious mononucleosis is uncommon, it does occur, mostly in young children; in these cases, a characteristic clinical picture and a rising titer of antibody to selected EBV antigens establishes the diagnosis of heterophile negative infectious mononucleosis
WBC differential	Patients with mononucleosis typically have a mild to moderate leukocytosis after the first week, with more than 60% of the WBCs as lymphocytes and 10%–20% of all lymphocytes being atypical; the maximum percentage of atypical lymphocytes appears between days 5 and 10 after the onset of symptoms, with a decrease to normal by approximately 3 weeks in most patients

EBV, Epstein–Barr virus.

hepatitis, colitis, pneumonitis, and retinitis, particularly in severely immunocompromised patients. CMV is also the most common congenital viral infection. It affects approximately 40,000 infants born each year in the United States. Hematogenous spread appears to be responsible for transmission of the virus to the fetus. Most congenital infections occur when the mother has a primary CMV infection during the pregnancy. Neonates can also acquire the infection from maternal breast milk. Approximately 10% of infants congenitally infected with CMV are symptomatic at birth. Common sites of involvement are liver, spleen, lungs, and central nervous system (CNS). Because specific antiviral therapy is available for treatment of these infants, rapid detection of CMV infection is necessary. Although most congenitally infected infants are asymptomatic at birth, approximately 10–15% of these will develop later problems such as hearing loss and other neurologic problems. In children and young adults, primary CMV infection can cause a mononucleosis-like illness.

> CMV is the most common congenital viral infection. It affects approximately 40,000 infants born each year in the United States.

Diagnosis

The detection of CMV in blood and tissues generally correlates with active disease, but detection of CMV in urine is often not diagnostic of active CMV disease, even in immunocompromised patients. Quantitative PCR assays of CMV DNA in blood correlate with the likelihood of severe infection. Congenital CMV infection is established when CMV is isolated from the urine of neonates less than 3 weeks of age. CMV isolation from respiratory secretions of bone marrow transplant recipients is likely to be clinically significant because interstitial pneumonia is a complication of bone marrow transplantation. In AIDS patients, asymptomatic shedding of CMV in respiratory secretions does not correlate with active infection. CMV serology is used to determine whether donors and/or recipients are latently infected with CMV. This has important implications for preventing subsequent infections. Diagnostic testing for CMV is summarized in **Table 5–8**.

Parvovirus B19

Description

Parvovirus B19 is a small single-stranded DNA virus that is transmitted by respiratory droplets. It is a common cause of infection in children in whom it causes a distinctive rash known as fifth disease. In adults, it often causes a significant arthropathy. An unusual feature of this virus is that it replicates in erythroid precursor cells and causes a temporary cessation of RBC production until the virus is cleared by the immune system. In normal hosts this has little, if any, consequence, but in patients who have a chronic hemolytic anemia such as sickle cell disease

TABLE 5–8   Laboratory Testing for Cytomegalovirus (CMV)

Laboratory Test	Result/Comment
Conventional cell culture	Detection of CMV infection typically requires 7–28 days with conventional viral inoculation of cell cultures; CMV can be isolated from a variety of specimens including blood, bronchoalveolar lavage fluid, urine, and tissue
Shell vial assay	This is a modification of the conventional cell culture methodology for more rapid viral detection; viruses are detected earlier using this technique than conventional cell culture because the specimen is inoculated onto the monolayer of cultured cells by low-speed centrifugation; this enhances the infectivity of the cultured cells; this assay can often provide a positive result in 1–2 days
CMV antigen testing	A test is available for the identification of CMV antigen in polymorphonuclear leukocytes using a monoclonal antibody directed at a specific CMV protein; the assay is semiquantitative and permits monitoring response to therapy
Enzyme immunoassay(EIA)	This test is used to detect antibodies to CMV; seroconversion from negative to positive or a significant rise in anti-CMV IgG titer provides evidence of infection; assays for anti-CMV IgM are available, but detection of anti-CMV IgM does not always indicate primary infection because the IgM can persist for up to 18 months; most adults are seropositive and therefore serologic tests have limited utility for diagnosis
Polymerase chain reaction (PCR)-based detection of CMV	DNA- and RNA-based detection is available for the detection of CMV in peripheral blood leukocytes and tissues; quantitative assays are important for diagnosis of active infection in immunosuppressed patients

or hereditary spherocytosis, the parvovirus B19 infection causes a transient aplastic crisis in which there is a profound drop in the hematocrit. Parvovirus B19 can cause a chronic anemia in immunocompromised patients who are unable to clear the virus. Intrauterine infection of the fetus can also cause a severe anemia that leads to congestive failure and hydrops fetalis.

Diagnosis

Acute parvovirus infection can be confirmed by demonstration of IgM antibodies or detection of viral DNA by PCR. During a transient aplastic crisis, the reticulocyte count decreases to <0.1% even as the hematocrit is declining.

ENDOCARDITIS: INFECTION OF THE HEART

Description

The clinical features of infectious endocarditis, a microbial infection of the valvular or nonvalvular endothelium of the heart, depend on the type of organism, location, and type of valve. Acute infective endocarditis can present with temperatures ≥103°F, shaking chills, rapid worsening of valve function, and a variety of septic embolic complications. Subacute bacterial endocarditis is characterized by a low-grade or absent fever (as a result of infection by low virulence organisms), and a variety of nonspecific signs and symptoms such as anorexia, weight loss, and malaise. Acute bacterial endocarditis typically occurs on native heart valves. It is most often caused by virulent organisms such as *S. aureus*, beta-hemolytic streptococci, and less commonly by *S. lugdunensis*, enterococci, and *S. pneumoniae*. Subacute bacterial endocarditis is usually caused by viridans group streptococci, enterococci, and fastidious gram-negative rods from the oral cavity. Several difficult-to-grow organisms are associated with "culture-negative" endocarditis. Prosthetic valve endocarditis is often caused by coagulase-negative staphylococci but can also be caused by *S. aureus*, other skin flora, enteric gram-negative rods, and fungi.

There are a number of risk factors for endocarditis, particularly in the acute form. These include diabetes, alcoholism, intravenous drug use, malignancy, infections in other sites, and

The clinical features of infectious endocarditis, a microbial infection of the valvular or nonvalvular endothelium of the heart, depend on the type of organism, location, and type of valve.

TABLE 5–9 Evaluation of the Patient with Infective Endocarditis

Differentiating Clinical Features	Acute Infective Endocarditis	Subacute Infective Endocarditis
Temperature	>102°F	<102°F
Osler nodes	No	Yes
Janeway lesions	Yes	No
Roth spots (in eye exam)	No	Yes
Laboratory tests		
Organisms most often detected in blood culture	Highly virulent pathogens such as *Staphylococcus aureus, Streptococcus pneumoniae, Pseudomonas aeruginosa*, often from a recognizable focus of infection	Organisms of lower virulence such as viridans streptococci, enterococci, and *Streptococcus bovis*; many other organisms can cause infective endocarditis, but are difficult to identify because they may require selective media or long periods for growth
Urinalysis and urine culture	The presence of hematuria and a pathogenic organism in a urine culture, in the appropriate clinical context, is consistent with acute infective endocarditic	Urinalysis reveals hematuria, pyuria, RBC casts, bacteriuria, and proteinuria
Complete blood count findings		
Erythrocyte sedimentation rate	<50 mm/hour	>50 mm/hour
Anemia (normochromic, normocytic)	No	Yes
Markedly elevated WBC count	Yes	No
Transesophageal echocardiography	>90% sensitivity in detecting vegetations on cardiac valves; it is also capable of identifying valvular perforation, regurgitation, and abscess formation in many patients	>90% sensitivity in detecting vegetations on cardiac valves

immunosuppression. Anatomic defects also predispose patients to the development of infectious endocarditis. Such defects include mitral valve prolapse, congenital or rheumatic heart disease, and calcific aortic stenosis. The worst prognosis among patients with valvular disease is associated with those who have aortic valve involvement. The mitral valve, however, is the most frequently involved. Most individuals with endocarditis are between 45 and 60 years of age.

Diagnosis

The clinical and laboratory features of acute and subacute bacterial endocarditis are different (**Table 5–9**). It should be noted, however, that patients can present with a syndrome of intermediate severity between acute and subacute endocarditis, usually as a result of infection by organisms of intermediate virulence, such as *Enterococcus* species, *Haemophilus* species, and *Streptococcus bovis*. Laboratory confirmation of infective endocarditis usually involves isolation of the same organism from multiple blood cultures. Organisms are more likely to be isolated from blood cultures in patients who have acute bacterial endocarditis because they have a high-grade persistent bacteremia. If 3 sets of blood cultures are obtained, the blood cultures are positive in more than 99% of patients who have not received antibiotics. At least 2 sets of blood cultures should be obtained by separate venipunctures at presentation. The erythrocyte sedimentation rate is a nonspecific test that is almost always elevated in cases of endocarditis, but it is useful for monitoring the response to therapy. It is not uncommon to obtain negative blood cultures in patients who meet the clinical and echocardiographic criteria for infectious endocarditis. Many of these "culture-negative" cases are due to prior antibiotic therapy. Others are caused by fastidious organisms. In the past, the "HACEK" group of oral gram-negative rods was linked to culture-negative endocarditis, but these organisms are readily detected by modern blood culture systems. More recently, interest has focused on *Coxiella burnetii*, *Bartonella* spp., *Tropheryma whipplei*, and *Brucella* spp. as potential causes of "culture-negative" endocarditis. These agents can be detected by a combination of serologic and molecular methods.

Laboratory confirmation of infective endocarditis usually involves isolation of the same organism from multiple blood cultures. Organisms are more likely to be isolated from blood cultures in patients who have acute bacterial endocarditis because they have a high-grade persistent bacteremia.

INFECTIONS OF THE CENTRAL NERVOUS SYSTEM

Overview

Many organisms can produce an infection within the CNS. The major sites of infection are the meninges and brain parenchyma. Most organisms gain access to the CNS by hematogenous spread or by direct extension from an adjacent site. Bacterial infections can cause acute meningitis or may lead to formation of a brain abscess. Viral infections can present as meningitis or encephalitis, but often both sites are involved and the infection is more appropriately described as meningoencephalitis. Both fungi and mycobacteria can cause chronic meningitis while several parasites can cause intracerebral mass lesions. Each of these syndromes is often associated with specific organisms, information that can be used to guide the diagnostic workup. Rational test ordering based on clinical presentation is particularly important in patients with CNS infections since diagnostic specimens are difficult to obtain and are often present in limited quantities. **Table 5–10** provides information on organisms that are frequently described causes of meningitis and/or encephalitis.

Acute Bacterial Meningitis

Description

Bacterial meningitis may present as a progressive illness over several days, or as a fulminant process that develops within hours. There is no single clinical sign that is pathognomonic of meningitis. Adolescents and adults typically present with combinations of fever, headache, nuchal rigidity, and other meningeal signs, and a decreased level of consciousness that can range from lethargy to coma; however, these findings are not present in all patients. Neonates and infants often present with nonspecific signs such as irritability, while nausea and vomiting are frequent complaints in children. Confusion, often without fever, is a common presenting sign in the elderly.

In most cases, the bacteria responsible for meningitis are acquired through the upper respiratory tract and then invade the blood. From the blood, they can then seed the meninges. There are a variety of factors that increase the risk for development of meningitis. These include splenectomy, sickle cell disease, cerebrospinal fluid leak, fistula or shunt, recent neurosurgical procedure, and infection contiguous to the CNS.

The organisms responsible for acute bacterial meningitis are highly dependent on the age of the patient and the clinical setting. *S. agalactiae* (group B strep [GBS]), *E. coli*, or *Listeria monocytogenes* are responsible for most cases of neonatal and infant meningitis. *S. pneumoniae* and *N. meningitidis* are responsible for most cases of community-acquired bacterial meningitis in children and adults (widespread vaccination for *Haemophilus influenzae* type b has nearly eliminated this previous childhood scourge). Elderly patients are at increased risk of infection with *L. monocytogenes* and aerobic gram-negative rods. In contrast, staphylococci and gram-negative rods are major causes of CNS shunt infections and postneurosurgery nosocomial infections. Knowledge of these patterns is important when deciding on empiric antibiotic therapy.

Diagnosis

Examination and culture of CSF is essential. There is usually a markedly elevated WBC count with a preponderance of neutrophils, elevated protein, and decreased glucose (relative to the blood level). Gram stain of CSF reveals the causative organism in 70% to 90% of cases of pneumococcal and meningococcal meningitis. The percentage is generally lower for other bacteria. Bacterial culture is essential in all cases because it has the greatest sensitivity and specificity. Patients who have rapidly progressive or severe disease frequently receive a dose of antibiotics before a CSF specimen can be collected. Although this may cause a false-negative culture, it should have little or no effect on the cell count and differential, protein, glucose, and Gram stain. Immunoassays that detect *S. pneumoniae* and *N. meningitidis* capsular antigens in CSF are useful in these patients with partially treated meningitis, but they are *not* more sensitive than a Gram stain.

Many organisms can produce an infection within the CNS. The major sites of infection are the meninges and brain parenchyma. Most organisms gain access to the CNS by hematogenous spread or by direct extension from an adjacent site.

TABLE 5–10   Laboratory Evaluation for Meningitis and Encephalitis

Disease/Organism	Age of Highest Incidence	Higher Incidence in	Culture Available?	Smear used in Diagnosis of CSF	Other Tests of Potential Use
Bacterial Meningitis					
Group B *streptococcus* (*Streptococcus agalactiae*)	<1 month	Neonates	Yes	Gram stain	Rapid antigen detection, mainly useful for partially treated infection
Streptococcus pneumoniae	All ages >3 months	Immunocompromised	Yes	Gram stain	Rapid antigen detection, mainly useful for partially treated infection
Escherichia coli and other gram-negative bacteria (75% of *E. coli* cases are K1 strains)	<1 month and >60 years	Immunocompromised	Yes	Gram stain	Rapid antigen detection for *E. coli* K1, mainly useful for partially treated infection
Listeria monocytogenes	<1 month and >60 years	Immunocompromised	Yes	Gram stain	
Haemophilus influenzae type b	1 month to 5 years	Immunocompromised; unvaccinated	Yes	Gram stain	Rapid antigen detection, mainly useful for partially treated infection
Neisseria meningiditis	1 month	Patients with complement deficiencies	Yes	Gram stain	Rapid antigen detection, mainly useful for partially treated infection
Mycobacteria, especially *M. tuberculosis*	≥1 month	Immunocompromised	Yes	Acid-fast stain (rarely positive)	Nucleic acid amplification
Treponema pallidum	Adults	Tertiary syphilis patients	No	None	Several tests for syphilis available (see the section "Syphilis")
Pseudomonas aeruginosa	All ages	Neurosurgical postoperative patients	Yes	Gram stain	
Staphylococcus aureus	All ages	Neurosurgical postoperative patients	Yes	Gram stain	
Coagulase-negative staphylococci	All ages	Neurosurgical postoperative patients	Yes	Gram stain	
Other streptococci	All ages	Neurosurgical postoperative patients	Yes	Gram stain	
Fungal Meningitis					
Cryptococcus neoformans	Adults	Immunocompromised	Yes	India ink	Rapid antigen detection, much more sensitive than India ink
Coccidioides immitis	Adults	Immunocompromised; those living in the southwestern United States, parts of Latin America	Yes	Calcofluor smear	Serologic testing of serum and CSF
Histoplasma capsulatum	Adults	Immunocompromised; those living in the Ohio, Mississippi, and St. Lawrence river valleys, and the Great Lakes region	Yes	Calcofluor smear	Serum test for antibody to organism; tissue biopsy; urine, serum, or CSF antigen test

Continued next page—

TABLE 5–10 **Laboratory Evaluation for Meningitis and Encephalitis (continued)**

Disease/Organism	Age of Highest Incidence	Higher Incidence in	Culture Available?	Smear used in Diagnosis of CSF	Other Tests of Potential Use
Viral Meningitis/Encephalitis/Meningoencephalitis					
Enteroviruses (includes Echovirus and Coxsackie virus)	All ages including infants	Late summer and early fall	Yes—viral culture using throat swab, CSF, and stool	None	PCR of CSF specimen is the preferred diagnostic test
Herpes simplex virus-1	All ages including infants	Those in direct contact with infected body fluids	Culture of CSF in neonates only or culture of brain biopsy	None	PCR of CSF specimen is the preferred diagnostic test; serologic testing; histochemical staining of brain biopsy
Herpes simplex virus-2	Neonates	Those in direct contact with infected body fluids	Culture of CSF in neonates only or culture and histochemical staining of brain biopsy	None	PCR of CSF specimen is the preferred diagnostic test; serum test for antibody to virus
Cytomegalovirus	All ages	Immunocompromised	Shell vial culture of CSF or tissue	None	Serum test for antibody to virus; antigen detection in circulating WBCs; PCR of CSF
Arboviruses	Peak age group varies for the different viruses in this group	Depending on the virus in the group, specific geographic regions and seasons for higher infection rates because transmission is by insects, usually mosquitoes or ticks	Rarely useful	None	Serum and/or CSF tested for antibody to selected viruses (e.g., West Nile)
Rabies virus	All ages	Individuals bitten or scratched by rabies-prone animal	Rarely useful	None	Immunofluorescence of brain biopsy specimen; testing of serum for antibodies to virus
Measles virus	Childhood	Nonvaccinated individuals recently exposed to measles infection	Rarely useful	None	Testing of serum for antibodies to virus
Mumps virus	Childhood	Nonvaccinated individuals recently exposed to mumps infection	Yes—viral culture of throat swab, CSF, and urine	None	Testing of serum for antibodies to virus
HIV	Adults	Patients with AIDS or unexplained opportunistic infections	Rarely useful	None	Assays for diagnosis and monitoring of HIV
Varicella zoster virus	All ages	Immunocompromised; exposure to recent varicella zoster infection	Yes—viral culture	None	Testing of serum for antibodies to virus; PCR of CSF specimen
Epstein–Barr virus	Children, adolescents, and young adults	Recent exposure to individual with infectious mononucleosis	Rarely useful	None	Serologic testing of serum; PCR of CSF specimen

CSF, cerebrospinal fluid; KOH, potassium hydroxide; PCR, polymerase chain reaction.

Acute Viral Meningitis

Description

Viral meningitis (often described as aseptic meningitis due to the absence of bacteria) presents with fever, headache, and meningeal signs. There may be a mildly decreased level of consciousness. At least 75% of these infections are caused by members of the Enterovirus family that includes the Coxsackie and Echo viruses. Arboviruses (arthropod-borne viruses), HSV-2, HIV, and many other viruses can also cause this syndrome. Both Enterovirus and Arbovirus infections exhibit seasonal variation; most cases occur in the summer and early fall. Viral meningitis is usually a self-limited illness with a generally good prognosis. This is fortunate since there are currently no clinically useful antiviral drugs that are active against the Enteroviruses and Arboviruses. The clinical diagnosis of viral meningitis is often not clear-cut because there can be parenchymal involvement leading to varying degrees of encephalitis (see below). In addition, several other conditions can cause a similar clinical syndrome. These include partially treated bacterial meningitis, neoplastic diseases that have spread to the meninges, and immune-mediated diseases. It is important to identify these conditions because each of them is treatable and requires specific therapy.

Acute bacterial meningitis must be differentiated from viral and fungal meningitis. There is a significant difference in the CSF findings between viral and bacterial meningitis (**Table 5–11**).

> Viral meningitis (often described as aseptic meningitis due to the absence of bacteria) presents with fever, headache, and meningeal signs. At least 75% of these infections are caused by members of the Enterovirus family that includes the Coxsackie and Echo viruses.

Diagnosis

CSF analysis usually reveals an elevated WBC count with a preponderance of mononuclear cells, elevated protein, and a normal glucose. Identification of the causative agent is best achieved through the use of specific nucleic acid amplification tests or immunoassays; routine viral culture has a relatively poor yield in most cases. Many clinical or reference laboratories offer RT-PCR assays for Enteroviruses, HSV, and West Nile virus. Immunoassays for detection of IgM and IgG are used to detect other viruses. Bacterial culture and cytopathology examination may be indicated if the diagnosis is unclear.

Chronic Meningitis

Description

Patients suffering from chronic meningitis usually present with a variety of signs including low-grade fever, headache, lethargy, confusion, nausea, vomiting, and stiff neck that develop over a period of 1 to 4 weeks. Fungi and mycobacteria are responsible for many cases of chronic meningitis. The encapsulated yeast, *C. neoformans*, is 1 of the most common causes, particularly in patients with depressed cell-mediated immunity due to HIV infection or immunosuppressive therapy. *C. neoformans* is acquired by inhalation that usually causes an asymptomatic pulmonary infection. These organisms then spread to the CNS by the hematogenous route. *Coccidioides* spp., a dimorphic fungus that is prevalent in the southwestern United States, is also acquired

TABLE 5–11   Typical Cerebrospinal Fluid (CSF) Findings in Meningitis[a]

	Normal	Bacterial	Viral	Fungal or Tuberculous
WBC (count/mL)	0–5	>100	100–1000	100–500
Neutrophils (% of total WBC)	0–15	90	<50[b]	<50
Glucose (mg/dL)	45–65	<40	45–65	30–45
CSF/blood glucose ratio	0.6	<0.4	0.6	<0.4
Protein (mg/dL)	20–45	>150	50–100	100–500

CSF, cerebrospinal fluid.

[a]Data from Segretti J, Harris AA. Acute bacterial meningitis. *Infect Dis Clin North Am.* 1996;10:797.

[b]The percentage of neutrophils can be elevated during early stages of infection.

by inhalation and has a predilection for infecting the meninges and CNS. Immunosuppressed patients who harbor *Mycobacterium tuberculosis* are at increased risk of CNS tuberculosis (TB). Neoplastic and immune-mediated diseases can also cause chronic meningeal symptoms and it is important to distinguish between these conditions and infection.

Diagnosis

The diagnosis of chronic meningitis requires evaluation of the CSF. Typically there are an increased number of mononuclear cells, mildly elevated protein, and normal glucose (except in TB). Immunoassays for *C. neoformans* capsular polysaccharide can be performed in less than an hour, have a very high sensitivity and specificity, and are superior to visual examination of India ink preparations. Fungal culture should also be performed. If the patient is at increased risk of disseminated TB (i.e., purified protein derivative [PPD]-positive or a history of pulmonary TB), then the CSF should be tested for mycobacteria. AFB smears are quite insensitive. PCR of CSF can provide early confirmation of *M. tuberculosis* infection in many cases. However, culture should still be performed to obtain an isolate for susceptibility testing.

Encephalitis

Description

Viral encephalitis is an infection of the brain parenchyma that can produce permanent neurologic damage or death in persons of all ages. A higher incidence of viral encephalitis is found in young children, the elderly, and persons with impaired immunity. For some viruses, there is a seasonal variation for infection. Most of the viruses that produce encephalitis enter the CNS via the hematogenous route. In its mildest form, viral encephalitis can present with fever and headache, and in its most severe form as an acute fulminating disorder with seizures and death. Prominent clinical findings include altered level of consciousness, altered mental status, headache, seizures, and other signs of neurologic dysfunction. The most important cause of sporadic encephalitis is HSV-1 that often causes permanent neurologic damage or death. Fortunately there is effective antiviral therapy for HSV encephalitis that can prevent most of these complications if given early in the infection. Arboviruses transmitted by mosquitoes are responsible for periodic epidemics of encephalitis. A dramatic example of this phenomenon was the appearance of West Nile virus in the eastern United States in the summer of 1999 and its subsequent spread across the country during the next 4 years. Arboviral encephalitis is usually a self-limited infection. Most patients recover, but a significant number have persistent neurologic symptoms. Amebas such as *Naegleria* should also be considered in the differential diagnosis of encephalitis since they require specific therapy.

> Viral encephalitis is an infection of the brain parenchyma that can produce permanent neurologic damage or death in persons of all ages. The most important cause of sporadic encephalitis is HSV-1 that often causes permanent neurologic damage or death.

Diagnosis

The diagnosis of viral encephalitis includes evaluation of CSF. In patients with viral encephalitis, there is a predominantly lymphocytic pleocytosis, with a slight to moderate elevation of CSF protein, and no change in glucose content from normal. However, there are variations, depending on the virus that produces the encephalitis. Some of the agents can produce CSF findings that mimic those of bacterial meningitis (e.g., pleocytosis with an increased number of neutrophils), particularly during the early stages of infection. The diagnosis of HSV encephalitis should be confirmed with a PCR assay of CSF that detects HSV DNA. This test is very sensitive and specific. Because of the severity of HSV infections and the availability of effective treatment, it should be performed on any patient with suspected encephalitis. Viral culture of CSF is insensitive and should not be routinely performed. Encephalitis caused by other viruses is often diagnosed by detection of viral nucleic acid or virus-specific IgM and IgG in serum or CSF.

Table 5–10 presents the laboratory evaluation for meningitis and encephalitis by disease and/ or organism. Organisms not listed in the table also may cause CNS infections. Chapter 2 provides descriptions of many of the tests mentioned in the table.

Brain Abscess

Description

A brain abscess is a focal lesion and therefore presents differently from meningitis and encephalitis. The most common clinical presentation is persistent, worsening headache. More than half of patients will have focal neurologic deficits but only half have fever. Bacterial abscesses can result from hematogenous dissemination or extension from an adjacent site. The most common organisms are viridans group streptococci, *Haemophilus* spp., and anaerobic gram-negative rods. If the patient is immunosuppressed, then the abscess could be caused by *Aspergillus* and other fungi, *Nocardia* spp. and *Mycobacterium* spp., and *Toxoplasma gondii*. Neurocysticercosis, a mass lesion that results from infection with the pork tapeworm *Taenia solium*, often presents as new onset seizures in an adult.

Diagnosis

Unlike other CNS infections, examination of CSF is unlikely to yield useful information and even performing a lumbar puncture may be contraindicated. The initial diagnosis is usually based on CT and MRI findings. Identification of the causative agent is important for guiding therapy. This usually requires stereotactic biopsy of the abscess to obtain material for microscopic examination and culture. Serologic assays performed on serum may be helpful in the diagnosis of *Toxoplasma* infections and neurocysticercosis.

BONE INFECTIONS/OSTEOMYELITIS

Description

Osteomyelitis is an infection of the bone characterized by progressive, inflammatory destruction of the bone tissue. Osteomyelitis can be classified by the route of infection (hematogenous, contiguous spread, direct traumatic, or surgical inoculation), the site of infection, the type of patient, or duration of infection (acute or chronic). Hematogenous osteomyelitis is most common in prepubertal children, where it usually involves the long bones, and older adults where it usually involves the vertebrae. Less common sites of osteomyelitis include the sternoclavicular and sacroiliac joints, and symphysis pubis. Children with acute osteomyelitis appear ill with fever, chills, localized pain, and leukocytosis. In contrast, adults with vertebral osteomyelitis often have a subacute course with slowly worsening back pain and little or no fever or leukocytosis. Hematogenous osteomyelitis is usually caused by a single organism. *S. aureus* accounts for half of cases. Other frequently encountered organisms are streptococci and enterobacteriaceae in neonates, gram-negative rods in the elderly, *Salmonella* spp. in patients with sickle cell disease, *Pseudomonas aeruginosa* in intravenous drug users, and *Candida* spp. in patients with intravascular catheters. TB and brucellosis can cause vertebral osteomyelitis in patients who have been exposed to these organisms.

> Osteomyelitis caused by a contiguous focus of infection often results from an injury associated with an open fracture or following surgery for reconstruction of bone.

Osteomyelitis caused by a contiguous focus of infection often results from an injury associated with an open fracture or following surgery for reconstruction of bone. It is also common in patients with poorly controlled diabetes mellitus due to peripheral neuropathy and vascular insufficiency. This form of osteomyelitis is found almost exclusively in the foot and starts insidiously in areas of traumatized skin. The infection of the skin may be easily overlooked as the organism makes its way to the bones in the toes, metatarsal heads, and tarsal bones. Unlike hematogenous osteomyelitis, these contiguous focus infections are usually polymicrobial involving combinations of staphylococci, streptococci, enterococci, and gram-negative rods. Additional classes of organisms may be present in the wound if the injury site was contaminated with soil. With between 500,000 and 1,000,000 hip replacements per year worldwide, infections associated with prosthetic joints are also common (see the section "Infections of the Joints")

TABLE 5–12   Organisms Associated with Osteomyelitis and Populations at Risk

Organism	Population with Highest Incidence or Predisposing Condition
Staphylococcus aureus	All ages, including infants and children; most frequent organism causing osteomyelitis
Salmonella spp.	Sickle cell disease patients; immunocompromised individuals
Pseudomonas aeruginosa	Intravenous drug abusers; those with a puncture wound to the foot; patients with urinary catheters
Aerobic streptococci	Patients with bites, diabetic foot lesions, or decubitus ulcers
Anaerobic streptococci	Patients with foreign body-associated infections such as those induced by prosthetic joints (chronic infection), bites, diabetic foot lesions, or decubitus ulcers
Mycobacterium tuberculosis	Patients with a history of pulmonary tuberculosis; immunocompromised individuals
Fungal species (includes *Candida* and *Aspergillus*)	Patients with catheter-related fungemia; intravenous drug abusers; immunocompromised individuals

Diagnosis

Imaging techniques can be used to detect osteomyelitis in the early phase and reveal the extent of damage to bones and joints. Definitive diagnosis requires biopsy and culture of the infected tissue in most cases. This permits an accurate identification of the organisms responsible for the osteomyelitis. In some situations, the organisms suspected of causing osteomyelitis may be identified from the culture of synovial fluid, blood, or biopsy of contiguous lesions. Microbiologic culture of blood or contiguous tissue does not definitively identify the organism in the bone, but it may provide a strong indication of the organisms responsible for the osteomyelitis.

Table 5–12 lists the organisms most likely to cause osteomyelitis and identifies the populations at risk for infection by the named organisms.

INFECTIONS OF THE JOINTS

Description

The mainstays of the laboratory investigation for a joint infection are synovial fluid Gram stain and culture to identify infecting organisms, and polarized microscopy of the synovial fluid to identify crystals in crystal-induced arthritis.

Acute pain and swelling in the joint can be produced by infectious agents, crystals of monosodium urate or other compounds, and a variety of less common causes. Because some organisms can destroy cartilage in a matter of days, the diagnosis of infectious arthritis must be made quickly. Organisms can seed the joint through the hematogenous route (via intravenous drug abuse, indwelling catheters, endocarditis, or direct inoculation from intra-articular injections or arthroscopy), or from a contiguous site of infection, especially the bones and bursae. Septic arthritis can resemble a variety of noninfectious processes, but an acutely inflamed joint should be considered septic until proved otherwise. Septic arthritis is most often monoarticular with polyarticular involvement in less than 20% of the cases.

Diagnosis

The mainstays of the laboratory investigation for a joint infection are synovial fluid Gram stain and culture to identify infecting organisms, and polarized microscopy of the synovial fluid to identify crystals in crystal-induced arthritis. It should be noted, however, that crystal-induced and infectious arthritis can coexist. Synovial fluid WBC counts consistent with infection are ≥50,000 μL^{-1}, with more than 90% as neutrophils. **Table 5–13** summarizes the organisms associated with joint infection and the relevant clinical features for each infection.

TABLE 5–13   Evaluation for Organisms Associated with Infections of the Joints

Organism	Population with Highest Incidence and/or Predisposing Conditions	Clinical Features	Laboratory Tests
Staphylococcus aureus	Damaged joint; cutaneous abscess; intravenous drug abuse; prosthetic joint	Most common cause of septic arthritis; can produce rapid destruction of the joint	Gram stain of synovial fluid is positive in majority of cases
Selected streptococcal species (excluding *Streptococcus pneumoniae*)	Diabetes mellitus	Second most common cause of septic joint after *S. aureus*; from benign to severe, depending on the specific organism and predisposing conditions	Gram stain and culture of synovial fluid and blood cultures reveal infecting organism in majority of cases
Coagulase-negative staphylococci	Prosthetic joint	Inflammation and tenderness around a prosthetic joint	Gram stain and culture of synovial fluid, with blood cultures, may reveal organism
Neisseria gonorrhoeae	Young adults	May have genitourinary findings of gonococcal infection; dermatitis and synovitis not uncommon	Gram stain of synovial fluid is positive in 25%–30% of cases; synovial fluid culture is positive in 25%–50% of cases; blood culture is positive in 10%–15% of cases
Gram-negative bacilli (pathogens include *Pseudomonas aeruginosa, Serratia, Klebsiella,* and *Enterobacter,* which may be specific for certain joints)	Immunocompromised patients; urinary or biliary tract infection; intravenous drug abusers (especially for *Pseudomonas*); prosthetic joint; SLE and sickle cell disease (especially for *Salmonella*)	Up to 20% of septic arthritis cases are caused by gram-negative organisms	Gram stain of synovial fluid reveals organisms in about 50% of cases; culture of synovial fluid and blood also may lead to organism identification
Streptococcus pneumoniae	Splenic dysfunction	Accounts for <5% of septic arthritis cases	Gram stain and culture of synovial fluid and blood cultures reveal infecting organism in majority of cases
Mycobacterial species (includes *M. tuberculosis* and *M. marinum*)	Earlier tuberculous infection reactivated by age or immunosuppression	Up to 50% of patients with *M. tuberculosis* joint involvement also have pulmonary tuberculosis	Culture of synovial fluid or synovial tissue may reveal organism
Fungal species (pathogens include *Sporothrix, Cryptococcus, Blastomyces, Coccidioides,* and *Candida*)	Alcoholism; myeloproliferative disorders	*Sporothrix* is the most common cause of fungal arthritis; *Cryptococcus* and *Blastomyces* infections may be associated with adjacent osteomyelitis; blastomycosis arthritis may be associated with pulmonary infection	Repeated cultures of synovial fluid and tissue are often required for identification of the organism; a calcofluor fungal smear of synovial fluid may be helpful
Borrelia burgdorferi (Lyme disease agent)	Patients with Lyme disease or history of tick exposure	Intermittent attacks of swelling in a large joint	One of several tests for Lyme disease (see the section "Lyme Disease")

SLE, systemic lupus erythematosus.

INFECTIONS OF THE SKIN AND ADJACENT SOFT TISSUE

Overview

Many different organisms can produce infections of the skin and soft tissue. Clinical manifestations and severity vary widely and include aggressive, fast-moving infections such as necrotizing fasciitis, abscesses that require incision and drainage, chronic superficial fungal infections, and rashes that can be caused by local or systemic viral infections. A brief description of infections associated with particular organisms is provided in **Table 5–14**. The diagnostic information to identify infecting organisms is also included in the table. Lyme disease and *Bartonella* infections

TABLE 5-14   Selected Skin and Soft Tissue Infections

Skin/Soft Tissue Infection	Description	Predisposing Condition(s)	Etiologic Agent(s)	Clinical Findings	Laboratory Diagnosis
Candida infections of the mouth, skin, nails, and vagina	Superficial infection of the skin, nails, and mucous membranes by species of the genus *Candida*; examples of infections include oral candidiasis, vaginal candidiasis, and chronic mucocutaneous candidiasis	Oral candidiasis (thrush) commonly seen in infants and in munosuppressed patients, such as those with AIDS, diabetes mellitus, and long-term steroid therapy; chronic mucocutaneous candidiasis seen in patients with reduced delayed-type hypersensitivity and those with defects in neutrophil function	*Candida albicans* most common; other species include *C. krusei* and *C. tropicalis*	Oral candidiasis: painless, confluent white plaques on the oral and pharyngeal mucosa, particularly on the tongue and in the mouth; chronic mucocutaneous candidiasis: persistent circumscribed hyperkeratotic skin lesions, crumbling dystrophic nails; vaginal candidiasis: pruritic white plaques on the vaginal mucosa	Demonstration of pseudohyphae from *Candida* on wet smear with confirmation by culture; *Candida* grows within tissue in both yeast and pseudohyphal forms; final identification of *Candida* species requires culture and biochemical tests
Furuncle	Acute bacterial infection of perifollicular skin, usually from preexisting folliculitis	Skin areas subject to friction and perspiration, poor hygiene, occupational exposure to grease or oil, malnutrition, alcoholism, and immunosuppression	*Staphylococcus aureus*	Indurated, dull red tender nodule with central purulent core on the face, buttocks, perineum, breast, and/or axilla	Diagnosis usually made clinically; Gram stain and culture of suppurative lesion support the clinical diagnosis
Carbuncle	Coalescence of interconnected furuncles; involves subcutaneous tissue with drainage at multiple sites	For untreated furuncles, complications include bacteremia, endocarditis, and osteomyelitis	*Staphylococcus aureus*	Multiple abscess formations separating connective tissue septae with drainage to surface along hair follicles	Diagnosis usually made clinically; Gram stain and culture of suppurative lesion support the clinical diagnosis
Superficial folliculitis	Infection of hair follicles of the skin	Poor hygiene, occupational exposure to oils and solvents	*Staphylococcus aureus* most common	Single or multiple superficial, dome-shaped, pruritic pustules at the ostium of hair follicles on the scalp, back, and/or extremities	Diagnosis usually made clinically; Gram stain and bacterial cultures support the clinical diagnosis
Hot tub folliculitis	Infection of hair follicles of the skin	Whirlpools and hot tubs with low chlorine, high pH, and high water temperatures	*Pseudomonas aeruginosa*	Small erythematous pruritic papules topped by pustules in areas submerged in hot water	Clinical diagnosis supported by bacterial culture and Gram stain of infected pustule or water source
Paronychia	Infection of the nail folds	Minor trauma causing break in the skin, as produced by splinters	Acute: staphylococci, beta-hemolytic streptococci, gram-negative enteric bacteria Chronic: *Candida albicans*	Tender, red swollen areas extending around the nail fold with or without pus	Clinical diagnosis supported by bacterial and/or fungal cultures of infected areas
Impetigo contagiosa (nonbullous)	Localized purulent infection of the skin	Underprivileged children (2–5 years old) living in warm, humid climates; preexisting superficial abrasions from insect bites, trauma, and other causes	Group A beta-hemolytic streptococci and *S. aureus*	Small superficial vesicles that form pustules rupture, forming characteristic yellow-brown "honey-colored" crusted lesions	Clinical diagnosis supported by culture/Gram stain of base of early lesion positive for staphylococci and/or streptococci; anti-DNase B and anti-hyaluronidase titers may be elevated

Continued next page—

TABLE 5-14   Selected Skin and Soft Tissue Infections (continued)

Skin/Soft Tissue Infection	Description	Predisposing Condition(s)	Etiologic Agent(s)	Clinical Findings	Laboratory Diagnosis
Bullous impetigo	Localized purulent infection of the skin causing bullous lesions	Occurs in newborns and younger children on nontraumatized skin of the buttocks, perineum, trunk, and/or face	Usually due to S. aureus producing exfoliative toxins	Begins as small vesicles that quickly enlarge to form bullae with clear fluid that rupture and leave a brownish black crust	Clinical diagnosis supported by culture/ Gram stain of base of lesion or clear fluid from bullae showing staphylococci
Ecthyma	A variant of impetigo on the lower extremities causing punched-out ulcerative lesions	May occur de novo or secondary to preexisting superficial abrasions such as insect bites; occurs in children and elderly most often	Usually group A beta-hemolytic streptococci	"Punched-out" ulcers with yellow crust extending into dermis, typically on lower extremities	Clinical diagnosis supported by culture and Gram stain of base of lesion that is positive for streptococci
Staphylococcal scalded skin syndrome (SSSS)	Widespread bullae and exfoliation as a severe manifestation of an infection by S. aureus strains producing exfoliative exotoxins	Higher incidence in newborns and younger children	S. aureus producing exfoliative exotoxins	Scarlatiniform rash with widespread tender bullae with clear fluid; bullae rupture, resulting in separation of skin; exfoliation exposes large areas of red skin	Diagnosis usually made clinically
Erysipelas	Acute inflammation of superficial layers of the skin with lymphatic involvement	Occurs most often in infants, young children, and elderly; those with skin ulcers, local trauma/abrasion, and eczematous lesions; increased susceptibility in sites with impaired lymphatic drainage	Group A beta hemolytic streptococci; rarely, group B, C, G streptococci and S. aureus	5%–20% facial, 70%–80% lower extremity; painful bright red edematous indurated lesions with raised border, well demarcated from uninvolved skin; regional lymphadenopathy common	Difficult to culture group A streptococci from lesion; up to 20% of throat cultures positive for group A strep; blood culture positive in 5% of cases
Cellulitis	Diffuse suppurative inflammation of skin and subcutaneous tissues	Occurs in sites of previous tissue damage such as operative wounds, ulcers, and focal trauma; increased incidence in intravenous drug abusers	Nonimmunosup-pressed hosts: commonly group A beta-hemolytic streptococci; less commonly S. aureus; group B and G streptococci in patients with lower extremity edema; Gram-negative rods in immunosuppressed patients; Pasteurella in cat and dog bites	Localized, painful, erythematous, warm lesions, poorly demarcated from uninvolved skin; regional lymphadenopathy may be present; bacteremia and gangrene may occur if untreated	Gram stain/culture of purulent exudate from advancing edge may reveal etiologic agent; blood cultures positive in 25% of cases
Erythrasma	Superficial chronic bacterial infection of the skin	More common in males, obese patients, and patients with diabetes mellitus	Corynebacterium minutissimum	Slowly spreading pruritic, red brown macules with scales— affecting axillae, groin, and toes	Gram-stained imprints of skin lesions reveal gram-positive bacilli; examination of skin under Wood's lamp reveals distinctive red coral fluorescence
Synergistic necrotizing cellulitis (nonclostridial anaerobic cellulitis)	A variant of necrotizing fasciitis (see following entities) involving skin, muscle, subcutaneous tissue, and fascia	Diabetes mellitus, obesity, advancing age, cardiac, and renal disease	Mixture of anaerobes (anaerobic streptococci and Bacteroides most commonly) and facultative bacteria (Klebsiella, E. coli, Proteus)	Acute onset of tender skin ulcers in lower extremity draining foul-smelling red-brown ("dishwater") pus, with underlying gangrene of subcutaneous tissue and muscle; tissue gas in 25% of patients; systemic toxicity is significant	Culture/Gram stain of exudate aspirated from lesion

Continued next page—

TABLE 5-14   Selected Skin and Soft Tissue Infections (continued)

Skin/Soft Tissue Infection	Description	Predisposing Condition(s)	Etiologic Agent(s)	Clinical Findings	Laboratory Diagnosis
Necrotizing fasciitis (Type I)	A deep-seated, severe necrotizing infection of the subcutaneous tissue, resulting in progressive destruction of superficial and, in some cases, deep fascia and fat	Diabetes mellitus, alcoholism, parenteral drug abuse; occurs at sites of trauma such as an insect bite, and following laparotomy performed in the presence of perineal soiling, decubitus ulcers, and perirectal abscesses	At least 1 anaerobic species (most commonly *Bacteroides* or *Peptostreptococcus*) along with a facultative anaerobic species such as streptococci or gram-negative enteric bacilli such as *E. coli, Enterobacter, Klebsiella,* and *Proteus*	Sudden onset of tender, warm, erythematous, well-demarcated cellulitis, usually involving the lower extremity, abdominal wall, perianal, and/or groin areas; sequential skin color changes from red-purple to patchy blue-gray over several days; within 3–5 days, skin breakdown occurs with bullae, a seropurulent exudate, frank cutaneous gangrene, and skin anesthesia; high fevers and systemic toxicity with early shock and organ failure common	Surgical exploration required to distinguish from cellulitis; leukocytosis, thrombocytopenia, azotemia, and increased serum levels of creatine kinase (CK) may be present; Gram-stained smears of exudates reveal a mixture of organisms; blood cultures are frequently positive; subcutaneous gas and soft tissue swelling detectable on radiographs
Necrotizing fasciitis (Type II) (also known as hemolytic streptococcal gangrene)	A deep-seated, severe, necrotizing infection of the subcutaneous tissue, resulting in progressive destruction of superficial and, in some cases, deep fascia and fat	Occurs in 50% of patients with streptococcal toxic shock syndrome; predisposing factors also include diabetes mellitus, long-term steroid therapy, cirrhosis, peripheral vascular disease, a recent history of minor trauma, stab wounds, and surgical procedures	Group A streptococci, either alone or in combination with other species, most commonly *S. aureus*	Sudden onset of tender, warm, erythematous well-demarcated cellulitis, usually involving the lower extremity, abdominal wall, perianal and groin areas; sequential skin color changes from red-purple to patchy blue-gray over several days; within 3–5 days, bullae develop with seropurulent exudate, frank cutaneous gangrene, and skin anesthesia; high fevers and systemic toxicity with early shock and organ failure	Surgical exploration required to distinguish from cellulitis; leukocytosis, thrombocytopenia, azotemia, and increased serum levels of creatine kinase (CK) may be present; Gram-stained smears of exudate reveal gram-positive cocci in chains; surgical debridement provides tissue for culture and Gram stain; subcutaneous gas and soft tissue swelling present on radiograph
Clostridial anaerobic cellulites	A necrotizing clostridial infection of devitalized subcutaneous tissue with rare involvement of deep fascia or muscle	Dirty or inadequately debrided traumatic wounds; preexisting localized infection; contamination of surgical wounds	Clostridial species, usually *Clostridium perfringens*	Localized edema of wound site; thin, foul-smelling drainage of wound with minimal pain, extensive gas formation in tissues, and frank crepitant cellulites	Gram stain of drainage shows numerous blunt-ended, thick, gram-positive bacilli and variable numbers of neutrophils; soft tissue radiographic films show abundant gas
Clostridial myonecrosis (gas gangrene)	Rapidly progressive infection characterized by muscle necrosis and systemic toxicity caused by potent clostridial exotoxins	Wounds associated with trauma and open fractures such as gunshot wounds; intestinal and biliary tract surgery	*Clostridium perfringens* accounts for 80% of cases; other species include *C. septicum, C. novyi,* and *C. sordelli;* the toxins released by these organisms are responsible for much of the morbidity and mortality associated with these infections	Sudden onset of severe pain at the site of a wound with rapid progression to localized tense edema and pallor; crepitance is a late finding and is neither a sensitive nor a specific feature; as the lesion progresses, the skin progresses to magenta or brown discoloration with brown serosanguinous discharge and "mousey" odor	Surgical exploration critical in demonstrating devitalized muscle tissue; CT scan shows gas in the muscle and in fascial planes with soft tissue swelling; Gram stain of exudate shows typical gram-positive or gram-variable rods with spores and lysed or absent neutrophils; with C perfringens, organism shows typical boxcar appearance without spores on Gram stain, "double-zone hemolysis" on anaerobic blood plate, and lecithinase activity (alpha-toxin); elevated CK, LDH, and myoglobin due to myonecrosis

Continued next page—

TABLE 5–14 **Selected Skin and Soft Tissue Infections (continued)**

Skin/Soft Tissue Infection	Description	Predisposing Condition(s)	Etiologic Agent(s)	Clinical Findings	Laboratory Diagnosis
Spontaneous or nontraumatic gas gangrene	Rapidly progressive infection characterized by muscle necrosis and systemic toxicity caused by *Clostridium septicum*	Hematologic malignancies, colon cancer, diabetes mellitus, peripheral vascular disease; commonly with no obvious portal of entry; not associated with traumatic or surgical wounds	Most cases due to *C. septicum*	Sudden onset of pain and localized swelling of extremity, followed by discoloration, blister formation, and crepitance; associated fever, abdominal pain, vomiting, and diarrhea	Surgical exploration critical in demonstrating myonecrosis; CT scan shows gas in the muscle and fascial planes with soft tissue swelling; Gram stain of exudate shows typical gram-positive or gram-variable rods with spores and lysed or absent neutrophils; elevated CK, LDH, and myoglobin due to myonecrosis

CK, creatine kinase; CT, computed tomography; LDH, lactate dehydrogenase.

TABLE 5–15 **Laboratory Evaluation for Lyme Disease**

Laboratory Test	Results/comments
Enzyme linked immunoassay (EIA)— total antibodies	Detects serum IgM and IgG that react with a sonicated extract of *B. burgdorferi*. Used as a screening test in a 2-step algorithm because of the potential for false-positive reactions. EIA can also be used to determine CSF/serum indices
Indirect immunofluorescence assay (IFA)	This assay also detects serum antibodies against *B. burgdorferi*. It has been replaced by EIAs in most laboratories
Western blot analysis	This assay detects serum antibodies to specific antigens of *B. burgdorferi* as a qualitative yes/no answer. Careful adherence to quality control procedures is very important. The results should be interpreted according to CDC guidelines: a positive IgG blot is defined as the presence of antibodies that react with at least 5 out of 10 specific proteins; a positive IgM blot is defined as the presence of antibodies that react with at least 2 out of 3 specific proteins. Western blots can also be performed on CSF
Anti-C6 EIA	A recently developed EIA that detects antibodies against a highly immunogenic, highly conserved epitope of *B. burgdorferi*. More specific than routine EIAs but not quite as specific as the 2-tiered algorithm
PCR analysis	May be useful for testing CSF or joint fluid in selected cases

CSF, cerebrospinal fluid; PCR, polymerase chain reaction.

are discussed in **Tables 5–15** and **5–16**. A number of other infectious diseases, such as syphilis and herpes simplex infections, also have skin manifestations and are more fully described elsewhere in this chapter.

Acute Bacterial Infections

Abscesses, infected wounds, and cellulitis are common acute infections of the skin. The most common organisms are *S. aureus*, beta-hemolytic streptococci (groups A and B), other streptococci and staphylococci, and several gram-negative rods. Certain underlying conditions, such as diabetes and peripheral vascular disease, predispose to polymicrobial infections involving gram-positive cocci and gram-negative rods.

Cat/dog and human bite wounds are commonly infected with the above organisms but they are also associated with specific organisms (*Pasteurella multocida* and *Eikenella corrodens*, respectively).

TABLE 5–16   Evaluation for Cat-Scratch Disease and Bacillary Angiomatosis

Infection	Description	Predisposing Conditions	Etiologic Agents	Clinical Findings	Laboratory Diagnosis
Cat-scratch disease	Regional lymphadenopathy that develops 2–3 weeks after contact with a cat in the presence of a scratch or eye lesion; culture or laboratory data are needed to identify the organism; a lymph node biopsy has a characteristic morphology	History of contact with cat	*Bartonella henselae*	Regional lymphadenopathy approximately 2 weeks after contact with a cat that persists for 2–4 months, usually as part of a mild illness in most cases	Lymph node biopsy with characteristic appearance; Warthin–Starry stain may reveal bacilli, but only a small percentage of specimens; indirect immunofluorescence test or enzyme immunoassay may be useful to measure serologic responses; PCR for *B. henselae* DNA is also available
Bacillary angiomatosis	A disease with unique vascular lesions caused by infection with small gram-negative organisms of the genus *Bartonella*	AIDS patients, especially those with low CD4 cell counts; history of contact with cat	*Bartonella henselae*	Cutaneous lesions: papular red nodules that may enlarge to form large pedunculated lesions with a vascular appearance; subcutaneous lesions: 1 or more deep nodule(s) with normal appearing or erythematous overlying skin; nodules may erode through the surface; bacillary angiomatosis legions also can occur in bones, spleen, gastrointestinal tract, respiratory tract, lymph nodes, bone marrow, and CNS	Skin biopsy with a characteristic vascular proliferation and numerous bacilli by Warthin–Starry stain; organisms can be isolated from blood using special isolator tubes and grown in culture

CNS, central nervous system; PCR, polymerase chain reaction.

Necrotizing fasciitis (usually caused by *streptococcus pyogenes*) and clostridial myonecrosis (also known as gas gangrene) are uncommon, but they are life-threatening infections that require prompt surgical and medical intervention.

Lyme Disease

Description

The causative agent of Lyme disease is *Borrelia burgdorferi*, which is spread by the bite of a tick of the genus *Ixodes*. Lyme disease is the most common vector-borne infection in North America and in Europe. It tends to go unnoticed by many patients because the associated influenza-like symptoms are not specific for the disease. Within days to weeks of infection, a distinctive skin rash, known as erythema migrans, appears. It is important to treat the patient at the time that this rash appears to prevent subsequent potential neurologic, cardiac, or musculoskeletal complications.

> The causative agent of Lyme disease is *Borrelia burgdorferi*, which is spread by the bite of a tick of the genus *Ixodes*. Lyme disease is the most common vector-borne infection in North America and in Europe.

Diagnosis

Unlike many infections, this laboratory diagnosis is rarely based on culture of *B. burgdorferi*. This is because there are few organisms in clinical specimens, and these organisms require specialized media for growth with prolonged incubation. Therefore, the diagnosis rests upon a characteristic clinical picture supported by positive serologic tests consistent with the infection. In patients who present with erythema migrans, the diagnosis is straightforward. However, for many patients with vague symptoms and equivocal serologic test results, it is difficult to make a definitive diagnosis. Serologic testing for Lyme disease is a 2-step process involving a screening enzyme-linked immunoassay (ELISA), followed by a confirmatory immunoblot (see Chapter 2 for a description of these assays). There are several important issues regarding the serologic assays to detect Lyme disease:

- The serologic tests are not entirely specific for Lyme disease.
- Serum samples collected in the early stage of the disease may contain no antibodies to the organism because there is little or no antibody production in many patients until 3 to 4 weeks after the onset of the illness.
- The immune response is variable, and treatment with antibiotics can reduce the magnitude of the response.

Cross-reactivity between the antigens from *B. burgdorferi* and antigens from other organisms may occur. For example, false-positive serologic reactions for Lyme disease have been reported in patients with RMSF, leptospirosis, and syphilis. False-positive reactions can also occur in some patients with autoimmune diseases.

PCR-based assays for detection of *B. burgdorferi* DNA may be useful for testing joint fluid or CSF. Only properly validated assays should be used since in a low-prevalence population (i.e., patients with nonspecific symptoms and no history of a tick bite), the positive predictive value can be very low. A summary of the different assays currently available for diagnosis of Lyme disease is provided in **Table 5–15**.

Cat-Scratch Disease and Bacillary Angiomatosis
Descriptions
Several organisms of the genus *Bartonella* were found to be associated with human disease in the 1990s when they were identified as the etiologic agents in cat-scratch disease and bacillary angiomatosis. Most cases of cat-scratch disease are caused by *B. henselae* (other *Bartonella* spp. and *Afipia felis* may account for a small percentage of these cases). Initially a papule or pustule forms at the site of the scratch, but most individuals seek medical attention several weeks later because of the development of a regional lymphadenopathy (mainly in the neck or upper extremity). In most cases, it resolves spontaneously, although in rare cases severe complications can occur, including encephalitis, conjunctivitis, and neuroretinitis. Bacillary angiomatosis is a disorder in which there are distinctive and occasionally lethal vascular proliferative responses in the skin, the bones, and other organs. Bacillary angiomatosis is most commonly diagnosed in individuals infected with HIV.

> Several organisms of the genus *Bartonella* were found to be the etiologic agents in cat-scratch disease and bacillary angiomatosis.

Diagnosis
A further description of cat-scratch disease and bacillary angiomatosis and recommendations for their diagnosis are included in **Table 5–16**. Serologic tests and PCR-based tests may be useful to support the histopathologic findings from lymph node biopsies in cat-scratch disease and from skin biopsies in bacillary angiomatosis. *Bartonella* spp. are difficult to culture.

Fungal Infections
Fungal infections of the skin can be characterized as superficial, cutaneous, and subcutaneous. Infections caused by fungi such as *Malassezia* spp. are limited to the superficial layers of the skin and can result in patchy alteration of pigmentation. The more invasive cutaneous infections caused by dermatophytes and subcutaneous infections are discussed in the following sections.

Descriptions
The dermatomycoses (also known as ringworm) are skin infections caused by dermatophytes. These organisms are closely related fungi that invade keratinous tissues such as skin, hair, and the fur of animals. The dermatophytes are classified into 3 genera, *Epidermophyton*, *Microsporum*, and *Trichophyton*. Dermatophyte infections are named according to the anatomic location (in Latin) for the body site, following the word "tinea." For example, tinea pedis is

a dermatophyte infection of the foot. The diagnosis of a dermatophyte infection is made by microscopic examination of a scraping of the lesion and by culturing the specimen on selective agar that inhibits the growth of commensal bacteria and other fungi. When organisms are successfully grown in culture, they are identified to the species level by colony and microscopic morphology.

Sporotrichosis is a chronic infection characterized by nodular lesions in cutaneous and subcutaneous tissues and adjacent lymphatics. This infection is caused by *Sporothrix schenckii*, a dimorphic fungus that is typically introduced by traumatic implantation into the skin (e.g., during gardening). Sporotrichosis commonly displays a lymphocutaneous pattern as it tracks up the lymphatic system in the hand and arm. Rare manifestations include pulmonary and disseminated infections. Histologic examination of a specimen will often reveal granulomatous inflammation, but organisms are rarely seen. Therefore, diagnosis depends on culturing the specimen to permit microbiologic isolation of the *S. schenckii* organisms.

Mycetoma is a chronic infectious disease that involves cutaneous and subcutaneous tissues, fascia, and bone, and remains localized. It is characterized by draining sinuses, with aggregates of the etiologic agent in the pus draining from the sinuses. The fungi that produce the mycetomata are associated with woody plants and soil. The organisms are usually introduced by traumatic inoculation into the skin. A tumor-like deforming disease can develop during subsequent years if untreated. Dozens of fungal organisms have been documented as causes of mycetoma. In the United States, the most common agent is *Pseudoallescheria boydii*. The asexual form of this organism is known as *Scedosporium apiospermum*. Other fungi predominate in tropical and subtropical areas. The fungal elements are most often found in the center of a suppurative and granulomatous lesion that develops in a deep site and extends out to the skin for drainage. Draining sinuses appear in essentially all patients within 1 year of the initial trauma. Identification of the causative agent is made by fungal smear and culture of the material draining from the sinus tracts. Clinically similar infections are caused by filamentous gram-positive bacteria in the genus *Nocardia*. It is important to identify the infecting agent because the therapy for fungi is very different from that used for bacteria.

Chromomycosis is a subcutaneous infection by organisms originating in the soil, with only rare cases of dissemination. It is rarely seen in the United States. The lesions typically appear on the lower extremities. They are pink, scaly papules that expand to form a superficial nodule, and their presence suggests the diagnosis. Examination of the lesions microscopically in potassium hydroxide (KOH) or calcofluor white preparations can be diagnostic. Without therapy, which is usually surgical, the scaly papules grow to form nodules with a verrucous and friable surface.

Diagnosis

A further description of the infections and the tests used to identify the associated organisms are included in **Table 5–17**.

Viral Infections with Prominent Skin Manifestations

Overview

Viral infections can cause a variety of macular, papular, or vesicular rashes. Many of these typically occur in the pediatric age range and may be associated with systemic signs and symptoms. Enteroviruses and parvovirus B19 are discussed in other sections.

Varicella Zoster Viral Infection

Description

Primary infection with VZV causes chickenpox, a vesicular rash that occurs predominantly on the trunk, scalp, and face. This disease is usually self-limited, with the symptoms resolving after 7 days. Varicella can also produce pneumonia, with pulmonary symptoms manifested approximately 4 days after the varicella rash. After primary infection, the virus enters the latent phase and remains in sensory ganglia. On reactivation, which occurs in a minority of adults, it produces herpes zoster, a vesicular rash that occurs along a dermatome distribution. The incidence of varicella has been declining since the introduction of a live virus vaccine.

Primary infection with varicella zoster virus causes chickenpox, a vesicular rash that occurs predominantly on the trunk, scalp, and face. This disease is usually self-limited, with the symptoms resolving after 7 days.

TABLE 5-17   Evaluation for Superficial, Cutaneous, and Subcutaneous Fungal Infections

Disease/dermatomycosis	Etiologic Agent(s)	Clinical Findings	Anatomic Pathology	Microbiology
Tinea capitis (scalp ring worm)	*Trichophyton, Microsporum*	Pruritic, scaly, erythematous lesions associated with alopecia on the scalp	Skin biopsies usually not necessary; if performed, hyphae may be visible in biopsy material	Wet hair or skin smears treated with KOH or calcofluor white reveal hyphae; culture on selective agar that contains cycloheximide
Tinea barbae	*Trichophyton verrucosum*	Pustular lesions in bearded areas	Skin biopsies usually not necessary; if performed, hyphae may be visible in biopsy material	Wet hair or skin smears treated with KOH or calcofluor white reveal hyphae; culture on selective agar that contains cycloheximide
Tinea corporis (body ring worm)	*Epidermophyton, Microsporum,* or *Trichophyton*	Sharply demarcated skin lesions on trunk and/or legs that contain pustules or papules and have prominent edges	Skin biopsies usually not necessary; if performed, hyphae may be visible in biopsy material	Wet hair or skin smears treated with KOH or calcofluor white reveal hyphae; culture on selective agar that contains cycloheximide
Tinea cruris ("jock itch")	*Trichophyton rubrum* or *Epidermophyton floccosum*	Localized rash with scaly lesions that involve anterior aspect of thighs; pustules and papules may be present	Skin biopsies usually not necessary; if performed, hyphae may be visible in biopsy material	Wet hair or skin smears treated with KOH or calcofluor white reveal hyphae; culture on selective agar that contains cycloheximide
Tinea manum	*Trichophyton rubrum*	Dry infection of the palmar surface of the hand	Skin biopsies usually not necessary; if performed, hyphae may be visible in biopsy material	Wet hair or skin smears treated with KOH or calcofluor white reveal hyphae; culture on selective agar that contains cycloheximide
Tinea pedis (athlete's foot)	*Trichophyton rubrum, Trichophyton mentagrophytes,* or *Epidermophyton floccosum*	Pruritic foot lesions that may peel and crack and form vesicles or pustules	Skin biopsies usually not necessary; if performed, hyphae may be visible in biopsy material	Wet hair or skin smears treated with KOH or calcofluor white reveal hyphae; culture on selective agar that contains cycloheximide
Tinea versicolor (pityriasis)	*Malassezia furfur*	Hypopigmented or hyperpigmented macules on trunk or proximal limbs	Skin biopsies may demonstrate yeast forms with short hyphae	Round yeast forms and short hyphae visible by direct microscopy of lesion scrapings
Sporotrichosis (usually involves cutaneous and subcutaneous tissues and adjacent lymphatics)	*Sporothrix schenkii*	Papulonodular, erythematous lesions in distal extremities; secondary lesions along lymphatic channels	Skin biopsies of involved lesions reveal a granulomatous response and, in some cases, cigar-shaped yeast forms	Skin lesions may be cultured; blood cultures may be positive if sporotrichosis is multifocal
Mycetoma (madura foot)	Madurella, *Pseudallescheria boydii,* other species	Foot or hand infection that extends from skin into deeper tissue; indurated swelling and multiple sinus tracts draining pus that contains aggregates of the fungus causing the disease	Hyphae may be visible in tissue or drainage using various stains; deep biopsies are preferred	Causative species inferred from organisms in sinus tract drainage
Chromomycosis (also known as chromoblastomycosis and many other names)	*Fonsecaea pedrosoi;* other species	Verrucous, cauliflower-like skin lesions, often pruritic; may result in secondary infection or lymphedema	Sclerotic bodies may be visible in stained tissue	Sclerotic bodies may be visible in exudates; culture confirmation recommended with Sabouraud's agar

KOH, potassium hydroxide.

TABLE 5–18   Evaluation for Varicella Zoster Virus (VZV) Infection

Laboratory Tests	Results/Comments
Viral culture	Vesicular fluid is the sample; the results are typically available within 7–21 days
Direct immunofluorescence assay	Cells at the base of a vesicular lesion are scraped from the skin and applied to a slide for direct immunofluorescent staining for VZV; the detection of VZV from any source is always clinically significant as no asymptomatic shedding of this virus is known to occur
Antibody detection assays (includes enzyme immunoassay, fluorescent anti-membrane antibody assay, latex agglutination assay, and complement fixation test)	These tests are used to confirm immunity to VZV, which may be important to know before and during pregnancy because a number of fetal anomalies are associated with VZV infection during pregnancy; the anomalies depend largely on the gestational age of the fetus at the time of infection
PCR analysis	Amplification of VZV DNA from a CSF specimen supports the diagnosis of VZV encephalitis

CSF, cerebrospinal fluid; PCR, polymerase chain reaction.

Diagnosis

Chickenpox and herpes zoster are diagnosed clinically in most cases because of the characteristic presentation of the diseases. Laboratory tests for the VZV virus, although they represent the gold standard for diagnosis, are typically unnecessary. Cutaneous lesions may be evaluated for the presence of VZV by direct immunofluorescence. Serologic testing is often important to determine whether an individual has ever been infected with VZV. Assays for VZV infection are summarized in **Table 5–18.**

Measles (Rubeola) and Rubella
Description

Rubeola and rubella infections are often confused because of the similarity in their names and similar clinical manifestations. Measles (or rubeola) is a highly contagious childhood disease characterized primarily by fever and a rash. The primary portal of entry for the rubeola virus is the upper respiratory tract. Approximately 14 days after exposure to the rubeola virus, a characteristic measles rash appears, and within 1 to 2 additional days there is a measurable amount of antibody to rubeola virus in the bloodstream. The leading cause of death in patients with measles is secondary bacterial pneumonia. Rubella, also known as German measles, is most often a mild illness in children and young adults. It is widely recognized as a dangerous infection in early pregnancy when an infection of the fetus can cause congenital abnormalities. Rubella is characterized by a rash and an enlargement of lymph nodes. Like the rubeola virus, the portal of entry of rubella virus is most often the respiratory tract. The availability of vaccines against measles and rubella has greatly decreased the incidence of these infections in the United States.

Diagnosis

The laboratory diagnosis of measles or rubella can be important for epidemiologic surveillance purposes and to limit its transmission to susceptible individuals. The laboratory diagnosis is usually based on detecting virus-specific IgM in serum or isolation of the virus from urine or respiratory specimens.

Within 24 to 48 hours of the development of a rash, antibodies to rubella become detectable. Primary infection stimulates production of antibodies that confer lifelong immunity, which exists during pregnancy. It is for this reason that the presence of antibodies to rubella is desirable before initiating pregnancy. The antibodies can be demonstrated in a serologic test that indicates

TABLE 5–19 **Laboratory Evaluation for Measles and Rubella**

Laboratory Tests	Results/Comments
Serology	Virus-specific IgM is defectable in serum a few days after appearance of rash; seroconversion or 4-fold rise in IgG in convalescent serum also supports the diagnosis; presence of IgG provides evidence of immunity
Culture	Specimens suitable for culture include nasopharyngeal secretions, urine, blood, or other sterile sites; these viruses can be difficult to grow

exposure to the rubella virus. Serologic testing is an important component of the evaluation of a pregnant woman with the clinical signs and symptoms of rubella. **Table 5–19** summarizes the laboratory evaluation for rubeola and rubella.

EYE INFECTIONS

Description and Diagnosis

Infectious agents play a prominent role in many diseases of the eye. **Table 5–20** describes the infections of the eye according to anatomic site of infection within the eye. Many organisms that produce eye infections are described in detail in other sections of this chapter. The microbiologic isolation and tests for identification of the organisms listed in **Table 5–20** as causative for disease are presented in other sections of this chapter.

INFECTIONS OF THE LARYNX, PHARYNX, MOUTH, EAR, ORBIT, AND SINUSES

Description and Diagnosis

Table 5–21 describes the infections of the pharynx, larynx, mouth, ear, orbit, and sinuses. Because there are such a large number of organisms that produce these infections, a brief description of the infections and their associated organisms is presented in **Table 5–21**. For similar reasons, the diagnostic studies useful in identifying the disease and its causative organisms are also provided in the table.

INFECTIONS OF THE LUNG AND PLEURAE

Overview

Many categories of organisms can cause pneumonia and other types of pulmonary infections. It is very important to consider the clinical setting when evaluating and managing a patient with pneumonia because the types of organisms that are responsible depend on whether or not specific risk factors are present.

Community-acquired pneumonia is commonly caused by *S. pneumoniae*, *Mycoplasma pneumoniae*, respiratory viruses, *H. influenzae*, and *Legionella* spp. In contrast, hospital-associated and ventilator infections are likely to be caused by multidrug-resistant organisms including *Klebsiella pneumoniae*, *P. aeruginosa*, *Acinetobacter baumanii* complex, and MRSA. *P. aeruginosa*, *Burkholderia cepacia*, and MRSA are also important causes of lung infections in patients with cystic fibrosis. Travel and/or exposure history can be an important clue in patients with persistent pulmonary signs and symptoms, as they may have TB or dimorphic fungal infections (described below). Patients with depressed cell-mediated immunity (e.g., transplant recipients or HIV infection) are at increased risk of *Pneumocystis* and CMV infections. Patients who have prolonged neutropenia from chemotherapy, for example, are at increased risk of invasive infections caused by *Aspergillus* spp. and other fungi.

Table 5–22 describes the infections of the lung and pleurae. The many different lung infections are grouped into bacterial, fungal, parasitic, and viral diseases. There are 2 major challenges

It is very important to consider the clinical setting when evaluating and managing a patient with pneumonia because the types of organisms that are responsible depend on whether or not specific risk factors are present.

TABLE 5–20   Infections of the Eye and Causative Organisms

Infection	Clinical Features/Definition	Causative Organisms
Eyelid infections		
Hordeolum	An acute infection of either a meibomian gland or a gland of Zeis, also known as a sty	*Staphylococcus aureus*
Chalazion	A chronic granuloma on a meibomian gland	*S. aureus*
Marginal blepharitis	Diffuse inflammation of the eyelid margins	*S. aureus* has been implicated
Infections of the lacrimal system		
Dacryoadenitis	Inflammation of the lacrimal gland	*S. aureus* most common; next most common is *Chlamydia trachomatis*, and rarely *Neisseria gonorrhoeae*
Canaliculitis	An inflammation of the canaliculi	*Actinomyces israelii*
Dacryocystitis	An infection of the lacrimal system occurring as a result of outflow obstruction in the nasolacrimal duct	Acute: *S. aureus*, *Streptococcus pyogenes*, *Streptococcus pneumoniae* in infants, *Haemophilus* spp. in children Chronic: *Actinomyces*, *Aspergillus*, and *Candida*
Conjunctivitis	Infection of the conjunctiva; a very common ocular infection	
Viral	More common than bacterial conjunctivitis in developed countries	Adenovirus is the most common virus, with herpes simplex virus, influenza A virus, enterovirus 70, and coxsackie virus as other causative agents
Bacterial (nonchlamydial)	Hyperacute bacterial conjunctivitis is the most severe form of conjunctivitis	Hyperacute: *Neisseria gonorrhoeae* common, but also *N. meningitidis* and *Corynebacterium diphtheriae* Acute: *S. aureus*, *Streptococcus pneumoniae*, *Haemophilus influenzae* in children, *Streptococcus pyogenes* and *Haemophilus aegyptius*; gram-negative bacillary infections are rare Chronic: *S. aureus* is the most common agent with *Moraxella lacunata* and *Moraxella catarrhalis* also causative
Chlamydial	Two distinct presentations exist—*C. trachomatis* infection is a leading cause of blindness in endemic areas of the world while *chlamydia*-induced inclusion conjunctivitis is a relatively benign infection	See the section "Chlamydial Infections"
Infectious keratitis	Infection of the cornea; can lead to loss of vision because of corneal scarring or because of progression to perforation and endophthalmitis	
Viral	Keratitis is almost always unilateral and may affect any age group	Herpes simplex virus is the most common cause of corneal ulcers in the United States
Bacterial	Bacteria causing conjunctivitis may invade the cornea following minor trauma to the corneal epithelium; contact lens wear is a predisposing factor for bacterial keratitis	Coagulase-negative staphylococci, *S. aureus*, *Pseudomonas aeruginosa*, *S. pneumoniae*, and viridans streptococci
Fungal	This is a rare entity accounting for less than 2% of infectious keratitis cases	*Aspergillus*, *Candida*, and *Fusarium* are the most common, with geographic variation
Parasitic	Most cases are in contact lens wearers	*Acanthamoeba* is the most common cause of parasitic keratitis in industrialized countries
Endophthalmitis	Infection of the vitreous; a severe ocular infection with significant permanent impairment of vision as a result of the infection	
Postoperative	This occurs in most patients 1–3 days after cataract surgery	Coagulase-negative staphylococci, *S. aureus*, gram-negative bacilli, streptococci, and *Haemophilus influenzae*

Continued next page—

TABLE 5-20 Infections of the Eye and Causative Organisms (continued)

Infection	Clinical Features/Definition	Causative Organisms
Posttraumatic	The onset is rapid for virulent bacteria; onset is over weeks to months for fungal organisms	Coagulase-negative staphylococci, *Bacillus*, gram-negative bacilli, and fungi
Endogenous	This form of endophthalmitis does not follow surgery or trauma	*S. aureus*, streptococci, gram-negative bacilli, *Candida*
Uveitis	Infection of the iris, retina, choroid, or sclera	
Anterior		
Viral		Herpes simplex 1 virus, varicella zoster virus, cytomegalovirus
Bacterial	Usually bilateral when associated with secondary syphilis	*Treponema pallidum* (syphilis)
Posterior		
Viral		Cytomegalovirus, herpes simplex virus, varicella zoster virus
Bacterial		*Treponema pallidum* (syphilis) is rare; *Mycobacterium tuberculosis* also rare
Fungal		*Candida, Cryptococcus, Histoplasma*
Parasitic		*Toxoplasma gondil, Pneumocystis carinil, Toxocara canis*

TABLE 5-21 Infections of the Larynx, Pharynx, Mouth, Ear, Orbit, and Sinuses

Disease or Pathogen	Clinical Findings	Histopathology/ Radiology	Microbiology Testing	Common Pathogens
Laryngeal infections				
Laryngitis, acute	Hoarseness and occasional aphonia are associated with upper respiratory infections	Histopathologic and radiographic studies are not useful for routine diagnosis	Diagnosis usually on clinical features	Influenza viruses, rhinoviruses, adenovirus, parainfluenza viruses, *Streptococcus pneumoniae*, *Haemophilus influenzae*, and *Streptococcus pyogenes*
Laryngitis, tuberculous (laryngeal tuberculosis) (also see the section "Tuberculosis")	Cough, wheezing, hemoptysis, dysphagia, odynophagia; laryngeal lesions vary from ulcers to exophytic masses	Granulomatous changes and acid-fast organisms may be observed in laryngeal biopsy material; chest radiographs may reveal pulmonary tuberculosis	Laryngeal biopsy may be submitted for mycobacterial smears and culture; blood cultures may be positive for mycobacteria	*Mycobacterium tuberculosis* (highly infectious)
Pharyngeal and oral infections				
Herpes gingivostomatitis	Painful, ulcerating vesicles in oral mucosa; fever, fetid breath, cervical adenopathy, drooling; usually in children less than 5 years old	Rapid diagnosis with Giemsa- or Wright-stained smears from lesion by identifying multinucleated giant cells (less sensitive than culture); Tzanck preparation	Rapid antigen detection of moist lesion scrapings may be positive (less sensitive than culture); lesions may be cultured, usually for 24–48 hours; serologic tests of acute and convalescent sera may aid in diagnosis	Herpes simplex virus is the agent of primary infection

Continued next page—

TABLE 5–21   Infections of the Larynx, Pharynx, Mouth, Ear, Orbit, and Sinuses (continued)

Disease or Pathogen	Clinical Findings	Histopathology/ Radiology	Microbiology Testing	Common Pathogens
Herpes labialis, recurrent	Painful, ulcerating vesicles beginning on the outer lip (usually lower lip); fever usually absent	Rapid diagnosis with Giemsa- or Wright-stained smears from lesion by identifying multinucleated giant cells (less sensitive than culture)	Rapid antigen detection in moist lesion scrapings may be positive (less sensitive than culture); lesions may be cultured, usually for 24-48 hours; serologic tests not useful	Herpes simplex virus is the agent of recurrent disease
Oral thrush (oral candidiasis)	Creamy white patches on the tongue and oral mucosa that bleed easily when scraped	Histopathologic studies are not useful for routine diagnosis	KOH or Gram-stained smears of oral lesions reveal pseudohyphae and yeast forms	*Candida albicans*
Streptococcal pharyngitis ("strep throat")	Pharyngeal pain, odynophagia, fever, chills, headache; anterior cervical adenopathy; purulent exudates, edema, and erythema in posterior pharynx	Histopathologic studies are not useful for routine diagnosis	Rapid antigen detection by throat swab (less sensitive than culture); routine culture of throat (posterior pharynx) swab is most sensitive	*Streptococcus pyogenes* (group A streptococci); groups C and G streptococci cause milder pharyngitis; infections of the throat by respiratory viruses may mimic strep throat clinically
Neisseria gonorrhoeae infection of the pharynx (see the section "Gonorrhea"				
Diphtheria	In its mildest form, asymptomatic carriage of organisms; formation of tough membrane over pharyngeal surface; also can cause skin lesions and damage to multiple organs	Histopathologic studies are not useful for routine diagnosis	Organisms from lesion can be grown in culture	*Corynebacterium diphtheriae*
The "common cold"	Nasal discharge and sinus congestion; often with pharyngeal and sinus pain; may be febrile with chills and headache	Not useful	Testing to rule out a bacterial infection, usually by culture of a throat swab specimen, is often performed when pharyngeal pain is present	Rhinovirus, coronavirus, and adenovirus, among others
Ear, orbit, and sinus infections				
Otitis externa	Pruritic and painful outer ear, with an edematous and erythematous ear canal	If invasive otitis externa present, CT or MRI of head is useful for monitoring bone or tissue infection	Wound or external auditory canal specimens for Gram stain and culture	Pseudomonas aeruginosa (swimmer's ear), *Staphylococcus aureus*, and *Streptococcus pyogenes*
Otitis media	Ear pain, otorrhea, hearing loss with fever, irritability, headache, lethargy, anorexia, and vomiting	Histopathologic and radiographic studies are not useful for routine diagnosis	Diagnosis usually on clinical features; tympanic fluid obtained by tympanocen-tesis may be cultured	*Streptococcus pneumoniae*, *Haemophilus influenzae*, *Moraxella catarrhalis*, *Streptococcus pyogenes*, *Staphylococcus aureus*, and selected viruses
Orbital cellulitis	Proptosis and eye pain; eyelid swelling, redness, warmth, tenderness	Cranial CT scan of sinuses and orbit may identify abscesses	Blood, conjunctival, and wound specimens for Gram stain and culture	*Staphylococcus aureus*, *Streptococcus pyogenes*, *Haemophilus influenzae*, and *Streptococcus pneumoniae*

Continued next page—

TABLE 5–21 Infections of the Larynx, Pharynx, Mouth, Ear, Orbit, and Sinuses (continued)

Disease or Pathogen	Clinical Findings	Histopathology/ Radiology	Microbiology Testing	Common Pathogens
Periorbital cellulitis	Eyelid pain, swelling, and erythema with low-grade fever	Sinus radiographs or CT scan may exclude sinus disease	Blood, conjunctival, and wound specimens for Gram stain and culture	*Haemophilus influenzae* and anaerobic bacteria
Sinusitis (acute)	Persistent upper respiratory symptoms; purulent nasal discharge, fever, facial pressure or pain, facial erythema or swelling, and nasal obstruction	For complicated cases, CT scanning of paranasal sinuses is method of choice—presence of an air-fluid level correlates with bacterial infection	Usually a clinical diagnosis; sinus puncture aspirates are specimen of choice for Gram stain and culture; endoscopic sampling of exudates less likely to identify pathogens	*Streptococcus pneumoniae, Haemophilus influenzae,* and rhinoviruses

CT, computed tomography; KOH, potassium hydroxide; MRI, magnetic resonance imaging.,

TABLE 5–22 Infections of the Lung and Respiratory Tract

Pathogen	Clinical Findings	Histopathology and Radiology	Microbiology Testing	Other Tests
Bacterial infections				
Bordetella pertussis (whooping cough)	Paroxysmal, nonproductive cough; low-grade fever, rhinorrhea; vomiting may follow cough	CXR may show pneumonia with consolidation	Cultures and/or PCR from nasopharyngeal specimens	Peripheral blood lymphocytosis often present
Burkholderia cepacia	Causes respiratory distress or progressive respiratory failure with high fever in cystic fibrosis patients (especially females)	CXR may show widespread infiltrates	Sputum from lower respiratory tract for Gram stain and culture with special media	
Moraxella catarrhalis	Tracheitis, bronchitis, sinusitis, and otitis media can all occur	In most cases, CXR findings are not prominent	Gram stain and culture from respiratory specimens	Serologic tests not useful
Chlamydia pneumoniae (TWAR agent)	Pharyngitis, hoarseness, fever, mild pneumonitis; atypical pneumonia, especially in the elderly	CXR usually reveals single subsegmental lesion; pleural effusion may be evident	*Chlamydia* culture possible but requires specialized cell lines; PCR assays for direct detection are being developed	IgM and IgG serologic tests for antibody to the organism may be useful for diagnosis
Coxiella burnetii (Q fever)	Causes atypical pneumonia with fever, severe headache, chills, sweats, myalgias; associated with exposure to livestock	CXR often shows multiple rounded opacities	Culture and PCR only performed in specialized or reference laboratories	IgM and IgG serologic tests for antibody to the organism most useful for initial diagnosis; normal WBC count; liver transaminases; elevated smooth muscle autoantibodies often present
Klebsiella pneumoniae	Bronchitis, bronchopneumonia, or lobar pneumonia; "currant jelly" sputum; frequent complications such as abscess and empyema	CXR may reveal pattern of pneumonia and identify complications, if they arise	Sputum from lower respiratory tract for Gram stain and culture	
Haemophilus influenzae (nontypeable)	Pneumonia with fever, productive cough; often exacerbates chronic bronchitis	CXR may show interstitial or bronchopneumonia, or pneumonia with consolidation	Sputum or other lower respiratory tract specimen for Gram stain and culture	

Continued next page—

TABLE 5–22   Infections of the Lung and Respiratory Tract (continued)

Pathogen	Clinical Findings	Histopathology and Radiology	Microbiology Testing	Other Tests
Legionella pneumophila (also see the section "*Legionella* Infections")	Atypical pneumonia with slightly productive cough, fever, and chest pain; diarrhea often present	CXR typically shows alveolar infiltrates; pleural effusions common	Respiratory specimens cultured on selective media; urinary antigen test is rapid and sensitive	Hyponatremia often present; PCR and serologic tests may be useful for diagnosis
Mycobacterium avium-intracellulare (atypical mycobacteria)	In the non-HIV-infected patient, pulmonary disease with productive cough, fever, weight loss, and occasionally hemoptysis	CXR mimics reactivation tuberculosis with cavitation	Sputum from lower respiratory tract specimen for acid-fast stain or culture	In HIV-infected population, must distinguish atypical mycobacteria form *M. tuberculosis* infection
Mycobacterium tuberculosis (see the section on "Tuberculosis")				
Mycoplasma pneumoniae	Often causes an upper respiratory tract infection with fever, malaise, headache, and nonproductive cough; may cause atypical pneumonia	CXR may show extensive infiltrates, out of proportion with symptoms	Difficult to diagnose by microbiologic culture; cultures require 1–4 weeks for growth with special media; negative by Gram stain	IgM and IgG tests are useful (may require acute and convalescent serum); can also be used for diagnosis
Pseudomonas aeruginosa	Causes pneumonia in elderly, hospitalized, and cystic fibrosis patients; may be fulminant with chills, fever, dyspnea, excessive purulent sputum, and cyanosis	CXR may reveal diffuse bronchopneumonia; in bacteremic pneumonia, alveolar and interstitial infiltrates with cavitation may be seen	Sputum from lower respiratory tract for Gram stain and culture; blood cultures may be positive	Mucoid isolates often obtained from cystic fibrosis patients; a leading cause of nosocomial pneumonia
Staphylococcus aureus	Pneumonia with fever, purulent sputum	CXR shows infiltrates, consolidation, abscesses, pleural effusions, and/or loculations	Sputum from lower respiratory tract for Gram stain and culture; pleural fluid or empyema if present should be cultured; blood cultures may be positive	Empyema is a frequent complication that requires drainage; pleural fluid very purulent with many neutrophils
Streptococcus agalactiae (group B streptococci)	Causes pneumonia in neonates and elderly; fever present; apnea, tachypnea, grunting, and cyanosis in neonates	CXR in neonates may show pulmonary infiltrates, often similar to hyaline membrane disease	Sputum from lower respiratory tract for Gram stain and culture; for neonates, serum and urine rapid antigen detection may be useful	Pregnant carrier females may be screened by culture of vaginal or cervical swab specimens
Streptococcus pneumoniae	Productive cough with rust-tinged sputum, fever, shaking chills, and pleuritic chest pain	CXR may show subsegmental infiltrations; segmental or lobar consolidation may be present	Sputum from lower respiratory tract for Gram stain and culture; blood cultures may yield organisms	Peripheral blood leukocytosis frequent; empyema is an uncommon complication
Streptococcus pyogenes (group A streptococci)	Abrupt onset of pneumonia with fever, chills, dyspnea, pleurisy, and blood-tinged sputum	CXR reveals bronchopneumonia with consolidation	Sputum from lower respiratory tract for Gram stain and culture; blood cultures may be positive	Empyema is a frequent complication
Fungal infections (see the section "Dimorphic Fungi and Other Fungal Infections")				
Pneumocystis (see the section "*Pneumocystis jirovecii* Pneumonia")				

Continued next page—

TABLE 5–22   Infections of the Lung and Respiratory Tract (continued)

Pathogen	Clinical Findings	Histopathology and Radiology	Microbiology Testing	Other Tests
Viral infections				
Adenovirus	Pharyngitis or tracheitis with cough, fever, sore throat, and rhinorrhea; interstitial pneumonia may develop; diarrhea also may be present	Adenoviral eosinophilic inclusions may be visible in lung biopsies if they are obtained	Adenoviral culture from respiratory specimens; rapid viral antigen detection may be useful	With serologic testing, a 4-fold rise in titer is consistent with new infection
Cytomegalovirus (CMV)	Interstitial pneumonitis with nonproductive cough, fever, dyspnea, and hypoxia	CXR shows interstitial pneumonia; nodules or cavities may be seen; lung biopsies reveal CMV inclusions ("owl's eye" cells)	Viral cultures from respiratory and blood specimens; CMV antigenemia detection useful for diagnosis of disseminated disease	PCR assays are available for direct detection of CMV in blood and cerebrospinal fluid
Hantavirus	Fever, severe myalgias, headache, tachypnea, and shortness of breath; rapidly progressive to hypotension, respiratory failure, and shock	CXR shows rapid progression to bilateral interstitial edema and diffuse alveolar disease; pleural effusions often present	Immunohistochemistry or PCR using blood or lung biopsy may confirm infection	IgM serologic tests by capture enzyme immunoassay or Western blot are diagnostic methods of choice
Influenza A or B virus	Fever, chills, myalgias, headaches, dry cough; primary viral pneumonia may occur	CXR may show bilateral infiltrates	Viral culture; direct viral antigen detection may be useful	RT-PCR assays performed on nasopharyngeal (NP) specimens
Parainfluenza viruses 1, 2, 3, and 4	Upper respiratory tract infections, otitis media, conjunctivitis, and pharyngitis; may cause croup or bronchiolitis	CXR is negative in cases with no pulmonary involvement	Viral culture; direct viral antigen detection may be useful	RT-PCR performed on NP specimen
Respiratory syncytial virus (usually infants and young children)	Pneumonia or bronchiolitis; fever, paroxysmal cough, dyspnea	CXR may show interstitial infiltrates or hyperinflation	Viral culture; rapid viral detection may be useful	RT-PCR performed on NP specimen
Pleural empyema: most common organisms found are *Streptococcus pneumoniae*, *Staphylococcus aureus*, *Haemophilus influenzae*, *Streptococcus pyogenes*, *Pseudomonas aeruginosa*, *Klebsiella pneumoniae*, and *Bacteroides*	Chest pain, chills, persistent fever, right sweats	Thoracic CT scan usually permits definitive diagnosis; ultrasound distinguishes solid lesions from pleural fluid collections; CXR may show pleural fluid accumulations in lateral decubitus views	Pleural or empyema fluid should be cultured for aerobic and anaerobic organisms	Peripheral blood leukocytosis usually present; pleural fluid values often show fluid pH below 7, glucose below 40 mg/dL, and LDH exceeding 1,000 IU/L

CXR, chest radiograph; LDH, lactate dehydrogenase; PCR, polymerase chain reaction; CT, computed tomography.

in the laboratory diagnosis of pulmonary infections. First, it can be difficult to obtain respiratory specimens that are not contaminated with oropharyngeal flora. This is particularly true of expectorated sputum. It is 1 of the reasons why this type of specimen is routinely screened microscopically for the presence of squamous epithelial cells to determine whether it is a true lower respiratory specimen. The other problem is that there is no single test that detects all of the potential respiratory pathogens. While routine Gram stain and sputum culture readily detects *S. pneumoniae*, common gram-negative rods, and *S. aureus*, separate cultures and/or test methods are required to detect *Legionella*, mycobacteria, fungi, respiratory viruses, CMV, and *Pneumocystis*. These are discussed in more detail in the following sections.

Tuberculosis

Description

TB is a major cause of morbidity and mortality around the world and remains a major challenge for public health officials. Approximately one-third of the world's population is estimated to be infected with the causative agent, *M. tuberculosis*. This slow-growing acid-fast bacterium continues to be an important concern in industrialized countries because of the development of drug-resistant strains and a growing population of immunosuppressed patients who are at increased risk of TB. Although it can infect a variety of organs, *M. tuberculosis* primarily causes pulmonary disease. It is usually acquired by inhalation of infectious aerosolized droplets. The majority of primary infections are asymptomatic; however, the organisms are not completely eliminated. This leads to a quiescent phase known as latent tuberculosis infection (LTBI). Otherwise healthy individuals with LTBI have an approximately 10% lifetime risk of developing secondary or reactivation pulmonary TB. Prophylaxis of asymptomatic-infected individuals reduces the risk of subsequent reactivation TB.

Clinical features of active pulmonary TB include fever, night sweats, weight loss, productive cough, and hemoptysis in later stages of the disease. Radiographic studies often show cavitary lung lesions, usually in the lung apices. It is important to realize that immunosuppressed patients who develop active TB often have atypical clinical presentations and can have nonspecific radiographic changes. Before the epidemic of HIV infection in the United States, approximately 85% of newly diagnosed infections with TB were limited to the lung, with 15% involving nonpulmonary sites or both pulmonary and nonpulmonary sites. With advanced HIV infection, less than half the cases are limited to pulmonary involvement. Extrapulmonary TB commonly involves the lymph nodes, pleura, genitourinary tract, bones and joints, meninges, peritoneum, and pericardium.

Early identification of patients with active pulmonary TB is crucial for preventing transmission of this serious infection to other patients and healthcare workers. Treatment of active TB caused by sensitive strains requires combination therapy for 6 months. Multidrug-resistant and extremely resistant *M. tuberculosis* (MDR-TB and XDR-TB, respectively) are more difficult to treat and have a poorer outcome.

> Approximately one-third of the world's population is estimated to be infected with the causative agent, *M. tuberculosis*. Early identification of patients with active pulmonary TB is crucial for preventing transmission of this serious infection to other patients and healthcare workers.

Diagnosis

There are 2 categories of laboratory tests for TB: those that detect latent infection and those that detect active disease. Skin testing with PPD detects previous exposure to *M. tuberculosis*. A delayed-type hypersensitivity response to the *M. tuberculosis* antigens (mediated by T cells) leads to induration at the site of injection. One problem with the PPD test is that individuals who have been vaccinated with BCG (bacille Calmette–Guerin) can also have a positive reaction. BCG is derived from *M. bovis*, a member of the *M. tuberculosis* complex, and is widely used outside the United States. Recent advances in immunology and genomics have led to the development of alternatives to the PPD test, such as interferon-gamma release assays (IGRAs). Peripheral blood or purified mononuclear cells are incubated with antigenic peptides that are unique to *M. tuberculosis* (i.e., they are not present in BCG) and then an immunoassay is performed to measure production of interferon-gamma. The IGRAs are at least as sensitive as the PPD and are more specific since BCG vaccination does not produce a false-positive result.

The diagnosis of secondary TB depends on detection of *M. tuberculosis* in clinical samples. This testing is particularly important since the PPD and IGRAs can be negative in patients with active TB. Acid-fast staining of sputum specimens (using either a fuchsin (red) stain or a fluorescent stain) enables visualization of the mycobacteria in ~70% of cases of pulmonary TB. Detection of mycobacteria in sputum using an AFB stain provides only presumptive evidence pulmonary TB in the presence of characteristic radiologic findings. The presence of *M. tuberculosis* must be confirmed by culturing the organism in liquid and/or solid media or by using nucleic acid amplification techniques (NAATs). Modern automated liquid culture systems routinely detect growth of *M. tuberculosis* in 1 to 2 weeks versus 4 to 6 weeks with traditional culture on solid media. These systems also make it possible to perform rapid susceptibility testing in liquid culture for first-line antituberculous drugs. The NAATs make possible same-day confirmation of smear-positive specimens, which contain relatively large numbers of organisms. Culture remains the gold standard for detecting *M. tuberculosis* in smear-negative specimens.

Table 5–23 includes the clinical and laboratory information relevant to the diagnosis of pulmonary, CNS, genitourinary, and disseminated TB.

TABLE 5-23 Evaluation for Tuberculosis (TB)

	Pulmonary Tuberculosis	CNS Tuberculosis	Genitourinary Tuberculosis	Disseminated Tuberculosis
Clinical findings	Symptoms range from none to fever with productive cough and dyspnea; hemoptysis indicates presence of advanced disease	Fever, unremitting headache, nausea, and malaise; in the United States, elderly are frequently affected; where TB is common, it primarily affects children aged 1–5 years	Most common site for extrapulmonary TB is the kidney; dysuria, frequency, and hematuria are common; women may present with a chronic pelvic inflammatory process, menstrual irregularities, or sterility; men may present with an enlarging scrotal mass	More likely to occur in HIV-positive individuals; may be present without miliary pattern in chest radiographs; patient may present with fever, weight loss, and anorexia
Tests				
PPD	In the presence of compatible radiologic and clinical findings, a positive PPD in an unvaccinated patient suggests TB	In the presence of compatible radiologic and clinical findings, a positive PPD in an unvaccinated patient suggests TB	In the presence of compatible radiologic and clinical findings, a positive PPD in an unvaccinated patient suggests TB	In the presence of compatible radiologic and clinical findings, a positive PPD in an unvaccinated patient suggests TB
Microscopy	Acid-fast bacilli in sputum smears permit rapid diagnosis; sensitivity is variable, but increases with the number of specimens examined (up to 4)	Acid-fast bacilli in smears of CSF lead to identification of 20% or less of CNS TB cases; sputum samples also should be tested	Both urine and sputum samples should be examined, as a smear from a urine sample may not have detectable acid-fast bacilli	Urine, lymph node, liver, bone marrow, and sputum smears have low sensitivity for organism detection
Mycobacterial culture	Culture from sputum specimen on liquid and solid media is the most sensitive method; for pediatric cases, multiple gastric lavage specimens can be used; liquid culture with DNA probe hybridization enables rapid TB confirmation	Culture of CSF may reveal organisms in CNS TB cases	Urine specimens for mycobacterial culture are positive in 60%–80% of cases, though it is more likely to be positive in men than in women	Culture may be performed using bone marrow, liver, urine, and sputum specimens
Nucleic acid amplification	Very useful for rapid detection of TB but does not replace culture	May provide a rapid diagnosis but cannot replace culture	Utility not well defined	Sputum specimens may be used for amplification
Other findings	Pleural fluid, if present, is an exudate (not a transudate) with mononuclear cells	With lumbar puncture, there may be an increased opening pressure and 100–1,000 cells/μL of CSF (mostly mononuclear cells) and elevated CSF protein	In the appropriate clinical setting, TB may be considered if negative routine urine cultures show WBCs in acid urine	Impaired function of infected organs may be noted in routine laboratory tests of those organ systems
Radiology	Chest radiograph may detect adenopathy, effusion, cavitation or nodule; in HIV-infected patients, the chest radiograph is less likely to show typical changes	If TB is established in the brain, it may produce a mass, or "tuberculoma," visible by CT scan	40%–75% of cases have a positive chest radiograph; other radiologic studies are not very useful	Chest radiograph may be normal and repeat testing may prove useful; CT scan or MRI may be useful to detect TB in extrapulmonary sites such as the brain or vertebrae
Anatomic pathology	Caseating granulomas may be observed in biopsies of enlarged lymph nodes	Biopsy may be diagnostic	Renal biopsy may be helpful to identify genitourinary lesions	If bronchial washings do not provide diagnosis, granulomas in bone marrow or liver biopsy may be diagnostic

CNS, central nervous system; CSF, cerebrospinal fluid; CT, computed tomography; MRI, magnetic resonance imaging; PPD, purified protein derivative.

Other nontuberculous mycobacteria, including slow-growing organisms such as *M. avium* complex and *M. kansasii*, and rapid growers, such as *M. abscessus*, can cause chronic pulmonary disease in both normal and immunocompromised hosts.

Legionella Infections

Description

Legionella pneumophila is a fastidious, slow-growing gram-negative rod. *Legionella* species are widespread in the environment and are a cause of community-acquired pneumonia. They are usually found in surface or potable water and are associated with moist environments. Approximately 10,000 to 15,000 cases of *Legionella* pneumonia occur each year in the United States. Most cases occur sporadically, but outbreaks have been associated with aerosolized transmission from cooling towers, evaporative condensers, potable hot water lines, showers, respiratory therapy equipment, decorative fountains, and whirlpool spas. Outbreaks in healthcare facilities are especially worrisome because of the large population of patients with compromised immunity or impaired pulmonary function who are at increased risk of severe *Legionella* infections.

Legionella infections can present as subclinical infections, nonpulmonary disease, pneumonia, and extrapulmonary inflammatory disease. Most patients with *Legionella* pneumonia present with a broad spectrum of symptoms, ranging from mild cough to widespread pulmonary infiltrates and multisystem failure. Patients with *Legionella* pneumonia may also experience hemoptysis, diarrhea, and a change in mental status.

Diagnosis

The diagnosis of legionellosis can be easily missed because the organisms are not detected on routine Gram stain (*Legionella* stains very poorly) and culture of sputum. A sputum Gram stain showing mostly neutrophils, without associated bacteria, should raise suspicion of Legionnaire disease or other atypical pneumonia. *L. pneumophila* serogroup 1 infections, which account for most community-acquired legionellosis, can be readily diagnosed using rapid immunoassays that detect a *Legionella* antigen that is excreted in urine. These tests detect 80% to 90% of cases and have good specificity. Another advantage is that they remain positive for several weeks, even after the patient has been started on antibiotics. Bacterial culture is the gold standard for the diagnosis of *Legionella* infection. Cultures from sputum, bronchoalveolar lavage (BAL), and/or lung tissue may require 4 to 5 days of growth for isolation of *Legionella* colonies. The sensitivity for organism detection is greater with a BAL specimen than with an expectorated sputum specimen. Isolation of *Legionella* from specimens requires the use of a charcoal-based bacteriologic medium, with the addition of antibiotics if the specimens are from nonsterile sites. The isolation and identification of *Legionella*, in association with pneumonia, is diagnostic for *Legionella* pneumonia. Direct fluorescent antibody tests of respiratory specimens are no longer recommended because they are relatively insensitive, and the specificity is greatly dependent on the experience of the individual performing the test. PCR testing and serology also may be useful in diagnosis of *Legionella* infections.

Table 5–24 summarizes the laboratory tests relevant to diagnosis of the *Legionella* infections.

Nocardiosis

Description

Nocardia spp. are aerobic gram-positive actinomycetes that are found worldwide in soil and decaying organic matter. Nocardiosis is chiefly an opportunistic infection, particularly in patients with impaired cell-mediated immunity such as hematopoietic malignancies, HIV/AIDS, those receiving immunosuppressive therapy, and transplant recipients. Pulmonary nocardiosis is the most common presentation. It can exhibit the full spectrum of acute or chronic pulmonary infection, including pneumonia and abscess formation. Other clinical manifestations include anorexia, productive cough, pleurisy, dyspnea, hemoptysis, and weight loss.

Primary *Nocardia* infection in the lung, skin, or soft tissue may erode into blood vessels and spread hematogenously to a variety of different organs. *Nocardia* have a well-recognized predilection for invasion into the CNS.

TABLE 5-24 **Evaluation of Patients for Legionnaire Disease**

Laboratory Test	Result
Bacteriologic culture	This is the "gold standard" test that requires special media for growth and isolation of the *Legionella* organisms
Urinary antigen	Detects only *Legionella* serogroup 1; overall sensitivity is 60%–80% because serogroup 1 represents 60%–80% of Legionnaire pneumonia cases; within serogroup 1, the sensitivity compared to culture is ≥95%
Direct fluorescent antibody test	Generally performed on colonies isolated from bacteriologic plates; less useful on respiratory specimens and lung biopsies due to lower sensitivity and specificity
Serology	Rising titers of antibody to *Legionella* may be useful in documentation of disease in culture-negative cases
PCR analysis	Amplification of *Legionella* DNA from respiratory specimens is a means to detect all *Legionella* pathogens—useful in selected situations

PCR, polymerase chain reaction.

TABLE 5-25 **Evaluation for Nocardiosis**

	Pulmonary Nocardiosis	Cutaneous/ Subcutaneous Nocardiosis	CNS Nocardiosis	Systemic Nocardiosis
Microbiology	Gram stain, modified acid-fast stain, or aerobic culture may generate a positive result from sputum and bronchial specimens; selective agar increases yield	Gram stain, modified acid-fast stain, or aerobic culture may generate a positive result from specimens obtained from fistulas, abscesses, or skin biopsies	Aerobic culture may generate a positive test in CSF specimens or aspirates of cerebral masses; Gram stain or modified acid-fast stain may reveal filamentous bacteria	Testing is most useful for cases involving CNS and lungs; blood culture may be positive if processed to maximize organism recovery; specimens from sites of suspected involvement may be used for smears and aerobic cultures
Anatomic pathology	Biopsies of large cavitary lesions in the lung may reveal organisms	Biopsies of skin lesions may reveal organisms	Fine needle aspirate of cerebral mass may reveal organisms	Biopsies of affected organs or tissues may reveal organisms

CNS, central nervous system; CSF, cerebrospinal fluid.

Diagnosis

Detection of the organism can be accomplished by microscopic examination of specimens combined with culture. Gram staining may reveal filamentous gram-positive rods with or without branching. They are also partially acid-fast; that is, they are positive on a modified acid-fast stain (which uses a less stringent decolorizer) but are negative on a regular acid-fast stain. *Nocardia* spp. are slowly growing organisms and may be difficult to recover. Traditionally they were identified based on biochemical reactions. More recently introduced DNA-based methods reveal that many of organisms that would previously have been identified as *Nocardia asteroides* are separate species with distinct antibiotic susceptibility profiles.

The laboratory information for diagnosis of nocardiosis in different anatomic sites is provided in **Table 5-25**.

Pneumocystis jirovecii Pneumonia

Description

Pneumocystis spp. are single-cell organisms that were originally described as protozoans, but phylogenetic analysis indicates that they are more appropriately classified with the fungi. These

TABLE 5–26 **Evaluation for *Pneumocystis jirovecii*[a]**

Type of Infection	Specimen	Laboratory Test	Results/Comments
Pneumocystis pneumonia	BAL fluid, induced sputum, or lung biopsy	Microscopy using special stains is the standard method for diagnosis of *Pneumocystis* pneumonia	Fluorescently labeled monoclonal antibodies can detect cysts and trophic forms. Gomori methenamine silver (GMS) stain only detects cyst walls; Giemsa stain only detects trophic forms
Extrapulmonary *Pneumocystis* infection	Lymph node, spleen, bone marrow, or liver	Microscopy using special stains	Organisms can be detected with GMS or fluorescent antibodies; they do not stain with hematoxylin and eosin

[a]In older literature, this organism is referred to as *P. carinii* (see *Emerg Infect Dis.* 2009;15:506).

organisms are a well-recognized cause of pulmonary infection in patients with profoundly impaired cell-mediated immunity. These infections were originally attributed to *P. carinii* (which is found in rats), but it is now known that human infections are caused by the morphologically similar *P. jirovecii*. From the beginning of the HIV epidemic in the early 1980s until 1993, *P. jirovecii* was the indicator infection for more than 20,000 newly diagnosed cases of AIDS in the United States reported to the Centers for Disease Control and Prevention. It has become much less common since the introduction of highly active antiretroviral therapy. In a small number of cases, *Pneumocystis* can also cause extrapulmonary infections.

Diagnosis

Pneumocystis spp. cannot be cultured in vitro. Laboratory diagnosis depends on identification of the organism in stained preparations of clinical specimens, most often induced sputum or BAL fluid. These are concentrated onto a slide by cytocentrifugation. Other specimens include transbronchial or open lung biopsies. The *Pneumocystis* life cycle includes trophozoite and cyst stages. The most sensitive method for detecting these forms is staining the preparation with fluorescently labeled monoclonal antibodies. Other stains that are sometimes used are Giemsa (stains trophozoites and intracystic stages) and GMS (stains cyst walls). PCR analysis of respiratory specimens may be useful in the diagnosis of *Pneumocystis*, but it is not widely available.

Table 5–26 summarizes the laboratory information that supports a diagnosis of *P. jirovecii* infection.

> The dimorphic fungi grow as filamentous molds in the environment but transform into yeast (or related forms) in infected tissue.

Dimorphic Fungi and Other Fungal Infections
Description

The dimorphic fungi grow as filamentous molds in the environment but transform into yeast (or related forms) in infected tissue. The most important members of this group are *H. capsulatum* and *Coccidioides* spp. These organisms are usually acquired by inhalation, but they can disseminate and cause systemic infections.

H. capsulatum is endemic along the Mississippi and Ohio river valleys, as well as in parts of Central America and the Caribbean region. Most infections are asymptomatic or subclinical; however, inhalation of large quantities of spores or hyphal fragments can cause symptomatic lung infection that requires antifungal therapy. As with TB, primary infection with *H. capsulatum* is contained by the cell-mediated immune response. However, the organism may not be eradicated. *H. capsulatum* infection in patients with underlying lung disease can lead to chronic progressive pulmonary histoplasmosis that must be treated to prevent further lung damage. Patients who have depressed cell-mediated immunity (due to underlying disease or immunosuppressive therapy) are at a risk of developing disseminated histoplasmosis. This form of the disease may present with nonspecific findings such as fever, weight loss, and hepatosplenomegaly, and it is fatal if untreated. Patients who harbor *H. capsulatum* and receive drugs that inhibit TNF or its receptor are at a high risk of developing disseminated infection.

Coccidioides spp. are endemic in the southwestern United States (*C. immitis* in the central valley of California and *C. posadasii* in Arizona). The life cycle of *Coccidioides* is similar to *H. capsulatum* except that it forms spherules in infected tissue and it tends to involve the meninges in immunosuppressed patients.

Immunosuppressed patients are susceptible to a variety of other fungal lung infections, including *Aspergillus* spp. and other septate molds, nonseptate molds such as *Mucor* and *Rhizopus*, and the encapsulated yeast *C. neoformans*.

Diagnosis

Diagnostic tests for *H. capsulatum* include fungal culture, immunoassays that detect a fungal cell wall antigen, and serology. Culture is the gold standard, but fungal growth is usually not detected for 1 to 2 weeks. Serology is useful for patients with chronic pulmonary histoplasmosis, but it is relatively insensitive for diagnosis of disseminated histoplasmosis. The antigen test performed on serum or urine is particularly useful for diagnosing disseminated disease. Coccidioidomycosis is diagnosed by serology and/or culture depending on the clinical presentation. The diagnosis of dimorphic fungal infections can also be confirmed by demonstration of characteristic structures in biopsy specimens. Currently the diagnosis of other fungal lung infections relies on culturing respiratory secretions and/or histopathologic examination of biopsy specimens. A serum assay that detects a galactomannan antigen produced by *Aspergillus* spp. is useful in the diagnosis of invasive pulmonary aspergillosis.

The clinical findings associated with systemic mycotic infections are shown in **Table 5–27** along with the microbiologic evaluation and histopathology findings.

Respiratory Virus Infections
Description

Many different viruses can cause upper and lower respiratory infections. Respiratory syncytial virus (RSV) and influenza viruses cause large numbers of infections in the winter months. RSV is the major cause of bronchiolitis in infants, and it can also cause serious infections in the elderly. Influenza is often thought of as an infection of adults (in whom it causes a syndrome characterized by rapid onset of fever, headache, and myalgias followed by upper respiratory symptoms). However, it also commonly infects children and may resemble RSV. Primary influenza pneumonia is a rare but dangerous form of the infection. More commonly, the typical influenza syndrome described above is followed several days later by a secondary bacterial pneumonia. Parainfluenza viruses classically cause croup (tracheobronchitis), the clinical manifestations of which often overlap those caused by RSV and influenza. Other important respiratory viruses include adenoviruses, metapneumovirus, and corona viruses, including the agent of SARS. Because of the availability of antiviral agents that target influenza viruses, it has become important to establish the specific cause of virus-like respiratory particularly in severely ill patients and those with underlying cardiac and pulmonary diseases. Identification of the cause of severe respiratory infections may also be needed for infection control activities. Immunosuppressed patients are susceptible to all of the viruses described above. They are also at increased risk of developing CMV pneumonitis.

Diagnosis

The common respiratory viruses can be identified by detecting specific viral antigens in nasopharyngeal specimens (aspirates, washes, or swabs). Rapid tests for influenza can provide an answer in less than 30 minutes, but their sensitivity is only 50% to 70% (specificity is >90%). Immunofluorescent assays in which a slide preparation is stained with labeled antibodies are much more sensitive. However, they are more labor intensive and require a skilled observer. Isolation of respiratory viruses requires proper specimen collection to prevent the loss of viability of the viruses before arrival in the laboratory. Traditional viral culture methods are sensitive, but respiratory viruses typically require 3 to 10 days in culture before they can be detected. Centrifugation-enhanced culture, in which the organisms are centrifuged onto the cultured cells, can detect viruses in 1 to 2 days. Commercially available multiplexed nucleic acid amplification assays (e.g., RT-PCR) can detect several respiratory viruses in <12 hours and rival or exceed the sensitivity of viral culture.

Laboratory methods for detecting respiratory viruses are summarized in **Table 5–22**.

The common respiratory viruses can be identified by detecting specific viral antigens in nasopharyngeal specimens (aspirates, washes, or swabs). Rapid tests for influenza can provide an answer in less than 30 minutes, but their sensitivity is only 50% to 70% (specificity is >90%).

TABLE 5–27   Evaluation for Systemic Mycotic Infections

Pathogen	Clinical Findings	Microbiology	Histopathology
Dimorphic fungi[a]			
Blastomyces dermatitidis (occurs in parts of central and eastern United States)	Chronic pneumonia with productive cough, hemoptysis, weight loss, and pleurisy; may be associated with verrucous or ulcerative skin lesions, subcutaneous nodules, osteolytic bone lesions, arthritis, prostatitis, and epididymitis	Broad-based budding yeasts may be visible in wet mounts of sputum or exudates; organism forms branching septate hyphae with microconidia in culture at 30°C, identification is usually confirmed by DNA hybridization; serologic tests have little utility	Broad-based budding yeasts in tissues; microabscesses and pyogranulomas may be present in tissue
Coccidioides spp. (common in the southwest United States)	Influenza-like syndrome or pneumonia; also may cause erythema nodosum or erythema multiforme, meningitis, and disseminated disease	Endospores or spherules may be visible in wet mounts of sputum or exudates; organism forms arthroconidia in culture at 30°C, identification is usually confirmed by DNA hybridization; serologic tests are useful in both pulmonary and disseminated diseases	Spherules with endospores may be visible within tissue; pyogenic and granulomatous (may be caseous) responses can be found in tissue
Histoplasma capsulatum (common in the Ohio and Mississippi river valleys)	Influenza-like syndrome or pneumonia; chronic progressive pulmonary infection in patients with underlying lung disease; and disseminated disease	Budding yeast or intracellular forms within macrophages may be seen in respiratory specimens; organism forms branching septate hyphae with tuberculate macroconidia in culture at 30°C, identification is usually confirmed by DNA hybridization; serologic tests are useful in pulmonary disease; antigen detection in serum and urine is particularly useful in disseminated disease	Yeasts may be seen intracellularly within macrophages and/or extracellularly as budding forms; epithelioid granulomas may be present
Paracoccidioides brasiliensis (restricted to Central and South America)	Respiratory symptoms such as productive cough and chest pain; fever, weight loss, ulcerative granulomas of buccal, nasal, or gastrointestinal mucosa may occur	Wet preps of sputum or pus may reveal multiple budding yeast; organism forms branching septate hyphae in culture at 30°C, identification usually confirmed by exoantigen tests or DNA-based assays	Multiple budding yeasts detectable in tissues; microabscesses and granulomas also may be present in tissue
Filamentous fungi			
Aspergillus spp.	Aspergilloma (fungus ball) in preexisting cavity; invasive pulmonary aspergillosis with fever, dyspnea, and chest pain; and disseminated disease	Calcofluor white stains of respiratory or biopsy material may reveal septate hyphae; culture isolates are usually identified by colonial and microscopic morphology; the serum galactomannan assay is useful for early detection of invasive pulmonary aspergillosis	Septate hyphae with 45° branching are visible in tissues
Mucor/Rhizopus	Invasive pulmonary disease similar to aspergillosis; rhinocerebral mucormycosis begins with facial pain and headache, can progress to invasion of the orbit and CNS	Calcofluor white stains of nasal or respiratory specimens may reveal broad nonseptate hyphae; organisms generally grow rapidly in culture but can be difficult to isolate from tissue	Broad, nonseptate hyphae with right-angle branching can be seen in tissue; often associated with necrosis

Continued next page—

TABLE 5–27   Evaluation for Systemic Mycotic Infections (continued)

Pathogen	Clinical Findings	Microbiology	Histopathology
Yeasts			
Candida spp.	Mucosal infections such as thrush, esophagitis, vaginitis, and disseminated disease	KOH/calcofluor preps of mucosal scrapings may reveal budding yeast, pseudohyphae, or hyphae; *Candida* grows well on routinely used agar and blood culture media	Yeast, pseudohyphae, or hyphae can be seen in infected tissue
Cryptococcus neoformans	Meningitis, pneumonia, skin lesions (in disseminated disease)	Antigen detection by latex agglutination of CSF is the most sensitive of the available tests; India ink smear may detect yeasts; confirmatory culture using CSF is recommended	Narrow-based budding yeasts may be visible in tissue (capsule stains with mucicarmine)

ᵃThe dimorphic fungi can undergo reversible transition between mold forms and yeast forms. They grow as molds in the environment but replicate as yeast (or spherules) in infected tissue.

INFECTIONS OF THE GASTROINTESTINAL TRACT

Overview

Although many organisms can cause infectious gastroenteritis, the clinical setting usually makes it possible to focus on a small group of likely pathogens. This is particularly important since no one laboratory test can detect all of the potential agents, which include viruses, bacteria, and parasites. Key factors to consider are whether the infection was acquired in the community or in a healthcare facility, duration of symptoms, travel history, and whether the patient is immunosuppressed.

Viruses Inducing Gastroenteritis
Description

In immunocompetent hosts, the majority of cases of community-acquired self-limited nausea, vomiting, and/or diarrhea are caused by viruses (primarily rotaviruses, enteric adenoviruses, and noroviruses). Laboratory testing is usually not performed unless there are large outbreaks that have epidemiological significance, for example, outbreaks on cruise ships or in healthcare facilities. Rotavirus-infected patients may be asymptomatic or have the signs and symptoms of acute gastroenteritis. Most cases of adenovirus-induced gastroenteritis are milder than those produced by rotavirus. However, in neonates, adenovirus can cause a fatal disseminated infection. Although Enteroviruses are usually acquired by fecal–oral transmission, they generally cause systemic infections; gastroenteritis is not a prominent clinical manifestation. CMV, especially in immunocompromised patients, can produce an explosive, watery diarrhea.

Diagnosis

Table 5–28 summarizes the clinical, radiologic, histopathologic, and laboratory findings associated with the gastrointestinal illnesses produced by rotavirus, adenovirus, CMV, and noroviruses.

Aerobic Bacterial Infections
Description and Diagnosis

Community-acquired diarrhea accompanied by abdominal pain or systemic symptoms should be evaluated for a select group of bacterial pathogens, consisting of *Salmonella* spp., *Shigella* spp., *Campylobacter* spp., Shiga toxin-producing *E. coli*, and *Yersinia* spp. Recent travel or consumption of raw shellfish would raise the possibility of *Vibrio* spp. All of these organisms are very unlikely to be the cause of gastroenteritis after a patient has been hospitalized for more than 3 days. Mycobacterial infections would need to be considered in profoundly immunosuppressed patients.

Community-acquired diarrhea accompanied by abdominal pain or systemic symptoms should be evaluated for a select group of bacterial pathogens, consisting of *Salmonella* spp., *Shigella* spp., *Campylobacter* spp., Shiga toxin-producing *E. coli*, and *Yersinia* spp.

TABLE 5–28   Evaluation for Viral Infections of the Gastrointestinal Tract

Pathogen	Clinical Findings	Histopathology and Radiology	Microbiology
Rotavirus	Watery diarrhea, fever, vomiting (mostly in infants and young children in winter)	Histopathologic evaluation is not useful for routine diagnosis	Direct antigen detection in stool specimens by enzyme immunoassay; viral culture is difficult
Adenovirus	Watery diarrhea in infants; fever	Histopathologic evaluation is not useful for diagnosis	The gastrointestinal adenoviruses are not culturable, but an enzyme immunoassay may be used to detect adenovirus infection in stool samples
Cytomegalovirus (CMV) (in immunosuppressed patients)	Explosive diarrhea (may be watery or bloody); fever	Colonic biopsies may reveal viral inclusions and inflammation (colitis)	CMV may be cultured from colonic biopsies
Norwalk virus (noroviruses)	Nonbloody diarrhea, vomiting, myalgias, and low-grade fever	Histopathologic evaluation is not useful for routine diagnosis	RT-PCR is the method of choice for detecting noroviruses in clinical specimens

Table 5–29 describes some of the more common bacterial infections of the gastrointestinal tract. Many of these organisms also can produce infections outside of the gastrointestinal tract.

Clostridium difficile and Other Clostridial Infections

Descriptions

C. difficile infection is frequently implicated in antibiotic-associated diarrhea and is responsible for most cases of pseudomembranous colitis, a potentially life-threatening condition that requires combined medical and surgical intervention. Antibiotics frequently implicated include ampicillin, amoxicillin, cephalosporins, and clindamycin. In *C. difficile* colitis, there is a disruption of the normal bacterial flora of the colon by the antibiotic treatment, after which there is colonization by *C. difficile* organisms. Colonization of the gastrointestinal tract occurs by the oral–fecal route. *C. difficile* elaborates toxins A and B that induce fluid secretion, mucosal damage, and intestinal inflammation and produces heat-resistant spores that persist for months in the environment. The organisms can be cultured from floors, toilets, bed pans, bedding, and all sites where patients with diarrhea from *C. difficile* infection have recently been treated.

> *C. difficile* infection is frequently implicated in antibiotic-associated diarrhea. *C. difficile* elaborates toxins A and B that induce fluid secretion, mucosal damage, and intestinal inflammation and produces heat-resistant spores that persist for months in the environment.

C. difficile infection is typically acquired in the hospital by both infants and adults. Neonates have an asymptomatic colonization, and most are resistant to the toxic effects of *C. difficile* infection. Adults can also be asymptomatically colonized. Symptomatic *C. difficile* infection usually presents with mild to moderate diarrhea and lower abdominal cramping. Symptoms often begin with antibiotic therapy, but may be delayed for several weeks after antibiotic therapy is initiated. Patients who go on to develop pseudomembranous colitis experience more severe diarrhea, abdominal tenderness, and systemic symptoms. Patients with advanced disease may present with a fulminant life-threatening colitis that must be treated promptly to avoid perforation of the bowel wall.

Histotoxic clostridial species, particularly *C. septicum*, have been linked to neutropenic enterocolitis. This is seen in patients with gastrointestinal or pelvic malignancies who have neutropenia and develop fever, abdominal pain, and diarrhea.

Diagnosis

Table 5–30 summarizes the evaluation of patients for *C. difficile* colitis, *C. perfringens*-induced food poisoning, and clostridial neutropenic enterocolitis.

Protozoal Infections

Description

Protozoa are a very diverse group of unicellular eukaryotic organisms that can be free-living or parasitic. Many have 2 morphologic stages—trophozoites and cysts. Trophozoites, which

TABLE 5–29 **Evaluation for Bacterial Infections of the Gastrointestinal Tract and for Peritonitis**

Pathogen	Clinical Findings	Histopathology and Radiology	Microbiology	Additional Diagnostic Information
Bacterial infections				
Campylobacter jejuni	Acute enteritis with diarrhea (may be watery or bloody), fever, and abdominal pain; Guillain–Barre syndrome may occur 2–3 weeks following diarrhea	Histopathologic evaluation is not routinely useful	Fecal wet mounts may reveal darting motility of organisms; Gram-stained fecal smears have a sensitivity of 50%–75%; stool cultures for C. *jejuni* must be incubated under microaerophilic condition	Leukocytes and erythrocytes often present in fecal smears; anti-GM1 ganglioside antibodies may be detected in post-*Campylobacter* Guillain–Barre syndrome
Escherichia coli	Watery or bloody diarrhea; hemolytic uremic syndrome (HUS) may be associated with gastrointestinal infection by shiga toxin-producing isolates (e.g. 0157: H7)	Histopathologic evaluation is not usually useful for diagnosis	Routine stool cultures are useful for suspected O157:H7 isolates; special growth media may be required	For HUS strains, O and H serotyping may be performed with cultured isolates; the shiga toxin can be detected by immunoassay
Mycobacterium avium-intracellulare (in AIDS patients)	Watery diarrhea, abdominal pain, nausea, vomiting, weight loss, and night sweats	Lymph node, liver, or bone marrow biopsies may reveal acid-fast organisms; small bowel biopsies not routinely performed	Blood cultures are the most likely to yield organisms; stool or sputum cultures lack sensitivity and are not routinely useful	Gastrointestinal symptoms precede disseminated mycobacterial disease in AIDS patients
Salmonella enteritidis or *typhimurium* (salmonellosis)	Nonbloody diarrhea, fever, nausea, vomiting, and abdominal cramping	Histopathologic evaluation is not usually useful for diagnosis	Routine stool cultures are useful; blood cultures rarely positive (less than 5%)	Serotyping of culture isolates is useful for epidemiologic purposes; fecal smears usually have neutrophils
Salmonella typhi or *paratyphi* (enteric or typhoid fever)	Fever, abdominal pain, hepatosplenomegaly, diarrhea, "rose spots," weakness, and weight loss	Histopathologic evaluation is not usually useful for diagnosis	Routine stool cultures are useful; blood cultures are 50%–70% sensitive; bone marrow cultures are 90% sensitive; duodenal fluid collected by intestinal string can be used for cultures	Serologic tests are generally not useful
Shigella (shigellosis; bacillary dysentery)	Dysentery with abdominal pain and bloody diarrhea	Histopathologic evaluation is not usually useful for diagnosis	Routine stool cultures used to detect organism	Direct fecal smears often contain abundant neutrophils; serologic tests are not useful
Vibrio cholerae	Mild or explosive watery diarrhea; dehydration may be severe	Histopathologic evaluation is not usually useful for diagnosis	Motile vibrios may be visible in fresh fecal smears; stool cultures should include selective media	Serotyping of organisms may be performed
Yersinia enterocolitica	Enterocolitis with diarrhea, abdominal pain, and fever; reactive polyarthritis and erythema nodosum may occur after diarrhea	Histopathologic evaluation is not usually useful for diagnosis	Stool cultures on selective media are necessary to permit growth of organisms for identification	Serologic tests for arthritis may be useful for assessing patients with polyarthritis

Continued next page—

TABLE 5-29   Evaluation for Bacterial Infections of the Gastrointestinal Tract and for Peritonitis (continued)

Pathogen	Clinical Findings	Histopathology and Radiology	Microbiology	Additional Diagnostic Information
Clostridium difficile (antibiotic-associated colitis) and *Clostridium perfringens* (food poisoning)	See Table 5.30			
Peritonitis				
Primary peritonitis (usually in children or patients with cirrhosis)	Fever, abdominal pain, nausea, vomiting, and diarrhea	Histopathologic evaluation is not usually useful for diagnosis	Gram stain and culture of peritoneal (ascitic) fluid is most likely to identify (in order of likelihood)—*E. coli*, *Klebsiella pneumoniae*, *Streptococcus pneumoniae*, enterococci	Typically, peritoneal fluid protein is low (<3.5 g/L) and peritoneal fluid leukocyte count is elevated (usually >1,000/μL) with neutrophils predominant
Secondary peritonitis (due to perforation, appendicitis, cholecystitis)	Signs of sepsis with fever, tachycardia, tachypnea, and hypotension	Histopathologic evaluation is not useful; abdominal ultrasound or CT scan may be useful for evaluation and identification of suspected intra-abdominal abscesses	Gram stain and culture of peritoneal fluid or aspirated abscess material usually reveals mixed aerobic and anaerobic flora; *E. coli*, *Bacteroides fragilis*, and *Candida albicans* commonly found	Peritoneal fluid studies less definitive in this setting; peripheral blood leukocytosis often present

CT, computed tomography.

TABLE 5-30   Evaluation for Clostridial Infections of the Gastrointestinal Tract

Diagnostic Test	*Clostridium difficile* Colitis	Food Poisoning With *Clostridia perfringens*, Type A	Neutropenic Enterocolitis Caused by *Clostridia septicum* and Other Organisms
Endoscopy with biopsy of suspicious lesions	Invasive and expensive; usually reserved for more severe cases	Not useful	Endoscopy is typically not performed, but if a sample of the bowel is removed, it will show the characteristic inflammation and/or necrosis
Tests for toxins by immunoassay or other method	The presence of toxins A or B in diarrheal stools establishes the diagnosis of *C. difficile* colitis; the tissue culture test for toxin B demonstrates a cytopathic effect from the filtrates of the diarrheal stool; with sensitivities of 70%–95%, false-negative results can occur with these tests for a variety of reasons; therefore, a negative test does not rule out *C. difficile*	Various tests are available to detect the enterotoxin responsible for the toxic effect of *C. perfringens* in food poisoning; these tests are performed in public health laboratories	Not routinely performed
Stool cultures	Most sensitive method; requires special media and must confirm that isolates produce toxin; patients may be asymptomatically colonized; DNA amplification may be a useful alternative	Stool samples are not cultured; 10^6 spores per gram of stool or 10^5 organisms per gram of suspected food source supports the diagnosis of food poisoning with *C. perfringens*; these tests are performed in public health laboratories	Not typically performed; because bacteremia may be produced in this illness, blood cultures for the clostridial organisms can be collected

are metabolically active feeding forms of the organism, may encyst within a protective coating to tolerate harsh environments. The cyst is a dormant form of the protozoan, and can re-emerge as a trophozoite (for asexually reproducing organisms) when exposed to favorable conditions. For protozoa that multiply by sexual reproduction, a zygote is formed from the fusion of 2 gametes. Encystation of a zygote produces an oocyst that may contain 2 or more sporocysts, each with its own cyst wall. Sporocysts contain sporozoites, infective forms of the organism.

The intestinal protozoa are divided into 5 main groups that differ in terms of epidemiology and clinical presentation. Several of the groups contain pathogenic as well as nonpathogenic species. Although the latter do not require treatment, their presence indicates that the individual has been exposed to oral–fecal contamination.

- **Flagellates:** Pathogenic species include *Giardia lamblia* and *Dientamoeba fragilis*. *Giardia* is the most common intestinal parasite in the United States. Sources of infection include ingestion of contaminated water and person-to-person transmission in daycare centers. *Giardia* can cause diarrhea, abdominal cramps, bloating and flatulence. Symptoms often persist for more than 1 week.
- **Amebas:** *Entamoeba histolytica* is a major cause of intestinal infections worldwide, particularly in tropical areas with limited sanitation facilities. Most infections in the United States are acquired elsewhere. Clinical manifestations range from asymptomatic colonization to diarrhea, amebic colitis/dysentery, or extraintestinal abscess formation (usually in the liver). The diagnosis of amebiasis is complicated by the fact that *E. histolytica* is morphologically indistinguishable from the nonpathogenic *E. dispar*. Other nonpathogenic amebas include *E. coli* and *Endolimax nana*.
- **Coccidia:** Human pathogens include *Cryptosporidium* spp., *Cyclospora* spp., and *Isospora belli*. These organisms are members of the apicomplexans family and are related to the tissue parasites *T. gondii* and *Plasmodium* spp. *Cryptosporidium* spp. are a relatively common cause of infection in the United States. Outbreaks have been caused by contamination of drinking water or recreational water such as pools or water parks. *Cryptosporidium* usually causes a self-limited diarrhea in immunocompetent hosts, but it can cause severe persistent diarrhea in AIDS patients. *Cyclospora* spp. have caused outbreaks linked to imported food, such as raspberries. *Isospora* infections are usually only diagnosed in immunosuppressed patients.
- **Ciliates:** *Balantidium coli* is the only pathogenic ciliate.
- **Microsporidia:** Although these organisms are included in the section on protozoans, recent phylogenetic analysis indicates that they are more closely related to the fungi. *Enterocytozoon bienusi* causes self-limited diarrhea in normal hosts and chronic diarrhea in AIDS patients in whom it can also spread to the biliary tract. *Encephalitozoon* spp. can cause diarrhea and a variety of extraintestinal infections in immunosuppressed hosts.

Diagnosis

Most intestinal protozoa are detected by examination of stained stool specimens. Sensitive immunoassays are available for detecting antigens produced by *Giardia* and *Cryptosporidium*. Serology can be useful for diagnosing invasive *E. histolytica* since *E. dispar* does not trigger an antibody response. **Table 5–31** describes infections produced by selected pathogenic protozoa. Protozoal infections are commonly found within the gastrointestinal tract but, as noted in the table, many other organs and tissues can be infected.

Intestinal Helminth Infections

Description

Helminth (worm) infections in humans constitute a significant percentage of the global burden of illness caused by infectious diseases. The helminths are multicellular organisms that are divided into 3 groups: round worms (nematodes), tapeworms (cestodes), and flukes (trematodes). Helminths are typically enclosed by a protective coat, inside of which may be differentiated organ systems for digestion, neuromuscular control, and reproduction. Many helminths have complex

The intestinal protozoa are divided into 5 main groups that differ in terms of epidemiology and clinical presentation. Most intestinal protozoa are detected by examination of stained stool specimens.

TABLE 5-31   Evaluation for Protozoal Infections

Pathogen	Clinical Findings	Histopathology and Radiology	Microbiology	Comments
Microsporidia				
Encephalitozoon and *Enterocytozoon*: microsporidiosis	Chronic, watery diarrhea; dehydration, weight loss, fever, abdominal pain, and vomiting	Spores are visible in duodenal or biliary aspirates, or within enterocytes in small intestinal biopsies; electron microscopy may be helpful	Chromotrope-based staining of stool specimens may be used to detect spores	D-Xylose and fat malabsorption are common; serologic tests are not useful
Amoebae				
Entamoeba histolytica	Infection may be asymptomatic or present as acute amebic or fulminant colitis with bloody diarrhea	Cysts or trophozoites may be demonstrated in colonic scrapings or biopsies; if amebic liver abscess is suspected, abdominal imaging by ultrasound or CT scan should be performed	Cysts or trophozoites may be visible in stool specimens	Serologic tests may be used in detection of an amebic liver abscess or intestinal amebiasis
Naegleria fowleri	Causes primary meningoencephalitis with abrupt onset of headaches, fever, nausea, vomiting, and pharyngitis; may be rapidly progressive	Brain biopsy not routinely recommended because CSF yields organisms, even though brain biopsy also may reveal organisms	Fresh CSF examination (wet mount) for motile trophozoites; may be Giemsa-stained; brain biopsies may be cultured	Purulent CSF with no bacteria is common; children or young adults exposed to fresh water are at risk
Acanthamoeba	Causes keratitis with ocular pain and corneal ulceration; also causes granulomatous amebic encephalitis (GAE)	Corneal biopsies may reveal organisms in patients with keratitis; brain or skin biopsy of nodules or ulcers required for diagnosis of GAE	Giemsa, Gram, or calcofluor-stained smears of corneal scrapings may reveal amoebae; culture of organisms from corneal scrapings or brain tissue is possible	Organism is not isolated from CSF; keratitis can be subacute or chronic and is often associated with soft contact lens use
Ciliates				
Balantidium coli	Infection may be asymptomatic or may cause severe diarrhea or dysentery; diarrhea may persist for weeks to months prior to development of dysentery	*B. coli* can invade the colonic mucosa, with consequent ulcer formation; in such cases, the organism is visible on histologic section	Wet preparation examination of fresh concentrated stool will demonstrate the trophozoite and cyst forms; the organisms are large and frequently can be seen under low magnification	These organisms do not stain well, making recognition and identification on a permanent stained smear very difficult
Flagellates				
Giardia lamblia	Acute or chronic watery diarrhea; nausea, anorexia, low-grade fever, and chills	Trophozoites may be identified by endoscopic brush cytology, mucosal smears, or histopathologic examination of small intestinal biopsy	Cysts or trophozoites may be visible in stool specimens; direct antigen detection is also useful	
Leishmania: cutaneous and mucosal leishmaniasis	Erythematous papules, nodules, or ulcers; regional lymphadenopathy and fever	Identification of organisms in touch preparations and sections of skin biopsy specimens	Organisms from skin biopsy specimens may be cultured in liquid media	Serum antibody titers are not useful

Continued next page—

TABLE 5-31 Evaluation for Protozoal Infections (continued)

Pathogen	Clinical Findings	Histopathology and Radiology	Microbiology	Comments
Leishmania: visceral leishmaniasis (kala-azar)	Fever, malaise, weight loss, hepatomegaly, splenomegaly	Fine needle aspiration of the spleen for touch preparation and culture is >96% sensitive; organisms may be visible in bone marrow aspirates	Specimens obtained by fine needle aspiration of spleen, liver, and bone marrow may be cultured	High serum antibody titers are present in immunocompetent persons with visceral leishmaniasis
Trichomonas vaginalis	Vaginitis with excessive discharge, dysuria, and dyspareunia	Visible on pap smear; histopathologic evaluation has no established role in the diagnosis of trichomonal infections	Trichomonads may be observed in wet mounts of vaginal secretions (60% sensitivity); endocervical or urethral cultures are most sensitive (exceed 90% sensitivity)	Abundant neutrophils are present in vaginal wet mounts; serologic tests are not useful and lack sensitivity and specificity
Trypanosomiasis, African (sleeping sickness caused by *Trypanosoma brucei*)	Chancre, intermittent fevers, lymphadenopathy, pruritic rash, and meningoencephalitis	Histopathologic evaluation lacks sensitivity	Trypomastigotes visible in peripheral blood smears, chancre fluid, lymph node or bone marrow aspirates	WBCs in CSF and an elevated CSF IgM titer are useful for diagnosis of meningoencephalitis
Trypanosomiasis, American (Chagas disease caused by *Trypanosoma cruzi*)	Chronic illness highlighted by cardiac disease (cardiomyopathy) and embolic phenomena; lymphadenopathy and chagoma occur in acute disease	Histopathologic evaluation of heart or other tissues lacks sensitivity	In acute disease, parasites may be detected in peripheral blood or buffy coat smears; lymph node, bone marrow aspirates, pericardial fluid, or CSF also may be examined	IgG serologic tests are used to diagnose chronic Chagas disease; PCR-based detection using peripheral blood specimens is in development
Coccidia				
Cryplosporidium parvum and *C. hominis*	Watery, cholera-like diarrhea, abdominal pain, nausea, fever, and fatigue	Organisms may be visible in small intestine biopsies, though many infections may be missed due to sampling variation	Oocysts may be detected in concentrated specimens with acid-fast stain or DFA; direct fecal antigen tests may detect organism	Serologic tests are not useful
Cyclospora cayetanensis	Watery diarrhea and constipation, nausea, anorexia, abdominal cramping, and weight loss	Jejunal biopsy may show inflammation, villous atrophy, or crypt hyperplasia; organisms may be detected with acid-fast stain	Oocysts are visible in fresh stool; variable appearance with acid-fast stain of stool specimen; oocysts show blue-green autofluorescence when excited at 365 nm	Serologic tests are not available
Isospora belli	Profuse, watery diarrhea; abdominal pain, cramping, weight loss, and low-grade fever; may be especially severe in HIV-infected patients	Intestinal biopsies may reveal organisms in sections	Oocysts are visible in wet smears of fresh or preserved stool; oocysts stain red with acid-fast stain	Serologic tests are not available
Toxoplasma gondii	Lymphadenopathy or mononucleosis-like syndrome in immunocompetent adults; encephalitis, pneumonitis, or chorioretinitis in immunosuppressed individuals; chorioretinitis and/or neurologic findings in congenital infections	Tachyzoites often visible in endomyocardial biopsies of heart transplant recipients; lymph node pathology is characteristic; brain biopsies lack sensitivity	Tachyzoites often visible in CSF, amniotic fluid, or bronchoalveolar lavage fluid; antigens from the organism may be detectable in the serum; PCR may identify *T. gondii* DNA in respiratory or amniotic specimens	Serologic tests remain the standard for diagnosis to determine recent vs chronic infection; however, serologic studies lack sensitivity in immunocompromised patients

CSF, cerebrospinal fluid; CT, computed tomography; PCR polymerase chain reaction; DFA, direct fluorescent antibody life cycles that involve 2 or more hosts. Helminths develop into adult worms and/or undergo sexual reproduction in the definitive host, and they do not develop past the larval stage in intermediate hosts. Infections in humans usually result from ingestion of eggs, penetration of intact skin by infective larvae, or bites by insect vectors. Many helminth life cycles involve a stage in which the larvae migrate through tissue. This migration can be relatively asymptomatic but can also have serious clinical consequences depending on the type of helminth. These principles are illustrated by the following 2 examples.

The definitive host for *Echinococcus granulosis* (a tapeworm) is the dog, which harbors the adult tapeworm in its intestinal tract and excretes eggs in the feces. When an intermediate host, such as sheep or humans, ingests these eggs, the eggs hatch in the intestinal tract and larvae penetrate the intestinal wall and eventually form slowly expanding cysts in visceral organs such as the liver or lungs.

Strongyloides stercoralis is 1 of the several nematodes that are acquired when infective larvae present in warm moist soil penetrate human skin. The larvae migrate through tissue into the venous circulation and are transported to the lungs where they invade the alveoli, are coughed up and swallowed, and then develop into mature worms in the intestinal tract. The adult worms produce larva that are shed in feces into the environment where they can complete their life cycle. Unlike other nematodes, however, *S. stercoralis* larvae can also penetrate the gut wall or perianal skin and initiate an autoinfective cycle that results in persistent low-level infection even after the host has left an endemic area. If an infected patient subsequently receives immunosuppressive therapy, particularly with corticosteroids, the patient can develop life-threatening *Strongyloides* hyperinfection syndrome in which nematode larvae migrate into the lungs and extraintestinal tissues.

Diagnosis

Infections with intestinal helminths are usually diagnosed by detection of eggs or larvae in feces. For many of the helminths, the identification of the organism is based on the morphologic characteristics of the organism and/or the eggs. These characteristics include size, shape, and thickness of the egg wall, special structures such as knobs and spines, and the developmental stage of the egg contents (e.g., undeveloped, developing, or embryonated).

Important information in the evaluation of a patient infected with helminths includes a history of possible exposure to the organism. Eosinophilia is commonly observed in patients with helminth infections due to larval migration through tissues. The clinical findings, mode of transmission to humans, aspects of microbiologic and serologic testing, and relevant radiologic findings for selected helminth infections are presented in **Table 5–32**.

Food Poisoning

Nausea and vomiting that occurs 1 to 8 hours after eating can be caused by ingestion of bacterial toxins that are already present in the food rather than by infection of the intestinal tract. The most common causes are enterotoxins produced by *S. aureus* (found in contaminated dairy and bakery products) and *Bacillus cereus* (found in reheated fried rice). The condition is self-limited. *C. perfringens* food poisoning results from the ingestion of food containing at least 10^8 enterotoxin-producing organisms. Often these are foods that have become grossly contaminated from storage over long periods at ambient temperature. This is particularly true of animal protein foods, such as cooked meats and gravies. Most individuals experience watery diarrhea with abdominal cramps (*B. cereus* can cause a similar syndrome). Fatalities are extremely rare, with spontaneous resolution of symptoms within 6 to 24 hours.

Botulism
Description

Botulism is a neuroparalytic disease produced by potent toxins derived from *Clostridium botulinum*. The toxins block the release of the neurotransmitter acetylcholine at peripheral cholinergic synapses. The most common cause of botulism in humans is ingestion of preformed toxins in food contaminated with *C. botulinum*. Food products identified as sources of outbreaks include home-canned vegetable products, fish products preserved by a variety of methods, and sausage

TABLE 5-32 Evaluation for Helminth Infections of the Gastrointestinal Tract

Pathogen	Clinical Findings	Mode of Transmission to Humans	Microbiology and Serology Testing	Radiology
Tapeworms *(Cestodes)*				
Diphyllobothrium latum (fish tapeworm)	Diarrhea and abdominal pain; intestinal obstruction, vitamin B_{12} deficiency, and pernicious anemia	Ingestion of cysts in freshwater fish	Characteristic operculate eggs or proglottids (segments of the organism) may be present in examination of feces	Radiograph contrast studies of intestine may reveal intraluminal filling defect
Echinococcus granulosus and *Echinococcus multilocularis*	Abdominal pain with hepatomegaly; confusion and headaches if CNS is involved	Ingestion of eggs; often hand-to-mouth transmission after contact with an infected surface	Serologic tests available to assess exposure	Cysts in tissue such as liver, lung, or brain may be visible by radiograph, ultrasound, or CT scan
Taenia saginata (beef tapeworm)	Abdominal discomfort, diarrhea, and intestinal obstruction	Ingestion of the organisms in contaminated beef	Spherical eggs or gravid proglottids (segments of the organism) often present in feces	Not useful
Taenia solium (pork tapeworm)	Subcutaneous nodules, headaches, generalized seizures if CNS is involved; higher incidence in Central American immigrants	Ingestion of cysts in infected pork or ingestion of eggs (shed by human carrier)	Proglottids (segments of the organism) may be visible in stool	Cystic lesions with tissue displacement may be visible on head CT or MRI scan
Roundworms *(nematodes)*				
Ascaris lumbricoides	Loeffler syndrome (simple pulmonary eosinophilia) in lungs with dyspnea, cough, and rales; eosinophilia in blood; intestinal obstruction or obstructive jaundice	Ingestion of embryonated eggs; often hand-to-mouth transmission after contact with contaminated soil or surface	Ovoid eggs usually present in examination of feces; developing or adult worms may be present in feces	Transient, shifting infiltrates may be visible in Loeffler syndrome patients by chest radiograph
Enterobius vermicularis (pinworm)	Usually children are infected; perianal and perineal pruritus	Ingestion of eggs; often hand-to-mouth transmission after scratching perianal area or contact with contaminated surface; infection also may occur by inhalation of airborne eggs in dust or by retroinfection through the anus	Cellulose tape test performed in which tape adheres to eggs in perianal folds; eggs transferred to slide for microscopy; anal swabs also useful	Not useful
Filariae (*Wuchereria bancrofti* for elephantiasis and *Onchocerca volvulus* for onchocerciasis)	Elephantiasis (lymphatic filariasis)—lower extremity swelling and fevers; Oonchocerciasis (river blindness)—cutaneous nodules and blindness	Injection of larvae—during mosquito bite for *Wuchereria* bancrofti and during black fly bite for *Onchocerca* volvulus	Microfilariae may be visible in thick peripheral blood smears; skin specimens may reveal microfilariae	Not useful
Hookworms (*Ancylostoma duodenale* and *Necator americanus*)	Intense pruritus, vesicular rash, Loeffler-like syndrome, abdominal pain, bloody diarrhea, and iron deficiency anemia	Skin penetration by larvae, often through the feet in contact with contaminated soil	Partially embryonated eggs present in feces; larvae may be present in feces	Not useful

Continued next page—

TABLE 5–32 **Evaluation for Helminth Infections of the Gastrointestinal Tract (continued)**

Pathogen	Clinical Findings	Mode of Transmission to Humans	Microbiology and Serology Testing	Radiology
Strongyloides stercoralis	Chronic infection-abdominal pain, intermittent urticarial rash, peripheral blood eosinophilia; Hyperinfection (immunosuppressed patient)-colitis, abdominal distention, respiratory distress, shock	Larvae penetration of skin or colon; organism persists due to autoinfective cycle	First-stage larvae are often visible in feces; larvae may be present in sputum or duodenal aspirates	Radiograph contrast studies of intestine may reveal duodenal edema, ulcers, or strictures; miliary nodules or reticular opacities may be present on chest radiograph
Trichinella spiralis	Gastroenteritis, fever, eosinophilia, myositis, and circumorbital edema following ingestion of raw pork or raw bear meat (trichinosis)	Ingestion of larvae in contaminated meat products	Larvae may be detected in sediment from digested muscle tissue; antibodies to organism may be detected with serologic tests	Not useful
Trichuris trichiura (whip-worm)	Diarrhea, dysentery, and abdominal cramping; rectal prolapse may occur	Ingestion of embryonated eggs through hands, food, or drink contaminated by contact with infected soil or surfaces	Barrel-shaped eggs visible in feces	Not useful
Flukes (trematodes)				
Fasciolopsis buski (intestinal fluke)	Abdominal discomfort; travel or residence in Asia	Ingestion of metacercariae (larval form of organism) in aquatic plants	Ellipsoidal eggs in feces or bile	Not useful
Liver flukes (Fasciola hepatica and Clonorchis sinensis)	Hepatomegaly, cholangitis, hepatitis; F. hepatica is worldwide; C. sinensis more common in Southeast Asian immigrants	Ingestion of metacercariae (larval form of organism) in aquatic plants (for F. hepatica) and in freshwater fish (for C. sinensis)	Ellipsoid or ovoid eggs present in feces	With F hepatica, hepatic nodules or linear tracks may be visible by CT scan
Paragonimus westermani (lung fluke)	Cough with brownish sputum, intermittent hemoptysis, pleuritic chest pain, and eosinophilia	Ingestion of metacercariae (larval form of organism) in crayfish or freshwater crabs	Ovoid eggs are present in feces and, less commonly, in sputum	Characteristic pulmonary findings by radiograph and CT scan
Schistosoma haematobium (blood fluke)	Hematuria, granulomatous disease of the bladder, bladder carcinoma, and secondary bacterial urinary tract infections	Penetration of intact human skin by cercariae (larval form of organism), often during bathing, swimming, or washing clothes in contaminated water	Eggs often visible in microscopic examination of the urine	Obstruction, hydronephrosis, or filling defects may be observed by renal ultrasonography or intravenous pyelography
Schistosoma japonicum (blood fluke)	Nausea, vomiting, hemoptysis, melena, hepatosplenomegaly, portal hypertension, and esophageal varices	Penetration of intact human skin by cercariae (larval form of organism) often during bathing, swimming, or washing clothes in contaminated water	Round to ovoid eggs in feces	Not useful
Schistosoma mansoni (blood fluke)	Nausea, vomiting, hemoptysis, melena, hepatosplenomegaly, portal hypertension, and esophageal varices	Penetration of intact human skin by cercariae (larval form of organism) often during bathing, swimming, or washing clothes in contaminated water	Lateral-spined eggs in feces that may be bloody or mucus-laden	Not useful

CNS, central nervous system; CT, computed tomography; MRI, magnetic resonance imaging.

TABLE 5–33   Laboratory Evaluation for Botulism

Laboratory Test	Positive Result
Mouse bioassay	This is the reference method for the detection of botulinum toxin; aliquots of serum, feces, food extract, gastric fluid, or culture supernatant are injected intraperitoneally into mice; control mice are injected with aliquots of the various samples containing botulinum antitoxin; the mice are observed for the toxic effects of the botulism toxin; if the mice receiving the botulinum antitoxin do not develop signs of botulism and the mice not receiving the antitoxin do develop signs, the diagnosis is established
Bacterial culture	The organism can be cultured anaerobically; the isolates must be shown to contain toxins by the bioassay
Enzyme immunoassays	Assays are now available for detecting the neurotoxins elaborated by *Clostridium botulinum*, though the sensitivity is lower than the mouse bioassay

and ham preserved by salting rather than heating and then consumed without cooking. Infant botulism, which affects children up to 35 weeks of age only, is a result of colonization of the intestinal tract by *C. botulinum* after the ingestion of viable spores. Wound botulism can occur when *C. botulinum* contaminates deep wounds and secretes the toxin.

Patients suffering from botulism typically present with muscle weakness, difficulty in speaking and swallowing, and blurred vision. Such patients can progress to symmetric descending weakness and paralysis that can affect the diaphragm. Constipation, nausea and vomiting, and abdominal cramping are also common presentations. Botulism toxin can be neutralized by antisera raised against it, but the use of antitoxin may not reverse existing neuroparalysis. Recently there has been concern about the potential use of botulinum toxin as a bioweapon.

Diagnosis

The laboratory confirmation of human botulism is established by detection of the toxin in the serum or stool of an affected patient or in a sample of food consumed prior to onset of the illness. These assays are only available in public health laboratories. Animal assays are still used because they can detect very low levels of toxin. Isolation of *C. botulinum* from stools, gastric samples, or wound specimens, in combination with the appropriate clinical signs and symptoms for botulism, also establishes the diagnosis. For wound botulism, both serum and wound specimens should be tested for the presence of toxin and organisms. For infant botulism, stool samples are required for analysis.

The laboratory diagnosis is described in **Table 5–33**.

PYELONEPHRITIS AND URINARY TRACT INFECTIONS

Description

UTIs can be divided into 3 categories:

- uncomplicated infections of the lower urinary tract involving the bladder and/or urethra
- uncomplicated infections of the upper urinary tract, or pyelonephritis, involving the ureters, renal pelvis, and kidney
- complicated UTIs involving various sites within the urinary tract

Acute symptomatic uncomplicated lower UTIs are common in women. The typical symptoms are painful urination (dysuria), urgency, and frequency. Approximately 80% of these infections are caused by *E. coli*. Uropathogenic *E. coli* are genetically distinct from other intestinal strains and possess virulence factors that facilitate colonization of the urinary tract epithelium. Other enteric gram-negative rods, such as *Proteus* spp. and *Klebsiella* spp., and gram-positive cocci including *Staphylococcus saprophyticus* and enterococci can cause uncomplicated UTIs. The high incidence of UTIs in women is probably due to the relatively short length of the urethra

Acute symptomatic uncomplicated lower UTIs are common in women. The typical symptoms are painful urination (dysuria), urgency, and frequency. Approximately 80% of these infections are caused by *E. coli*.

TABLE 5–34   Evaluation for Urinary Tract Infection (UTI)

Laboratory Test/Clinical Feature	Uncomplicated Lower Urinary Tract Infection	Uncomplicated Pyelonephritis	Complicated Urinary Tract Infection
Site of infection	Bladder and urethra	Ureters, renal pelvis, and kidney	Varies
Risk factors	Intercourse and diaphragm/spermicide use	Includes risk factors for both uncomplicated lower UTI and complicated UTI	Structural or functional abnormalities in the urinary tract
Symptoms	Frequency, urgency, and dysuria	Frequency, urgency, dysuria, flank pain, and fever	Depends on the site of infection
Level of pyuria	>5 WBC per high-power field using a fresh urine specimen or a positive leukocyte esterase dipstick test result	>5 WBC per high-power field using a fresh urine specimen or a positive leukocyte esterase dipstick test result	>5 WBC per high-power field using a fresh urine specimen or a positive leukocyte esterase dipstick test result
Level of bacteriuria (CFU)	For women without symptoms, >10^5 CFU/mL on 2 consecutive specimens; for women with symptoms, ≥10^2 CFU/mL; for men with symptoms, >10^3 CFU/mL	>10^4 CFU/mL	≥10^5 CFU/mL

CFU, colony-forming unit.

and its proximity to the anus and the genital tract. Risk factors for uncomplicated lower UTI in young, sexually active women include intercourse and diaphragm and spermicide use. UTIs are uncommon in men until after the age of 50 years. UTIs in children are also more common in females. They can be associated with constipation, incomplete or infrequent voiding, sexual abuse, and anatomic defects within the urinary tract.

Acute uncomplicated pyelonephritis (upper UTI) is usually due to an ascending infection that begins in the bladder. The main clinical features are fever and chills, nausea, vomiting, and abdominal pain. Costovertebral angle tenderness is usually present. The majority of these infections are caused by *E. coli*. Risk factors for pyelonephritis include the presence of renal stones, obstruction of urine outflow, vesicoureteral reflux, pregnancy, anatomic abnormalities of the kidney and urinary tract, and urinary catheterization. Intrarenal infections are often the result of hematogenous dissemination of *S. aureus* or *Candida* spp.

Complicated UTI refers to infections in patients with a variety of underlying conditions such as anatomic or functional urologic abnormalities, stones, or obstruction. Imaging studies are often useful for identifying the underlying problem. Other predisposing factors are indwelling catheters or urologic instrumentation, immunosuppression, renal disease, and diabetes. These infections are typically caused by hospital-acquired bacteria including *Klebsiella* spp., *Proteus* spp., *Morganella morganii*, *P. aeruginosa*, enterococci, staphylococci, and yeast.

Asymptomatic bacteriuria occurs in 3% of women; of these, 10% will develop UTIs. A higher incidence of UTIs is found in the elderly population where 10% to 15% of women older than 60 years suffer from recurrent UTIs.

> The laboratory diagnosis of a UTI involves tests to detect WBCs in the urine (pyuria) and tests to detect bacteria in the urine (bacteriuria).

Diagnosis

The laboratory diagnosis of a UTI involves tests to detect WBCs in the urine (pyuria) and tests to detect bacteria in the urine (bacteriuria).

Rapid detection of WBCs and bacteria in the urine can be performed using a urine dipstick. The WBCs are detected with a dipstick pad containing leukocyte esterase reagents and some bacteria can be detected by their ability to convert nitrate to nitrite (see Chapter 18 for a discussion of urinalysis). WBCs and bacteria also can be identified and counted in a microscopic analysis of the urine. A urine WBC count of >5 leukocytes per high-power field is defined by most authors as significant pyuria. The level of bacteriuria in the 3 categories of UTIs varies.

Urine culture is the gold standard for the diagnosis of UTIs, although it may not be necessary for uncomplicated outpatient UTIs. Unlike most other specimen types, urine is always cultured using a quantitative procedure because interpretation of the results depends on both the type and

TABLE 5–35   Infections of the Male Genital Tract

Site of Infection	Common Causative Organisms
Seminal vesicles	Gram-negative bacilli and *Neisseria gonorrhoeae*
Epididymis	Chlamydia, gram-negative bacilli, *N. gonorrhoeae, Mycobacterium tuberculosis*
Prostate gland	Gram-negative bacilli, enterococci (and staphylococci), and *N. gonorrhoeae*

TABLE 5–36   Laboratory Evaluation for Mumps

Laboratory Tests	Results/Comments
Serology	A positive mumps IgM assay is useful for diagnosis of acute mumps infection. Measurement of a mumps IgG seroconversion (from negative to positive) in acute and convalescent specimens or a 4-fold rise in mumps IgG titer also supports the diagnosis
PCR	RT-PCR is useful for detecting viral RNA in oropharyngeal secretions (e.g., parotid duct fluid), urine, and CSF
Culture	Mumps virus grows slowly; it can be isolated from oropharyngeal secretions, urine, and CSF. Typing of viral isolates is important for epidemiologic studies

the number of organisms in the specimen. Because urine passes through the distal urethra, which is colonized with a variety of gram-negative rods and other organisms, isolation of bacteria from a midstream clean catch urine specimen does not automatically establish the presence of infection. Significant bacteriuria is often defined as the presence of $\geq 10^5$ colony-forming units (CFU)/mL; however, many patients with a urethral syndrome can have lower counts. The presence of 3 or more organisms with none predominating indicates contamination, and a new specimen should be collected. Rapid specimen transport and refrigeration of stored specimens is important because bacteria can replicate in urine that is left at room temperature, unless a preservative is used, leading to overgrowth of contaminants and inaccurate colony counts. A summary of the laboratory evaluation for UTI is presented in **Table 5–34**.

INFECTIONS OF THE MALE GENITAL TRACT

Description and Diagnosis

Epididymitis is most often caused by a sexually transmitted disease such as gonorrhea or *Chlamydia* infection (discussed in a later section). However, it can also be caused by enteric gram-negative rods or *Pseudomonas* in patients with underlying urinary tract disease.

Acute bacterial prostatitis presents with urinary tract symptoms, a tender prostate, and is often accompanied by systemic findings such as fever. Chronic infection of the prostate due to gram-negative rods or gram-positive cocci is often asymptomatic, but it can serve as a source of recurrent symptomatic bacteriuria. Chronic pelvic pain syndromes have also been attributed to chronic prostatitis, but often the etiology is unclear. Granulomatous prostatitis caused by extrapulmonary TB or systemic fungal infections produces nodular lesions that can mimic prostatic carcinoma. Histologic examination of a biopsy specimen would distinguish these possibilities. **Table 5–35** provides an association between site of infection in the male genital tract and common causative organisms.

The most common infection of the testicle is viral orchitis that is usually caused by mumps or Coxsackie viruses. Mumps is an acute viral disease that causes painful enlargement of the salivary glands, particularly the parotid glands. The virus is transmitted via respiratory droplets. Orchitis in postpubertal males is often due to mumps, although the incidence is low due to vaccination. Laboratory diagnosis is important for epidemiologic investigations. The laboratory tests for mumps are summarized in **Table 5–36**.

The most common infection of the testicle is viral orchitis that is usually caused by mumps or Coxsackie viruses.

TABLE 5–37   Infections of the Female Genital Tract

Disease/Condition	Common Etiologic Agent(s)	Clinical Features	Laboratory Diagnosis
Vulvovaginitis	*Candida albicans, Trichomonas vaginalis*	Pruritus, irritation, external dysuria, vaginal discharge (especially with *T. vaginalis*)	Microscopy after treating specimen with 10% KOH to reveal yeast and hyphal forms; wet mount to detect motile trichomonads; culture; nucleic acid detection
Vaginosis	Polymicrobial (multiple anaerobes and *Garderella vaginalis*)	Vaginal odor, vaginal discharge	Vaginal discharge pH > 4.5; "fishy" odor after addition of 10% KOH; "clue cells" (vaginal epithelial cells coated with coccobacilli) on wet mount; or Gram stain with decreased gram-positive rods and increased gram-negative or variable coccobacilli
Cervicitis, pelvic inflammatory disease (PID)	*Chlamydia trachomatis, Neisseria gonorrheae*	Cervicitis is often asymptomatic; PID is associated with lower abdominal pain, vaginal discharge, dysuria, and dyspareunia; long-term sequelae can include infertility and ectopic pregnancy	Culture or nucleic acid amplification of *N. gonorrheae* and *C. trachomatis* from cervical swab; nucleic acid amplification of urine also useful but less sensitive

INFECTIONS OF THE FEMALE GENITAL TRACT

Description and Diagnosis

Infections of the female genital tract include vaginitis, vaginosis, and cervicitis/pelvic inflammatory disease (infection of the uterus, fallopian tubes, and adjacent structures). As with infections of the male genital tract, many of these infections are due to sexually transmitted diseases that are discussed in a later section.

The primary symptom of vaginitis is pruritus that can be accompanied by a discharge. The most common cause is the yeast *Candida albicans*. *Trichomonas vaginalis* (a protozoan) can cause a similar syndrome. The chief complaint in bacterial vaginosis is vaginal odor. In the past this condition was ascribed to overgrowth of *Gardnerella vaginalis*, but the current view is that it results from a disruption of the normal vaginal flora in which lactobacilli (gram-positive rods) are largely replaced by a mixture of gram-negative coccobacilli.

Table 5–37 briefly describes the etiologic agents, clinical features, and laboratory diagnosis of vaginitis, vaginosis, and pelvic inflammatory disease. Genital herpes and other sexually transmitted diseases are discussed in a subsequent section.

Organisms that infect or colonize the female genital tract can also cause infections of the newborn. Beta-hemolytic streptococci belonging to Lancefield group B (GBS) are also known as *S. agalactiae*. These organisms often asymptomatically colonize the gastrointestinal and female genital tracts; however, they are also an important cause of neonatal sepsis and meningitis (*E. coli* capular type K1 is another common cause of this type of infection). Risk factors associated with early onset neonatal infection include maternal colonization with GBS, premature rupture of membranes, chorioamnionitis, and previous delivery of an infected infant. Pregnant women are routinely screened during the third trimester at 35 to 37 weeks for colonization with GBS. This can be done by culture of vaginal and rectal swabs or nucleic acid amplification. Women who are colonized (or have the risk factors listed above) are given antibiotics during delivery to prevent neonatal infections. *Chlamydia trachomatis, Neisseria gonorrheae*, and *Herpes simplex* can also be transmitted to the newborn during delivery and cause serious infections.

SEXUALLY TRANSMITTED DISEASES

Syphilis

Description

Syphilis is a multisystem infectious disease that has prominent dermatologic and neurologic manifestations. It is caused by *Treponema pallidum*, a thin elongated bacterium known as a spirochete. *T. pallidum* is typically spread through contact with infectious lesions during sexual

The primary symptom of vaginitis is pruritus that can be accompanied by a discharge. The most common cause is the yeast Candida albicans. Trichomonas vaginalis (a protozoan) can cause a similar syndrome.

activity. Transmission occurs in about one-third of patients exposed to early syphilis. Primary skin lesions, also known as chancres, usually develop within 3 weeks after initial exposure. Primary syphilis is the stage defined by the presence of lesions at the site of inoculation. Secondary syphilis is the stage of hematogenous dissemination of *T. pallidum*, with widespread physical findings and constitutional signs and symptoms. The signs and symptoms include rash, alopecia, condylomata lata, and shallow painless ulcerations of mucous membranes known as "mucous patches." Even in the absence of treatment, the signs of primary and secondary syphilis spontaneously resolve, and patients enter a latent stage of infection. Manifestations of tertiary syphilis develop in approximately 30% of untreated patients after a variable period of latency. The manifestations of tertiary syphilis involve cardiovascular and/or neurologic and ophthalmic abnormalities. Neurologic involvement, however, is not limited to patients in the tertiary stage of the disease. The clinical manifestations of neurosyphilis include meningitis, general paresis, and tabes dorsalis. Congenital syphilis can occur in newborns whose mothers have syphilis.

The number of cases of primary and secondary syphilis in the United States was relatively stable from the early 1960s to the mid-1980s with 20,000 to 30,000 cases per year. With the appearance of AIDS and the decline of public health programs, the number of cases of primary and secondary syphilis in the United States increased to more than 50,000 by 1990; however, by 2000 it had declined by 80%. More recently there has been a gradual increase in the number of cases.

Diagnosis

T. pallidum organisms are too narrow to be visualized by standard light microscopy, but they can be seen by darkfield microscopy. This technique requires considerable expertise to distinguish *T. pallidum* from nonpathogenic treponemes and other artifacts, and currently it is rarely available.

T. pallidum cannot be cultured on microbiologic media. As a result, serologic testing is the most widely used approach for the diagnosis of syphilis. Two types of tests are routinely used. Nontreponemal screening tests for syphilis include the Venereal Disease Research Laboratory (VDRL) and rapid plasma reagin (RPR) tests. These assays detect antibodies that react with an antigen composed of cardiolipin and other lipids. A single reactive test requires supplemental historical, clinical, or laboratory information to provide a diagnosis of syphilis, as there are many biological causes of a false-positive VDRL or RPR.

Positive screening test results are routinely confirmed with more specific tests that detect antibodies that react with *T. pallidum* antigens (i.e., treponemal tests). The fluorescent treponemal antibody absorption test (FTA-ABS) uses indirect immunofluorescence to detect the binding of the patient's antibodies to *T. pallidum* organisms fixed onto a microscopic slide (the patient's serum is first preabsorbed with a nonpathogenic treponeme to increase the specificity of the test). The microhemagglutination assay for *T. pallidum* test (MHA-TP) measures the ability of serum antibodies to agglutinate RBCs that are coated with formalin-fixed *T. pallidum*. Because these assays are more expensive and/or technically demanding than the screening tests, they have traditionally been used to confirm a positive nontreponemal test rather than being used for initial evaluation. The introduction of high-throughput EIAs utilizing *T. pallidum* antigens has led to a reevaluation of the standard testing algorithm.

The treponemal tests are specific and sensitive, but they do not distinguish current infection from past infection. Although the nontreponemal tests are less specific, they are still very useful because changes in the antibody titer are used to monitor the response to therapy.

Diagnosis of syphilis in newborns is complicated by the fact that they can have substantial quantities of anti-treponemal IgG as a result of transfer of this IgG from the maternal circulation to the fetus. A serologic diagnosis of congenital syphilis in the neonate, therefore, can only be made if anti-treponemal IgM, made by the fetus, is found in the neonatal circulation.

The laboratory tests used in the diagnosis of primary, secondary, latent and tertiary, and congenital syphilis are shown in **Table 5–38**.

Gonorrhea

Description

Gonorrhea, an infection with the organism *Neisseria gonorrhoeae*, is a major cause of morbidity as a sexually transmitted disease, primarily because of complications of the initial infection. These complications include ascending pelvic infections in women, epididymo-orchitis in men,

T. pallidum cannot be cultured on microbiologic media. As a result, serologic testing is the most widely used approach for the diagnosis of syphilis. Nontreponemal screening tests for syphilis include the Venereal Disease Research Laboratory (VDRL) and rapid plasma reagin (RPR) tests. Positive screening test results are routinely confirmed with more specific tests that detect antibodies that react with *T. pallidum* antigens.

TABLE 5–38 **Evaluation of Syphilis**

Laboratory Test	Primary Syphilis	Secondary Syphilis	Latent and Tertiary Syphilis	Congenital Syphilis
Dark-field microscopy (from wet prep of exudate obtained directly from chancre or lesion)	In early primary stage, when other tests are less sensitive, this test is useful	If exudative secondary stage lesions are present, this test is useful	Exudative lesions are absent, so this test cannot be performed	Exudative lesions are absent, so this test cannot be performed
Rapid plasma reagin test (RPR)	Lag in nonspecific serological response results in markedly reduced sensitivity in primary syphilis	Rapid, inexpensive screening test; incidence of biological false-positivity ranges from 0.3% to 1%; positive results must be confirmed by other antitreponemal serology tests; useful for treatment follow-up by assessing titer of antibody	Screening test for both latent and tertiary stages; VDRL recommended over RPR to diagnose neurosyphilis when using a CSF specimen	Maternal IgG antibodies cross placenta, rendering test ineffective
Venereal Disease Research Laboratory test (VDRL)	Lag in nonspecific serological response results in markedly reduced sensitivity in primary syphilis	Rapid, inexpensive screening test; incidence of biological false-positivity ranges from 0.3% to 1%; positive results must be confirmed by antitreponemal serologies; useful for treatment follow-up by assessing titer of antibody	Screening test for both latent and tertiary stages; positive CSF VDRL (sensitivity 30%–70%) is sufficient to diagnose neurosyphilis, but negative CSF VDRL does not exclude diagnosis	Maternal IgG antibodies cross placenta, rendering test ineffective
Fluorescent treponemal antibody test with absorptions (FTA-ABS)	Used as a confirmatory diagnostic test or in lieu of RPR or VORL; sensitivity of 80%–85% in primary syphilis	Useful as a confirmatory diagnostic test in RPR- or VDRL-positive patients; overall sensitivity is approximately 98%; FTA-ABS test fails to distinguish syphilis from other treponematoses (such as yaws and pinta); this test is not useful to follow effectiveness of treatment	Useful as a confirmatory diagnostic test in RPR- or VDRL-positive patients; overall sensitivity is approximately 98%, but it is reduced in late latent phase	There is a useful modification of the standard test that detects only neonatal or infant IgM antitreponemal antibody, known as the IgM FTA-ABS assay
Microhemagglutination assay for *Treponema pallidum* (MHA-TP)	Useful as confirmatory diagnostic test or in lieu of RPR or VDRL; sensitivity of 80%–85% in primary syphilis	Useful as confirmatory diagnostic test in RPR- or VDRL-positive patients; does not distinguish syphilis from other treponematoses; not useful for treatment follow-up	Useful as confirmatory diagnostic test in RPR- or VDRL-positive patients; sensitivity reduced in late latent phase	Maternal antitreponemal IgG antibodies cross placenta, rendering test ineffective
Enzyme immunoassay for specific detection of anti-*T. pallidum* IgM	Useful as confirmatory diagnostic test, especially in untreated primary syphilis	Not useful because IgM level diminishes several weeks after infection	Not useful because serum IgM levels are negligible in latent and chronic infection	This test is useful for making the diagnosis, because, unlike IgG, maternal IgM does not cross the placenta
Enzyme immunoassay for specific detection of anti-*T. pallidum* IgG	Useful as confirmatory diagnostic test, confirmatory, especially in untreated primary syphilis	Useful as confirmatory diagnostic test, with sensitivity approaching 100% regardless of VDRL status	Useful as confirmatory diagnostic test, with sensitivity approaching 100% regardless of VORL status	Maternal antitreponemal IgG antibodies cross placenta, rendering test ineffective

TABLE 5-38   Evaluation of Syphilis (continued)

Laboratory Test	Primary Syphilis	Secondary Syphilis	Latent and Tertiary Syphilis	Congenital Syphilis
Western blot to detect anti-*T. pallidum* IgM	Useful as confirmatory diagnostic test especially in untreated primary syphilis; IgM becomes detectable 2 weeks after first chancre appears	Not useful because IgM level fades several weeks after infection	Not useful because serum IgM levels are negligible in latent and chronic infection	This test is useful in diagnosis, as maternal IgM does not cross the placenta
Western blot to detect total anti-*T. pallidum* IgG	May be useful as a confirmatory diagnostic test, though FTA-ABS and MHA-TP are simpler and more rapid	May be useful as a confirmatory diagnostic test in RPR- or VDRL-positive patients; overall sensitivity of approximately 90% and specificity of 100%	May be useful as a confirmatory diagnostic test in RPR- or VDRL-positive patients	Maternal antitreponemal IgG antibodies cross placenta, rendering test ineffective

and disseminated gonococcal infections in women and men. Infants born to untreated mothers can also develop ophthalmia neonatorum. The clinical symptoms of gonorrhea include dysuria, urethral and/or vaginal discharge, and pelvic pain. Gonorrhea is generally more symptomatic in men than in women. Clinical features include urethral discharge and mucopurulent cervicitis, respectively. Untreated asymptomatic individuals serve as a reservoir for *N. gonorrhoeae*. Transmission from males to females is more efficient than in the reverse direction. Pharyngeal infections of *N. gonorrhoeae* are typically asymptomatic.

The incidence of gonorrhea in the United States peaked in 1978 and declined approximately 75% through the late 1990s. Since then it has leveled off. Most cases are reported in men because they are more symptomatic than women. Individuals with gonorrhea have a high rate of other sexually transmitted diseases and therefore require complete screening. Ascending pelvic infections that occur in 10% to 20% of acutely infected women can result in infertility and ectopic pregnancy.

Diagnosis

The gold standard for diagnosis continues to be growth of the organism in culture. *N. gonorrhoeae* requires a nutrient-rich selective agar for successful culture and an incubation period of up to 48 hours for colony formation. Due to the fastidious nature of the organism, false-negative results frequently occur as a result of poor specimen handling and delayed transport. As a result of these limitations, nucleic acid amplification is now widely used to diagnose gonorrhea. These NAAT assays are as sensitive as culture when performed on cervical or male urethral swabs and provide rapid results. Several of the assays are also approved for use on urine, although the sensitivity is less for this type of specimen. These assays have high specificity but caution must be used when interpreting positive results in a low prevalence population. Culture is still recommended for nongenital sites. The samples collected for analysis depend on the site most likely to be infected and the sex of the patient (**Tables 5–39** and **5–40**).

> *N. gonorrhoeae* requires a nutrient-rich selective agar for successful culture and an incubation period of up to 48 hours for colony formation. Due to the fastidious nature of the organism, false-negative results frequently occur as a result of poor specimen handling and delayed transport.

Chlamydial Infections
Description

Chlamydiae are gram-negative, nonmotile, obligate intracellular bacteria. *C. trachomatis* is the most common cause of sexually transmitted disease in North America. It is also the agent of trachoma, a major cause of preventable blindness worldwide. *Chlamydophila pneumoniae* causes a respiratory infection that is similar to *Mycoplasma* infection. *C. psittaci*, which is common in certain birds and can be spread to humans via aerosolized feces, causes psittacosis, a respiratory and/or systemic infection.

C. trachomatis produces up to 4,000,000 infections each year in the United States as a sexually transmitted disease. Groups at increased risk for *C. trachomatis* infection include men or women who have had a new sexual partner or more than 1 sexual partner in the past year and sexually

TABLE 5–39 Sample Collection Site by Patient Type for *Neisseria gonorrhoeae*

Specimen	Patient
Urine[a]	Symptomatic (or at-risk) male or female
Urethral exudate	Symptomatic male
Urethral swab if no exudate can be expressed	Symptomatic male
Anorectal and pharyngeal swab	Male or female with rectal or pharyngeal exposure
Conjunctival swab	Infant with conjunctivitis
Blood and synovial fluid	Male or female patient presenting with arthritis and/or dermatitis and suspected of prior gonococcal infection
Swab from endocervical canal and possibly anal canal, urethra, and pharynx	Female suspected of infection

[a]For nucleic acid amplification, not culture.

TABLE 5–40 Evaluation for *Neisseria gonorrhoeae* Infection

Laboratory Test	Result/Comment
Gram stain and culture	Gram-negative kidney-bean-shaped diplococci (within neutrophils and extracellular) on Gram stain; the sensitivity of Gram stain smears for detection of gonorrhea varies from 40% to 95% depending on the patient and the site of collection
Culture of the organism	The gold standard method, usually requires 1–2 days to become positive; it is not 100% sensitive, especially when there are delays in specimen collection and transport
DNA probe tests	These tests provide rapid turnaround time because there is no need to grow the organism in culture; a disadvantage is the lack of an isolate for subsequent susceptibility testing; these tests have largely been supplanted by amplification which is more sensitive
DNA amplification tests	These tests provide direct detection of *N. gonorrhoeae* and/or *C. trachomatis* in clinical specimens using polymerase chain reaction (PCR), strand displacement amplification (SDA), or transcription mediated reaction (TMA); these tests provide rapid results but are costly; their major advantages are that they can be used with urine specimens and swab specimens, are the most sensitive assays available, and have a high specificity (≥98%)

active women using barrier contraceptive methods. Approximately one-third of infected males and half of infected females may have asymptomatic or mild infections. Subclinical infection and scarring of the fallopian tubes with subsequent infertility is 1 of the major complications of *Chlamydia* infections. *C. trachomatis* can also infect newborns during delivery and cause conjunctivitis and pneumonia. Lymphogranuloma venereum (LGV), a disease characterized by tender inguinal lymphadenopathy and often proctitis, is caused by specific serovars of *C. trachomatis*.

Diagnosis

Direct detection of chlamydial DNA using NAAT assays is now the preferred method for diagnosing genital *C. trachomatis* infections due to the high sensitivity and specificity of these assays. These tests use PCR, strand displacement amplification (SDA), or transcription-mediated amplification (TMA) to amplify *C. trachomatis* genes. They have largely replaced other nonculture methods such as antigen detection.

TABLE 5–41   Evaluation of the Patient for Chlamydial Infection

Laboratory Test	Chlamydia trachomatis	Chlamydia psittaci	Chlamydia pneumoniae
Culture of the organism	Organisms commonly require 48–72 hours to grow in cultured cells; the intracytoplasmic inclusions are best visualized with fluorescein-conjugated monoclonal antibodies	Organisms commonly require 5–10 days to grow in cultured cells; the intracytoplasmic inclusions are best visualized with fluorescent antibodies	Organisms are difficult to grow in cultured cells; in positive cultures, the intracytoplasmic inclusions are best visualized with fluorescent antibodies
Microscopic examination of stained smear from potentially infected site	Useful in the diagnosis of acute neonatal inclusion conjunctivitis (sensitivity >90%)	Not useful	Not useful
Direct immunofluorescence (DIF) of sample from potentially infected site	Test performed in minutes but the result is dependent on the skill of the person performing the assay; most useful for cervical and urethral specimens	Not specific for C. psittaci	Not specific for C. pneumoniae
Enzyme-linked immunoassay (EIA) using sample from potentially infected site	Less sensitive and less specific in cervical infections than the DIF test for detection of C. trachomatis; has generally been replaced by molecular methods	Cross-reactions with normal respiratory flora limit its utility	Cross-reactions with normal respiratory flora limit its utility
Serologic test using complement fixation (CF) technique	Not useful for the detection of trachoma, neonatal infections, inclusion conjunctivitis, and genital infections	Useful in the diagnosis of psittacosis if there is a 4-fold increase in titers between acute and convalescent serum samples	Useful in the diagnosis of primary infection if there is a 4-fold increase in titers between acute and convalescent serum samples
Serologic test using Immunofluorescence technique	Salpingitis and epididymitis often result in higher titers than superficial infections; women generally have higher titers than men	Useful in the diagnosis of psittacosis if there is a rising IgG titer	Method most often used in the diagnosis of C. pneumoniae infections; a 4-fold rise in titer, a single IgM titer of >1:16, or an IgG titer of >1:512 suggests infection
Nucleic acid probe assay	Commercial direct hybridization assay available for diagnosis of C. trachomatis; approximately as sensitive and specific as the best antigen detection methods; less sensitive than nucleic acid amplification	Commercial kits not available	Commercial kits not available
Nucleic acid amplification assays: polymerase chain reaction (PCR), strand displacement amplification (SDA), and transcription-mediated amplification (TMA)	Several commercial assays currently available for C. trachomatis detection; a major advantage is that these tests can be performed with urine specimens as well as swab specimens; these assays are more sensitive than the other methods	Commercial kits not available	Commercial assays available for C. pneumaniae (and Mycoplasma pneumoniae) from respiratory specimens, with the preferred specimen being a nasopharyngeal aspirate or throat swab; bronchoalveolar lavage and sputum specimens are also acceptable

Diagnosis of a chlamydial infection also can be made on the basis of a positive culture of the organism from infected sites. This requires cells in which the organism proliferates and is a labor-intensive procedure. Careful sample collection and specimen transport are important in the maintenance of viable organisms for culture. Although culture is less sensitive than NAAT assays, it is still used in medicolegal situations. Commercial NAAT assays may be positive in patients with LGV, but they do not distinguish specific LGV serovars nor are they currently approved for rectal specimens. Serologic tests for anti-*Chlamydia* antibodies involving complement fixation or immunofluorescence detect anti-chlamydial IgG or IgM in the serum and are sometimes used to support the diagnosis of LGV.

Table 5–41 summarizes the tests available to diagnose *Chlamydia* infections.

TABLE 5–42 **Evaluation for Herpes Simplex Viral Infection**

Laboratory Test	Positive Result
Viral culture	Viral culture continues to be the standard method for the diagnosis of mucocutaneous HSV infection; PCR has supplanted viral culture for the diagnosis of HSV infection in the central nervous system; the greatest likelihood for recovery of virus for culture is when a vesicular or pustular lesion is sampled within 72 hours of its appearance; a negative result for a culture does not rule out HSV infection and it may be necessary to take multiple cultures of many lesions before a diagnosis can be conclusively established
Smear with Tzanck preparation	Intranuclear inclusions and multinucleated giant cells in the Tzanck preparation support a diagnosis of HSV infection; the sensitivity of this test for HSV infection is approximately 65%, and, therefore, the diagnosis of HSV infection should be supported by the results of other tests; this assay cannot distinguish between HSV type 1, HSV type 2, and varicella zoster virus infections
Direct fluorescent antibody preparation	Direct fluorescent antibody staining of cells from skin lesions, when positive, provides rapid results; however, a negative result does not rule out infection; direct fluorescence assays can distinguish between HSV type 1 and HSV type 2
Serologic assay for antibodies to HSV	HSV-2 infection can be detected with type-specific enzyme immunoassays or immunoblots that detect antibodies to glycoprotein G; other serologic assays cannot distinguish HSV-1 and HSV-2; a negative result does not exclude HSV, particularly during a primary infection
Polymerase chain reaction	The PCR assay has become the gold standard for the diagnosis of encephalitis and meningitis from HSV infection because it is much more sensitive than culture for detection of virus; because HSV encephalitis in newborns responds to therapy if it is initiated early in the course of the disease, the diagnosis of HSV encephalitis by PCR using cerebrospinal fluid is particularly important; PCR is not useful for the routine diagnosis of cutaneous HSV lesions

HSV, herpes simplex virus; PCR, polymerase chain reaction.

Herpes Simplex Virus Infections

Description

Herpes Simplex Viruses can be subdivided into HSV type 1 and type 2. Oral herpes infections, which are typically present as cold sores, are primarily caused by HSV-1. Genital herpes infections are primarily caused by HSV-2.

HSV is a double-stranded DNA virus surrounded by a lipid envelope and is usually transmitted by person-to-person contact. The virus initially causes a productive infection of epithelial cells and then establishes a latent infection in sensory ganglia for the lifetime of the host. It can later reactivate and produce active infections. The classic pattern of infection is a group of recurring vesicles on an erythematous base; however, HSV infection is often asymptomatic, and lesions occur in a minority of infected patients. Individuals infected with HSV are potentially contagious, whether or not lesions are visible. HSVs can be subdivided into HSV type 1 and type 2. Oral herpes infections, which are typically present as cold sores, are primarily caused by HSV-1. Genital herpes infections are primarily caused by HSV-2. It is estimated that 50,000,000 individuals in the United States have genital HSV infection. Transmission of genital herpes occurs during sexual contact, which is not limited to intercourse. Genital HSV-2 infection is much more likely to recur and have asymptomatic virus shedding than HSV-1 infection. Neonatal herpes may be acquired when the infant comes into contact with HSV, typically through an infected birth canal (it can also be acquired from caregivers infected with HSV). Neonatal herpes can present as a severe disseminated infection predominantly affecting the liver and lungs, as a localized CNS infection, or as a skin and mucous membrane infection.

Diagnosis

The laboratory diagnosis of HSV depends on the type of infection and specimen (see **Table 5–42**). Viral culture of vesicle fluid is useful for patients who present with genital lesions. The presence of HSV-2 infection between recurrences can be confirmed by performing type-specific serologic tests that detect antibodies to glycoprotein G. PCR testing of CSF is superior to all other methods for the diagnosis of CNS HSV infections.

REFERENCES

Aguero-Rosenfeld ME, et al. Diagnosis of lyme borreliosis. *Clin Microbiol Rev.* 2005;18:484–509.

Allos BM. *Campylobacter jejuni* infections: update on emerging issues and trends. *Clin Infect Dis.* 2001;32:1201–1206.

Arnon SS, et al. Working Group on Civilian Biodefense. Botulinum toxin as a biological weapon: medical and public health management. *JAMA.* 2001;285:1059–1070.

Ashley RL. Performance and use of HSV type-specific serology test kits. *Herpes.* 2002;9:38–45.

Assi MA, et al. Systemic histoplasmosis: a 15-year retrospective institutional review of 111 patients. *Medicine (Baltimore).* 2007;86:162–169.

Baron EJ, et al. Prolonged incubation and extensive subculturing do not increase recovery of clinically significant microorganisms from standard automated blood cultures. *Clin Infect Dis.* 2005;41:1677–1680.

Bartlett JG. Clinical practice. Antibiotic-associated diarrhea. *N Engl J Med.* 2002;346:334–339.

Bauer TM, et al. Derivation and validation of guidelines for stool cultures for enteropathogenic bacteria other than *Clostridium difficile* in hospitalized adults. *JAMA.* 2001;285:313–319.

Baum S. Adenovirus. In: Mandell GL, Douglas RG, Bennett JE, Dolin R, eds. *Mandell, Douglas, and Bennett's Principles and Practice of Infectious Diseases.* 6th ed. New York: Elsevier/Churchill Livingstone; 2005:1835–1841.

Berbari EF, et al. Infective endocarditis due to unusual or fastidious microorganisms. *Mayo Clin Proc.* 1997;72:532–542.

Bisno AL, Stevens DL. Streptococcal infections of skin and soft tissues. *N Engl J Med.* 1996;334:240–245.

Bortolussi R. Listeriosis: a primer. *CMAJ.* 2008;179:795–797.

Boulware DR, et al. Maltreatment of *Strongyloides* infection: case series and worldwide physicians-in-training survey. *Am J Med.* 2007;120:545.e1–e8.

Brandt ME, Warnock DW. *Histoplasma, Blastomyces, Coccidioides,* and other dimorphic fungi causing systemic mycoses. In: Murray PR, Baron EJ, Jorgensen JH, Pfaller MA, Landry ML, eds. *Manual of Clinical Microbiology.* 9th ed. Washington, DC: ASM Press; 2007:1857–1873.

Bryant RE, Salmon CJ. Pleural empyema. *Clin Infect Dis.* 1996;22:747–762.

Centers for Disease Control and Prevention. Sexually transmitted diseases treatment guidelines, 2006. *MMWR.* 2006;55(No. RR-11):1–93.

Chapman AS, et al. Diagnosis and management of tickborne rickettsial diseases: Rocky Mountain spotted fever, ehrlichioses, and anaplasmosis—United States: a practical guide for physicians and other health-care and public health professionals. *MMWR Recomm Rep.* 2006;55:1–27.

Chon CH, et al. Pediatric urinary tract infections. *Pediatr Clin North Am.* 2001;48:1441–1459.

Cunha BA, et al. Acute infective endocarditis. Diagnostic and therapeutic approach. *Infect Dis Clin North Am.* 1996;10:811–834.

de Louvois J. Acute bacterial meningitis in the newborn. *J Antimicrob Chemother.* 1994;34(suppl A):61–73.

Didier ES, Weiss LM. Microsporidiosis: current status. *Curr Opin Infect Dis.* 2006;19:485–492.

Duff P. Maternal and perinatal infection. In: Gabbe SG, Niebyl JR, Simpson JL, eds. *Obstetrics: Normal & Problem Pregnancies.* 5th ed. New York, NY: Churchill Livingstone; 2007:1233–1248.

Dumler JS, et al. Ehrlichioses in humans: epidemiology, clinical presentation, diagnosis, and treatment. *Clin Infect Dis.* 2007;45:S45–S51.

Durand ML. Eye infections. In: Betts RF, Chapman SW, Penn RL, eds. *Reese and Betts' A Practical Approach to Infectious Diseases.* Philadelphia, PA: Lippincott Williams & Wilkins; 2003:222–250.

Edelstein PH, Cianciotto NP. *Legionella.* In: Mandell GL, Douglas RG, Bennett JE, Dolin R, eds. *Mandell, Douglas, and Bennett's Principles and Practice of Infectious Diseases.* 6th ed. New York: Elsevier/Churchill Livingstone, 2005:2711–2724.

Edwards MS, Baker CJ. *Streptococcus agalactiae* (group B streptococcus). In: Mandell GL, Douglas RG, Bennett JE, Dolin R, eds. *Mandell, Douglas, and Bennett's Principles and Practice of Infectious Diseases.* 6th ed. New York: Elsevier/Churchill Livingstone, 2005:2423–2434.

Enright AM, Prober CG. *Herpesviridae* infections in newborns: Varicella zoster virus, herpes simplex virus, and cytomegalovirus. *Pediatr Clin North Am.* 2004;51:889–908.

Espy MJ, et al. Real-time PCR in clinical microbiology: applications for routine laboratory testing. *Clin Microbiol Rev.* 2006;19:165–256.

Essig A. *Chlamydia* and *Chlamydophila.* In: Murray PR, Baron EJ, Jorgensen JH, Pfaller MA, Landry ML, eds. *Manual of Clinical Microbiology.* 9th ed. Washington, DC: ASM Press; 2007:1021–1035.

Farthing MJG. Giardiasis. *Gastroenterol Clin North Am.* 1996;25:493–515.

Fenollar F, Raoult D. Molecular diagnosis of bloodstream infections caused by non-cultivable bacteria. *Int J Antimicrob Agents.* 2007;30:7–15.

Fishman JA. Infection in solid-organ transplant recipients. *N Engl J Med.* 2007;357:2601–2614.

Fleming RV, et al. Emerging and less common fungal pathogens. *Infect Dis Clin North Am.* 2002;16:915–933.

Florin TA, et al. Beyond cat scratch disease: widening spectrum of *Bartonella henselae* infection. *Pediatrics.* 2008;121:e1413–e1425.

Fox JD. Nucleic acid amplification tests for detection of respiratory viruses. *J Clin Virol.* 2007;40(suppl 1): S15–S23.

Fraser IP, et al. Case records of the Massachusetts General Hospital. Case 32-2006. A 3-year-old girl with fever after a visit to Africa. *N Engl J Med.* 2006;355:1715–1722.

Fredricks DN, et al. Molecular identification of bacteria associated with bacterial vaginosis. *N Engl J Med.* 2005;353:1899–1911.

Freedman DO, et al. Spectrum of disease and relation to place of exposure among ill returned travelers. *N Engl J Med.* 2006;354:119–130.

García HH, et al; Cysticercosis Working Group in Peru. *Taenia solium* cysticercosis. *Lancet.* 2003;362: 547–556.

Gasquet S, et al. Bacillary angiomatosis in immunocompromised patients. *AIDS.* 1998;12:1793–1803.

Gea-Banacloche J, et al. West Nile virus: pathogenesis and therapeutic options. *Ann Intern Med.* 2004;140:545–553.

Glaser CA, et al. Beyond viruses: clinical profiles and etiologies associated with encephalitis. *Clin Infect Dis.* 2006;43:1565–1577.

Gradon JD. Space-occupying and life threatening infections of the head, neck and thorax. *Infect Dis Clin North Am.* 1996;10:857–878.

Gray LD, Fedorko DP. Laboratory diagnosis of bacterial meningitis. *Clin Microbiol Rev.* 1992;5:130–145.

Gupta R, et al. Genital herpes. *Lancet.* 2007;370:2127–2137.

Gwaltney JM. Clinical significance and pathogenesis of viral respiratory infections. *Am J Med.* 2002;112:13–18.

Hall CB. Respiratory syncytial virus and parainfluenza virus. *N Engl J Med.* 2001;344:1917–1928.

Hay RJ. Yeast infections. *Dermatol Clin.* 1996;14:113–124.

Heilpern KL, Lorber B. Focal intracranial infections. *Infect Dis Clin North Am.* 1996;10:879–898.

Herwaldt BL. *Cyclospora cayetanensis*: a review, focusing on the outbreaks of cyclosporiasis in the 1990s. *Clin Infect Dis.* 2000;31:1040–1057.

Hines J, Nachamkin I. Effective use of the clinical microbiology laboratory for diagnosing diarrheal diseases. *Clin Infect Dis.* 1996;23:1292–1301.

Ho M. The history of cytomegalovirus and its diseases. *Med Microbiol Immunol.* 2008;197:65–73.

Hurt C, Tammaro D. Diagnostic evaluation of mononucleosis-like illnesses. *Am J Med.* 2007;120:911. e1–911.e8.

Jarzembowski JA, Young MB. Nontuberculous mycobacterial infections. *Arch Pathol Lab Med.* 2008;132:1333–1341.

Johnson CC, et al. Peritonitis: update on pathophysiology, clinical manifestations, and management. *Clin Infect Dis.* 1997;24:1035–1045.

Johnson RT. Acute encephalitis. *Clin Infect Dis.* 1996;23:219–224.

Jones MK, McManus DP. Trematodes. In: Murray PR, Baron EJ, Jorgensen JH, Pfaller MA, Landry ML, eds. *Manual of Clinical Microbiology.* 9th ed. Washington, DC: ASM Press; 2007:2175–2187.

Kauffman C, et al. Clinical practice guidelines for the management of sporotrichosis: 2007 update by the Infectious Diseases Society of America. *Clin Infect Dis.* 2007;45:1255–1265.

Kelly CP, LaMont JT. *Clostridium difficile*—more difficult than ever. *N Engl J Med.* 2008;359:1932–1940.

Klein JO. Otitis media. *Clin Infect Dis.* 1994;19:823–832.

Krieger JN. Prostatitis, epididymitis, and orchitis. In: Mandell GL, Douglas RG, Bennett JE, Dolin R, eds. *Mandell, Douglas, and Bennett's Principles and Practice of Infectious Diseases.* 6th ed. New York: Elsevier/Churchill Livingstone, 2005:1381–1386.

Lalvani A. Diagnosing tuberculosis infection in the 21st century. *Chest.* 2007;131:1898–1906.

Lederman ER, Crum NF. A case series and focused review of nocardiosis: clinical and microbiologic aspects. *Medicine (Baltimore).* 2004;83:300–313.

Lednicky JA. Hantaviruses. a short review. *Arch Pathol Lab Med.* 2003;127:30–35.

Leeflang MM, et al. Galactomannan detection for invasive aspergillosis in immunocompromised patients. *Cochrane Database Syst Rev.* 4 2008:CD007394.

Li E, Stanley SL. Protozoa: amebiasis. *Gastroenterol Clin North Am.* 1996;25:471–492.

Linde A. Diagnosis of Epstein–Barr virus-related diseases. *Scand J Infect Dis Suppl.* 1996;100:83–88.

Lorber B. Gas gangrene and other *Clostridium*-associated diseases. In: Mandell GL, Douglas RG, Bennett JE, Dolin R, eds. *Mandell, Douglas, and Bennett's Principles and Practice of Infectious Diseases.* 6th ed. New York: Elsevier/Churchill Livingstone, 2005:2828–2838.

Mahmoud AA. Strongyloidiasis. *Clin Infect Dis.* 1996;23:949–952.

Mandell LA, et al.; Infectious Diseases Society of America; American Thoracic Society. Infectious Diseases Society of America/American Thoracic Society consensus guidelines on the management of community-acquired pneumonia in adults. *Clin Infect Dis.* 2007;44(suppl 2):S27–S72.

Marshall MM, et al. Waterborne protozoan pathogens. *Clin Microbiol Rev.* 1997;10:67–85.

McClean KL, Sheehan GJ, Harding GK. Intraabdominal infection: a review. *Clin Infect Dis.* 1994;19: 100–116.

McCormack WM. Pelvic inflammatory disease. *N Engl J Med.* 1994;330:115–119.

McPherson T, Nutman TB. Filarial nematodes. In: Murray PR, Baron EJ, Jorgensen JH, Pfaller MA, Landry ML, eds. *Manual of Clinical Microbiology.* 9th ed. Washington, DC: ASM Press; 2007:2156–2165.

Moran GJ, et al. Methicillin-resistant *S. aureus* infections among patients in the emergency department. *N Engl J Med.* 2006;355:666–674.

Murdoch DR, et al. Clinical presentation, etiology, and outcome of infective endocarditis in the 21st century: the International Collaboration on Endocarditis—prospective cohort study. *Arch Intern Med.* 2009;169:463–473.

Murray HW, et al. Advances in leishmaniasis. *Lancet.* 2005;366:1561–1577.

Naktin J, Beavis KG. *Yersinia enterocolitica* and *Yersinia pseudotuberculosis. Clin Lab Med.* 1999;19: 523–536.

Nataro JP, et al. *Escherichia, Shigella,* and *Salmonella.* In: Murray PR, Baron EJ, Jorgensen JH, Pfaller MA, Landry ML, eds. *Manual of Clinical Microbiology.* 9th ed. Washington, DC: ASM Press; 2007:670–687.

Ng VL, et al. Extrapulmonary pneumocystosis. *Clin Microbiol Rev.* 1997;10:401–418.

Pai M, et al. Systematic review: T-cell-based assays for the diagnosis of latent tuberculosis infection: an update. *Ann Intern Med.* 2008;149:177–184.

Perfect JR, Casadevall A. Cryptococcosis. *Infect Dis Clin North Am.* 2002;16:837–874.

Petric M, et al. Role of the laboratory in diagnosis of influenza during seasonal epidemics and potential pandemics. *J Infect Dis.* 2006;194(suppl 2):S98–S110.

Pioro MH, Mandell BF. Septic arthritis. *Rheum Dis Clin North Am.* 1997;23:239–258.

Queiroz-Telles F, et al. Subcutaneous mycoses. *Infect Dis Clin North Am.* 2003;17:59–85.

Ribes JA, Vanover-Sams CL, Baker DJ. Zygomycetes in human disease. *Clin Microbiol Rev.* 2000;13: 236–301.

Rick M, et al. *Plasmodium* species (malaria). In: Mandell GL, Douglas RG, Bennett JE, Dolin R, eds. *Mandell, Douglas, and Bennett's Principles and Practice of Infectious Diseases.* 6th ed. New York: Elsevier/Churchill Livingstone; 2005:3121–3144.

Rotbart HA. Enteroviral infections of the central nervous system. *Clin Infect Dis.* 1995;20:971–981.

Sack K. Monarthritis: differential diagnosis. *Am J Med.* 1997;102(1A):30S–34S.

Sande MA, Gwaltney JM. Acute community-acquired bacterial sinusitis: continuing challenges and current management. *Clin Infect Dis.* 2004;39(suppl 3):S151–S158.

Saubolle MA, et al. Epidemiologic, clinical, and diagnostic aspects of coccidioidomycosis. *J Clin Microbiol.* 2007;45:26–30.

Schantz PM. Tapeworms (cestodiasis). *Gastroenterol Clin North Am.* 1996;25:637–653.

Segreti J, Harris AA. Acute bacterial meningitis. *Infect Dis Clin North Am.* 1996;4:797–809.

Sheorey H, et al. Nematodes. In: Murray PR, Baron EJ, Jorgensen JH, Pfaller MA, Landry ML, eds. *Manual of Clinical Microbiology.* 9th ed. Washington, DC: ASM Press;2007:2144–2155.

Sia IG, Berbari EF. Infection and musculoskeletal conditions: osteomyelitis. *Best Pract Res Clin Rheumatol.* 2006;20:1065–1081.

Small PM, Fujiwara PI. Management of tuberculosis in the United States. *N Engl J Med.* 2001;345:189–200.

Sobel JD. What's new in bacterial vaginosis and trichomoniasis? *Infect Dis Clin North Am.* 2005;19: 387–406.

Sobel JD. Vulvovaginal candidosis. *Lancet.* 2007;369:1961–1971.

Stamm WE, Hooton TM. Management of urinary tract infections in adults. *N Engl J Med.* 1993;329: 1328–1334.

Storch GA. Diagnostic virology. In: Knipe DM, Howley PM, eds. *Fields' Virology.* 5th ed. Wolters Kluwer; 2007:565–604.

Summerbell RC, et al. *Trichophyton, Microsporum, Epidermophyton,* and agents of superficial mycoses. In: Murray PR, Baron EJ, Jorgensen JH, Pfaller MA, Landry ML, eds. *Manual of Clinical Microbiology.* 9th ed. Washington, DC: ASM Press; 2007:1874–1897.

Swarts MN, Pasternack MS. Cellulitis and subcutaneous tissue infections. In: Mandell GL, Douglas RG, Bennett JE, Dolin R, eds. *Mandell, Douglas, and Bennett's Principles and Practice of Infectious Diseases.* 6th ed. New York: Elsevier/Churchill Livingstone; 2005:1172–1194.

Taylor-Robinson D. Infections due to species of *Mycoplasma* and *Ureaplasma:* an update. *Clin Infect Dis.* 1996;23:671–682.

Thielman NM, Guerrant RL. Clinical practice. Acute infectious diarrhea. *N Engl J Med.* 2004;350:38–47.

Thomas CF Jr, Limper AH. *Pneumocystis* pneumonia. *N Engl J Med.* 2004;350:2487–2498.

Thomson RB Jr, Bertram H. Laboratory diagnosis of central nervous system infections. *Infect Dis Clin North Am.* 2001;15:1047–1071.

Tunkel AR, Scheld WM. Acute meningitis. In: Mandell GL, Douglas RG, Bennett JE, Dolin R, eds. *Mandell, Douglas, and Bennett's Principles and Practice of Infectious Diseases.* 6th ed. New York: Elsevier/Churchill Livingstone; 2005:1083–1126.

Vannier E, Gewurz BE, Krause PJ. Human babesiosis. *Infect Dis Clin North Am.* 2008;22:469–488.

Weinstein MP, et al. The clinical significance of positive blood cultures in the 1990s: a prospective comprehensive evaluation of the microbiology, epidemiology, and outcome of bacteremia and fungemia in adults. *Clin Infect Dis.* 1997;24:584–602.

Whitley RJ. Herpes simplex encephalitis: adolescents and adults. *Antivir Res.* 2006;71:141–148.

Wicher K, et al. Laboratory methods of diagnosis of syphilis for the beginning of the third millennium. *Microbes Infect.* 1999;1:1035–1049.

Wilson ML, Gaido L. Laboratory diagnosis of urinary tract infections in adult patients. *Clin Infect Dis.* 2004;38:1150–1158.

Wolf J, Daley AJ. Microbiological aspects of bacterial lower respiratory tract illness in children: atypical pathogens. *Paediatr Respir Rev.* 2007;8:212–219.

Young NS, Brown KE. Parvovirus B19. *N Engl J Med.* 2004;350:586–597.

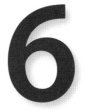
Toxicology[1]

Sheila Dawling and Michael Laposata

CHAPTER OUTLINE

INTRODUCTION

Toxicology testing can be divided into 2 main categories. One is the monitoring of the concentration of therapeutic drugs to limit the toxicity of medications with a narrow margin of safety. The second category is the monitoring for drugs of abuse and environmental toxins. Most of the chapters in this textbook are organized by disease, rather than the tests used to diagnose the disease. In toxicology, with the vast number of therapeutic drugs, drugs of abuse, and environmental toxins, the diseases associated with exposure or overdose are too numerous to count. For this reason, and the need to present the fundamental principles of toxicology in a laboratory medicine textbook, this chapter is organized by drugs and divided into 2 major sections—therapeutic drug monitoring (TDM) and monitoring for drugs of abuse and environmental toxins (**Figure 6–1**).

---

[1]Dr. Jane Yang provided content for this chapter in the previous edition. Sheila Dawling and Michael Laposata have revised the chapter for the new edition.

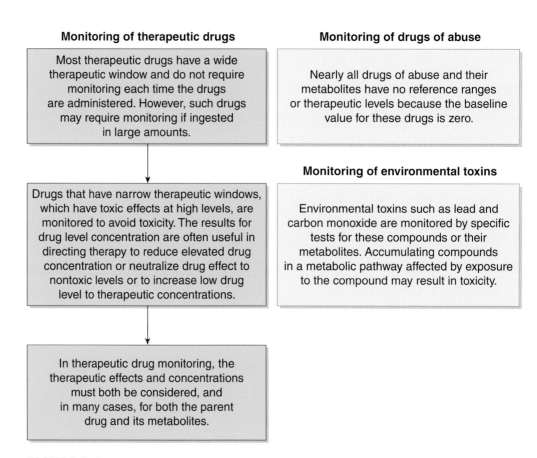

FIGURE 6–1 Considerations in therapeutic drug monitoring, drugs of abuse monitoring, and environmental toxin monitoring.

THERAPEUTIC DRUG MONITORING

Overview of Therapeutic Drug Monitoring

TDM is the practice of measuring the concentration of a drug or its metabolite (usually in blood, but occasionally in other fluids such as urine and oral fluids) to aid in the correct dosing of that drug and/or to assess patient compliance with their prescribed regimen. The goal of TDM is to increase the likelihood of a therapeutic effect and avoid or minimize adverse effects. **Table 6–1** lists the commonly monitored drugs. Patients do not require monitoring for most drugs. However, for a limited group of agents, TDM plays an essential role in establishing the appropriate therapeutic dosing regimen.

Prior to the 1960s, drug dosing was entirely empirical. For certain agents, this trial-and-error approach yielded wide variations in patient response with a very high incidence of toxicity. Since then, physicians have learned to avoid many of these adverse drug reactions through TDM that has been enabled by the development of assays and the establishment of therapeutic ranges for many pharmaceutical compounds.

The goal of therapeutic drug monitoring is to increase the likelihood of a therapeutic effect and avoid or minimize adverse effects. Patients do not require monitoring for most drugs.

Indications for Therapeutic Drug Monitoring

Patient conditions and drug characteristics determine whether an agent is a potential candidate for therapeutic monitoring (**Table 6–2**). The most common indication is a low margin of safety or therapeutic index. Another indication for TDM is significant pharmacokinetic variability. Such variability may be caused by drug interactions, genetic variation in drug metabolism, metabolism by nonlinear kinetics, physiologic conditions such as pregnancy and aging, and underlying diseases that alter the effective amount of drug delivered to the body. In addition, when patient

TABLE 6-1 **Commonly Monitored Drugs**

Methotrexate
Tacrolimus (FK-506) Cyclosporine
Lithium
Antibiotics • Gentamycin • Tobramycin • Vancomycin
Tricyclic antidepressants • Amitriptyline • Desipramine • Doxepin • Imipramine • Nortriptyline
Antiepileptics (first generation) • Phenytoin • Phenobarbital • Carbamazepine • Valproic acid
Antiepileptics (second generation) • Lamotrigine • Levetiracetam • Oxcarbazepine
Other therapeutic agents • Buprenorphine • Clonazepam • Digoxin • Methadone

TABLE 6-2 **Indications for Therapeutic Drug Monitoring**

The prescribed drug has a low margin of safety; that is, toxic blood drug concentrations or dosages are only slightly greater than therapeutic ones (a narrow therapeutic index)
To evaluate patient compliance with their prescribed drug regimen
The drug does not act via irreversible inhibition ("hit and run" effect)
Symptoms of underlying disease are difficult to distinguish from drug toxicity
The treatment goal is not an objectively measured end-point (such as blood pressure)
The prescribed drug has significant pharmacokinetic variability as a result of: • Interindividual metabolic capacity • Nonlinear (zero-order) drug kinetics • Frequent drug–drug interactions • Physiologic conditions (e.g., aging, pregnancy) • Underlying disease state (e.g., liver or renal impairment)

compliance is in question, drug monitoring may be used to demonstrate the presence or absence of the prescribed agent. Finally, a suitable drug assay must exist to practice TDM, and there usually must be some established blood therapeutic reference range and/or a quantitative value that has been correlated with efficacy and/or toxicity. In some cases, urine or oral fluid samples are used to evaluate patient compliance (the most common examples are monitoring buprenorphine, methadone, and oxycodone compliance).

TDM is performed by measuring the concentration of a drug and/or its major metabolite(s), usually in patient serum or plasma. By using blood levels to guide drug therapy, certain assumptions about the pharmacokinetic properties of that drug are made. For instance, it is assumed that a proportional relationship exists between the plasma or serum concentration and the pharmacologic effect. For obvious practical reasons, only blood levels of the drug are measured and not concentrations in tissues where the drug is active. In some well-defined instances, drug concentrations in urine may be useful. These instances involve assessing if a patient has started to re-use a drug of abuse after a period of abstinence (see the section "Selected Drugs of Abuse and Substances Abused by Excess Intake").

Pharmacokinetic Principles

Zero-order versus First-order Kinetics

Most but not all drugs are eliminated by first-order (or linear) kinetics. This means that a constant fraction of drug is eliminated per unit time. These drugs have a constant biological half-life, and changes in dose will generally cause predictable changes in blood levels. Other drugs are eliminated by zero-order (or nonlinear) kinetics, such that a constant amount of drug is eliminated per unit time. Typically, metabolism by zero-order kinetics occurs when elimination pathways for that drug have been saturated. Under these circumstances, the biological half-life is not constant but depends on drug concentration. As a result, small increments in dose may cause disproportionately large increments in blood levels. Due to their lack of a predictable dose–response relationship, drugs that follow zero-order kinetics often require monitoring.

> Most but not all drugs are eliminated by first-order (or linear) kinetics. This means that a constant <u>fraction</u> of drug is eliminated per unit time. Other drugs are eliminated by zero-order (or nonlinear) kinetics, such that a constant <u>amount</u> of drug is eliminated per unit time.

Steady-state Concentration

In TDM, serum drug levels (peak, trough, or random) are most often determined only after steady state has been achieved. Steady state is the condition that occurs when the amount of drug entering the system equals the amount being eliminated. Steady-state levels are used in relation to the target concentration range to dictate any necessary changes in dosing. Assuming first-order kinetics, 5 half-lives are required after initiation of drug therapy to reach nearly complete (97%) steady state (5 half-life rule). Five half-lives are also required for nearly complete clearance of a drug after the termination of therapy, and for attaining a new steady state whenever a dosing regimen has been changed.

Drug Absorption

When considering clinical monitoring questions, factors affecting drug absorption, distribution, metabolism, and elimination must be considered. The route of drug administration and the formulation of the drug will affect the rate and extent of drug absorption. For example, oral drug absorption is affected by many factors including drug solubility in enteral fluid, the acid–base characteristics of the drug, the lipid solubility of the drug, interferences with absorption by food, destruction of the drug by gastrointestinal flora, co-administration of other drugs—especially antacids, cholestyramine, and other resin-binding agents—blood flow to the gastrointestinal tract, and gastrointestinal transit time. Some orally delivered drugs are also subject to a significant "first pass effect," whereby they are largely metabolized by the liver to inactive compounds before reaching the systemic circulation. Significant variability in drug absorption is a common indication for TDM.

Drug Metabolism and Elimination

Drug metabolism typically renders nonpolar lipophilic drugs into more polar, water-soluble compounds for elimination. The liver is the primary site for drug metabolism. Genetic variants, age, cirrhosis, and other hepatic conditions may adversely affect drug metabolism and thus predispose a patient to toxicity. Many drugs are hepatic enzyme inducers or inhibitors and thus can influence the rate of their own metabolism, as well as the metabolism of many other drugs. Elimination of many polar, nonlipophilic drugs is achieved primarily through renal excretion, which is dependent on adequate renal function and renal blood flow. Other parameters relevant to elimination through the kidneys include urine pH and the properties of the drug itself, such as pKa and molecular size. Other less common pathways of drug elimination are via feces, sweat, and respiration. Drug clearance is the theoretical volume of plasma that is completely cleared of a drug per unit time. Importantly, clearance is the sum of all elimination mechanisms—hepatic, renal, biliary, and any other—that apply for a particular drug. Patients with impaired drug clearance may need more frequent monitoring.

Binding of Drugs to Proteins

Protein binding is another consideration in TDM. Binding to plasma proteins occurs to some extent for most drugs, with bound and free (unbound) drugs existing in equilibrium. Although it is only the free drug fraction that is biologically active, most laboratory assays measure the total drug concentration, that is, the sum of the bound and the unbound drugs. Several factors can cause changes in plasma proteins and, consequently, affect free drug levels. For example, hypoalbuminemia, which occurs in the elderly and in patients with cirrhosis, may cause an increased free drug fraction in the setting of nonelevated total drug levels. The presence of uremia also may elevate the free drug fraction by displacing drugs from albumin.

Drug Interactions and Dose Adjustments

Drug interactions also cause displacement of bound drug. The clinical significance of the interaction is likely to be increased when both drugs are highly protein bound (80% or more), when 1 of the drugs has a higher binding affinity, and/or when 1 of the drugs is present in higher quantity than the other. Dosing adjustments may be required in these instances. Displacement of bound drug does not inevitably lead to an increased free drug level, because free drug is subject to increased metabolism and elimination. Finally, increases in plasma proteins may occur as an acute phase response or during pregnancy, and consequently, higher dosing may be necessary. In all these situations, caution must be used when interpreting total drug levels, and obtaining free drug levels may be useful (see text that follows).

Laboratory Methods

Currently, most clinical laboratories utilize immunoassays for the rapid and quantitative measurement of drugs. Immunoassays utilize synthesized drug conjugate (drug attached to an enzyme or fluorescein molecule) and specific antibodies that bind both free or protein-bound drug (in patient serum) and drug conjugate (see Chapter 2). Typically, patient serum and a known amount of drug conjugate are incubated with antibody. Antibody binding results in blocking enzyme activity or in enhancing fluorescence polarization. By measuring enzyme activity or fluorescence polarization, the amount of drug in the patient serum or urine is quantitated. Chemiluminescent immunoassays offering superior sensitivity are just emerging onto the market. Other immunological methods such as ELISA or CEDIA (which involves enzyme activation by subunit assembly in the presence of drug) are less commonly used. More complex laboratory techniques, such as chromatography with ultraviolet or mass spectral detection, also may be used for drug measurements. As stated, only *total* drug concentrations are routinely measured. Free drug levels require a more time-consuming and expensive ultracentrifugation step to separate the protein-bound drug from the free drug. Free drug concentrations are typically lower than total drug concentrations by a factor of 2- to 20-fold, so more sensitive assays are required.

Specimen Collection

The appropriate specimen for therapeutic drug measurements is usually serum or plasma. Most laboratories do not accept gel separator tubes as the gel interferes with drug recovery. Tacrolimus, sirolimus, and cyclosporine levels are measured using whole blood due to their considerable concentration in RBCs, which are removed in the preparation of serum. EDTA-anticoagulated blood is the appropriate sample for these 3 drug measurements. Urine samples are frequently used to evaluate patient compliance in cases of therapeutic administration of buprenorphine, methadone, and several opiates (including oxycodone). A significant problem with urine samples is that they are subject to adulteration by the patient, in order to confound result interpretation by a clinician. (See the section "Specimen Collection and Laboratory Analysis.")

The appropriate specimen for therapeutic drug measurements is usually serum or plasma. A significant problem with urine samples is that they are subject to adulteration by the patient, in order to confound result interpretation by a clinician.

In general, *trough* levels are drawn just prior to the next dose and are used to evaluate the likelihood of a *therapeutic* effect. *Peak* levels are drawn at varying times, depending on the particular drug, and are used typically to assess *toxicity* risk. More specific recommendations are given for individual drugs (see text that follows).

Selected Commonly Monitored Drugs

Selected individual drugs and their relevant TDM issues are presented in this section and in **Table 6–3**. There are many drug interactions that increase or decrease the effects of the drugs mentioned in the following subsections. Information on drug interactions should be obtained before administering these compounds and when a standard dose is subtherapeutic or toxic.

Methotrexate

Methotrexate is a folate antagonist used in the treatment of a wide variety of neoplasms. Dose-related toxicity is common with high-dose methotrexate therapy (defined as >1 g/m^2 or 20 mg/kg). Adverse effects include renal failure, myelosuppression, hepatic toxicity, neurotoxicity, gastrointestinal toxicity, and death. Toxicity correlates with serum methotrexate concentration and duration of exposure. Patients with poor hydration, renal insufficiency, pleural effusion, ascites, or gastrointestinal obstruction are at increased risk for toxicity. Adverse effects of methotrexate are ameliorated by administration of leucovorin, a reduced folate. Serial methotrexate levels are used to guide the appropriate dosing and duration of leucovorin rescue following high-dose methotrexate administration.

Tacrolimus

Tacrolimus, also known as FK-506, is a potent immunosuppressant with the ability to reverse acute allograft rejection in transplant patients. Monitoring of whole blood concentrations is indicated because of its wide inter- and intraindividual pharmacokinetic variability and its narrow therapeutic index. Adverse effects include nephrotoxicity, and neurotoxicity characterized by light sensitivity, tingling in the palms, and tinnitus.

Tacrolimus undergoes hepatic metabolism to at least 9 metabolites, some of which also have immunosuppressant activity. Some metabolites possess cross-reactivity in tacrolimus immunoassays. Therefore, these assays may overestimate tacrolimus (parent drug) concentrations in situations where elimination is impaired and when metabolites accumulate, as in cholestasis. It is unclear whether toxicity is due to the parent compound, its metabolites, or both. Also, patients who have received mouse monoclonal antibodies, such as in cancer therapy, may have inaccurate results for tacrolimus using immunoassays. HPLC with tandem mass spectrometry is increasingly being used to circumvent these problems.

Cyclosporine

Cyclosporine is an immunosuppressant used in transplant patients and in patients with autoimmune disease. Its pharmacokinetics are highly variable. There is a poor correlation between dose and blood concentration. Factors that influence cyclosporine potency include liver function, dietary fat content, age, and drug interactions. Cyclosporine toxicity is characterized by nephrotoxicity, tremor, hypertension, and hepatotoxicity.

Low trough concentrations may indicate subtherapeutic immunosuppression and may be associated with increased risk of rejection. Some studies suggest that nephrotoxicity occurs more often with high trough concentrations. The identification of nephrotoxicity in renal transplant patients is especially difficult. Some metabolites cross-react in cyclosporine immunoassays, and there may be overestimation of cyclosporine (parent drug) concentrations if elimination is impaired and metabolites accumulate. Mouse monoclonal antibodies may cause unreliable results for cyclosporine using immunoassays. HPLC with tandem mass spectrometry is increasingly being used to circumvent these problems. Cyclosporine levels must be interpreted in conjunction with other laboratory test results and clinical findings to discriminate between toxicity and rejection. The only definitive method for differentiating graft rejection from cyclosporine-induced nephrotoxicity is renal biopsy.

TABLE 6-3   Therapeutic Drug Monitoring for Commonly Monitored Drugs

Drug	Monitoring Recommendations	Specimen Collection Tube and Instructions	Suggested Therapeutic Range	Special Considerations
Methotrexate	24, 48, 72 hours after bolus; then daily until below cytotoxic levels	5 mL red top; wrap in foil to protect from light; indicate time past bolus	<10 μmol/L at 24 hours <1 μmol/L at 48 hours <0.4 μmol/L at 72 hours	Monitoring guidelines are for high-dose therapy (>20 mg/kg) only
Tacrolimus (FK-506)	Trough levels, 12 hours postdose	3 mL purple top	5–20 ng/mL	Cross-reactivity with its metabolites in immunoassays
Cyclosporine	Trough levels, 12 or 24 hours postdose	3 mL purple top; avoid drawing from line of administration	Transplant of: (1) Liver: 400–800 ng/mL (2) Heart: 150–300 ng/mL (3) Kidney: (a) <3 months: 150–250 ng/mL, (b) >3 months: 100–200 ng/mL	Ranges depend on organ transplanted and time since transplant
Aminoglycosides	Peak: (1) IV: 30–60 minutes postdose (2) IM: 60–90 minutes postdose (3) Trough: 30 minutes prior to next dose	5 mL red top	Gentamicin—peak: 5–10 μg/mL, trough: <2.0 μg/mL Tobramycin—peak: 4–8 μg/mL, trough: <2.0 μg/mL	Guidelines for conventional dosing only (not low-dose therapy or pulse therapy)
Vancomycin	Either peak or trough, once per day	5 mL red top	Peak: 30–40 μg/mL, trough: 5–10 μg/mL	Frequency of monitoring dependent on clinical situation
Phenytoin	Peak for toxicity is 4–5 hours after dose; trough for monitoring	5 mL red top	10–20 μg/mL	Pertains to assay that measures total drug (free + bound)
Phenobarbital	Trough	5 mL red top	15–50 μg/mL	Steady state attained in 2–3 weeks
Carbamazepine	Peak level for toxicity is 2–4 hours after dose; trough for monitoring	5 mL red top	4–12 μg/mL	Not helpful for idiosyncratic toxicities
Clonazepam	Peak for toxicity is 4 hours after dose; trough for monitoring	1 mL red or green top	20–60 μg/mL	
Lamotrigine	Peak for toxicity is 2–4 hours after dose; trough for monitoring	1 mL red or green top	3–14 μg/mL	
Levetiracetam	Peak for toxicity is 1 hour after dose; trough for monitoring	1 mL red or green top	5–30 μg/mL	
Oxcarbazepine	Peak MHD for toxicity is 4–6 hours after dose; trough for monitoring	1 mL red or green top	15–35 μg/mL MHD	
Valproic acid	Trough is not well defined	5 mL red top	50–100 μg/mL	Upper limit of therapeutic range
Tricyclic antidepressants	Steady state occurs in about 5 days; 10–14 hours after once per day dosing; 4–6 hours after twice per day dosing	5 mL red top	[a]Amitriptyline: 120–250 μg/L Desipramine: 150–300 μg/L [a]Doxepin: 150–250 μg/L [a]Imipramine: 150–250 μg/L Nortriptyline: 50–150 μg/L	Measure sum of parent and active metabolite for drugs noted with "a" in box at left
Lithium	10–14 hours after dose; then biweekly or weekly until steady state; then every 1–3 months	5 mL red top	0.5–1.5 mmol/L (avoid green top tubes)	Toxicity may occur at <1.5 mmol/L, especially in patients who show chronic toxicity
Digoxin	8 hours after PO dose; 12 hours after IV dose; and at steady state (1 week after initiation)	5 mL red top	0.9–2.0 ng/mL	Specimen collection time is crucial to avoid falsely high levels; STAT levels occasionally necessary

IM, intramuscular; IV, intravenous; PO, oral.

[a]Measure the sum of parent and active metabolite, that is, (amitriptyline + nortriptyline), (imipramine + desipramine), and (doxepin + desmethyldoxepin).

Antibiotics

Aminoglycosides

Gentamicin, tobramycin, and amikacin are aminoglycoside antibiotics. Ototoxicity and nephrotoxicity from aminoglycosides are related to dose and duration of exposure. Numerous factors, such as renal and cardiac function, age, liver disease, and obesity, affect the pharmacokinetic properties of aminoglycosides. Because of the many patient factors, as well as the low margin of safety and high incidence of dose-related toxicity, aminoglycoside levels are usually indicated in conjunction with renal function monitoring to minimize toxicity. In patients with normal renal function and without underlying disease, the indication for drug monitoring is less well defined.

Vancomycin

Vancomycin is a tricyclic glycopeptide antibiotic with significant dose-related nephrotoxicity and ototoxicity. The practice of measuring vancomycin levels emerged from the guidelines for aminoglycoside monitoring. However, the necessity for vancomycin monitoring is controversial, because a good correlation between serum vancomycin levels and efficacy or toxicity has yet to be definitively demonstrated. Adult patients with normal renal function may not require routine monitoring. Indications for monitoring include impaired or changing renal function, concomitant use of nephrotoxic drugs, altered volume of distribution (as in a burn injury victim), prolonged vancomycin use, higher than usual doses, and use in neonates, children, pregnant women, and patients with malignancy.

Antiepileptics

Antiepileptics are frequently monitored to establish the dose necessary to maintain a therapeutic level, where the goal is seizure prophylaxis at a minimum dose to avoid side effects. The concentration of drug in the blood also may be used to evaluate patient compliance to explain refractory cases. Trough levels are typically used to establish minimum effective dose. When toxicity is suspected, peak or random levels may be obtained.

> Antiepileptics are frequently monitored to establish the dose necessary to maintain a therapeutic level, where the goal is seizure prophylaxis at a minimum dose to avoid side effects.

Phenytoin (Dilantin®)

Phenytoin (or its pro-drug phosphenytoin) is a widely used anticonvulsant with nonlinear kinetics and wide interindividual variability in dose requirement. Phenytoin toxicity includes ataxia, tremor, lethargy, seizure exacerbation, and neuropsychiatric changes. Phenytoin use in certain populations requires special consideration. Neonates and the elderly have decreased clearance. On the other hand, children metabolize phenytoin more rapidly than adults, and therefore, dose adjustment is necessary at various ages. Phenytoin is highly protein-bound, and conditions such as renal failure, liver disease, burn injury, and age will affect the amount of free drug by altering the amount of plasma protein.

Extensive protein binding also predisposes phenytoin to significant interactions with other drugs, such as valproic acid, which are also highly albumin-bound. Co-administration of valproic acid and phenytoin is common and may cause a decrease in total phenytoin. Valproic acid displaces phenytoin from albumin, which causes a transient increase in free phenytoin, but this free phenytoin is readily metabolized and cleared. The overall effect is usually a decrease in total phenytoin with an unchanged level of free phenytoin. Therefore, in the absence of renal and hepatic insufficiency, measurement of free phenytoin levels is not usually necessary.

Phenobarbital and Primidone (Mysoline®)

Phenobarbital and primidone are used to treat all types of seizures except absence (petit mal) seizures. The major active metabolite of primidone is phenobarbital. Clearance of both primidone and phenobarbital is prolonged in neonates, the elderly, and patients with hepatic and renal dysfunction. Furthermore, phenobarbital is a potent hepatic enzyme inducer, and on that basis may affect the levels of many other drugs. Concurrent valproic acid use significantly decreases phenobarbital clearance.

Carbamazepine (Tegretol®)

The anticonvulsant carbamazepine is used not only for seizures, but also for treatment of trigeminal neuralgia and bipolar disorder. Monitoring of carbamazepine levels is useful due to its slow and unpredictable absorption. Age and hepatic function affect drug clearance. Dose-related toxic effects include blurred vision, paresthesias, ataxia, nystagmus, and drowsiness. Carbamazepine is metabolized to the active metabolite, carbamazepine 10,11-epoxide. Children are known to accumulate the epoxide metabolite and, as a result, may present with toxicity in the setting of nonelevated carbamazepine levels. With chronic therapy, carbamazepine induces its own metabolism, and dosing adjustment becomes necessary.

Valproic Acid (Depakane®, Depakote®)

Valproic acid is used to treat all types of seizures. It is also used in the treatment of migraines and bipolar disorder. Valproic acid has a narrow therapeutic index. Dose-related adverse effects involve primarily central nervous system (CNS) depression. The average half-life of valproic acid is about 12 to 16 hours, but there is significant interindividual variability, and use of a sustained-release formulation is popular. In addition, its half-life is prolonged in neonates and in patients with liver dysfunction. Extensive protein binding accounts for the increased valproic acid toxicity observed in patients with uremia and cirrhosis.

Lamotrigine (Lamictal®)

Lamotrigine is used in adjunctive therapy in the treatment of generalized tonic–clonic seizures, and increasingly as monotherapy in partial seizures to replace conventional enzyme-inducing anticonvulsants. Common adverse effects are dizziness, ataxia, blurred vision, nausea, and vomiting. The drug is extremely well absorbed, and metabolized in the liver to inactive glucuronide metabolites that are renally excreted. The half-life is 24 to 32 hours, but this is reduced to 12 to 15 hours if phenytoin or carbamazepine are co-ingested. Lamotrigine binds to plasma albumin (approximately 55%), and co-administration of valproic acid displaces lamotrigine and increases its half-life to about 60 to 72 hours. More recently, lamotrigine is being used for neuropathic relief of chronic pain. Of the newer anticonvulsants, lamotrigine has the best established therapeutic range and is often monitored. HPLC is usually used as immunoassays are not yet available.

Oxcarbazepine (Trileptal®)

Oxcarbazepine is a pro-drug related to carbamazepine. It is almost immediately and completely metabolized to the active drug 10-hydroxy-10,11-dihydrocarbamazepine (MHD). Further metabolism produces a variety of metabolites that are renally excreted, and MHD accumulates in renal failure. MHD has a half-life of 8 to 10 hours, which is decreased by co-administration of enzyme-inducing anticonvulsants. MHD is about 40% bound to plasma albumin, and in contrast to carbamazepine shows linear kinetics. Toxic effects include hyponatremia, dizziness, ataxia, tremor, nausea, and vomiting. HPLC is usually used as immunoassays are not yet available.

Levetiracetam (Keppra®)

Levetiracetam is approved for adjunctive therapy of partial onset seizures. It is readily and completely absorbed, and only minimally distributed and protein-bound (<10%). Its half-life is about 6 to 8 hours and is highly dependent on renal function. Toxic effects include decreased hematocrit, neutropenia, somnolence, and dizziness. Because of its wide therapeutic index, linear kinetics, and lack of kinetic interaction with other anticonvulsants, monitoring is not usually indicated in otherwise healthy patients. HPLC is usually used as immunoassays are not yet available.

Antidepressants
Tricyclic Antidepressants

Tricyclic antidepressants are monitored for multiple reasons. There is significant interindividual variation in metabolism and elimination, such that standard dosing results in therapeutic levels in less than half of patients. Genetic variation accounts for some of this variability. The fraction of "poor metabolizers" is about 17% of Caucasians and 5% of other ethnic groups. Other indications for monitoring include a narrow therapeutic index, multiple drug interactions, and patient compliance.

Tricyclic antidepressants have a low margin of safety and cause anticholinergic toxicity, seizures, and arrhythmias in overdose. Although the correlation between toxicity and blood level is poor, there are general guidelines. Levels in excess of 500 µg/L may be associated with anticholinergic toxicity (flushing, tachycardia, fever, dilated pupils, dry mucous membranes, urinary retention, and absent bowel sounds). Cardiotoxicity is more likely to occur at levels greater than 1,000 µg/L in acute overdose.

Lithium

Lithium is a univalent cation most commonly used to treat bipolar disorder. Lithium monitoring is useful due to its narrow therapeutic index and the wide interindividual variation in dose requirement.

Excretion of lithium is primarily renal. Children have increased clearance, while the elderly have decreased clearance. Lithium excretion parallels sodium excretion. Therefore, patients on stable doses of lithium may become toxic in states of sodium conservation such as fever, excessive sweating, lack of fluid intake, and diarrhea.

Toxicity is usually associated with levels in excess of 1.5 mmol/L. However, toxicity may occur at lower levels, especially in cases of chronic toxicity. Lithium overdose is characterized by lethargy, weakness, slurred speech, ataxia, tremor, and myoclonic jerks. Severe toxicity may result in seizure, hyperthermia, and coma. Management of patients who have ingested sustained-release lithium preparations is difficult, and serum measurements play a crucial role in the decision to instigate hemodialysis or whole bowel irrigation. Analytical methods involve the use of ion-specific electrodes, and color reactions.

Later-generation Antidepressants

Fluoxetine was the first selective serotonin-reuptake inhibitor used to treat depression. Fluoxetine monitoring is useful when patient compliance is in question. Further monitoring is not likely to be beneficial since fluoxetine has a wide therapeutic index, and there is a poor correlation between blood levels and clinical response. Fluoxetine is metabolized by the liver to the active metabolite norfluoxetine.

Other serotonin-reuptake inhibitors/later-generation antidepressants—such as sertraline (Zoloft®), paroxetine (Paxil®), fluvoxamine (Luvox®), citalopram (Celexa®), quetiapine (Seroquel®), trazodone (Deseryl®), and venlafaxine (Effexor®)—do not require routine monitoring due to their wide therapeutic indices.

Other Therapeutic Agents

Digoxin

> Drug of abuse testing (DAT) includes testing for the use of illicit drugs, potentially addictive or harmful therapeutic drugs and agents used in drug withdrawal/treatment programs.

Digoxin is a commonly used drug in the treatment of heart failure and arrhythmias, and it has a low therapeutic index. There is significant interindividual variation in digoxin absorption and distribution along with prolonged clearance in patients with impaired renal function. Digoxin overdose is characterized by gastrointestinal distress, confusion, visual changes, hyperkalemia, and life-threatening cardiac toxicity. Such overdoses may be treated with an antidigoxin antibody antidote. Such treatment typically renders subsequent blood digoxin concentrations unreliable. Blood digoxin immunoassays are generally less reliable than immunoassays for other therapeutic agents. Interferences with digoxin immunoassays are frequently reported. These interferences are frequently referred to as Digoxin-like immunoreactive substance ("DLIS") ones.

DETECTION OF DRUGS OF ABUSE AND ENVIRONMENTAL TOXINS

Overview of Drugs of Abuse

Drug of abuse testing (DAT) includes testing for the use of illicit drugs (e.g., cocaine and phencyclidine), potentially addictive or harmful therapeutic drugs (e.g., benzodiazepines, opiates, and amphetamine), and agents used in drug withdrawal/treatment programs (e.g., buprenorphine

TABLE 6–4   Detection Times Post Last Drug Use for Commonly Abused Substances

Urine DAT Name	Time (days)	Comments
Amphetamines	2–4	
Barbiturates	1 to >5	Depends on barbiturate
Benzodiazepines	2 to >8	Depends on benzodiazepine
Cocaine metabolite	2 to >7	Heavy users may remain positive for 6–10 days using sensitive immunoassays with a 150 ng/mL cut-off
Methadone	1–4	
Opiates	2 to >5	Heavy users may remain positive for up to 7–8 days
Phencyclidine	7–14	
Propoxyphene	2–8	
THC (marijuana)	20–30	

and methadone). The goal of DAT is to detect past exposure or use of a drug. Quantitative levels of a drug or its metabolite in fluids are not required. It is only necessary to know if the analyte is above (i.e., "present") or below (absent) a defined cut-off concentration.

The ideal DAT test for illicit or addictive drugs would detect any use of a substance, as far in the past as possible. Thus, DAT assays are usually designed to detect either the parent drug of interest or a metabolite with a longer half-life. The classic example of this strategy involves cocaine. The half-life of cocaine in blood is less than 60 minutes. Testing for cocaine in blood would be a very poor strategy for maximizing detection of drug use, since cocaine blood levels typically become undetectable 4 to 5 hours after drug ingestion. Hence, virtually all DAT cocaine tests are designed to detect cocaine's principal metabolite, benzoylecgonine, which has an 8-hour serum half life. In this way, cocaine abuse can be detected several days after use. **Table 6–4** lists the typical time after drug use that immunoassays are capable of detecting the parent drug and/or metabolites.

Another strategy to maximize the "window" for detection of past drug use is to analyze the most concentrated sample readily available. Typically, drugs and their metabolites are much more concentrated in urine than serum, analogous to endogenous compounds such as urea and creatinine. Urine is the specimen of choice for virtually all DAT testing because of its high concentrations and ready availability. Use of meconium can detect in utero exposure of a fetus to drugs from as early as the sixth month of gestation. In DAT, the clinical utility of other specimen types such as hair or nails has not been clearly demonstrated, but these samples may be useful for testing for environmental toxins.

Virtually all DAT testing is initially performed using immunoassays on urine specimens. Typically these assays detect many drugs in a class, and are not specific for an individual drug. A listing of drugs detected in common "class-specific" or "compound-specific" immunoassays is shown in **Table 6–5**. These immunoassays are easily adapted for use on both central laboratory automated analyzers and point-of-care devices. Employing a capture antibody that recognizes a part of the molecule shared by many drugs in a class allows for a single assay to detect many members of a particular drug family.

Samples that test positive in an initial immunoassay test are then tested using a more specific, sensitive chemical method if the testing is carried out for legal, forensic, insurance, or pre-employment reasons. This second-level or "confirmatory" testing employs a liquid or gas chromatographic separation prior to mass-spectrometric detection and confirmation of the identity of a drug or metabolite. This confirmatory testing is very expensive and time-consuming, and is not usually performed on clinical samples, especially those from hospital emergency wards, as results of the confirmatory testing do not contribute to the immediate care of a patient as they are most often not available for several days.

The goal of Drug of abuse testing is to detect past exposure or use of a drug. Quantitative levels of a drug or its metabolite in fluids are not required. It is only necessary to know if the analyte is above (i.e., "present") or below (absent) a defined cut-off concentration.

TABLE 6–5   Characteristics of Common Tests for Drugs of Abuse

DAT Name	Specificity	Drug Class Targeted	Typical Cut-off (Range) Level	Causes of False-Positives	Common Drugs Typically Detected	Comments
Primary tests						
Amphetamines	Class	Amphetamines	1000 (300–2000) ng/mL	Isometheptine Heptaminol Seligeline Propylhexadrine	Amphetamine, methamphetamine MDMA ("ecstasy")	Pseudoephedrine no longer interferes with current immunoassays
Barbiturates	Class	Barbiturates	300 (100–500) ng/mL	–	Butalbital, barbital, secobarbital, phenobarbital	
Benzodiazepines	Class	Benzodiazepines	200 (100–300) ng/mL	Oxaprozin	Diazepam, chlordiazepoxide, alprazolam, oxazepam	Many assays are insensitive to clonazepam and lorazepam
Cocaine	Compound	Cocaine metabolites	150 (100–300) ng/mL	–	Cocaine metabolites	True false-positives are quite rare, despite information on the Internet
Opiates	Class	Morphine and related compounds	300 (300–2000) ng/mL	Quinoline antibiotics	Heroin, morphine, codeine, hydromorphone, hydrocodone	Oxycodone and oxymorphone are poorly detected. Methadone use does not cause a positive test
Phencyclidine	Compound	Phencyclidine	25 (10–25) ng/mL	Dextromethorphan, tramadol	Phencyclidine	
THC	Compound	Cannabinoids	50 (20–100) ng/mL	See comments	Marijuana and hashish use	Nexium use may cause false-positives with some immunoassays
Adjuvant tests						
Buprenorphine	Compound	Buprenorphine and buprenorphine-3-glucuronide	5–10 ng/mL	–	Buprenorphine	Used to assess compliance and/or drug diversion
Methadone	Compound	Methadone	300 (200–500) ng/mL	–	Methadone	Used to assess compliance and/or drug diversion
Oxycodone	Compound	Oxycodone	100 (100–300) ng/mL	–	Oxycodone, oxymorphone	Used to assess compliance/diversion and/or cause of a positive opiate test
6-Monoacetyl-morphine	Compound	Heroin metabolite	10 ng/mL	–	Heroin use	Specific for heroin use, negating the "poppy-seed" defense. Used to assess cause of a positive opiate test

The lack of confirmatory testing on clinical samples can lead to significant test misinterpretation unless the clinician and/or clinical laboratory scientist maintain an active dialog regarding the likely causes of false-positives. Many laboratories append a positive urine immunoassay result on a laboratory report with popular causes of false-positives.

Some typical causes of false-positive DAT results are listed in **Table 6–5**. It is important to know that causes of false-positives can be very different from one laboratory manufacturer's reagents to another. Therefore, a clinician should know the characteristics of the drug tests being used at the laboratory he/she uses. **Table 6–5** also lists the typical specificity of the primary DAT tests (compound- or class-specific), the typical cut-off concentration that distinguishes a positive from a negative, and other information.

Drugs of abuse should be undetectable in urine and serum. For these compounds, there is no reference or therapeutic range because the appropriate values are zero. There are a few exceptions, however. Ethanol is a drug that can be abused, but ingestion of low amounts of ethanol (1 to 2 drinks/day) is medically and legally acceptable.

When monitoring drugs of abuse, it is common to use a toxicology "screen." It is important to understand that screening for drugs of abuse does not detect every possible drug of abuse that the patient may have ingested. Rapid identification by the laboratory of a drug of abuse or therapeutic drug taken in excess amounts may permit effective treatment to reduce the toxic effect of the compound. Individual descriptions of acetaminophen overdose and excess alcohol ingestion are provided as specific examples. Concomitant ingestion of different drugs is very common and may play a role in monitoring drugs of abuse. For example, ethanol and cocaine are often ingested together, and patients ingesting these drugs together can form a toxic compound called cocaethylene.

Sometimes a positive DAT test is desired by the ordering physician. Examples are listed in the "Adjuvant Tests" section of **Table 6–5**. Both buprenorphine and methadone are used in the treatment of heroin detoxification. Both also can be sold by a patient for a monetary profit. A urine oxycodone test is also useful for monitoring compliance/possible diversion of this highly sought-after drug. Hence, patients prescribed these drugs are frequently monitored to assure that they are compliant with their drug regimen and not diverting the drug for other uses.

Specimen Collection and Laboratory Analysis

When evaluating a patient, it must be known whether a particular compound or its metabolites are best detected in urine, serum, or other body fluids.

- A urine sample is appropriate to screen for amphetamines, benzodiazepines, barbiturates, cannabinoids, cocaine metabolites, opiates, and their metabolites (including codeine and morphine), oxycodone, phencyclidine, and propoxyphene.
- A serum sample is needed to quantitate and assess the possible toxicity of alcohols, analgesics (including acetaminophen and salicylates), anticonvulsants, barbiturates, benzodiazepines, and selected other sedatives, should they be present.
- Other body fluids may prove useful in the following circumstances: in utero exposures may be evaluated by using meconium; vitreous humor may be collected in the postmortem examination; and hair and nails may be examined for long-term or historically timed exposure to certain drugs of abuse and environmental toxins; sweat and oral fluid are less prone to adulteration.

It is essential that specimens be collected at an appropriate time following ingestion and that the sample be properly preserved to limit false-positive or false-negative results. To obtain the peak level of a particular compound, it may be necessary to perform serial measurements over time because of delayed gastric emptying or prolonged absorption from sustained-release preparations. It is also not uncommon for blood levels to correlate poorly to the severity of toxicity because many compounds distribute in specific body compartments or become bound to a protein, and thereby become less detectable in laboratory assays.

An overwhelming percentage of all DAT tests are reported as "negative." The percent or absolute number of false-negative DAT tests is probably greater than false-positive ones. False-negative results can be caused by purposely adulterating a urine sample so that either the immunological or indicator reaction used in the immunoassay does not work, leading to a negative result no matter how much drug is present in the sample. Common household chemicals such as bleach, vinegar, Visine, sodium bicarbonate, Drano, soft drinks, or hydrogen peroxide are frequently added to a urine sample in an effort to cause false-negatives. Many of these additives work by altering a sample pH drastically, so that the pH of the final assay reaction mixture is no longer optimum. Such adulteration is easily detected by checking the pH of urine samples submitted for drug testing. Other adulterants available include glutaraldehyde or nitrites, but use of these is also easily detectable by drug-testing laboratories. Finally, sample substitution is perhaps the hardest to detect cause of false-negatives. Sources of drug-free urine are readily available via the Internet, and these materials are used by patients trying to avoid detection of their drug use. In nearly all standard tests, these materials act like normal, unadulterated human urine. Without close monitoring of a patient during urine sample collection, sample substitution is virtually undetectable by laboratory methods.

Selected Drugs of Abuse and Substances Abused by Excess Intake

The list of drugs and other compounds that can be abused is endless. A number of well-known substances are described in this section.

Amphetamines

Amphetamines are well-known drugs of abuse. Methamphetamine (crank, speed), 3,4-methylenedioxymethamphetamine (a derivative of methamphetamine, also known as MDMA or ecstasy), and several other amphetamine derivatives are used orally and intravenously as illicit drugs. A smokable form of methamphetamine is known as "ice." Amphetamine-like drugs also can be used as prescription medications for treatment of a variety of conditions and disorders. These include weight loss, narcolepsy, attention deficit disorders, and sinus congestion. Amphetamine-like drugs work primarily by activating the sympathetic nervous system via the CNS. Drugs in this class can produce toxicity at levels only slightly above the usual doses, but a high degree of tolerance can develop after repeated use. Patients who are intoxicated with amphetamine-like drugs present with CNS effects that can extend from euphoria to seizure and coma. More severe signs and symptoms are usually associated with greater amounts of drug ingestion. The acute peripheral manifestations extend from sweating and tremor to myocardial infarction, even if the coronary arteries are normal. Death in amphetamine users can be caused by ventricular arrhythmia. The ingestion of amphetamines and related drugs can be conclusively established by identification of these compounds in urine or in gastric samples. Quantitative serum levels often do not correlate with the severity of the signs and symptoms.

Barbiturates

Barbiturates are used clinically as hypnotic and sedative agents, for induction of anesthesia, and for treatment of epilepsy. Ultrashort-acting, short-acting, intermediate-acting, and long-acting barbiturates have different pharmacokinetic properties. All barbiturates cause a generalized depression of neuronal activity in the brain. The toxic dose of barbiturates depends on the specific barbiturate used, the route and rate of administration, and individual patient tolerance. Toxicity is likely to appear when the dose administered exceeds 5 to 10 times the hypnotic dose, but chronic use may result in marked tolerance. The patient with mild to moderate intoxication from an overdose of barbiturates often presents with lethargy, slurred speech, nystagmus, and ataxia. With greater amounts of drug ingestion, hypotension, coma, and respiratory arrest can occur. Barbiturates can be detected in both urine and serum as documentation of their ingestion.

Benzodiazepines

The many different benzodiazepines vary widely in potency, duration of effect, and the generation of active metabolites. Benzodiazepines produce a generalized depression of spinal reflexes and may cause coma. Death from benzodiazepine overdose is rare unless the drugs are used in combination with other compounds. Oral overdoses of diazepam (Valium®) have been reported in excess of 15 to 20 times the therapeutic dose without serious depression of consciousness. However, if the same drug is given at a much lower concentration with rapid intravenous injection, respiratory arrest can occur. Although there is variability among benzodiazepines, the onset of CNS depression is typically observed 30 to 120 minutes after ingestion. Drug levels can be obtained from both serum and urine specimens. However, because they are rarely of value in emergency management, they are often not obtained. Of the benzodiazepines, clonazepam, used in the treatment of absence seizures, is the most often monitored, especially in children, although most patients are managed without monitoring. There is very little evidence for a therapeutic window, probably because receptor effects do not mirror plasma concentrations, and tolerance does develop with continued use. HPLC is used, as immunoassays are not available.

Sources of drug-free urine are readily available via the Internet, and these materials are used by patients trying to avoid detection of their drug use. In nearly all standard tests, these materials act like normal, unadulterated human urine.

Cannabinoids

Cannabis derivatives include marijuana and hashish. Marijuana consists of the leaves and flowering parts of the plant *Cannabis sativa*. It is usually smoked in cigarettes or pipes, and can be added to food. Dried resin from the plant can be compressed into blocks to make hashish. The primary psychoactive cannabinoid in marijuana is delta-9-tetrahydrocannabinol (THC). THC is also available in capsule form as a treatment for emesis in patients being treated with chemotherapeutic agents and those undergoing treatment for glaucoma. The dose and time after consumption is significantly related to the effects of THC, which may be a stimulant, a sedative, or a hallucinogenic compound. A typical marijuana cigarette contains 1% to 3% THC, but some may contain up to 15% THC. Hashish contains 3% to 6% THC, and an oil that can be prepared from hashish has 30% to 50% THC. There is significant interindividual variability in the toxicity, which is influenced by prior experience with the drug and degree of tolerance. The clinical presentation of the patient after THC exposure can be almost anything, from euphoria and a heightened sensory awareness to impaired short-term memory, depersonalization, visual hallucinations, and acute paranoid psychosis. Documentation of exposure to THC is usually established by demonstration of the drug in the urine. Urine levels correlate poorly with the degree of intoxication. A urine test for cannabinoids may be positive for 10 to 25 days after the last exposure in moderate and heavy users. In fact, there are well-documented reports of true-positive test results in users more than 80 days after their last exposure to THC.

Cocaine

Cocaine may be sniffed into the nose, smoked, or injected intravenously. The "free base" form of cocaine is preferred for smoking because it volatilizes at a lower temperature and is not as easily destroyed by heat as the hydrochloride salt of the drug. Crack cocaine is a dried form of the drug that has been mixed in alkaline aqueous solution to generate the free base. Cocaine is abused by some individuals by combining it with heroin and injecting it as a "speed ball." The primary effects of cocaine are generalized sympathetic stimulation, very similar to that produced by amphetamines. There is also a depression of cardiovascular function as a result of decreased cardiac contractility. The toxic dose depends significantly on the tolerance of the individual to the drug, the route of administration, and whether the cocaine is administered with other compounds. A dose that produces only euphoria when swallowed or snorted can produce convulsions and cardiac arrhythmias when rapidly injected intravenously or smoked. The initial euphoria from exposure to cocaine can be followed by anxiety, agitation, hyperactivity, and seizures, and with high doses, respiratory arrest can occur. When death results from cocaine abuse, it is usually caused by a fatal arrhythmia, status epilepticus, intracranial hemorrhage, or hyperthermia. Demonstration of exposure to cocaine can be provided by detection of cocaine and its metabolite benzoylecgonine in the urine.

Opiates and Opioids

Opiates are naturally occurring compounds from the juice of the poppy *Papaver somniferum*. Opioids include the naturally occurring opiates and their derivatives (morphine and codeine) and therapeutic synthetic opiods (dihydrocodeine, heroin, hydrocodone, hydromorphone, oxycodone, and oxymorphone). Many prescription medications contain opioids. Mixtures of aspirin or acetaminophen with an opioid compound, such as codeine, are in common use. Dextromethorphan is an opioid derivative that is used to suppress cough. This compound can be obtained without a prescription as it has no analgesic or addictive properties. Morphine is an opiate that is widely used in medicine to reduce pain. The best known drug of abuse in this category is heroin. In general, all opiates and opioids cause sedation and respiratory depression. Toxicity is related to respiratory failure that can lead to death. The toxic dose varies widely with the opioid administered, its route and rate of administration, and the individual's tolerance to the drug. Diagnosis of opiate intoxication may be established clinically when the typical signs and symptoms are present—pinpoint pupils, and respiratory and CNS depression—and these are reversed by administration of the opioid antagonist naloxone. Demonstration of exposure to some opioids can be made by qualitative screening for these compounds in the urine using rapid immunoassays. Establishing the presence of other opioids may need additional targeted immunoassays (such as methadone and propoxyphene, as well as fentanyl and buprenorphine

A urine test for cannabinoids may be positive for 10 to 25 days after the last exposure in moderate and heavy users. In fact, there are well-documented reports of true-positive test results in users more than 80 days after their last exposure to THC.

which are discussed below), or chromatographic techniques (for meperidine and tramadol). Levels of these compounds in the serum, however, are not usually determined because they correlate poorly with their clinical effects.

Oxycodone and Oxymoprhone (OxyContin®, Percocet®, Percodan®)

Oxycodone is synthesized from thebane, a natural constituent of opium. Oxycodone is available in a number of compound analgesics, with acetaminophen and aspirin. The persistence of the predilection for OxyContin abuse over the last decade has resulted in the manufacture of targeted immunoassays for this compound and its metabolite. These show minimal cross-reactivity with morphine and codeine, and with the other opioids. Side effects and treatment of overdose are as for opiates above.

Fentanyl (Actiq®, Duragesic®, and Sublimaze®)

Fentanyl is a synthetic opiate analgesic, about 80 times more potent than morphine and highly addictive. It is used acutely to treat severe pain, or pain after surgery, and also in the management of chronic pain in patients already tolerant to opiates. Its abuse potential is high, and the manufacture of fentanyl patches, lozenges, and most recently "lollipops" has increased abuse significantly. The most common street names are dance fever, friend, tango, cash, china girl, jackpot, and percopops. "China White" refers to a number of clandestinely produced fentanyl analogs, especially the highly potent and long-acting α-methylfentanyl. Co-ingestion of fentanyl with other drugs of abuse such as heroin or cocaine is particularly dangerous. Side effects and treatment of overdose are as for opiates above. Plasma levels correlate poorly with clinical effect because of tolerance, and it is difficult to detect because of the low concentrations present. Immunoassays for urine are just emerging onto the market.

Buprenorphine (Temgesic®, Suboxone®, and Subutex®)

Buprenorphine is a synthetic analgesic first marketed in the 1980s, with 20 to 40 times the potency of morphine, but less addiction potential. Buprenorphine undergoes extensive first-pass metabolism, and its appearance in rapidly acting high-dose sublingual and transdermal preparations undoubtedly contributed to its popularity as a recreational drug. The half-life is long, about 20 to 72 hours, with hepatic elimination producing a number of water-soluble metabolites. Its use is mainly in substitution treatment of opiate dependence, and to that end, Suboxone® is a preparation that also contains the antidote naloxone, since buprenorphine toxicity is not easily reversed due to the high affinity of the drug for the opiate receptor. Street names include "bupe" and "sub(s)." Plasma levels of buprenorphine correlate poorly with clinical effect because of tolerance, and it is difficult to detect because of the low concentrations present. Immunoassays for urine are just emerging onto the market.

Phencyclidine (PCP)

PCP is an anesthetic agent that became popular as an inexpensive street drug in the late 1960s. It is most often smoked, but it can be snorted, ingested orally, or injected. It is commonly used in combination with other illicit drugs. Ingestion of the compound produces a generalized loss of pain perception and can cause hallucinations, euphoria, and disinhibition. Ingestion of large amounts can produce death, often from self-destructive behavior or from complications of hyperthermia. Documentation of PCP ingestion can be established by demonstrating the presence of the drug in the urine. PCP levels in the serum are not clinically valuable because they do not correlate with the degree of intoxication.

Acetaminophen

When it is used in the recommended doses, it is not necessary to measure acetaminophen levels. However, excess intake of acetaminophen can be associated with severe liver injury.

Acetaminophen is a therapeutic drug used as an analgesic and an antipyretic. When it is used in the recommended doses, it is not necessary to measure acetaminophen levels. However, excess intake of acetaminophen can be associated with severe liver injury. Thus, acetaminophen is a representative of many compounds with a wide therapeutic window that does not require therapeutic monitoring when used in recommended doses. However, because toxicity can occur if the

TABLE 6-6   Laboratory Evaluation for Acetaminophen Toxicity

Laboratory Tests	Results/Comments
Laboratory monitoring of acetaminophen concentration	The importance of laboratory monitoring is related to the use of N-acetylcysteine as a treatment for the acetaminophen overdose; it is important that the neutralizing effect of N-acetylcysteine be provided before acetaminophen metabolites produce liver injury. To determine whether the acetaminophen ingestion is likely to cause liver toxicity, a 4-hour postingestion serum concentration should be obtained; the serum concentration of the drug will be used to determine if the patient is likely to experience liver injury and, if so, treated with N-acetylcysteine. If the first acetaminophen level is obtained more than 4 hours postingestion, a nomogram can be used (available in many textbooks) to determine if the acetaminophen level at that time postingestion is likely or not likely to be associated with liver injury
Liver function tests	Hepatic necrosis becomes evident 24–48 hours after the ingestion of the excess amount of acetaminophen if the patient is not treated; at that time, standard liver function tests such as AST (SGOT), ALT (SGPT), bilirubin, as well as the prothrombin time, can be used to assess the extent of liver injury

ALT, alanine aminotransferase; AST, aspartate aminotransferase; BUN, blood urea nitrogen. The prothrombin time is a good prognostic tool when used as an indicator of hepatic recovery.

upper limit of the window is exceeded, monitoring acetaminophen levels in patients with excess intake is critical, particularly since an antidote to the major toxic effect can be administered.

Acetaminophen is rapidly absorbed from the gastrointestinal tract. The plasma concentration reaches its highest level 30 to 60 minutes after a dose. One of the compounds resulting from acetaminophen metabolism is an oxidation product that is hepatotoxic. Normally this metabolite is detoxified by binding to glutathione in the liver. With excess intake of acetaminophen, the production of the toxic metabolite exceeds the amount of hepatic glutathione, and this permits the toxic metabolite to produce liver injury. Renal damage also may occur as a result of injury by the same compound.

The recommended daily dose of acetaminophen is no more than 4 g/day. A single dose of 10 to 15 g may produce liver injury. Fatal disease is usually associated with ingestion of ≥25 g of acetaminophen. Acetaminophen at slightly more than the recommended 4 g/day can produce hepatotoxicity when the patient has also ingested ethanol, and this response can be exacerbated if the patient had been fasting prior to ingestion of acetaminophen and ethanol, or takes another enzyme-inducing drug such as phenytoin. The ingestion of acetaminophen at greater than recommended doses produces corresponding elevations of acetaminophen in the blood, and the level of the drug in the blood correlates with the severity of hepatic injury.

Acute manifestation of excess acetaminophen intake typically occurs 2 to 3 hours after ingestion. Most often this includes nausea, vomiting, and abdominal pain. Cyanosis of the skin and fingernails may be observed as a result of methemoglobin generation from the overdose. The full extent of liver damage usually becomes apparent 2 to 4 days after drug ingestion. At that time, liver function test results, including the prothrombin time, become abnormal. A variety of associated abnormalities, including electrolyte disturbances, can occur if there is significant liver damage. Acute renal failure also may occur, even if liver failure is not observed.

Table 6-6 presents an overview of the laboratory evaluation for acetaminophen toxicity.

The recommended daily dose of acetaminophen is no more than 4 g/day. A single dose of 10 to 15 g may produce liver injury. Fatal disease is usually associated with ingestion of ≥25 g of acetaminophen.

Aspirin

Aspirin (acetylsalicylic acid) is a therapeutic drug in use for more than a century as an analgesic, antipyretic, anti-inflammatory, and antithrombotic agent. It is readily absorbed and rapidly metabolized by hydrolysis to salicylic acid. Peak concentrations occur within 1 to 2 hours with a therapeutic dose. Between 50% and 90% is bound to albumin in a dose-dependent manner. Further metabolism produces salicyluric and gentisic acids and glucuronide conjugates that are renally excreted. Aspirin is contained in many preparations, including those with other analgesics. When used in therapeutic doses, it is not necessary to measure levels. However, chronic salicylate poisoning (salicylism) carries a high morbidity (30%) and mortality (25%), and is difficult to diagnose without monitoring

TABLE 6–7   Laboratory Evaluation for Aspirin Toxicity

Laboratory Tests	Results/Comments
Detection of aspirin metabolites in urine by color test (Trinder's reagent); monitoring of serum salicylate concentration by enzymatic assay or immunoassay	The importance of these tests is to establish the diagnosis of poisoning. Since a number of preparations are available containing sustained-release aspirin, it is recommended that serial blood samples be drawn at 3-hour intervals to determine whether the drug concentration is still rising
	The Done nomogram interprets the serum salicylate concentrations taken at 6 hours after acute ingestion as follows: • <50 mg/dL: asymptomatic • 51–110 mg/dL: mild to moderate toxicity • >110 mg/dL: serious toxicity
	The use of the Done nomogram is unreliable when: • There has been a previous ingestion within 24 hours • Chronic poisoning (where concentrations >30 mg/dL indicate serious toxicity) • Enteric coated or sustained-release preparations have been ingested • Renal failure is present
	Treatment for aspirin overdose is symptomatic and supportive—administration of repeat doses of oral activated charcoal may be given in an attempt to prevent further absorption and increase fecal elimination. Bicarbonate is used to counteract the metabolic acidosis, and calcium and electrolytes are administered to prevent seizures and cardiac failure. Hemodialysis may be indicated at concentrations above 100 mg/dL (>40 mg/dL in chronic salicylism), and to support renal function and electrolyte balance
	Regular monitoring of renal function, blood gas and lactate, and coagulation assessment are important for patient care

levels since the patient may be too confused to give a reliable history. About 500 mg/kg as an acute dose is potentially lethal in comparison to a normal dose of 15 mg/kg. When taken in therapeutic doses, the half-life is 2 to 5 hours, but metabolism becomes saturated once the dose exceeds about 30 mg/kg, causing a delay in drug elimination. An early feature of toxicity is respiratory alkalosis through direct stimulation of the respiratory drive center, followed by vomiting. The later mechanism of toxicity is via uncoupling of oxidative phosphorylation, leading to ketosis, metabolic acidosis, and pyrexia, with further dehydration and electrolyte imbalance. Hematologic consequences arise that manifest as an increased prothrombin time, GI bleeding, and occasionally DIC.

Table 6–7 presents an overview of the laboratory evaluation for salicylate toxicity.

Alcohols: Ethanol, Methanol, Ethylene Glycol, and Isopropanol

Ethanol is the most common drug of abuse. Many patients presenting to hospitals with altered mental status suffer from excess ethanol intake. Ethanol is present not only in beverages, but also in many medications. Ethanol intoxication is associated with many different types of accidental injury, particularly those involving motor vehicles. Ethanol is rapidly absorbed from the gastrointestinal tract. It distributes into the total body water and diffuses freely into the tissues. It is metabolized by an oxidative pathway to acetaldehyde and acetic acid, and also, by a nonoxidative pathway to fatty acid ethyl esters. When the acetaldehyde is subsequently converted to acetic acid, acidosis can occur. The major enzyme for oxidation of ethanol to acetaldehyde is alcohol dehydrogenase, and a second enzyme is the cytochrome P-450 system. The P-450 enzymes can be induced to higher levels of activity by ethanol. On that basis, ethanol ingestion can alter the metabolism of a number of drugs, which are metabolized by this same system. When ethanol induces higher levels of cytochrome P-450 and is still present, ethanol can also compete with drugs normally metabolized by cytochrome P-450. When the ethanol is no longer present, but the enzyme is still induced, the metabolism of compounds that are acted upon by cytochrome P-450 is enhanced. This may increase or decrease the therapeutic and/or toxic effect of drugs.

Despite many years of investigation, the mechanism by which ethanol induces organ damage has not been clearly established. Although acetaldehyde has been implicated as a mediator

Ethanol is the most common drug of abuse. Many patients presenting to hospitals with altered mental status suffer from excess ethanol intake.

TABLE 6-8   Laboratory Evaluation for Ethanol Intake

Laboratory monitoring: acute intake	Blood ethanol level (see below)
Laboratory monitoring: chronic intake	Long-term markers of ethanol intake include elevated gamma glutamyl transferase (GGT), carbohydrate deficient transferring, and fatty acid ethyl esters
Liver function tests	AST (SGOT), ALT (SGPT), and bilirubin assess ethanol-induced liver injury (see Chapter 16 on liver disease for a discussion of cirrhosis)
Pancreatic function tests	Amylase and lipase can be used to assess ethanol-induced pancreatic injury (see Chapter 17 on pancreatic disorders for a discussion of pancreatitis)
Blood Ethanol Concentration (mg/dL) (Ranges Overlap Because of Person-to-person Variability)	**Influence of Blood Alcohol Concentration in Individuals Who Are Not Chronic Ethanol Abusers**
10–50	Sobriety
40–120	Euphoria
90–250	Excitement
180–300	Confusion
270–400	Stupor
350–500	Coma
>450	Death can be produced by ingestion of 300–400 mL of pure ethanol or 600–800 mL of 100 proof whiskey in <1 hour

Data from Dubowski KM. Alcohol determination in the clinical laboratory. *Am J Clin Pathol*. 1980;74:747–750.

of liver damage, it has not been widely accepted as causative agent of ethanol-induced pancreatic injury. More recently, fatty acid ethyl esters have been proposed as causative for ethanol-induced organ damage, especially in the pancreas. Peak blood ethanol levels occur 30 to 75 minutes after ethanol ingestion. Food ingestion can delay absorption. A useful rule of thumb is that 1 ounce of 80 to 100 proof spirits, 4 ounces of wine, or 12 ounces of beer increases the blood alcohol concentration by 25 to 30 mg/dL when ingested over a period of several minutes. The blood ethanol in a nonchronic alcoholic decreases at a rate of 15 to 25 mg/dL per hour once ethanol ingestion is discontinued. The blood ethanol levels required to induce fetal alcohol syndrome have not yet been determined. Pregnant women who abuse ethanol have a high risk of delivering an infant with fetal alcohol syndrome. These infants have prenatal growth retardation, dysfunction of the CNS, and characteristic craniofacial abnormalities. Because an acceptable lower limit of alcohol intake in pregnancy has not been defined, pregnant women are generally advised to abstain from ethanol.

The measurement of blood ethanol concentration can be performed by breath analysis, or more accurately, by an enzymatic assay for ethanol specifically or a gas chromatographic test that can measure ethanol, methanol, and isopropanol, individually (**Table 6–8**).

Methanol and isopropanol are also toxic, primarily as a result of their metabolism by alcohol dehydrogenase and other enzymes to their corresponding acids, as is the case for ethanol. A separate test must be performed to detect and quantitate ethylene glycol, a different alcoholic compound in this family. The clinical presentation, sources for ingestion, and laboratory detection and quantitation of methanol, ethylene glycol, and isopropanol are shown in **Table 6–9**.

Overview—Environmental Toxins

Monitoring of environmental toxins is a significant challenge because there are so many substances encountered in daily life, particularly in the workplace, that can produce illness and even fatality. Compounds that can be fatal include carbon monoxide, mercury, cyanide, mushroom poisons, and a variety of insecticides. Other compounds such as lead, which can be obtained from a variety of occupational and nonoccupational sources (such as paint chips), can produce

The measurement of blood ethanol concentration can be performed by breath analysis, or more accurately, by an enzymatic assay for ethanol specifically or a gas chromatographic test that can measure ethanol, methanol, and isopropanol, individually.

TABLE 6-9   Methanol, Ethylene Glycol, and Isopropanol Toxicity and Laboratory Monitoring

	Methanol	Ethylene Glycol	Isopropanol
Sources for ingestion	Methanol, methanol-contaminated alcohols, and antifreeze	Antifreeze	Rubbing alcohol
Time until onset of symptoms	12–48 hours	0.5–12 hours	Minutes
Fatal dose of the pure compound	60–250 mL in most cases	Approximately 100 g	Approximately 250 mL
Clinical features	Impaired vision up to blindness, vomiting, seizures, coma	Anuria, vomiting, seizures, coma	Vomiting, abdominal pain, hematemesis, melena, coma
Antidote administration	4MP; ethanol	4MP; ethanol	None (hemodialysis >400 mg/dL)
Laboratory monitoring			
Presence in blood	Yes	Yes	Yes
Osmolality [MOsm = (mg/dL alcohol)/(10 × molecular weight)]	Elevated	Elevated	Elevated
Hypoglycemia	Yes	Yes	No
Acidosis (blood pH)	Severe	Severe	Mild
Oxalate crystals (urine)	No	Yes (because ethylene glycol is metabolized to oxalate)	No
Anion gap	Large	Large	Normal

4MP, 4-methylpyrazole.

subclinical to life-threatening illness, depending on the amount ingested. Low-level exposure in children may produce serious disease but have less of an impact in adults. In some cases, the compound impairs the flux through a metabolic pathway. In these cases, accumulated metabolites that result from the blockade can be measured as a reflection of the toxic effects of the compound. An example of this is the effect of lead on heme synthesis, which is inhibited at a specific point in its synthetic pathway. A specific description is provided for carbon monoxide and lead as they are commonly encountered environmental toxins.

Carbon Monoxide

Description

Carbon monoxide poisoning is responsible for up to 4,000 deaths per year in the United States and is the leading cause of accidental and deliberate poisonings. Approximately 10% of the cases involve children. The heart, CNS, and lungs are the organs most immediately affected by the toxic effects of carbon monoxide. Carbon monoxide can also impair vision, hearing, and peripheral nerve conduction. The poisoning may be sublethal and in that setting may cause cardiac dysrhythmias, myocardial ischemia, headache, and a variety of other signs and symptoms. Survivors often suffer permanent, severe neurologic impairment.

The principal pathologic consequence of carbon monoxide poisoning is the binding of carbon monoxide to oxygen-binding sites in the hemoglobin molecule. When carbon monoxide reacts with normal hemoglobin, the configuration of the molecule is altered. It develops a greater affinity for oxygen, and this decreases its ability to deliver oxygen to the tissues and produces an ischemic effect. The binding of carbon monoxide to hemoglobin also results in the formation of

Carbon monoxide poisoning is responsible for up to 4,000 deaths per year in the United States and is the leading cause of accidental and deliberate poisonings. The principal pathologic consequence of carbon monoxide poisoning is the binding of carbon monoxide to oxygen-binding sites in the hemoglobin molecule.

TABLE 6–10   Clinical Presentation of Carbon Monoxide Toxicity

Carboxyhemoglobin Relative to Total Hemoglobin (%)	Clinical Findings in Adults[a]
0.1–0.9	Normal range for nonsmoking adults
10–30	As concentration elevates, increasingly severe headache and greater dyspnea on exertion
40–50	Very severe headache and dyspnea with tachycardia; may be fatal
60–70	Coma, seizures, often fatal
80	Rapidly fatal

[a]Children are more sensitive and can present differently.

TABLE 6–11   Laboratory Tests Used in the Evaluation of a Patient for Carbon Monoxide Poisoning

Laboratory Test	Comments
Carboxyhemoglobin (% relative to total hemoglobin)	See **Table 6–10**
CBC/relevant microbiology studies	Anemias and infections can increase the concentration of carboxyhemoglobin and should be identified if present
Indicators of ischemic damage to skeletal and cardiac muscle	Creatinine kinase, troponin I, troponin T, lactate dehydrogenase, and/or aldolase may be elevated; myoglobin may be detectable in the urine if there is muscle damage

carboxyhemoglobin (see below). A relatively small amount of carbon monoxide is generated normally in vivo, primarily from the degradation of hemoglobin and the release of carbon monoxide that is normally bound to hemoglobin.

The normal range for percent carboxyhemoglobin for adults is 0.1% to 0.9% of total hemoglobin. When hemolytic disease is present with increased breakdown of hemoglobin, the carboxyhemoglobin levels can increase to approximately 2%. Values at this level can have adverse clinical effects in patients with pre-existing heart disease. **Table 6–10** shows an approximation of percent carboxyhemoglobin relative to total hemoglobin, and corresponding clinical findings in adults. It should be noted, however, that there is a poor correlation between carboxyhemoglobin levels and clinical findings. Children are much more susceptible to acute carbon monoxide poisoning and have a different clinical picture that mimics gastroenteritis. Like adults, they can also have serious neurologic sequelae and myocardial ischemia. Patients are often unaware of their exposure to carbon monoxide because it is odorless and nonirritating. There is no pathognomonic feature of carbon monoxide intoxication. It is important to make the diagnosis of carbon monoxide poisoning rapidly to institute appropriate management and identify sources of carbon monoxide before other exposures can occur.

Diagnosis

Laboratory monitoring of carbon monoxide poisoning is performed by measurement of the carboxyhemoglobin levels. The patient also must be evaluated for possible underlying cause(s) of an increased carbon monoxide level, such as the presence of anemia, infection, and other clinical entities that increase endogenous carbon monoxide production. Because carbon monoxide can cause ischemic damage to skeletal and cardiac muscle, it also may be appropriate in some patients to determine whether ischemic muscle damage is present.

Table 6–11 presents information on the laboratory tests used in the evaluation of patients for carbon monoxide poisoning.

Laboratory monitoring of carbon monoxide poisoning is performed by measurement of the carboxyhemoglobin levels.

Lead

Description

Lead poisoning is primarily a disease of childhood. As understanding has increased about the toxicity of lead, the threshold for the definition of lead poisoning has decreased continuously for the past 20 years. Prior to 1970, lead poisoning (plumbism) was defined by blood levels greater than 60 μg/dL. In 1971, the threshold was lowered to 40 μg/dL. By 1975, the acceptable level was 25 μg/dL and since 1985, blood levels of 10 to 15 μg/dL have been recognized to impair cognitive and behavioral development. According to 1991 guidelines from the Centers for Disease Control and Prevention, the threshold for action for lead poisoning is 10 μg/dL. As recently as 1992, 17.2% of children in the United States between the ages of 6 months and 5 years were estimated to have a blood lead level in excess of 15 μg/dL, although this pales in comparison to those observed in developing countries. These children were primarily from low-income families in large urban settings. The sources of lead for these children included not only lead paint, but also lead-contaminated household dust, soil, and clothing from the workplace; the use of lead containing cookware; exposure to lead in storage batteries, and in fishing and curtain weights; and even lead-contaminated water from the use of lead solder in pipes. Some canned food also has been reported to contain lead. The use of lead-containing costume jewelry, medicines, and cosmetics (such as surma or kohl) in some cultures has been demonstrated to cause lead poisoning. Obviously it is important in the investigation of cases of lead poisoning to identify the precise source of lead being ingested so that exposure can be eliminated.

There is a significant effort nationally to screen children, particularly those between the ages of 6 months to 5 years who live in, or are frequent visitors to, deteriorated housing built prior to

> As understanding has increased about the toxicity of lead, the threshold for the definition of lead poisoning has decreased continuously for the past 20 years.

TABLE 6–12 **Laboratory Monitoring of Children for Lead Poisoning** (http://www.cdc.gov/nceh/lead/casemanagement/caseManage_chap3.htm, Summary of Recommendations for Children with Confirmed (Venous) Elevated Blood Lead Levels)

Blood Lead Level (μg/dL)				
10–14	**15–19**	**20–44**	**45–69**	**>70**
Lead education • Dietary • Environmental Follow-up blood lead monitoring	Lead education • Dietary • Environmental Follow-up blood lead monitoring Proceed according to actions for 20–44 μg/dL if: • A follow-up BLL[a] is in this range at least 3 months after initial venous test **or** • BLLs increase	Lead education • Dietary • Environmental Follow-up blood lead monitoring Laboratory work: • Hemoglobin or hematocrit • Iron status Environmental investigation Lead hazard reduction Neurodevelopmental monitoring Abdominal X-ray (if particulate lead ingestion is suspected) with bowel decontamination if indicated	Lead education • Dietary • Environmental Follow-up blood lead monitoring Laboratory work: • Hemoglobin or hematocrit • Iron status • FEP or ZPP Environmental investigation Lead hazard reduction Neurodevelopmental monitoring Abdominal X-ray with bowel decontamination if indicated Chelation therapy	Hospitalize and commence chelation therapy Proceed according to actions for 45–69 μg/dL

[a]BLL; Blood lead level
The following actions are **not** recommended at any blood lead level: searching for gingival lead lines; testing of neurophysiologic function; evaluation of renal function (except during chelation with EDTA); testing of hair, teeth, or fingernails for lead; radiographic imaging of long bones; X-ray fluorescence of long bones. For adults, it is recognized that accumulation of lead occurs, and blood lead concentrations <25 μg/dL do not require action.

1960. Exposure to lead at high doses can produce persistent seizures, mental retardation, and chronic behavioral dysfunction. Most of the retained lead is stored in the bones. However, it is also found in soft tissues and erythrocytes. Lead interferes with the enzymes required to synthesize heme, and on that basis produces anemia. Renal toxicity is also observed in some cases of chronic lead poisoning. Lead poisoning should be considered in children with developmental delay, behavioral disorders, seizures, learning disabilities, iron deficiency, hearing impairment, renal disorders, and in any child with recurrent vomiting and abdominal pain.

Diagnosis

The whole blood lead level reflects the lead burden of the body. For small children, a fingerstick sample is usually sent for analysis. If the blood lead level is greater than 10 μg/dL, testing of a sample taken by venipuncture is recommended to rule out surface contamination. If this "clean" specimen contains more than 10 μg/dL lead, parental education on possible exposure sources is instigated. While initial testing is often performed by anodic stripping voltammetry, for confirmation of concentrations above 40 μg/dL, atomic absorption or mass spectrometry is advisable. Free erythrocyte protoporphyrin (zinc protoporphyrin) is an alternate product of heme synthesis as a result of lead toxicity. The measurement of free erythrocyte protoporphyrin is, however, an insensitive screening test for lead exposure because it does not detect lead poisoning in children with lead levels between 10 and 25 μg/dL, and it identifies less than 50% of children with blood levels 25 μg/dL and higher. Its utility is primarily to indicate ongoing exposure. Because the anemia in lead poisoning may resemble iron deficiency anemia, studies for iron deficiency anemia (such as serum ferritin and the red cell distribution width in the complete blood count) should be obtained to differentiate the anemia of lead poisoning from iron deficiency anemia.

Table 6–12 describes the laboratory monitoring for children suspected of lead poisoning relative to the presenting blood lead level.

A portion of this chapter on TDM is also found in a newsletter to the physicians at the Massachusetts General Hospital in Clinical Laboratory Reviews, 1999;8:1.

> The whole blood lead level reflects the lead burden of the body. For small children, a fingerstick sample is usually sent for analysis. If the blood lead level is greater than 10 μg/dL, testing of a sample taken by venipuncture is recommended to rule out surface contamination.

REFERENCES

Braaten K, et al. Therapeutic drug monitoring. *Clin Lab Rev* (a publication of the Massachusetts General Hospital). 1999;8:1.

Committee on Environmental Health. Lead poisoning: from screening to primary prevention. *Pediatrics.* 1993;92:176.

Dasgupta A. Therapeutic drug monitoring of digoxin: impact of endogenous and exogenous digoxin-like immunoreactive substances. *Toxicol Rev.* 2006;25:273–281.

Doyle KM, et al. Fatty acid ethyl esters in the blood as markers for ethanol intake. *JAMA.* 1996;276:1152.

Ellenhorn MJ, et al. Alcohols and glycols. In: *Ellenhorn's Medical Toxicology: Diagnosis and Treatment of Human Poisoning.* 2nd ed. Philadelphia, PA: Williams & Wilkins; 1997:1127.

Ham RJ. The signs and symptoms of poor nutritional status. *Prim Care.* 1994;21:33.

Hammet-Stabler CA, et al. Laboratory guidelines for monitoring of antimicrobial drugs. *Clin Chem.* 1998;44:1129.

Hammond S, et al. Laboratory assessment of oxygenation in methemoglobinemia. *Clin Chem.* 2005;51:434–444.

Huestis MA, Cone EJ. Differentiating new marijuana use from residual drug excretion in occasional marijuana users. *J Anal Toxicol.* 1998;22:445–454.

Jacob RA, et al. Biochemical assessment of vitamins and trace minerals. *Clin Lab Med.* 1993;13:371.

Labbe RF, et al. Nutrition in the clinical laboratory. *Clin Lab Med.* 1993;13:313.

Laposata M. Fatty acid ethyl esters: short term and long-term serum markers of ethanol intake. *Clin Chem.* 1997;43:1527.

Leibovici L, Vidal L, Paul M. Aminoglycoside drugs in clinical practice: an evidenced based approach. *J Antimicrob Chemother.* 2009;63:246–251.

Linder MW, et al. Standards of laboratory practice: antidepressant drug monitoring. *Clin Chem.* 1998;44:1073.

Moeller KE, et al. Urine drug screening: practical guide for clinicians. *Mayo Clin Proc.* 2008;63:66–76.

Moyer TP, et al. Therapeutic drug monitoring. In: Burtis CA, Ashwood ER, eds. *Textbook of Clinical Chemistry.* 2nd ed. Philadelphia, PA: WB Saunders & Company; 1994:1094.

Oellerich M, Armstrong VW. The role of therapeutic drug monitoring in individualizing immunosuppressive drug therapy: recent developments. *Ther Drug Monit.* 2006;28:720–725.

Olson KR, ed. *Poisoning & Drug Overdose.* 2nd ed. Norwalk, CT: Appleton & Lange; 1994.

O'Malley GF. Emergency department management of the salicylate-poisoned patient. *Emerg Med Clin N Am.* 2007;25:333–346.

Patsalos PN, et al. Antiepileptic drugs—best practice guidelines for therapeutic drug monitoring: a position paper by the subcommission on therapeutic drug monitoring, ILAE Commission on Therapeutic Strategies. *Epilepsia.* 2008;49:1–38.

Rumack BH, et al. Acetaminophen overdose: 662 cases with evaluation of oral acetylcysteine treatment. *Arch Intern Med.* 1981;141:380.

Smilkstein MJ, et al. Efficacy of oral N-acetylcysteine in the treatment of acetaminophen overdose. *New Engl J Med.* 1988;319:1557.

Sullivan LE, Fiellin DA. Narrative review: buprenorphine for opioid-dependent patients in office practice. *Ann Intern Med.* 2008;148:662–670.

Tsunoda SM, et al. Optimising immunosuppressive therapy. *Clin Pharmacokinet.* 1996;30:108.

United States Center for Disease Control. http://www.atsdr.cdc.gov/csem/lead/; Accessed 17.04.09.

Valdes R Jr, et al. Standards of laboratory practice: cardiac drug monitoring. *Clin Chem.* 1998;44:1096.

Willie S, Cooreman S, Neels H, Lambert L. Relevant issues in the monitoring and the toxicology of antidepressants. *Crit Rev Clin Lab Sci.* 2008;45:25–89.

Diseases of Infancy and Childhood

Paul Steele

Paul Steele

LEARNING OBJECTIVES

1. Identify the clinical situations that indicate the need for prenatal testing of mother and/or infant, and the clinical consequences of premature birth.

2. Understand the rationale for selection of laboratory tests in neonatal screening programs.

3. Learn the assessment for diagnosis of Down syndrome and the clinical situations in which it is most often performed.

4. Learn the underlying defects that produce hemolytic disease of the newborn and cystic fibrosis and the laboratory test abnormalities associated with these disorders.

5. Learn the names of the diseases and the associated biochemical defects for the more commonly encountered or better characterized inborn errors of metabolism in the following categories:

   • amino acidurias not involving urea cycle enzymes;

   • amino acidurias involving urea cycle enzymes;

   • lysosomal storage diseases with impaired degradation of sphingolipids;

   • lysosomal storage diseases with impaired degradation of mucopolysaccharides;

   • lysosomal storage diseases with impaired degradation of glycogen.

CHAPTER OUTLINE

INTRODUCTION

It is difficult to precisely identify the diseases of infancy and childhood because many disorders that begin in childhood become clinically evident in adulthood if a long period of time is required to generate a pathologic lesion. The topics chosen for inclusion in this chapter are disorders presenting almost exclusively in childhood. However, they obviously represent only a small fraction of "childhood disorders." Many disorders in other sections of this book, such as hemophilia and numerous infections, occur or are diagnosed primarily in childhood. The chapter begins with an overview of prenatal and neonatal laboratory testing.

PRENATAL AND NEONATAL LABORATORY TESTING

Prenatal Testing and Screening

The disorders that can be diagnosed before birth number in the thousands. In families in which there is a history of a particular disorder, it is not uncommon to test prenatally for that particular disorder, often with DNA-based diagnostic tests. However, for the vast majority of families without a history of a specific illness, prenatal screening may be undertaken. A screen differs from a test in that it does not provide a definitive diagnosis but rather an assessment of the risk of a diagnosis. For most of these families, screening is preferred as an initial step because it is less invasive; for example, there are several maternal serum screening *assays* (see below) for fetal Down syndrome (also known as trisomy 21) but *testing* for fetal Down syndrome requires an invasive procedure such as chorionic villus sampling or collection of amniotic fluid. The decision to screen is a personal one for families and includes considerations such as parental age and desire to avoid having a diseased child.

Neonatal Screening

Neonatal screening was introduced as a means to detect disorders in which immediate treatment can result in the prevention of catastrophic consequences. For example, in phenylketonuria (PKU) and congenital hypothyroidism, if the disease is not quickly recognized and treated, mental retardation will result. One could apply a financial justification to neonatal screening programs, for example, for every dollar spent on the program, a certain number of dollars was saved in avoiding the medical and social expenses of a lifetime of caring for a retarded patient. The rationale for neonatal screening still includes these treatable and preventable disorders, but the cost of neonatal screening has decreased with improved technology, and now many states also test for disorders that are not preventable but that are treatable, or desirable to identify at an early age, including illnesses such as sickle cell anemia, congenital adrenal hyperplasia, and cystic fibrosis.

There is significant variability among the states in the United States in which tests are performed in newborn screening, which leads to disparities in the level of care for newborns. The American College of Medical Genetics has suggested that a national minimum standard be adopted that includes a core screen for 29 diseases. Of these, 23 disorders can be studied by liquid chromatography/tandem mass spectrometry (LC/MS/MS) that provides multiplexing (i.e., multiple diseases screened by a single test). These 29 tests include 9 organic acidemias (such as isovaleric acidemia), 6 amino acidurias (such as PKU), 5 disorders of fatty oxidation (such as medium-chain acyl CoA dehydrogenase deficiency (MCAD)), 3 hemoglobinopathies associated with hemoglobin S, and 6 other conditions including cystic fibrosis, congenital adrenal hyperplasia, and congenital hypothyroidism.

Practical considerations for a successful neonatal screening program include consideration of the fact that false-negatives may occur before 24 hours of age; thus, many babies discharged with their mother "early" may require a follow-up visit to obtain a heelstick sample for the blood spots that are used in this screening. Another consideration is that positive results for screening tests require follow-up testing to further investigate the patient because not all screening test positives are true-positives.

Neonatal screening was introduced as a means to detect disorders in which immediate treatment can result in the prevention of catastrophic consequences. There is significant variability among the states in the United States in which tests are performed in newborn screening, which leads to disparities in the level of care for newborns.

TABLE 7–1   **Routine Laboratory Screening for Inherited Metabolic Disease**

Laboratory Test	Specimen
Lactate	Blood, CSF if indicated
Pyruvate	Blood
Amino acids	Urine, blood, CSF if indicated
Organic acids	Urine
Reducing sugars	Urine
Glucose	Blood, urine, CSF if indicated
Ketones and pH	Urine
Liver enzymes, electrolytes, uric acid, ammonia	Blood
Acylcarnitine profile	Blood
Mucopolysaccharide screen	Urine

CSF, cerebrospinal fluid.

Neonatal Testing

The laboratory evaluation of an infant who appears clinically well in the first 24 hours of life but develops signs of illness on the second or third day may include:

- blood gases to detect metabolic acidosis/alkalosis
- urinalysis to detect ketonuria
- complete blood count to detect abnormalities in blood cells
- a blood glucose test to detect hypoglycemia
- a blood ammonia test to detect elevated ammonia
- liver function tests to detect hepatic dysfunction
- prothrombin time and partial thromboplastin time to detect coagulopathies
- blood lactate to detect lactic acidosis

Table 7–1 lists a number of screening laboratory tests that are typically ordered when there is suspicion that a neonate (or older child) is suffering from an inborn error of metabolism.

The results of these tests only suggest specific disorders, with additional testing required to identify a specific metabolic defect. Definitive tests to make a conclusive diagnosis of a metabolic disorder often involve the measurement of specific enzyme activities or various metabolites in a pathway. Because sepsis is often suspected, it must be ruled out in the sick infant if there are any signs or symptoms of infection.

A major cause of neonatal mortality and morbidity is preterm labor and delivery.

PREMATURITY

Description

A major cause of neonatal mortality and morbidity is preterm labor and delivery. Maternal infection, particularly bacterial infections involving genital, urinary, and other sites, is correlated with preterm labor and delivery. For example, the common entity of bacterial vaginosis, which involves overgrowth of gram-negative, anaerobic bacteria in the vagina, is associated with a risk of preterm labor and delivery. Conflicting information exists about the value of intervention, for example, antibiotic therapy.

Another cause of prematurity is iatrogenic, when the medical condition of the mother and/or fetus compels intervention to produce early delivery. The timing of such elective intervention for early delivery is influenced by the risk for fetal organ immaturity. Principal among these concerns is lung immaturity that is associated with the development of respiratory distress syndrome in the newborn.

Diagnosis

Risk of preterm delivery can be assessed by measurement of fetal fibronectin in cervical or vaginal fluid. This glycoprotein is produced by fetal membranes and appears in the cervix and vagina early in pregnancy as implantation develops, but normally disappears by week 20. Its reappearance in the third trimester often precedes labor and delivery. Its chief clinical value lies in its negative predictive value, that is, patients thought to be at risk for preterm labor who are negative for fetal fibronectin in their cervicovaginal fluid are very unlikely to deliver within 1 week of the laboratory result. The major barrier to the widespread use of fetal fibronectin is that clinical interventions to end preterm labor are only partially successful.

In those instances when fetal or maternal health dictates early delivery, there are several tests available to assess fetal lung maturity. A simple and inexpensive test is to count lamellar bodies in amniotic fluid, using the platelet channel in a conventional hematology automated analyzer. These lamellar bodies are surfactant-containing products of Type II pneumocytes. The finding of greater than 50,000 lamellar bodies per microliter of amniotic fluid predicts lung maturity. If fewer bodies are present, further testing on the amniotic fluid sample is warranted. This testing can include determination of a surfactant-to-albumin ratio known as TDx FLM II, identification of the presence of phosphatidyl glycerol (PG), and determination of the ratio of lecithin to sphingomyelin (L/S ratio). (See Chapter 14 on Respiratory Disease for additional information.)

DOWN SYNDROME

Description

Down syndrome is the most commonly encountered, clinically significant autosomal chromosome aberration affecting individuals beyond infancy. This genetic defect, which can be detected by cytogenetic analysis, is trisomy 21. More than 90% of Down cases occur as a result of meiotic nondisjunction. Down syndrome is characterized by mental retardation, cardiac malformations, malformations of the digestive tract, eyes, and ears, and the development of an Alzheimer-like disease process in later life.

The overall birth prevalence of Down syndrome is approximately 1 in 1,000 births. However, a woman's individual risk to deliver an infant with Down syndrome depends substantially on her age. The risk increases significantly past age 35 years, with an incidence in the range of 1:270 to 1:100 by age 40 years.

Screening and Diagnosis

The neonatal diagnosis of Down syndrome is clinical, with metaphase chromosome analysis on peripheral blood serving merely to confirm the diagnosis.

Noninvasive fetal screening for Down syndrome involves many more tests (**Table 7–2**) that are used in combination to develop a risk assessment of Down syndrome during pregnancy. Definitive diagnosis of fetal Down syndrome during pregnancy is established by an invasive test, namely metaphase analysis of cells from either chorionic villus sampling (typically limited to first trimester) or amniotic fluid collection. The decision to engage in fetal screening for Down syndrome or to move from screening tests to invasive diagnostic testing once a risk assessment is completed depends on patient preference. The invasive tests to assess for Down syndrome during pregnancy do carry a risk of miscarriage.

First-trimester screening typically consists of measurement of 2 analytes in maternal serum: pregnancy-associated plasma protein A (PAPP-A) and the free beta subunit of human chorionic gonadotropin (fβhCG); the former is low and the latter high in mothers carrying a Down syndrome fetus. A third part of first-trimester screening is ultrasound determination of nuchal translucency, which is increased as a result of fluid accumulation in the neck of a Down syndrome fetus. This first-trimester screening is associated with a sensitivity of approximately 85%, with a 5% false-positive rate. False-positives would be uncovered through definitive testing, that is, metaphase analysis on chorionic villus sampling or amniotic fluid. Nuchal translucency alone is not recommended in singleton pregnancy because its sensitivity is only about 70%. However, in multiple gestation pregnancies, the interpretation of maternal serum markers can be problematic, while the nuchal translucency test permits evaluation of each fetus.

TABLE 7–2   Laboratory Evaluation for Down Syndrome

Laboratory Test	Result/Comment
First-trimester screen	
Pregnancy-associated plasma protein A (PAPP-A)	Low in pregnancy with Down syndrome fetus
Free beta hCG	Elevated in pregnancy with Down syndrome fetus
Nuchal translucency	Ultrasound exam; permits evaluation of each fetus in multiple gestation pregnancy
Quadruple screen	Second-trimester screen
Alpha-fetoprotein (AFP)	Low in pregnancy with Down syndrome fetus; elevated with fetal neural tube defect
hCG	Elevated in pregnancy with Down syndrome fetus
Unconjugated estriol (UE3)	Low in pregnancy with Down syndrome fetus
Inhibin A	Elevated in pregnancy with Down syndrome fetus
Metaphase chromosome analysis	Diagnostic test; can be performed on chorionic villus sample, cells from amniotic fluid, and newborn blood

Second-trimester screening typically consists of the so-called quadruple screen of maternal serum, consisting of measurement of the following analytes: alpha-fetoprotein, unconjugated estriol (both decreased in mothers carrying a Down syndrome fetus), and total hCG and inhibin A (both increased in such mothers). The quadruple screen has a detection rate of approximately 81% with a 5% false-positive rate. An older test, the "triple screen" includes all of these second-trimester markers except inhibin A. It is characterized by higher false-positive rates and lower detection rates.

Combining first- and second -trimester screens can provide an even higher level of detection. One approach is to sequentially conduct the tests; that is, inform the patient of the results of the first-trimester screen as soon as they are available (this permits her to choose chorionic villus sampling for definitive diagnosis if indicated), and later perform the quadruple screen in the second trimester.

Three additional points are worthwhile to add about Down syndrome screening. First, the maternal serum results are typically described in the form of "multiples of the median" (or MoM); the normal range is highly dependent on several factors including gestational age, number of gestations, maternal weight, and race. Second, determination of nuchal translucency is highly operator-dependent and requires specific training. Third, the alpha-fetoprotein assay in the quadruple screen, if elevated, provides a measure of increased risk for neural tube defects such as spina bifida. These cases can be further studied by amniotic fluid collection, with assessment of acetylcholinesterase as well as alpha-fetoprotein (both elevated with neural tube defects) and high-resolution ultrasound examination.

INFECTIOUS DISEASES IN THE PERINATAL PERIOD

Description

A number of maternal infections affect the fetus and newborn. Bacterial vaginosis, sexually transmitted diseases, and others increase the risk of preterm labor. Rubella and syphilis are associated with congenital anomalies. Neonatal death has been linked to a number of infections, including cytomegalovirus (CMV), group B streptococcus, herpes simplex, *Listeria*, parvovirus, and others. Postnatal disease in the offspring occurs with many of these infections, as well as hepatitis B and C, human immunodeficiency disease (HIV), CMV, rubella, toxoplasmosis, and syphilis.

A number of maternal infections affect the fetus and newborn. Neonatal death has been linked to a number of infections, including cytomegalovirus (CMV), group B streptococcus, herpes simplex, *Listeria*, parvovirus, and others.

Screening and Diagnosis

Routine prenatal care is designed to screen for several of these infections, for the purpose of identifying patients who need intervention or identifying susceptibility in the mother. The results of these maternal screening tests may have implications for the fetus should maternal infection occur during pregnancy. An example of the latter is rubella serology screening of maternal serum. Routine testing also includes serologic testing for syphilis, hepatitis B and C, and HIV. Routine rectovaginal culture for group B streptococcus is performed late in the third trimester. Detection through nucleic acid testing and/or culture is carried out for *Chlamydia* and for gonorrhea in high-risk mothers, and for herpes simplex in mothers with genital lesions.

HEMOLYTIC DISEASE OF THE NEWBORN

Description

Hemolytic disease of the newborn (HDN), also known as erythroblastosis fetalis, is a syndrome in which the newborn becomes anemic from the destruction of his/her RBCs in utero. This RBC destruction is a result of maternal IgG antibodies formed against a red cell antigen, most commonly the Rh antigen (also known as D antigen), which are then delivered into the fetal circulation across the placenta. Antibody production by the mother, who is Rh-negative, results from exposure to Rh-positive fetal cells during pregnancy and, to a much greater extent, at delivery. Therefore, the women at greatest risk for delivering infants with HDN are Rh-negative mothers who conceive Rh-positive babies, and are in the second or subsequent pregnancies. It is general practice to identify risk of sensitization during pregnancy and treat the mother prophylactically by rapidly removing Rh-positive fetal cells through passive immunization with Rh immune globulin (which is almost always effective in preventing the mother's immune system from developing these alloantibodies); treatment is employed not only following delivery (when fetal to maternal bleeding is expected), but also during pregnancy itself.

Other red cell alloantibodies may be involved, although much less commonly. A form of HDN, usually mild, results from transplacental passage of IgG-class antibodies against A or B red cell antigens, to a Type A, B, or AB fetus. This disorder may occur with the first pregnancy, as it involves maternal antibodies that normally arise without the requirement of a previous pregnancy or incompatible blood transfusion.

Neonatal disease related to maternal antibody may occasionally involve targets other than RBC antigens; examples include neonatal alloimmune thrombocytopenic purpura (NAIT) with maternal anti-platelet antibodies and neonatal autoimmune disease with maternal autoantibodies.

Screening and Diagnosis

ABO/Rh typing is used in routine prenatal care to identify the mother's blood type. An antibody screen against a standard panel of red cells, employing the indirect antiglobulin method (see Chapter 2), is also routinely performed to determine if there are maternal alloantibodies (such as anti-Rh) that might be a threat to the fetus.

Testing for fetal blood type (which establishes presence or absence of fetal susceptibility in that pregnancy), as well as monitoring for fetal anemia and hyperbilirubinemia (the latter a consequence of the RBC destruction), typically requires invasive procedures such as amniocentesis (withdrawal of amniotic fluid) or cordocentesis (withdrawal of blood from the cord, in utero). Both of these carry some risk of pregnancy loss or fetal damage. A new, noninvasive approach is possible with genetic testing for the antigen genes. Genotyping of the father that reveals homozygosity of the antigen gene implies fetal antigen positivity. Heterozygosity in the father implies a 50% chance of fetal antigen negativity (in which case there would be absence of risk for HDN); confirmation of fetal antigen negativity can be accomplished by genotyping of fetal DNA that is present in maternal plasma. Titering the quantity of maternal antibody as a disease predictor in the fetus has been used, but the amount of antibody does not always correlate with the severity of the disease. Testing of amniotic fluid for bilirubin by spectrophotometric analysis can be performed to help manage the disease; fetuses at high risk of severe anemia, based on the amniotic fluid bilirubin, would be delivered if tests of fetal lung maturity on the amniotic fluid sample (see above) reveal a low risk of respiratory distress syndrome; otherwise, intrauterine blood

TABLE 7–3 Laboratory Evaluation of the Mother and Newborn for Hemolytic Disease of the Newborn (HDN)

	Result/Comment
To predict HDN during pregnancy	
Maternal ABO and Rh type	Provides screening for possible HDN risk
Maternal antibody screen	Detects many common anti-red cell antibodies
Maternal antibody titer	Significant elevation implies risk of HDN
Genotyping of father	Homozygosity for antigen gene implies fetal risk; heterozygosity for antigen gene requires further testing to assess fetal susceptibility
Genotyping of fetus	Presence of antigen gene can be assessed; specimen may be amniotic fluid or cord cells (both invasive) or maternal plasma
To assess for HDN during pregnancy	
ΔOD_{450}	Invasive; spectrophotometric assessment of bilirubin through assessment of change (delta) of optical density at 450 nm from expected to observed
Fetal hematocrit	Invasive; requires cordocentesis
Fetal middle cerebral artery flow	Noninvasive; peak velocity of systolic blood flow increases progressively with fetal anemia
To evaluate disease in the newborn	
Clinical findings	Infant may appear normal to very abnormal; jaundice is common; cardiorespiratory problems may occur; severely affected fetuses may die in utero or at delivery
Reticulocyte count	At 7 days of life, an elevated level is consistent with HDN
Nucleated red blood cells	A persistently high percentage of nucleated red blood cells is consistent with increased red blood cell production
Unconjugated bilirubin	Markedly elevated, but other entities, such as liver immaturity, can cause an increased unconjugated bilirubin in neonates
Haptoglobin	Low value indicates intravascular hemolysis
Hemopexin	Decreased value is consistent with hemolysis
Direct antiglobulin test	Positive result indicates maternal antibodies to red blood cells in the newborn circulation

transfusion and exchange could be performed. A noninvasive ultrasound test can detect fetal middle cerebral artery blood flow rates that correlate well with the presence of fetal anemia. This test has been shown to be more sensitive, specific, and accurate than the invasive amniotic fluid bilirubin measurement.

Laboratory evaluation of newborns for HDN includes blood count and direct antiglobulin test (DAT) on cord blood. The latter test detects the presence of immunoglobulin and/or complement deposited on the surface of red blood cells. See **Table 7–3** for a list of tests that are helpful in the laboratory evaluation of HDN.

CYSTIC FIBROSIS

Description

Cystic fibrosis is an autosomal recessive disease that results from a mutation in the cystic fibrosis transmembrane conductance regulator (CFTR) gene on the long arm of chromosome 7. The clinical presentation is dysfunction of exocrine glands, from abnormal chloride conduction across the apical membrane of epithelial cells, and subsequently chronic obstructive lung disease and exocrine pancreatic insufficiency. The most commonly found mutation in the CFTR gene is

Cystic fibrosis is an autosomal recessive disease that results from a mutation in the cystic fibrosis transmembrane conductance regulator (CFTR) gene on the long arm of chromosome 7.

TABLE 7–4   Laboratory Evaluation for Cystic Fibrosis

Laboratory Test	Result/Comment
Quantitative pilocarpine iontophoresis sweat chloride test	Sweat chloride concentration >60 mEq/L confirms the diagnosis, in the presence of supporting clinical and laboratory information; differential diagnosis for a positive sweat test result includes untreated adrenal insufficiency, hereditary nephrogenic diabetes insipidus, hypothyroidism, pancreatitis, and malnutrition
Genetic testing	Used for carrier testing, disease testing, and newborn screen follow-up testing
Duodenal fluid viscosity	Elevated
72 hour fecal fat level	Elevated
Fecal elastase	Decreased
Immunoreactive trypsinogen	Elevated in newborn screening test

ΔF508 (loss of a phenylalanine codon at position 508), and it is present in approximately 70% of cases. However, more than 1,300 mutations in this gene have been described, most of which are rare.

The incidence of cystic fibrosis is approximately 1 in 2,500 to 3,400 Caucasian births, 1 in 17,000 births from individuals of African descent, and 1 in 90,000 Asian births. As many as 1 in 30 Caucasians may be a carrier for cystic fibrosis.

Screening and Diagnosis

Extending an offer to screen the carrier status of couples planning for pregnancy is now recommended, especially for Caucasians (who are at highest risk) and those with a family history of disease. The carrier screen is a molecular genetic test designed to detect the most common mutations, typically around 23 in number.

Screening newborns for the disease is increasingly common. The usual approach is to screen blood spots for immunoreactive trypsinogen (IRT) and then follow up elevated values with either a multiple-mutation DNA test or repeat IRT on a new sample.

Laboratory evaluation for screen-positive patients includes the same test used in the assessment of patients clinically suspected of having the disease: quantitative sweat chloride. This analysis involves testing to determine whether the patient exhibits elevated levels of chloride in sweat samples; these samples are typically elicited with the use of pilocarpine and iontophoresis.

Genetic testing for disease detection (as opposed to screening) involves a larger number of mutation investigations, typically more than 75. If necessary, nucleotide sequencing of the gene can be performed; this procedure would typically be limited to the proband within a family; if an unusual mutation is found, other family members can be tested with sequencing of DNA from the involved exon rather than the entire gene. **Table 7–4** presents the laboratory evaluation of cystic fibrosis.

AMINO ACIDURIAS

Description and Diagnosis

Amino acidurias are defects in the metabolism of amino acids that lead to their accumulation. The primary amino acidurias are a result of an inherited enzyme defect within a degradative pathway for a specific amino acid, or in a transporter in the renal tubules that alter the reabsorption of the amino acid. Selected primary amino acidurias associated with impaired amino acid degradation are shown in **Table 7–5**. The defective enzymes and the amino acid or other

Amino acidurias are defects in the metabolism of amino acids that lead to their accumulation. The primary amino acidurias are a result of an inherited enzyme defect within a degradative pathway for a specific amino acid, or in a transporter in the renal tubules that alter the reabsorption of the amino acid.

TABLE 7–5 Selected Amino Acidurias

Disorder	Defective Enzymes	Amino Acid or Other Compound in Elevated Concentration (Most Prominent Ones)
For enzymes outside the urea cycle		
Phenylketonuria (multiple forms of the disorder with different enzyme deficiencies)	Phenylalanine hydroxylase Dihydropteridine reductase Defect in biopterin synthesis	Phenylalanine
Tyrosinemia (multiple forms of the disorder with different enzyme deficiencies)	Fumarylacetoacetate hydrolase Tyrosine aminotransferase	Tyrosine
Alkaptonuria	Homogentisic acid oxidase	Homogentisic acid
Homocystinuria (multiple forms of the disorder with different enzyme deficiencies)	Cystathionine β-synthase Methylenetetrahydrofolate reductase (MTHFR) Methyltransferase	Homocysteine
Histidinemia	Histidase	Histidine
Maple syrup urine disease	Branched-chain keto acid decarboxylase	Leucine, isoleucine, alloisoleucine, valine, and corresponding ketoacids (in acute attacks)
Nonketotic hyperglycemia	Block in glycine cleavage enzyme system	Glycine
Methylmalonic acidemia	Methylmalonyl-CoA mutase	Glycine and methylmalonic acid
Cystathioninuria	γ-Cystathionase	Cystathionine
Carnosinemia	Carnosinase	Carnosine
Hyperprolinemia (multiple forms of the disorder with different enzyme deficiencies)	Proline oxidase Δ^5-Pyrroline-5-carboxylic acid dehydrogenase	Proline
For enzymes within the urea cycle		
Citrullinemia	Argininosuccinate synthetase	Citrulline, ammonia, and alanine
Argininosuccinic aciduria	Argininosuccinate lyase	Argininosuccinic acid, and citrulline; ammonia after meals
Argininemia	Arginase	Arginine; ammonia after meals
Hyperornithinemia	Ornithine decarboxylase	Ornithine, glutamine, and alanine; ammonia after meals
Ornithine transcarbamylase deficiency	Ornithine transcarbamylase	Ammonia and glutamine
Carbamoylphosphate synthetase deficiency	Carbamoylphosphate synthetase	Ammonia, glycine, and glutamine

compound in elevated concentration are listed for the individual disorders. In contrast to primary amino acidurias, secondary amino acidurias are accumulations of amino acids that arise when the organs responsible for their elimination or degradation, notably the liver and kidney, are functionally impaired. The diagnosis of a primary amino aciduria may be made by demonstrating a decrease in a specific enzyme activity required for the metabolism of the amino acid or by finding the associated abnormality in the gene coding for the enzyme. The presence of characteristic clinical signs and symptoms for the individual disorders is highly contributory toward establishing a diagnosis. The different amino acidurias vary from essentially benign, with no apparent disease, to lethal disorders. Furthermore, the clinical features can vary widely within a single disease, because some of the amino acidurias have multiple forms and because different enzyme deficiencies can result in an elevation of the same amino acid.

TABLE 7–6   Selected Lysosomal Storage Disorders

The Compound Stored in the Lysosome and Associated Disease	Enzyme Deficiency
Sphingolipidoses[a]	
Niemann–Pick disease	Sphingomyelinase
Gaucher disease	β-Glucosidase
Krabbe disease	Galactosylceramide β-galactosidase
Metachromatic leukodystrophy	Arylsulfatase A
Fabry disease	α-Galactosidase (X-linked)
Tay–Sachs disease	β-N-Acetylglucosaminidase A
Sandhoff disease	β-N-Acetylglucosaminidase A and B
Generalized gangliosidosis	β-Galactosidase
Mucopolysaccharidoses (MPS)[b]	
Hurler syndrome	α-L-Iduronidase
Scheie syndrome	α-L-Iduronidase
Hunter syndrome	Iduronate sulfatases (X-linked)
Sanfilippo syndrome (multiple forms of the disorder with different enzyme deficiencies)	Heparan N-sulfatase α-N-Acetylglucosaminidase α-Glucosaminide-N-acetyltransferase N-Acetylglucosamine-6-sulfate sulfatase
Morquio disease (multiple forms with different enzyme deficiencies)	Galactosamine-6-sulfate sulfatase β-Galactosidase
Maroteaux–Lamy disease	Arylsulfatase B
Glucuronidase deficiency	β-Glucuronidase
Glycogen storage disorders[c]	
Pompe disease	α-Glucosidase

[a]Accumulation of sphingolipids (which includes sphingomyelins, glucosylceramides, galactosylceramides, sulfatides, and gangliosides) due to deficiencies of enzymes required for their degradation.

[b]Accumulation of mucopolysaccharides (glycosaminoglycans) due to enzyme deficiencies required for their degradation.

[c]Accumulation of glycogen due to an enzyme deficiency required for its degradation.

LYSOSOMAL STORAGE DISEASES

Description and Diagnosis

The lysosomal storage diseases result from the lysosomal accumulation of compounds that should otherwise be degraded by the enzymes in the lysosome. The diagnosis of a lysosomal storage disease is made by identifying the products stored in the tissues or excreted in the urine.

Lysosomal storage diseases, like the amino acidurias, are inborn errors of metabolism. The lysosomal storage diseases result from the lysosomal accumulation of compounds that should otherwise be degraded by the enzymes in the lysosome. The diagnosis of a lysosomal storage disease is made by identifying the products stored in the tissues or excreted in the urine. Demonstration of an enzyme deficiency is usually sufficient for diagnosis of a specific lysosomal storage disease. With some disorders, DNA analysis for the mutation producing the enzyme deficiency also can be performed. As with the amino acidurias, a number of lysosomal storage disorders have subtypes, because different enzyme deficiencies may result in the accumulation of similar or identical compounds. **Table 7–6** provides a list of selected lysosomal storage disorders grouped into those associated with impaired degradation of sphingolipids (the sphingolipidoses), mucopolysaccharides (the mucopolysaccharidoses—the more recently invoked term for mucopolysaccharide is glycosaminoglycan), and glycogen. Among the lysosomal storage diseases, Tay–Sachs, 1 of the sphingolipidoses, has been the most thoroughly studied. As a class of disorders, the lysosomal storage disorders are rare. The 1 with the highest prevalence is Gaucher disease, which affects 1 in 600 in the Ashkenazic Jewish population. Each lysosomal storage disorder has its own characteristic clinical features, and most signs and symptoms of these diseases are expressed early in life. Many of these disorders can even be diagnosed in utero or in the period immediately after birth. There is often an urgency to establish the diagnosis so that appropriate treatment can be instituted as soon as possible.

NEUROBLASTOMA

Description

Neuroblastoma is a solid tumor that affects infants and toddlers. It is the most common malignancy under 1 year of age, and most patients are diagnosed by age 2 years. It presents either as a mass, often in the abdomen or neck, or with signs and symptoms of tumor spread, including bone pain or spinal cord dysfunction. Neuroblastoma is 1 of the "small round cell" tumors of childhood, and it must be distinguished from other tumors of that type, which include lymphoma, rhabdomyosarcoma, Ewing's sarcoma, and primitive neuroectodermal tumor (PNET).

Diagnosis

Measurement of urinary catecholamines can be used to alert clinicians to the likelihood that an infant's tumor mass is a neuroblastoma, as the other "round cell tumors" listed above do not excrete catecholamines. Unlike pheochromocytoma (see Chapter 22 on Disorders), urinary metanephrines are not helpful, as neuroblastomas do not produce an abundance of epinephrine. For the evaluation of neuroblastoma, vanillylmandelic acid (VMA) and homovanillic acid (HVA) are typically measured in urine by high-performance liquid chromatography (HPLC) methodology.

The treatment of neuroblastoma patients can be followed with quantitation of VMA and HVA in their urine. Detection of metastases in bone marrow samples of these patients is challenging with histologic methods as there are often very few tumor cells, but molecular studies are now being brought to bear on these samples to detect minimal residual disease. Examples of assays being used for this purpose include reverse transcriptase-polymerase chain reaction (RT-PCR) for tyrosine hydroxylase (an enzyme involved in catecholamine synthesis) and for the proto-oncogene MYCN. The latter gene is of interest because its copy number has long been studied in neuroblastoma tumor samples. Amplification of MYCN is associated with a poorer prognosis in these patients.

> Neuroblastoma is a solid tumor that affects infants and toddlers. It is the most common malignancy under 1 year of age, and most patients are diagnosed by age 2 years. Measurement of urinary catecholamines can be used to alert clinicians to the likelihood that an infant's tumor mass is a neuroblastoma.

REFERENCES

American College of Medical Genetics. Newborn screening: toward a uniform screening panel and system. *Genet Med.* 2006;8(5):1s.

Christenson RH, Azzazy HME. Amino acids. In: Burtis CA, Ashwood ER, eds. *Tietz Textbook of Clinical Chemistry.* 3rd ed. Philadelphia, PA: WB Saunders; 1999:444.

Goldenberg RL, et al. Maternal infection and adverse fetal and neonatal outcomes. *Clin Perinatol.* 2005;32:523.

Malone FD, et al. First-trimester or second-trimester screening, or both, for Down's syndrome. *N Engl J Med.* 2005;353:2001.

O'Brien JF. Lysosomal storage disease. In: Burtis CA, Ashwood ER, eds. *Tietz Textbook of Clinical Chemistry.* 3rd ed. Philadelphia, PA: WB Saunders; 1999:1776.

Oepkes D, et al. Doppler ultrasonography versus amniocentesis to predict fetal anemia. *N Engl J Med.* 2006;355:156.

Rock MJ, et al. Newborn screening for cystic fibrosis in Wisconsin: nine-year experience with routine trypsinogen/DNA testing. *Pediatrics.* 2005;147:S73.

Tekesin I, et al. Assessment of rapid fetal fibronectin in predicting preterm delivery. *Obstet Gynecol.* 2005;105:280.

Ventolini G, et al. Changes in the threshold of fetal lung maturity testing and neonatal outcome of infants delivered electively before 39 weeks gestation: implications and cost-effectiveness. *J Perinatol.* 2006;26:264.

Wagner L, et al. Pilot study to evaluate MYCN expression as a neuroblastoma cell marker to detect minimal residual disease by RT-PCR. *J Pediatr Hematol Oncol.* 2006;28:635.

Blood Vessels

Michael Laposata

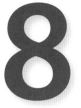

CHAPTER OUTLINE

INTRODUCTION

Because blood vessels are present in all organs and tissues, vascular disease is not restricted to a limited group of signs and symptoms. All organs and tissues are potential targets of injury in vascular disease, and most patients present with signs and symptoms indicative of injury to a specific organ or tissue, usually as a result of diminished blood flow. For example, if there is decreased blood flow to the heart, the patient presents with signs and symptoms related to cardiac dysfunction. The decrease in blood flow could be the result of a lesion that originates in the blood vessel wall, and therefore a vascular disease, or an obstruction by a blood clot inside the blood vessel. The disorders originating within the blood vessel wall include atherosclerotic vascular disease, hypertensive vascular disease, vasculitis, tumors, and aneurysms. Deep vein thrombosis (DVT), which is also discussed in this chapter, is not usually associated with primary disease in the blood vessel wall. A first time DVT is nearly always the result of clot formation inside a normal vein. However, if abnormal vein structure is present (such as congenital atresia of the inferior vena cava), it can predispose to DVT.

- Atherosclerotic vascular disease is 1 of the most predominant illnesses in the Western world. The goal of clinical laboratory testing is to identify the cause of atherosclerosis. This is usually related to excess dietary lipid or a disorder of lipid metabolism. This chapter provides information on disorders of lipid metabolism that lead to atherosclerosis.
- Hypertensive vascular disease is also common. The role of clinical laboratory testing is to determine if there is a correctable cause for hypertension. Because more than 90% of hypertension cases are "essential," there is no correctable cause. Treatment with antihypertensive medical therapy is important and beneficial, but it does not treat the underlying cause for hypertension in most cases. An example of a surgically correctable form of hypertension is one in which a tumor secretes a hormone responsible for the elevation of blood pressure. Removal of the tumor typically results in normalization of the blood pressure. The section on hypertensive vascular disease focuses on the correctable causes of hypertension and the laboratory tests useful in identifying them.
- Vasculitis represents a less commonly encountered group of disorders with inflammation in the blood vessel wall. Clinical laboratory testing has a limited role in establishing the diagnosis of a particular form of vasculitis. The diagnosis is made by the specific clinical features of the patient, the results of antineutrophil cytoplasmic antibody (ANCA) testing, and, on occasion, histopathologic review of a blood vessel biopsy specimen.

Atherosclerosis, hypertensive vascular disease, vasculitis, and DVT are discussed in the sections that follow.

ATHEROSCLEROSIS

Description

Atherosclerotic vascular disease is a major cause of mortality and morbidity in the Western world. It is the consequence of an accumulation of lipid in large arteries including the aorta and, thereby, a narrowing of the lumen of the arteries, which results in decreased blood flow. When an atherosclerotic plaque ruptures, a thrombus can form over the ruptured plaque and totally occlude blood flow. Atherosclerotic disease is vascular in origin in that lipid deposition and cell proliferation occur within the blood vessel wall. The end organ damage depends on the anatomic location of the occluded artery. It is not uncommon to have generalized atherosclerosis with multiple vascular beds affected.

The causes of atherosclerotic vascular disease include:

- Ingestion of excess or atherogenic dietary fat, which is primarily saturated fatty acids and cholesterol. This is the most common cause of atherosclerotic vascular disease.
- Primary lipid disorders, also known as primary hyperlipidemias, which result in an increase in either cholesterol, triglyceride, or both in the plasma. Many of these disorders are a result of genetic mutations that perturb the metabolism of cholesterol. They are not uncommon.
- Nonlipid disorders causing elevations in the concentration of plasma lipids, usually cholesterol and/or triglyceride. These are also called secondary hyperlipidemias. Disorders or conditions that adversely affect lipid metabolism include hypothyroidism, nephrotic syndrome, liver disease, diabetes, obesity, and alcohol abuse. Many medications can alter plasma lipid levels.
- Elevated levels of lipoprotein (a), also known as Lp(a) and pronounced "L-P-little a," with or without other lipid or lipoprotein abnormalities.
- Disorders that are associated with direct damage to the blood vessel wall, independent of lipid levels, such as very high circulating concentrations of homocysteine.

The initial approach to the patient for routine evaluation or for monitoring the status of atherosclerotic vascular disease is to determine if the patient has an elevation in serum or plasma cholesterol and triglyceride concentrations, and if so, to first determine if the cause is excess intake of dietary fat.

Diagnosis

The initial approach to the patient for routine evaluation or for monitoring the status of atherosclerotic vascular disease is to determine if the patient has an elevation in serum or plasma cholesterol and triglyceride concentrations, and if so, to first determine if the cause is excess intake of dietary fat. An elevated total cholesterol level (>200 mg/dL) prompts the need to determine the

TABLE 8-1   The Major Plasma Lipoproteins

Lipoprotein Class	Lipid Components of Core	Synonyms for Lipoprotein Classes	Predominant Apolipoproteins (Protein Components of the Lipoprotein Shell)
Chylomicrons	Triglycerides >> cholesterol esters	None	AI, AIV, B48, CII, CIII, E
Very low-density lipoproteins (VLDL)	Triglycerides > cholesterol esters	Pre-beta lipoproteins	B100, CII, CIII, E
Low-density lipoproteins (LDL)	Cholesterol esters > triglycerides	Beta lipoproteins	B100
High-density lipoproteins (HDL)	Cholesterol esters > triglycerides	Alpha lipoproteins	AI, AII, CII, CIII, E

From Executive summary of the third report of the National Cholesterol Education Program (NCEP) expert panel on detection, evaluation, and treatment of high blood cholesterol in adults (Adult Treatment Panel III). *JAMA*. 2001; 285: 2486–97.

TABLE 8-2   ATP III Classification of LDL, Total, and HDL Cholesterol (mg/dL)[a]

LDL cholesterol	
<100	Optimal
100–129	Near or above optimal
130–159	Borderline high
160–189	High
>190	Very high
Total cholesterol	
<200	Desirable
200–239	Borderline high
>240	High
HDL cholesterol	
<40	Low
>60	High

[a]ATP, Adult Treatment Panel; HDL, high-density lipoprotein; LDL, low-density lipoprotein.

From Executive summary of the third report of the National Cholesterol Education Program (NCEP) expert panel on detection, evaluation, and treatment of high blood cholesterol in adults (Adult Treatment Panel III). *JAMA*. 2001; 285: 2486–97.

plasma or serum concentrations of low-density lipoprotein (LDL) cholesterol (a high level is bad) and high-density lipoprotein (HDL) cholesterol (a high level is good). Nonfasting specimens are acceptable for total and HDL cholesterol determinations. Measurement of plasma or serum triglycerides requires a fasting specimen because recently ingested dietary fat (within the previous 8 to 10 hours) elevates the triglyceride level. The calculation of LDL cholesterol (see above) involves the triglyceride measurement and, therefore, also requires a fasting specimen. **Table 8-1** describes the lipoproteins that transport lipids in the plasma.

Table 8-2 describes the desirable, borderline, and undesirable serum or plasma lipid levels for total, LDL, and HDL cholesterol.

Table 8-3 presents the risk factors for atherosclerotic coronary artery disease that are not associated with laboratory test results. Decisions about patient management involve an assessment for both these risk factors and laboratory test results. As shown in **Table 8-4**, among the laboratory tests included in the evaluation, the LDL cholesterol level is the primary determinant for therapy. Patients with >2 risk factors are targeted to a lower LDL cholesterol level than those with <2 risk factors. Those with a history of myocardial infarction or angina (CHD in **Table 8-4**) are targeted to an even lower LDL level. The LDL cholesterol is calculated by subtracting the amount of HDL cholesterol and very low-density lipoprotein (VLDL) cholesterol

Nonfasting specimens are acceptable for total and HDL cholesterol determinations. Measurement of plasma or serum triglycerides requires a fasting specimen because recently ingested dietary fat elevates the triglyceride level. The calculation of LDL cholesterol involves the triglyceride measurement and, therefore, also requires a fasting specimen.

TABLE 8–3   Major Risk Factors (Exclusive of LDL Cholesterol) That Modify LDL Goals[a]

Cigarette smoking
Hypertension (blood pressure ≥140/90 mmHg or on an antihypertensive medication)
Low HDL cholesterol (<40 mg/dL)[b]
Family history of premature CHD (CHD in male first-degree relative <55 years; CHD in female first-degree relative <65 years)
Age (men ≥45 years; women ≥55 years)

[a]Diabetes is regarded as a coronary heart disease (CHD) risk equivalent. HDL, high-density lipoprotein; LDL, low-density lipoprotein.
[b]HDL cholesterol ≥60 mg/dL counts as a "negative" risk factor; its presence removes 1 risk factor from the total count.

From Executive summary of the third report of the National Cholesterol Education Program (NCEP) expert panel on detection, evaluation, and treatment of high blood cholesterol in adults (Adult Treatment Panel III). *JAMA*. 2001; 285: 2486–97.

TABLE 8–4   LDL Cholesterol Goals and Cutpoints for TLC and Drug Therapy in Different Risk Categories

Risk Category	LDL Goal (mg/dL)	LDL Level (mg/dL) at Which to Initiate TLC	LDL Level (mg/dL) at Which to Consider Drug Therapy
CHD or CHD risk equivalents (10-year risk >20%)	<100 (optional goal <70)	≥100	≥100 (<100: drug optional)[a]
2+ risk factors 10-Year risk 10%–20%	<130 (optional goal <100)	≥130	≥130 (100–129: consider drug options)
10-Year risk <10%	<130 (optional goal <100)	≥130	≥160
0–1 risk factor[b]	<160	≥160	≥190 (160–189: LDL-lowering drug optional)

CHD, coronary heart disease; HDL, high-density lipoprotein; LDL, low-density lipoprotein; TLC, therapeutic lifestyle changes.

[a]Some authorities recommend use of LDL-lowering drugs in this category if an LDL cholesterol level of <100 mg/dL cannot be achieved by TLC. Others prefer use of drugs that primarily modify triglycerides and HDL (e.g., nicotinic acid or fibrate). Clinical judgment also may call for deferring drug therapy in this subcategory.

[b]Almost all patients with 0–1 risk factor have a 10-year risk <10%; thus, 10-year risk assessment for patients with 0–1 risk factor is not necessary.

From Executive summary of the third report of the National Cholesterol Education Program (NCEP) expert panel on detection, evaluation, and treatment of high blood cholesterol in adults (Adult Treatment Panel III). *JAMA*. 2001; 285: 2486–97.

The metabolic syndrome is characterized by low HDL cholesterol, elevated triglycerides, abdominal obesity, small, dense LDL, insulin resistance, and an increased risk for diabetes mellitus type 2, atherosclerosis, and cardiovascular disease.

(which is the triglyceride/5) from the total cholesterol level, in a fasting specimen. The metabolic syndrome is characterized by low HDL cholesterol, elevated triglycerides, abdominal obesity, small, dense LDL, insulin resistance, and an increased risk for diabetes mellitus type 2, atherosclerosis, and cardiovascular disease. Therefore, high-risk patients with high triglycerides or low HDL cholesterol may benefit from adding fibrate or nicotinic acid therapy to their treatment regimen.

Figure 8–1 is a summary of the latest assessment of the 10-year risk for coronary heart disease. Point scores are established by the presence or absence of lipid and nonlipid risk factors. The point total is associated with the 10-year risk of coronary heart disease, with separate tables for men and women. **Table 8–5** shows the nutrient composition of the low fat diet recommended by the latest National Cholesterol Education Program (ATP-III).

Methods for reliable, direct measurement of LDL cholesterol are emerging. In most cases, the level of apolipoprotein B reflects the LDL cholesterol level, and the amount of apolipoprotein (A1) is proportional to the HDL cholesterol concentration, but the tests for the apolipoproteins are more expensive. For this reason, the levels of these 2 apolipoproteins are rarely determined, even though assays for their quantitation are available.

If a hyperlipidemia is present, treatment options include restriction of dietary fat, lipid-lowering medications, or both. If an elevation in cholesterol, triglyceride, or both is present and it is not linked to a dietary cause, the patient must be evaluated for other causes of primary and secondary hyperlipidemias. The number of different substances in the serum, other than total,

Estimate of 10-Year Risk for Men
(Framingham Point Scores)

Age (years)	Points
20–34	−9
35–39	−4
40–44	0
45–59	3
50–54	6
55–59	8
60–64	10
65–69	11
70–74	12
75–79	13

Total Cholesterol (mg/dL)	Points				
	Age (years) 20–39	Age (years) 40–49	Age (years) 50–59	Age (years) 60–69	Age (years) 70–79
<160	0	0	0	0	0
160–199	4	3	2	1	0
200–239	7	5	3	1	0
240–279	9	6	4	2	1
≥280	11	8	5	3	1

	Points				
	Age (years) 20–39	Age (years) 40–49	Age (years) 50–59	Age (years) 60–69	Age (years) 70–79
Nonsmoker	0	0	0	0	0
Smoker	8	5	3	1	1

HDL (mg/dL)	Points
≥60	−1
50–59	0
40–49	1
<40	2

Systolic BP (mm Hg)	Points If Untreated	Points If Treated
<120	0	0
120–129	0	1
130–139	1	2
140–159	1	2
≥160	2	3

Point Total	10-Year Risk (%)
<0	<1
0–4	1
5–6	2
7	3
8	4
9	5
10	6
11	8
12	10
13	12
14	16
15	20
16	25
≥17	≥30

Estimate of 10-Year Risk for Women
(Framingham Point Scores)

Age (years)	Points
20–34	−7
35–39	−3
40–44	0
45–59	3
50–54	6
55–59	8
60–64	10
65–69	12
70–74	14
75–79	16

Total Cholesterol (mg/dL)	Points				
	Age (years) 20–39	Age (years) 40–49	Age (years) 50–59	Age (years) 60–69	Age (years) 70–79
<160	0	0	0	0	0
160–199	4	3	2	1	1
200–239	8	6	4	2	1
240–279	11	8	5	3	2
≥280	13	10	7	4	2

	Points				
	Age (years) 20–39	Age (years) 40–49	Age (years) 50–59	Age (years) 60–69	Age (years) 70–79
Nonsmoker	0	0	0	0	0
Smoker	9	7	4	2	1

HDL (mg/dL)	Points
≥60	−1
50–59	0
40–49	1
<40	2

Systolic BP (mm Hg)	Points If Untreated	Points If Treated
<120	0	0
120–129	1	3
130–139	2	4
140–159	3	5
≥160	4	6

Point Total	10-Year Risk (%)
<9	<1
9–12	1
13–14	2
15	3
16	4
17	5
18	6
19	8
20	11
21	14
22	17
23	22
24	27
≥25	≥30

FIGURE 8–1 Summary of adult treatment panel III report to estimate the 10-year risk of coronary heart disease (CHD). From Executive summary of the third report of the National Cholesterol Education Program (NCEP) expert panel on detection, evaluation, and treatment of high blood cholesterol in adults (Adult Treatment Panel III). *JAMA*. 2001; 285: 2486–97.

TABLE 8–5   Nutrient Composition of the Therapeutic Lifestyle Changes (TLC) Diet

Nutrient	Recommended Intake
Saturated fat[a]	<7% of total calories
Polyunsaturated fat	Up to 10% of total calories
Monounsaturated fat	Up to 20% of total calories
Total fat	25%–35% of total calories
Carbohydrate[b]	50%–60% of total calories
Fiber	20–30 g/day
Protein	Approximately 15% of total calories
Cholesterol	<200 mg/day
Total calories[c]	Balance energy intake and expenditure to maintain desirable body weight/prevent weight gain

[a]*Trans* fatty acids are another LDL-raising fat that should be kept at a low intake.

[b]Carbohydrates should be derived predominantly from foods rich in complex carbohydrates including grains, especially whole grains, fruits, and vegetables.

[c]Daily energy expenditure should include at least moderate physical activity (contributing approximately 200 kcal/day).

LDL, and HDL cholesterol, and triglyceride, which have been proposed as markers of increased cardiovascular risk, exceeds 100. Elevated concentrations of homocysteine, C-reactive protein, and Lp(a) appear to reflect increased cardiovascular risk. The distribution of LDL subclasses, and possibly HDL and VLDL lipoprotein subclasses, also may ultimately be shown to be useful in the evaluation of patients for atherosclerotic vascular disease. The same can be said for apolipoprotein E isoforms. See **Table 8–6** for additional information on these markers.

Table 8–7 presents a classification of the hyperlipidemias by phenotype (I to IV). **Table 8–8** describes selected genetic primary hyperlipidemias that result in elevated or decreased plasma lipids and the etiologies of the disorders. Genetic abnormalities are much less common explanations for high blood lipid levels than excess intake of dietary fat. **Table 8–9** sorts the primary and secondary hyperlipidemias according to serum or plasma lipid abnormalities.

HYPERTENSION

Description

Hypertension is a very common chronic disease, particularly in Western countries. As many as 60 million Americans have high blood pressure. A commonly accepted definition of hypertension is a systolic reading >140 mmHg or a diastolic >90 mmHg on at least 3 occasions, with a minimum of 2 weeks between each of the 3 readings. In evaluating a patient with hypertension, 1 question is whether there is an identifiable cause for the hypertension or whether it is idiopathic or "essential." Another important question is whether the hypertension has resulted in damage to the organs commonly injured in hypertensive individuals, namely, the brain, the heart, and the kidneys.

To understand the causes of hypertension, it is necessary to understand the mechanism by which blood pressure is regulated (see Chapter 22 for a related discussion on adrenal gland hormones). In response to decreased arterial pressure from a variety of causes, there is decreased blood flow to the kidney, causing the kidney to secrete renin. Renin released within the renal circulation converts angiotensinogen to angiotensin I, which is subsequently converted to angiotensin II. This molecule acts on the adrenal cortex to release aldosterone. Aldosterone increases sodium retention by the kidney, and thereby expands the extracellular fluid volume and returns the blood pressure to normal. Any alteration in this pathway, such as an increase in aldosterone or a decrease in blood flow to the kidney, will activate the renin–angiotensin system, lead to inappropriate fluid accumulation, and increase the blood pressure. This is why many of the diseases producing hypertension listed in **Table 8–10** are associated with the kidney. The renal disorders that are associated with hypertension can be renovascular, in which case

A commonly accepted definition of hypertension is a systolic reading >140 mmHg or a diastolic >90 mmHg on at least 3 occasions, with a minimum of 2 weeks between each of the 3 readings.

TABLE 8–6 **Risk Factors for Atherosclerotic Coronary Artery Disease**[a]

Laboratory Test	Results/Comment
Total, LDL, and HDL cholesterol and triglycerides	See **Table 8–2** for lipid levels and associated risk: normal fasting TG is <150 mg/dL; borderline high is 150–199 mg/dL; high is 200–499 mg/dL; and very high is ≥500 mg/dL
Homocysteine	Very high homocysteine concentrations in the blood are associated with damage to the blood vessel wall
Lipoprotein (a) [Lp(a)]	Lp(a) is an LDL particle linked to a protein with repeating polypeptide units found in plasminogen; Lp(a) levels are predominantly genetically determined; there is evidence that an elevation in Lp(a) promotes thrombosis by inhibiting the generation of plasmin to lyse clots; it is currently acceptable to measure Lp(a) in the patient who has developed early coronary artery disease without other obvious risk factors, especially if there is a family history of the disorder
C-reactive protein by "ultrasensitive" test	Atherosclerosis has an inflammatory component and an elevated concentration of this marker of inflammation has shown promise as an indicator of cardiovascular risk; this test differs from the standard test for C-reactive protein in that it can measure further down into the low range of values
LDL subclasses	Small dense LDL appear to be more atherogenic than larger LDL particles
Apolipoprotein E isoforms	Apolipoprotein E is bound to several lipoproteins and mediates the binding of these lipoproteins to the LDL receptor and a separate receptor known as the LDL receptor-related protein; there are 3 major isoforms of apolipoprotein E known as E_2, E_3, and E_4; in an individual, there are 2 alleles coding for each isoform, so any combination of 2 of these alleles is possible; the most common is E_3E_3; individuals with 2 E_2 alleles have lipoproteins that bind less avidly to the LDL receptor; these patients may develop hyperlipidemia and are therefore at risk for coronary artery disease

HDL, high-density lipoproteins; LDL, low-density lipoproteins; TG, triglycerides.

[a]Excluding markers for hypercoagulable states presented in Chapter 11.

TABLE 8–7 **Hyperlipidemia Classification by Phenotype**

Phenotype	Lipoproteins in Increased Concentration	Lipids in Increased Concentration	Relative Incidence
I	Chylomicrons	Triglycerides	Rare
IIa	LDL	Cholesterol[a]	Common
IIb	LDL and VLDL	Triglycerides and cholesterol	Very common
III	Intermediate-density (between VLDL and LDL) lipoprotein, also known as IDL	Triglycerides and cholesterol	Rare
IV	VLDL	Triglyceride and in some cases cholesterol	Very common
V	VLDL and chylomicrons	Triglyceride and in some cases cholesterol	Common

HDL, high-density lipoproteins; LDL, low-density lipoproteins; VLDL, very low-density lipoproteins.

[a]Serum cholesterol, whether total, LDL, or HDL, represents the sum of cholesterol and cholesterol esters.

the blood flow to the kidney is decreased, or they can be parenchymal. Parenchymal diseases include chronic kidney infections, glomerulonephritis, and polycystic kidney disease, among many others. Most of these conditions are treatable, and treatment of the underlying disorder may reduce the hypertension. Abnormalities in the adrenal gland, such as a pheochromocytoma or an aldosterone-secreting tumor (discussed in Chapter 22), also can lead to hypertension, and may be surgically correctable.

TABLE 8–8   Selected Genetic Primary Hyperlipidemias[a]

Primary Hyperlipidemia	Risk for Coronary Artery Disease/Comment	Etiology
Familial hypercholesterolemia	Heterozygous: 2–3-fold elevation in LDL cholesterol with a 4-fold increase in risk of death from coronary artery disease; tendon and tuberous xanthomas; incidence is 1 in 500 in the United States Homozygous: more severe form than heterozygous disease with very high risk for coronary artery disease if left untreated; incidence is 1 in 1,000,000 in the United States	Deficiency of LDL receptor activity; hundreds of mutations identified producing null, transport defective, binding defective, internalization defective, and receptor recycling defective mutants
Familial defective apolipoprotein B-100	Increased risk for coronary artery disease; incidence unknown, but may be as high as 1 in 600; lower level of LDL cholesterol than in heterozygous familial cholesterolemia	Defect in apolipoprotein B-100 results in impaired binding to LDL receptor and elevated cholesterol levels in the serum or plasma
Familial hyperalphalipoproteinemia	HDL cholesterol elevated, usually to >75 mg/dL; reduced risk for coronary artery disease	Elevation in HDL cholesterol results in an antiatherogenic effect
Familial combined hyperlipidemia	Incidence may be as high as 1% in the United States; increased risk for coronary artery disease	Overproduction of VLDL by the liver and/or multiple inherited defects in lipoprotein metabolism
Familial dysbetalipoproteinemia	Uncommon disorder (1 in 5,000–10,000); increased risk for coronary artery disease; as an approximation, total cholesterol range is 250–770 mg/dL and range for triglycerides is 530–1,770 mg/dL; most patients are homozygous for apolipoprotein E_2	Impaired binding of apolipoprotein E_2 particles to receptors, possibly with a coexisting disorder that increases hepatic VLDL synthesis
Familial hypertriglyceridemia	Common disorder in which elevations in triglyceride levels are first expressed in puberty or early adulthood; patients also have hyperglycemia and hyperinsulinemia and are often obese; increased risk for coronary artery disease in majority of cases	Defect in VLDL catabolism or an overproduction of VLDL triglycerides in the liver
Familial lipoprotein lipase deficiency	Rare (1 in 1,000,000); presents with abdominal pain and hepatosplenomegaly usually in childhood; markedly elevated triglycerides and chylomicrons; pancreatitis can occur from elevated triglycerides	Defect in enzyme that degrades triglycerides in chylomicrons and in VLDL
Familial apolipoprotein CII deficiency	Similar to lipoprotein lipase deficiency	Lipoprotein lipase is activated by CII; therefore, CII deficiency results in lower activity of lipoprotein lipase
Familial hypoalphaproteinemia	Common (1 in 400–500); HDL cholesterol low at <30 mg/dL; increased risk for coronary artery disease	Lower HDL cholesterol results in decreased antiatherogenic activity
Lecithin cholesterol acyltransferase (LCAT) deficiency	Low HDL cholesterol levels; corneal opacities, hemolytic anemia, increased risk for coronary artery disease	Accumulation of nonesterified cholesterol in plasma and tissues from decreased activity of LCAT, which converts cholesterol to cholesterol esters
Tangier disease	Low HDL cholesterol levels; moderately increased risk for coronary artery disease; large orange tonsils; corneal opacities	Increased catabolism of HDL accounts for the low HDL levels

HDL, high-density lipoprotein; LDL, low-density lipoprotein.

[a]Excluding markers for hypercoagulable states presented in Chapter 11.

TABLE 8–9 Serum or Plasma Lipid Abnormalities Classified by the Lipid with the Abnormal Concentration

Lipid Class and Abnormality	Hyperlipoproteinemia Phenotype(s) in Category	Selected Disorders Associated with the Designated Lipid Abnormality[a]
Elevated cholesterol	IIa	Primary hyperlipidemias: • Familial hypercholesterolemia • Polygenic hypercholesterolemia • Familial defective apolipoprotein B-100 • Familial hyperalphalipoproteinemia Secondary hyperlipidemias: • Hypothyroidism • Nephrotic syndrome • Liver disease • Anorexia nervosa
Elevated cholesterol and elevated triglyceride (mixed hyperlipidemias)	IIb and III, and IV and V when cholesterol is elevated with triglyceride	Primary hyperlipidemias: • Excess dietary fat intake • Familial combined hyperlipidemias • Familial dysbetalipoproteinemia Secondary hyperlipidemias: • Hypothyroidism • Diabetes • Obesity • Anorexia nervosa • Liver disease
Elevated triglyceride	IV and V, but only when cholesterol is not elevated with triglyceride	Primary hyperlipidemias: • Familial hypertriglyceridemia • Familial lipoprotein lipase deficiency • Familial apolipoprotein CII deficiency Secondary hyperlipidemias: • Diabetes • Chronic renal disease • Alcohol abuse • Medications such as diuretics, beta blockers, and oral contraceptives
Decreased HDL cholesterol	None, it is a hypolipoproteinemia	Primary causes for low HDL cholesterol: • Familial hypoalphaproteinemia • Lecithin cholesterol acyltransferase (LCAT) deficiency • Tangier disease Secondary cause for low HDL cholesterol: • Decreased physical activity

HDL, high-density lipoprotein.

[a]See **Table 8–8** for descriptions of the primary lipid disorders in this column.

Diagnosis

The hypertensive patient undergoing evaluation is first studied using a number of routine tests including:

- complete blood count to determine if the patient is anemic or polycythemic;
- electrolyte measurements to measure the potassium and bicarbonate levels;
- creatinine concentration in plasma or serum and creatinine clearance to assess renal function;
- glucose (usually a fasting level) to diagnose diabetes, because diabetic patients have an approximately 2-fold higher incidence of hypertension than nondiabetic patients;
- urinalysis to detect the presence of diabetes by glucose in the urine; urinalysis also may indicate the presence of significant parenchymal disease in the kidney if proteinuria, hematuria, or pyuria are present.

TABLE 8-10   Evaluation of the Patient for Correctable Causes of Hypertension

Disorder	Tests Used in Formulating a Diagnosis
"Essential" hypertension	An array of tests is used to rule out causes of correctable hypertension described below
Drug-induced hypertension	Determination if history is positive for ingestion of sympathomimetics, corticosteroids, mineralocorticoids, vasopressin, or cocaine, among other drugs, which have a hypertensive effect
Renal and vascular causes of hypertension	
Renal artery stenosis	Renal angiogram consistent with stenosis; elevated plasma renin level (which can also be affected by salt intake and selected medications) in sample obtained from peripheral blood or renal vein
Chronic renal disease of multiple etiologies	Elevated BUN and creatinine
Polycystic kidney disease	Radiologic studies to confirm cystic disease of the kidney
Renin-secreting tumors (renal or extrarenal)	Elevated plasma renin activity, normal renal angiogram, low serum potassium, and elevated urinary aldosterone secretion
Coarctation of the aorta (decreased blood flow to kidney resulting from a defect in the aorta)	Angiography of the aorta
Adrenal causes of hypertension	
Primary aldosteronism	Low or borderline serum potassium and elevated urinary aldosterone secretion
17-alpha hydroxylase deficiency	Reduction in activity of 17-alpha hydroxylase (see Chapter 22); similar to primary aldosteronism but with virilization and precocious puberty in males
11-beta hydroxylase deficiency	Reduction in activity of 11-beta hydroxylase (see Chapter 22); similar to primary aldosteronism but with virilization and precocious puberty in males
Cushing syndrome	Tests for the diagnosis of different forms of Cushing syndrome (see Chapter 22)
Pheochromocytoma	Tests that demonstrate an excess of catecholamines (see Chapter 22)

BUN, blood urea nitrogen.

The tests to further investigate the cause of hypertension beyond the screening tests are more invasive, costly, or esoteric. These are noted in **Table 8–10**.

VASCULITIS

Description

Inflammation in the blood vessel wall is known as vasculitis. The large number of different vasculitides, which are sometimes overlapping in their clinical or anatomic characteristics, often makes the diagnosis of a specific form of vasculitis challenging. In general, a diagnosis is made by 1) the presence of characteristic clinical findings for the particular form of vasculitis and 2) inflammation within a specific size of blood vessels, as shown in **Table 8–11**. There are vasculitides that are infectious in origin that are not included in **Table 8–11**. Rocky Mountain spotted fever, syphilis, aspergillosis, herpes, and neisserial infections can all be associated with vasculitis. (See Chapter 5 for information on organisms and infections that can cause vasculitis.)

> Inflammation in the blood vessel wall is known as vasculitis. The large number of different vasculitides, which are sometimes overlapping in their clinical or anatomic characteristics, often makes the diagnosis of a specific form of vasculitis challenging.

Diagnosis

The laboratory testing is different for each of the vasculitides in **Table 8–11**. Some of the disorders will affect the kidney, and for those, monitoring of renal function is important. Others are associated with the presence of either antiproteinase 3 antineutrophil cytoplasmic antibodies (anti-PR3 ANCA) or antimyeloperoxidase antinuclear cytoplasmic antibodies (anti-MPO ANCA). The diagnosis of a particular form of vasculitis can be supported by a variety of other test results, as shown in **Table 8–11**.

TABLE 8-11   Laboratory Evaluation of the Patient for Noninfectious Causes of Vasculitis

Vasculitic Disorder	Vessels with Inflammation	Clinical Laboratory Testing
Giant cell (temporal) arteritis	Aorta and large- to medium-sized arteries	Elevated erythrocyte sedimentation rate (ESR) in most patients
Takayasu arteritis	Aorta and large- to medium-sized arteries	Elevated ESR in most patients; BUN, creatinine, and urinalysis to assess and monitor renal disease
Polyarteritis nodosa	Large- to medium-sized arteries; small arteries without pulmonary or glomerular involvement	Cases can be divided into those infectious in origin and ANCA negative vs those not associated with infections and antimyeloperoxidase ANCA positive
Kawasaki disease	Large- to medium-sized arteries; small arteries	Laboratory testing is not informative with self-limited form of the disease; if cardiac complications occur, tests for damage to cardiac muscle may be useful (see Chapter 9)
Wegener granulomatosis	Small arteries, arterioles, capillaries, venules, veins	Antiproteinase 3 ANCA detectable in the majority of patients with active disease; a smaller percentage have antimyeloperoxidase ANCA
Churg–Strauss syndrome	Small arteries, arterioles, capillaries, venules, veins	Antimyeloperoxidase ANCA detectable in most patients; eosinophilia
Microscopic polyangiitis	Small arteries, arterioles, capillaries, venules	Antimyeloperoxidase ANCA (more common) or antiproteinase 3 ANCA (less common) detectable in most cases; BUN, creatinine, and urinalysis to assess and monitor renal abnormalities
Henoch–Schönlein purpura	Arterioles, capillaries, venules	BUN, creatinine, and urinalysis to assess and monitor renal abnormalities
Essential cryoglobulinemic vasculitis	Arterioles, capillaries, venules	Serum cryoglobulin with identification of type and quantitation, if present (see discussion on cryoglobulinemia in Chapter 3)
Cutaneous leukocytoclastic angiitis	Capillaries, venules	May have underlying autoimmune, neoplastic, or infectious process or an accompanying vasculitis of a different type; laboratory testing is directed at detection of underlying diseases

ANCA, antineutrophil cytoplasmic antibody; BUN, blood urea nitrogen; ESR, erythrocyte sedimentation rate.

DEEP VEIN THROMBOSIS

Description

DVT is a common disorder. It has a high incidence in patients with 1 or more congenital or acquired risk factors for DVT. The acquired factors include trauma, immobilization, the postoperative state, antiphospholipid antibodies, malignancy, myeloproliferative disorder, pregnancy, and the postpartum state, among many others. The most commonly encountered congenital risk factors, described in detail in the section "Hypercoagulable States" in Chapter 11, include the factor V Leiden mutation that produces activated protein C resistance, the prothrombin G20210A mutation, and deficiencies of protein C, protein S, and antithrombin. The major concern for patients with DVT is the risk of embolism to the lungs (pulmonary embolism or PE). A lower extremity DVT, especially if it is small, is often asymptomatic. If the DVT has extended above the knee, patients are more likely to experience soft tissue swelling and discomfort, distention of the vein (a palpable "cord" on physical examination), Homan's sign (pain on dorsiflexion of foot), erythema, and warmth. Upper extremity (usually arm) DVTs are much less common than lower extremity (leg) DVTs.

> The major concern for patients with DVT is the risk of embolism to the lungs. A lower extremity DVT, especially if it is small, is often asymptomatic.

Diagnosis

Table 8–12 describes the tests for DVT, most of which are not performed in the clinical laboratory. PE is more completely discussed in Chapter 14. Discussion of arterial vascular disease, which is predominantly atherosclerotic, is covered in the section "Atherosclerosis" of this chapter and

TABLE 8–12   **Tests for the Diagnosis of Deep Vein Thrombosis (DVT)**

Tests for DVT	Description	Advantages	Disadvantages	Comments
Venography	Intravenous contrast injection is followed by radiographic examination of the vein; thrombosis is identified as a filling defect	Useful for both distal (below the knee) and proximal (above the knee) lower extremity DVT	Invasive; may predispose to thrombosis; expensive	Gold standard test for DVT diagnosis
Ultrasonography	Vein is visualized by ultrasound; then external compression is applied to the skin surface above the vein; normal veins collapse and thrombosed veins are not compressible	Useful for symptomatic proximal lower extremity DVT; noninvasive; highly specific	Less sensitive for asymptomatic DVT and distal lower extremity DVT	Most commonly used procedure for initial evaluation of the patient suspected of having a DVT
Computed tomography (CT) scan	Small, but not negligible amounts of X-rays are used to generate 3-dimensional images of the body	Convenient if already using CT for diagnosing pulmonary embolism	Intravenous contrast material usually required	
D-dimer measurement	D-dimer is a specific degradation product of cross-linked fibrin that is produced by physiologic fibrinolysis of thrombi	Simple blood test in a patient with a low risk for DVT or PE; using a sensitive method, a negative D-dimer test has a high negative predictive value in excluding DVT and PE	A positive result has to be confirmed by a more specific imaging test	Insensitive methods including manual latex agglutination must not be used to rule out DVT or PE

the section "Acute Myocardial Infarction" in Chapter 9. In addition to D-dimer testing to exclude DVT and PE (**Table 8–12**), D-dimer testing may be useful for predicting recurrent DVT after anticoagulation treatment for an initial DVT is completed.

REFERENCES

Allen NB, Bressler PB. Diagnosis and treatment of the systemic and cutaneous necrotizing vasculitis syndromes. *Med Clin North Am*. 1997;81:243.

Bachorik PS, et al. Lipids and dyslipoproteinemia. In: Henry JB, et al., eds. *Clinical Diagnosis and Management by Laboratory Methods*. 19th ed. Philadelphia, PA: WB Saunders; 1996:229.

Bates SM, Ginsberg JS. Treatment of deep-vein thrombosis. *New Engl J Med*. 2004; 351:268–277.

Bild DE, et al. Identification and management of heterozygous familial hypercholesterolemia: summary and recommendations from an NHBLI workshop. *Am J Cardiol*. 1993;72:1D.

Brown MJ. Hypertension. *BMJ*. 1997;314:1258.

Executive summary of the third report of the National Cholesterol Education Program (NCEP) Expert Panel on Detection, Evaluation, and Treatment of High Blood Cholesterol in Adults (Adult Treatment Panel III). *JAMA*. 2001;285:2486.

Ginsburg HN, Goldberg IJ. Disorders of lipoprotein metabolism. In: Fauci AS, et al., eds. *Harrison's Principles of Internal Medicine*. 14th ed. New York, NY: McGraw-Hill; 1998:2138.

Grundy SM, et al.; Coordinating Committee of the National Cholesterol Education Program. Implications of recent clinical trials for the National Cholesterol Education Program Adult Treatment Panel III guidelines. *Circulation*. 2004;110:227–239.

Horvath JR, Hoffman GS. Systemic vasculitis: pitfalls in diagnosis and treatment. *Hosp Med*. 1997;33:10.

Hunder G. Vaculitis: diagnosis and therapy. *Am J Med*. 1996;100(2A):37S.

Kwiterovich PO. Identification and treatment of heterozygous familial hypercholesterolemia in children and adolescents. *Am J Cardiol*. 1993;72:30D.

Palareti G, et al. D-dimer testing to determine the duration of anticoagulation therapy. *New Engl J Med*. 2006; 355:1780–1789.

Righini M, et al. D-dimer for venous thromboembolism diagnosis: 20 years later. *J Thromb Haemost*. 2008; 6:1059–1071.

Soutar AK. Familial hypercholesterolemia and LDL receptor mutations. *J Intern Med*. 1992;231:633.

Thomas SM, et al. Diagnostic value of CT for deep vein thrombosis: results of a systemic review and meta-analysis. *Clin Radiol*. 2008; 63:299–304.

Townsend RR, Di Pette DJ. Evaluation of elevated blood pressure. *Clin Lab Med*. 1993;13:287.

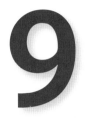

The Heart

Fred S. Apple

CHAPTER OUTLINE

INTRODUCTION

There are many forms of cardiac disease. This chapter briefly covers the role of biomarkers in acute myocardial infarction (AMI) and congestive heart failure (CHF). The large numbers of other cardiac diseases are not discussed in this chapter because of the relatively minor role of diagnostic clinical laboratory tests in these disorders.

ACUTE MYOCARDIAL INFARCTION

Description

The term AMI is defined as an imbalance between myocardial oxygen supply and demand, resulting in injury to and the eventual death of myocytes. When the blood supply to the heart is interrupted, necrosis of the myocardium results. Such necrosis is most often associated with a thrombotic occlusion superimposed on coronary atherosclerosis. It is now apparent that the process of plaque rupture and thrombosis is 1 of the ways in which coronary atherosclerosis progresses. Total loss of coronary blood flow results in a clinical syndrome associated with an ST segment elevation MI (STEMI). Partial loss of coronary perfusion, if severe, can lead to necrosis as well, which is generally less severe and is known as non-ST segment elevation MI (NSTEMI). Other events of still lesser severity may be missed entirely or called angina, which can range from stable to unstable. About 1.7 million patients are hospitalized each year in the United States with an acute coronary syndrome (ACS). Approximately 700,000 patients suffer from an initial AMI annually and another 500,000 from a recurrent AMI. Coronary heart disease causes 20% of all deaths and cardiovascular diseases up to 40%. Historically, most deaths caused by ischemic heart disease have been acute, but as our therapeutic abilities have improved, the disease is slowly becoming a more chronic one.

In many patients with AMI, no precipitating factor can be identified. The clinical history remains of substantial value in establishing a diagnosis. A prodromal history of angina can be elicited in 40% to 50% of patients with AMI. Of the patients with AMI presenting with prodromal symptoms, approximately one third have had symptoms from 1 to 4 weeks before hospitalization; in the remaining two thirds, symptoms predate admission by a week or less, with one third having had symptoms for 24 hours or less. The pain of AMI is variable in intensity and the discomfort is described as a squeezing, choking, vise-like, or heavy pain. It may also be characterized as a stabbing, knife-like, boring, or burning discomfort. Often the pain radiates down the left arm. In some instances, the pain of AMI may begin in the epigastrium and simulate a variety of abdominal disorders, which often causes AMI to be misdiagnosed as indigestion. In other patients, the discomfort of AMI radiates to the shoulders, upper extremities, neck, and jaw, again usually favoring the left side.

Diagnosis

The ideal marker of myocardial injury should 1) provide early detection of injury, 2) provide rapid diagnosis for an acute MI, 3) serve as a risk stratification tool in ACS patients, 4) assess the success of reperfusion after thrombolytic therapy, 5) detect reocclusion and reinfarction, 6) determine the timing of an infarction and infarct size, and 7) detect procedural-related perioperative MI during cardiac or noncardiac surgery. Ruling *out* AMI requires a test with high diagnostic specificity (preferred by the ER physician in the urgent care setting), whereas ruling *in* AMI requires a test with high diagnostic sensitivity (preferred by the cardiologist following admission). It is the function of the laboratory to provide advice to physicians about cardiac biomarker characteristics.

Until 2000, the diagnosis of AMI established by the World Health Organization (WHO) required at least 2 of the following criteria: 1) a history of chest pain, 2) evolutionary changes on the ECG, and/or 3) elevations of serial cardiac biomarkers (total creatine kinase [CK] and CKMB). It was rare for a diagnosis of AMI to be made in the absence of biochemical evidence of myocardial injury. A 2000 ESC/ACC consensus conference, updated in 2007 by the "Global Task Force for the Universal Definition of MI," has codified the role of biomarkers by advocating that the diagnosis be made from evidence of myocardial injury based on biomarkers of cardiac damage, preferably cardiac troponin (cTn) I or T, in the appropriate clinical situation of ischemic symptoms (**Table 9–1**). This guideline does not suggest that all increases of cTn should elicit a diagnosis of AMI, but only those associated with the appropriate clinical, ECG, and imaging findings. When cTn increases that are not caused by acute ischemia occur, the clinician is obligated to search for another etiology for the elevation, a number of which are shown in **Table 9–2**. The initial ECG is diagnostic of AMI in about 30% of AMI patients.

cTn testing is most useful when patients are having nondiagnostic ECG tracings. Patients with AMI can be categorized into 4 groups based on time of presentation. First, there is the group of patients who present early to the emergency department (ED), within 0 to 4 hours after the onset of chest pain, without diagnostic ECG evidence of AMI. For laboratory tests to be clinically useful, biomarkers of MI must be released rapidly from the heart into the circulation to provide sensitive and specific diagnostic information. Further the analytical assays using serum or plasma specimens must be rapid and sensitive enough to distinguish small changes within the reference interval. The second group includes those presenting 4 to 48 hours after the onset of chest pain, without evidence of AMI on ECG. In this group of patients, the diagnosis of AMI requires serial monitoring of both cardiac biomarkers and ECG changes. The third group presents more than 48 hours after the onset of chest pain or symptoms of ischemia with nonspecific ECG changes. The ideal biomarker of myocardial injury in this group would persist in the circulation for several days to provide a late diagnostic time window. The shortfall of such a marker might be its inability to distinguish recurrent injury from old injury. The fourth group includes those who present to the ED at any time after the onset of ischemic symptoms with clear ECG evidence of AMI. In this group, detection with serum biomarkers of myocardial injury is theoretically not necessary.

A 2000 ESC/ACC consensus conference, updated in 2007 by the "Global Task Force for the Universal Definition of MI," has codified the role of biomarkers by advocating that the diagnosis be made from evidence of myocardial injury based on biomarkers of cardiac damage, preferably cardiac troponin (cTn) I or T, in the appropriate clinical situation of ischemic symptoms.

TABLE 9–1 Criteria for Diagnosis of Acute Myocardial Infarction

The term myocardial infarction should be used when there is evidence of myocardial necrosis in a clinical setting consistent with myocardial ischemia. Under these conditions, any 1 of the following criteria meets the diagnosis for myocardial infarction:

1. Detection of rise and/or fall of cardiac biomarkers (preferably troponin) with at least 1 value above the 99th percentile of the upper reference limit (URL) together with evidence of myocardial ischemia with at least 1 of the following:
   - Symptoms of ischemia
   - ECG changes indicative of new ischemia (new ST-T changes or new left bundle branch block [LBBB])
   - Development of pathological Q waves in the ECG
   - Imaging evidence of new loss of viable myocardium or new regional wall motion abnormality

2. Sudden, unexpected cardiac death, involving cardiac arrest, often with symptoms suggestive of myocardial ischemia, and accompanied by a presumably new ST elevation, or new LBBB, and/or evidence of fresh thrombus by coronary angiography and/or at autopsy, but death occurring before blood samples could be obtained, or at a time before the appearance of cardiac biomarkers in the blood

3. For percutaneous coronary interventions (PCI) in patients with normal baseline troponin values, elevations of cardiac biomarkers above the 99th percentile URL are indicative of peri-procedural myocardial necrosis. By convention, increases of biomarkers greater than 3× 99th percentile URL have been designated as defining PCI-related myocardial infarction. A subtype related to a documented stent thrombosis is recognized

4. For coronary artery bypass grafting (CABG) in patients with normal baseline troponin values, elevations of cardiac biomarkers above the 99th percentile URL are indicative of peri-procedural myocardial necrosis. By convention, increases of biomarkers greater than 5× 99th percentile URL plus either new pathological Q waves or new LBBB, or angiographically documented new graft or native coronary artery occlusion, or imaging evidence of new loss of viable myocardium have been designated as defining CABG-related myocardial infarction

5. Pathological findings of an acute myocardial infarction

TABLE 9–2 Diagnoses of Increased Cardiac Troponin Without Overt Ischemic Heart Disease

Trauma (including contusion, ablation, pacing, and cardioversion)
Congestive heart failure—acute and chronic[a]
Aortic valve disease and HOCM with significant LVH[a]
Hypertension
Hypotension, often with arrhythmias
Postoperative noncardiac surgery patients who seem to do well[a]
Renal failure[a]
Critically ill patients, especially with diabetes, respiratory failure[a]
Drug toxicity, for example, Adriamycin, 5-FU, Herceptin, snake venoms[a]
Hypothyroidism
Coronary vasospasm, including apical ballooning syndrome
Inflammatory diseases, for example, myocarditis, for example, with parvovirus B19, Kawasaki disease, sarcoid, smallpox vaccination, or myocardial extension of PE
Post-PCI patients who appear to be uncomplicated[a]
Pulmonary embolism, severe pulmonary hypertension[a]
Sepsis[a]
Burns, especially if TBSA >30%[a]
Infiltrative diseases including amyloidosis, hemochromatosis, sarcoidosis, and scleroderma[a]
Acute neurologic disease, including CVA, subarachnoid bleeds[a]
Rhabdomyolysis with cardiac injury
Transplant vasculopathy
Vital exhaustion

HOCM, hypertrophic obstructive cardiomyopathy; LVH, left ventricular hypertrophy; 5-FU, 5-fluorouracil; PE, pulmonary embolus; PCI, percutaneous coronary intervention; TBSA, total surface body area; CVA, cardiovascular accident.

[a]Designations imply prognostic information has been reported.

TABLE 9–3   Analytical Characteristics of Representative Commercial Cardiac Troponin I and T Assays As Stated By Manufacturer

Company/Platform/Assay (Generation)	LoD (µg/L)	99th Percentile (µg/L)	10% CV (µg/L)
Abbott ARCHITECT	0.009	0.028	0.032
Abbott i-STAT	0.02	0.08	0.10
Beckman Access (2nd)	0.01	0.04	0.06
BioMerieux Vidas Ultra	0.01	0.01	NA
Inverness Biosite Triage	0.05	<0.05	NA
Ortho Vitros ES (2nd)	0.012	0.034	0.034
Radiometer AQT90	0.0095	0.023	0.039
Response Biomedical RAMP	0.03	<0.01	0.21
Roche Elecsys 2010 (4th)	0.01	<0.01	0.030
Siemens Centaur Ultra (2nd)	0.006	0.04	0.030
Siemens Stratus CS (2nd)	0.03	0.07	0.06

LoD, lower limit of detection; CV, coefficient of variation; NA, not available.

Data from: IFCC Committee on Standardization of Markers of Cardiac Damage, www.ifcc.org.

Cardiac Troponin

The contractile proteins of the myofibril include the regulatory protein troponin. Troponin is a complex of 3 protein subunits, troponin C (the calcium-binding component), troponin I (the inhibitory component), and troponin T (the tropomyosin-binding component) (TIC). The subunits exist in isoforms distributed between cardiac muscle and slow and fast twitch skeletal muscle. Troponin is localized primarily in the myofibrils (94% to 97%), with a smaller cytoplasmic fraction (3% to 6%). cTn subunits I and T have different amino acid sequences encoded by different genes allowing for their cardiac tissue specificity. Following myocardial injury, multiple forms are elaborated both in tissue and in blood. The multiple forms of cTnI include the T–I–C ternary complex, IC binary complex, and free I. Multiple chemical modifications of these 3 forms can occur, involving oxidation, reduction, phosphorylation and dephosphorylation, and both C- and N-terminal degradation. The conclusions from these observations are that immunoassays need to be developed in which the antibodies recognize epitopes in the stable region of cTnI and, ideally, demonstrate an equimolar response to the different cTnI forms that circulate in the blood.

> Troponin is a complex of 3 protein subunits, troponin C (the calcium-binding component), troponin I (the inhibitory component), and troponin T (the tropomyosin-binding component). Over the past 20 years, numerous manufacturers have developed monoclonal antibody-based diagnostic immunoassays for the measurement of Troponin I and Troponin T.

Analytical Methods for Measuring Cardiac Troponin

Over the past 20 years, numerous manufacturers have developed monoclonal antibody-based diagnostic immunoassays for the measurement of cTnI and cTnT. Assay times range from 5 to 30 minutes. **Table 9–3** shows analytical characteristics of representative assays approved by the FDA for patient testing. In clinical practice, 2 obstacles limit the ease for switching from 1 cTnI assay to another. First, there is currently no primary reference cTnI material available for manufacturers to use for standardizing assays. Second, assay concentrations fail to agree because of the different epitopes recognized by the different antibodies used. Therefore, standardization of cTnI assays remains elusive. For cTnT, there is only 1 manufacturer. Therefore, there are no standardization problems. In 2001, the IFCC Committee on Standardization of Markers of Cardiac Damage (C-SMCD) established recommended quality specifications for cTn assays. These specifications were intended for use by the manufacturers of commercial assays and by clinical laboratories using troponin assays to establish uniform criteria so that all assays could be evaluated objectively for their analytical qualities and clinical performance. Both analytical and preanalytical factors were addressed including: antibody selection, calibration materials, imprecision characteristics at clinical decision values, effects of storage time and temperature, glass versus plastic tubes versus gel separator tubes, the influence of anticoagulants, and whole blood measurements.

99th Percentile Reference Value as a Cutoff for Diagnosis of Acute Myocardial Infarction

Both the initial 2000 ESC/ACC redefinition of MI consensus document and the 2007 "Universal Definition of Myocardial Infarction" guideline are predicated on cTn monitoring, with detection of a rising and/or falling cTn, and with at least 1 value above the 99th percentile value. Using the 99th percentile value (compared to the older WHO criteria) has demonstrated an increase in the number of MIs in day-to-day clinical practice, EDs, epidemiologic studies, and clinical trials. The data suggest that the more analytically sensitive cTn tests result in greater rates of MI diagnosis and greater rates of cTn positivity compared with other biomarkers such as CKMB. Milder and smaller MIs will be detected. Clinical cases that were earlier classified as unstable angina will be given a diagnosis of MI because of an increased cTn. Further, procedure-related troponin increases (i.e., following angioplasty) will be labeled MI. The importance of small troponin increases has been confirmed by their association with a poor prognosis.

Several markers should no longer be used to evaluate cardiac disease. They include aspartate aminotransaminase (AST), total CK activity, CKMB isoforms, myoglobin, total lactate dehydrogenase (LD), and LD isoenzymes. These markers have poor specificity for the detection of cardiac injury because of their wide tissue distribution. Because CKMB have been utilized for so many years, some laboratories may continue to measure them to allow for comparisons with cTn over time before discontinuing use of the CKMB assay. Although it has been suggested that CKMB be used together with cTn to aid in the timing of the onset of myocardial injury, infarct sizing, or determination of reinfarction, at present there is no strong evidence to support dual testing for cTn and CKMB.

Several markers should no longer be used to evaluate cardiac disease. They include aspartate aminotransaminase (AST), total CK activity, CKMB isoforms, myoglobin, total lactate dehydrogenase (LD), and LD isoenzymes.

Role of Cardiac Troponin for Risk Outcomes Assessment

Patients with Ischemia

In the environment of preventive and evidence-based medicine, the use of cTnI or cTnT measured in patients with ischemia will allow clinicians to use markers as both exclusionary and prognostic indicators. The results will assist in determining who is more at risk for AMI and death, and thereby determine who may benefit from early medical or surgical intervention. Such patients benefit from the use of anticoagulant therapy and the use of platelet antagonists, and an early invasive strategy. The goal of monitoring cardiac markers in patients suggestive of ACS with and without AMI would be to effectively identify patients with unstable coronary disease and triage them to an appropriate therapeutic regimen. Optimal use of this strategy requires at least 2 blood samples for cTn measurement. General population screening of hospitalized patients with cTnI or cTnT is not recommended.

Patients with Nonischemic Presentations

Clinicians are often confronted with a clinical history of a patient without overt coronary artery disease and a low probability of myocardial ischemia. However, as a precautionary measure, serial cTns are ordered. When 1 or 2 of the serial cTn concentrations are found to be increased, the clinician would likely be confronted with the following concerns: 1) What does this increase mean in the clinical setting of a nonischemic patient? 2) Is this a false-positive finding resulting from an analytical error? 3) Why was this test ordered in the first place? As cTn assays with increasing low-end analytical sensitivity have been developed and marketed, the ability to detect minor degrees of myocardial injury in a variety of clinical conditions has widened and has led to a better understanding that cTn is not just a biomarker for MI, but a sensitive biomarker for myocardial injury. The 20% of suspected ACS patients who clinically do not rule in for MI, but display an increased cTn, represents patients with nonischemic pathologies (**Table 9-2**) in whom the mechanisms of injury are well defined (such as myocarditis, blunt chest trauma, and chemotherapeutic agents), and patients with increased cTn, in whom the mechanism of injury is not clear.

Orders for Serial Cardiac Troponin Testing

Blood samples should be drawn at presentation to the hospital (often this is hours after the index clinical symptom onset) and at least once more at 6 to 9 hours later. Occasionally a patient may require a 12- to 24-hour sample, if the earlier measurements are normal and the clinical suspicion of AMI is high. As the cTn concentration may remain increased 5 to 12 days after an AMI, after 2 positive values, it does not appear cost-effective to continually monitor cTn because a diagnosis is established. In patients where recurrent MI is suspected from clinical signs or symptoms following the initial MI, an immediate measurement (0 hour) and testing of 6- to 9-hour serial blood samples are recommended. It is reasonable to suspect recurrent infarction if there is a >20% increase in the second value as long as it exceeds the 99th percentile.

CONGESTIVE HEART FAILURE

Description

CHF is a condition in which there is ineffective pumping of the heart leading to an accumulation of fluid in the lungs. Typically, it results from a loss of cardiac tissue and subsequent function. It is defined as the pathophysiological condition in which an abnormality of cardiac function is responsible for the failure of the heart to pump sufficient blood to satisfy the requirements of the metabolizing tissues. In the United States, CHF is the only cardiovascular disease with an increasing incidence. The National Heart, Lung, and Blood Institute estimates that current prevalence is about 5 million Americans with CHF, with an incidence of approximately 400,000 new cases each year. CHF is the leading cause of hospitalization in individuals 65 years and older. Current prognosis is dependent on disease severity, but overall it is poor. The 5-year mortality is approximately 10% in mild CHF, 20% to 30% in moderate CHF, and up to 80% in end-stage disease.

Diagnosis

Natriuretic Peptides (NP) in Monitoring CHF

Two biomarkers have been well studied to assist in these clinical settings: B-type natriuretic peptide (BNP, pharmacologically active hormone) and N-terminal proBNP (NT-proBNP, not pharmacologically active peptide). Both blood peptides are derived from cleavage of the myocardial proBNP peptide following myocardial stress and/or fluid overload. In general, the clinical evidence for utilization of either biomarker is very similar, but each has subtle analytical and physiological differences, depending on the pathophysiology of an individual patient. In the course of this chapter, both are used interchangeable unless specifically noted.

The ACC/AHA practice guidelines for the evaluation and management of CHF indicate that the role of NP in the identification of CHF patients remains to be clarified. In contrast, the ESC has incorporated monitoring NPs into their practice algorithm at the time of patient presentation alongside the clinical history, physical examination, ECG, and chest X-ray. An abnormal NP finding would trigger an echocardiogram or other imaging modality. NP concentrations in patients diagnosed with CHF are substantially increased (>1,000 ng/L for either BNP or NT-proBNP) when compared with patients who have minor increases (<300 ng/L) because of left ventricular (LV) dysfunction without acute CHF. CHF is more common in patients with advanced chronic renal disease. BNP and NT-proBNP are secreted in a pulsatile fashion from cardiac ventricles with an approximate half-life for BNP of 22 minutes in blood, with the NT-proBNP half-life on the order of hours. While 1 mechanism of BNP clearance involves the renal parenchyma, the kidney is not thought to be the primary site for BNP clearance. The kidney more specifically affects NT-proBNP clearance. Thus, increases in BNP in hemodialysis patients are thought to represent both regulatory responses from the cardiac ventricle, resulting from increased wall tension, and a lack of renal clearance.

Importantly, NPs are not 100% specific for CHF. Increases have been described for other non-CHF etiologies involving filling pressure defects, including LV hypertrophy, inflammatory cardiac diseases, systemic arterial hypertension, pulmonary hypertension, acute and chronic renal failure, liver cirrhosis, and several endocrine disorders (e.g., hyperaldosteronism and Cush-

CHF is a condition in which there is ineffective pumping of the heart leading to an accumulation of fluid in the lungs. Two biomarkers have been well studied to assist in these clinical settings: B-type natriuretic peptide (BNP, pharmacologically active hormone) and N-terminal proBNP (NT-proBNP, not pharmacologically active peptide).

TABLE 9–4   Representative Commercial BNP and NT-proBNP Assays

BNP
1. Abbott ARCHITECT and AxSYM
2. Inverness Medical Biosite Triage
3. Beckman Coulter Access
4. Siemens (Bayer) Centaur

NT-proBNP
1. Roche Elecsys
2. Seimens (Dade Behring)
3. Ortho-Clinical Diagnostics
4. Response Biomedical
5. Mitsubishi

ing's syndrome). In CHF patients presenting to the ED, patients admitted trend to have higher BNP concentrations (>500 ng/L) versus those who are discharged (mean <300 ng/L) at triage. Linear relationships with increasing BNP/NT-proBNP levels and the severity of CHF (NYSHA classification I to IV) have been described. The largest prospective trial to date to evaluate the diagnostic value of BNP is "The *Breathing Not Properly* Multicenter Study," from which the level of BNP was found to be an independent predictor of CHF. Using a blood BNP cutoff concentration of 100 ng/L for CHF, there was a 90% clinical sensitivity and 75% clinical specificity, with an 81% accuracy. Without BNP monitoring, clinical judgment and traditional diagnostic methods demonstrated a diagnostic accuracy of only 74%. The knowledge of BNP reduced the proportion of patients in whom the clinician was uncertain of the diagnosis from 43% to 11%. Plasma BNP monitoring in the ED improved the treatment and evaluation of patients with early dyspnea, reducing the time to discharge and total cost of treatment. After an AMI, NP increases in proportion to the size of the infarction, prompting investigators to explore the role of screening BNP for detection of LV dysfunction. In post-MI patients, BNP concentrations are inversely correlated with LV ejection fraction. However, there is inconclusive evidence for the role of BNP screening for asymptomatic LV dysfunction in the general population.

Blood NP monitoring can be valuable in the diagnostic setting, where it will possibly improve the performance of nonspecialist clinicians in diagnosing CHF. In clinical practice, BNP monitoring can best be used as a "rule out" test for suspected cases of new CHF. It is not a stand-alone test and should not be a replacement for a full clinical assessment, including an echocardiogram when indicated. In the presence of a normal BNP or NT-proBNP, a diagnosis of CHF is highly unlikely if concentrations are <100 ng/L for BNP or <300 ng/L for NT-proBNP. Monitoring NP may be useful in 1) guiding therapy, 2) monitoring the course of the disease, and 3) providing useful risk stratification information. NPs have been shown to be an independent predictor of cardiovascular mortality in patients with both CHF and ACS over a 1-year period. Further, BNP or NT-proBNP monitoring may assist in identifying patients with a lower risk of readmission with the next 30 days before discharge.

> Blood NP monitoring can be valuable in the diagnostic setting. In the presence of a normal BNP or NT-proBNP, a diagnosis of CHF is highly unlikely.

Analytical Methods for Measuring Natriuretic Peptides

Table 9–4 shows the current FDA-approved assays for BNP or NT-proBNP. The commercial assays differ in standardization of measurements and antibodies used in the assay. Assays that use an antibody that recognizes the N-terminus labile region of BNP (Biosite, Beckman, and Abbott) demonstrate less analyte stability at room temperature (24 hours) than assays that use 1 of their antibodies recognizing the C-terminus (Siemens [Bayer]). The Roche NT-proBNP antibody configuration allows for 72 hours of sample stability at room temperature.

Reference Intervals: Medical Decision Cutoff Values

A number of clinical factors affect the BNP and NT-proBNP concentrations, most importantly age, gender, obesity, and renal function. Significant differences are observed between men and women (higher), and there are increasing concentrations with age by decade. For BNP and NT-proBNP, the significance of the results for these assays in relation to the degree of left ventricle dysfunction remains a debate. For both analytes, there is an inverse relationship between values and body mass index. For NT-proBNP, establishing reference intervals has been challenging. Review of both the FDA-approved US package insert and the European assay package insert reveals substantial differences in what concentrations are considered normal by age and sex. For BNP, a cutoff of 100 ng/L has been endorsed as demonstrating optimal sensitivity and specificity. For NT-proBNP, the FDA-approved package insert describes a 2-tier cutoff by age at—<75 years: 125 ng/L and >75 years: 450 ng/L. However, more evidence-based cutoffs have been derived from the PRIDE/ICON studies based on age and renal function, and are recommended as follows—age <50 years: >450 ng/L; age ≥50 years: >900 ng/L; all ages: best negative predictive value <300 ng/L; age <50 years and eGFR >60 mL/minute: 450 pg/mL, and eGFR ≤60 mL/minute: 1,200 ng/L; age ≥50 years and eGFR >60 mL/minute: 900 pg/mL, and eGFR ≤60 mL/minute: 1,200 ng/L.

Implications for Therapy Using Test Results for Natriuretic Peptides

Routine blood BNP or NT-proBNP testing is not warranted for making specific therapeutic decisions for patients with acute or chronic heart failure because of the still emerging and incomplete data as well as intra- and inter-individual variations. The concept of NP-guided management of heart failure is still being debated, and there is no general consensus in expert opinion regarding this issue.

Biological Variability

As BNP and NT-proBNP become more widely used to monitor CHF patients following therapy, questions have addressed the usefulness of serial monitoring in assisting the success of drug therapy. In a study of 11 patients with CHF, the biological variation for BNP and NT-proBNP was evaluated using 4 different assays. The findings indicated that a change of 130% for BNP and 90% for NT-proBNP is necessary before results of serially collected data can be considered clinically and statistically significant. For example, these findings imply that a decrease from approximately 500 to 250 ng/L would be necessary for a clinician to conclude that therapy was successful in improving CHF features. Clinicians without this knowledge may inappropriately assume that a decrease from an admission BNP value of 500 ng/L to a 24-hour post-admission value of 400 ng/L may have been a result of successful patient management. It has been suggested that following the admission BNP value, a second BNP value be obtained within 24 hours of discharge to optimize the diagnostic utility of BNP in the overall assessment of patients with CHF.

REFERENCES

Apple FS, et al. Quality specifications for B-type natriuretic peptide assays. *Clin Chem*. 2005;51:486–493.

Apple FS, et al. National Academy of Clinical Biochemistry and IFCC Committee for Standardization of Markers of Cardiac Damage laboratory medicine practice guidelines: analytical issues for biomarkers of heart failure. *Circulation*. 2007;116:e95–e98.

Apple FS, et al. National Academy of Clinical Biochemistry and IFCC Committee for Standardization of Markers of Cardiac Damage laboratory medicine practice guidelines: analytical issues for biomarkers of acute coronary syndromes. *Clin Chem*. 2007;53:547–551.

Morrow DA, et al. National Academy of Clinical Biochemistry practice guidelines: clinical characteristics and utilization of biomarkers in acute coronary syndromes. *Clin Chem*. 2007;53:552–574.

Panteghini M, et al. Quality specifications for cardiac troponin assays. *Clin Chem Lab Med*. 2001;39: 175–179.

Tang WHW, et al. National Academy of Clinical Biochemistry practice guidelines: clinical utilization of cardiac biomarker testing in heart failure. *Circulation*. 2007;116:e99–e109.

Thygesen K, et al., on behalf of the Joint ESC/ACCF/AHA/WHF Task Force for the redefinition of myocardial infarction. Universal definition of myocardial infarction. *J Am Coll Cardiol*. 2007;50: 2173–2195.

Wu AHB, et al. National Academy of Clinical Biochemistry laboratory medicine practice guidelines: use of cardiac troponin and B-type natriuretic peptide or N-terminal proB-type natriuretic peptide for etiologies other than acute coronary syndromes and heart failure. *Clin Chem*. 2007;53:2086–2096.

Diseases of Red Blood Cells

Daniel D. Mais

CHAPTER OUTLINE

ANEMIA

Definition

Anemia refers to a deficiency in red blood cells (RBC) and implies a decline in oxygen-carrying capacity. The complete blood count (CBC) provides several measures of red cell quantity, including RBC count, hemoglobin (Hb) concentration, and hematocrit (Hct) (see description of RBC indices later in this chapter). Hb concentration is the parameter most widely used to diagnose anemia, based on 1967 World Health Organization (WHO) recommendations (**Table 10–1**). This definition is not universally accepted, and numerous alternatives have been proposed over the years, usually suggesting slightly higher values and race-specific values. It is important to remember also that the normal ranges for Hb and Hct are different for infants, children, adult men, adult women, pregnant women, and the elderly. Attention to age- and gender-appropriate normal ranges is important in the evaluation of anemia.

TABLE 10–1　**WHO Definition of Anemia**

Group	Hemoglobin (g/dL)
Infants and children, 6 months–6 years	<11.0
Pregnant females	<11.0
Children, 6–14 years	<12.0
Nonpregnant adult females	<12.0
Adult males	<13.0

Anemia may present with pallor, fatigue, dyspnea, or evidence of poor tissue oxygenation (chest pain due to poor cardiac oxygenation and altered mental status due to poor cerebral oxygenation). Often, particularly when anemia is mild or the patient is otherwise healthy, anemia presents simply as an abnormal CBC.

Anemia stimulates several compensatory mechanisms. The cardiopulmonary system compensates by attempting to make the most of the blood it has by exchanging more gases (tachypnea), and circulating more volume (tachycardia). The marrow responds with increased erythropoiesis, stimulated by an increase in renal production of erythropoietin (EPO) in response to hypoxia. If the means to create mature red cells are intact (i.e., if the underlying cause of the anemia is not a production or maturation defect), then this response can usually succeed. In addition to making more erythrocytes, the marrow begins to release immature erythrocytes into the circulation. Many of these still contain a network of ribosomes and rough endoplasmic reticulum involved in the making of Hb, which identifies them morphologically as reticulocytes (**see description of reticulocyte counting later in this chapter**). Over the next 3 to 4 days, this reticulin network dissolves. In very brisk marrow responses, some red cells may be released that still contain a nucleus.

Differential Diagnosis

Identifying the cause of anemia is usually fairly straightforward. There are several strategies for reaching the diagnosis (**Tables 10–2** and **10–3**), 1 of which is illustrated in the algorithms (**Figures 10–1** to **10–4**). Examination of the peripheral smear is especially important, since numerous clues can be found there (**Table 10–4**). **Figures 10–5 to 10–23 show many of the abnormal morphologies and intracellular inclusions of RBC.**

The reticulocyte count is an important piece of information. When markedly elevated, this is usually noticeable in a Wright-stained peripheral blood smear. Reticulocytes appear as large, polychromatophilic red cells, and when these are numerous, the smear is often described as having polychromasia. Anemia due to a production defect is associated with a normal reticulocyte count. Such hyporegenerative anemias include iron deficiency anemia, anemia of chronic disease (ACD), lead poisoning, folate deficiency, B_{12} deficiency, myelodysplastic syndrome, aplastic anemia, and pure red cell aplasia. The megaloblastic anemias (folate and B_{12} deficiency) have a hemolytic component as well.

Regardless of the morphology or red cell size, anemia that is accompanied by reticulocytosis suggests either hemolysis or hemorrhage. An exception is a partially treated production defect, such as in the early treatment of iron, folate, or B_{12} deficiency. Hemorrhage is usually clinically apparent; however, significant blood loss into the retroperitoneum or pelvis may go unnoticed. In neonates, intracranial hemorrhage of sufficient quantity to cause anemia may occur. Both hemolytic and blood-loss anemia may eventually lead to depletion of iron, folate, or B_{12}, and they can present as a production defect. Paroxysmal nocturnal hemoglobinuria (PNH) is a hemolytic anemia that may transform to aplastic anemia.

Hemolytic anemias are those in which red cell survival, normally 120 days, is shortened. The premature destruction of erythrocytes may occur within the blood stream (intravascular

Identifying the cause of anemia is usually fairly straightforward. Examination of the peripheral smear is especially important. The reticulocyte count is an important piece of information.

TABLE 10-2   **Classification of Anemia by Pathophysiology**

Production Defect	Survival Defect
Proliferation defect Anemia of chronic disease Renal disease (low erythropoietin states) Fanconi anemia Blackfan–Diamond Syndrome Parvovirus Drugs or toxins	**Hemolysis** Hemoglobinopathies Immune hemolytic anemias Infectious causes of hemolysis Membrane abnormalities Metabolic abnormalities Mechanical hemolysis Drugs or toxins Wilson's disease
Maturation defect Vitamin B_{12} deficiency Folate deficiency Iron deficiency Sideroblastic anemia Lead poisoning	**Hemorrhage** **Hypersplenism**

TABLE 10-3   **Classification of Anemia by Mean Corpuscular Volume (MCV) and Red Blood Cell Distribution Width (RDW)**

	Normal RDW	High RDW
Low MCV	Anemia of chronic disease Thalassemia Hemoglobin E	Iron deficiency anemia Sickle cell disease
Normal MCV	Acute blood loss Anemia of chronic disease Low EPO states (renal failure)	Early nutritional (iron, B_{12}, folate) deficiency Sickle cell disease
High MCV	Aplastic anemia Liver disease Alcohol abuse	Folate and B_{12} deficiency Myelodysplasia Reticulocytosis (e.g., hemolysis)

EPO, erythropoietin.

hemolysis) or within the reticuloendothelial system (extravascular hemolysis). Intravascular hemolysis is caused by mechanical red cell trauma (microangiopathic hemolytic anemia [MHA] or mechanical heart valve), complement fixation on the red cell surface (e.g., ABO incompatibility), PNH, paroxysmal cold hemoglobinuria (PCH), snake envenomation, and infectious agents (malaria, babesiosis, and *Clostridium*). Extravascular hemolysis is much more common and is typical for all remaining causes of hemolysis. The causes of hemolysis may be inherited or acquired. Inherited forms of hemolytic anemia usually, but not always, present in early childhood (**Table 10–5**).

Hemolytic anemia presents with jaundice, fatigue, tachycardia, and pallor. Enhanced excretion of Hb breakdown products often leads to the development of pigmented gallstones. Intravascular hemolysis may present with dark urine and back pain. Leg ulcers are common in sickle cell disease and hereditary spherocytosis (HS). Splenomegaly is a common finding in extravascular hemolysis. Laboratory findings in support of hemolysis include increased unconjugated bilirubin, increased lactate dehydrogenase (LDH), and decreased haptoglobin. Reticulocytes, which are larger than mature red cells, are responsible for an unpredictability of the mean corpuscular volume (MCV). The blood smear may display helpful morphologic findings. Intravascular hemolysis is associated with hemoglobinuria and hemosiderinuria.

Laboratory findings in support of hemolysis include increased unconjugated bilirubin, increased lactate dehydrogenase (LDH), and decreased haptoglobin.

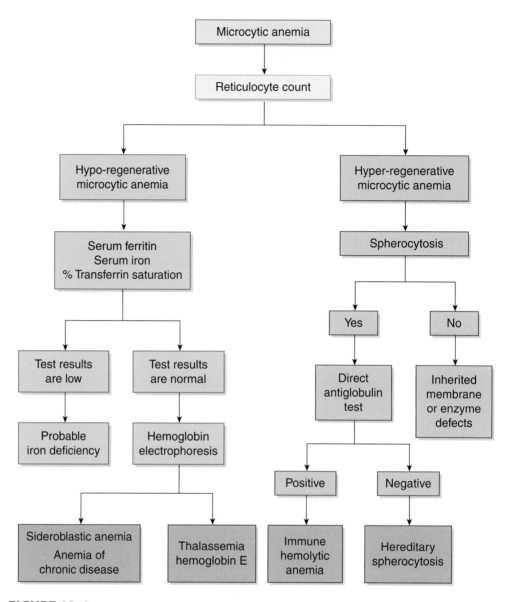

FIGURE 10–1 Diagnostic algorithm for microcytic anemia.

Acute Blood Loss

Description

Acute blood loss (hemorrhage) is seen most often as a result of surgery, trauma, or gastrointestinal pathology. Most often, hemorrhage is quite obviously present, but occasionally it is occult and internal (large retroperitoneal or pelvic hemorrhages). It can occur in the prehospital setting, and in that case its volume cannot be estimated.

The cardinal manifestations of acute blood loss—tachycardia, tachypnea, and hypotension—reflect not so much a decreased oxygen-carrying capacity as a decreased intravascular volume. A shift of water from the interstitial fluid compartment into the plasma leads to hemodilution and a lowered Hct.

Chronic slow blood loss is generally well tolerated and usually presents late in the disease process, as iron deficiency anemia. Acute blood loss is not the only form of anemia that can present abruptly. Causes other than hemorrhage that may present as rapid-onset severe anemia include intravascular hemolysis and acute exacerbations of a chronic compensated hemolytic anemia, such as in sickle cell disease (**Table 10–6**).

Most often, hemorrhage is quite obviously present, but occasionally it is occult and internal (large retroperitoneal or pelvic hemorrhages). Chronic slow blood loss is generally well tolerated and usually presents late in the disease process, as iron deficiency anemia.

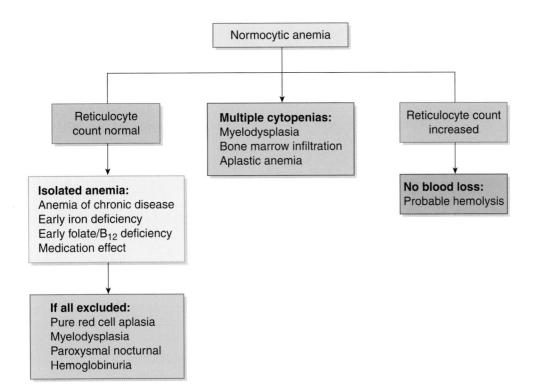

FIGURE 10–2 Diagnostic algorithm for normocytic anemia.

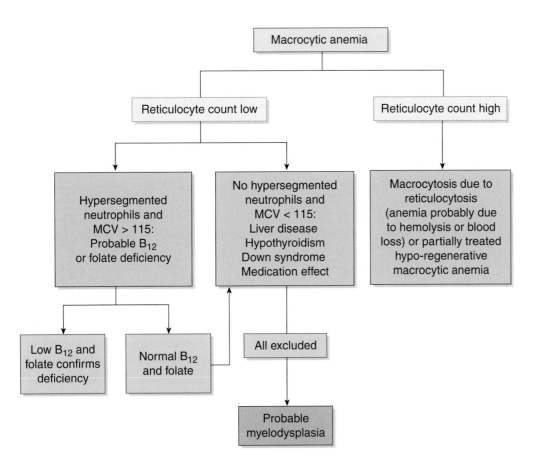

FIGURE 10–3 Diagnostic algorithm for macrocytic anemia.

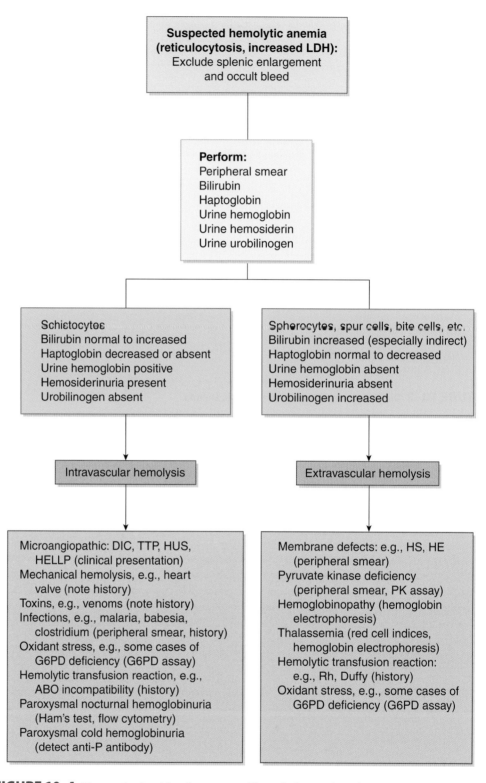

FIGURE 10–4 Diagnostic algorithm for suspected hemolytic anemia. Information enclosed in parentheses is important supplemental information needed to establish a diagnosis. DIC, disseminated intravascular coagulation; TTP, thrombotic thrombocytopenic purpura; HUS, hemolytic uremic syndrome; HELLP, hemolysis, elevated liver function tests, low platelets; G6PD, glucose-6-phosphate dehydrogenase deficiency; HS, hereditary spherocytosis; HE, hereditary elliptocytosis; PK, pyruvate kinase.

TABLE 10–4   Morphologic Findings in Red Cells

Finding	Definition	Associated Conditions
Basophilic stippling	Small blue dots in red cells, due to clusters of ribosomes	Hemolytic anemias Lead poisoning Thalassemia
Pappenheimer bodies	Larger, more irregular, and grayer than basophilic stippling, due to iron-containing mitochondria	Asplenia Sideroblastic anemia
Heinz bodies	Gray-black round inclusions, seen only with supravital stains (crystal violet)	Oxidative injury as found in G6PD deficiency or with unstable hemoglobins
Bite cells	Sharp bite-like defects in red cells where a Heinz body has been removed in the spleen. Both are due to denatured hemoglobin	Oxidative injury as found in G6PD deficiency or with unstable hemoglobins
Howell-Jolly bodies	Dot-like, dark purple inclusion	Asplenia
Cabot rings	Ring-shaped dark purple inclusion. Both represent a residual nuclear fragment	Asplenia
Target cells	Red cells with a dark circle within the central area of pallor, reflecting redundant membrane	Thalassemia Hemoglobin C Liver disease
Schistocytes	Fragmented red blood cells, with forms such as helmet-shaped cells, due to mechanical red cell fragmentation	Microangiopathic hemolytic anemias (MHA): DIC, TTP, HUS, HELLP. Mechanical heart valves
Dacrocytes (teardrop cells)	Teardrop or pear-shaped erythrocytes	Can be seen in thalassemia and megaloblastic anemia Often seen in myelophthisis
Echinocytes (burr cells)	Red blood cells that have circumferential undulations or spiny projections with pointed tips	Uremia Gastric cancer Pyruvate kinase deficiency
Acanthocytes (spur cells)	Red blood cells that have circumferential blunt and spiny projections with bulbous tips	Liver disease Abetalipoproteinemia McLeod phenotype
Spherocytes	Red cells without central pallor due to decreased red cell membrane	Immune hemolytic anemia Hereditary spherocytosis
Elliptocytes	Red cells twice as long as they are wide	Iron deficiency Hereditary elliptocytosis
Stomatocytes	Red cells whose area of central pallor is elongated in a mouth-like shape	Alcohol abuse Dilantin exposure Rh null phenotype (absence of Rh antigens) Hereditary stomatocytosis

See **Figures 10–5** to **10–23** for peripheral smears with abnormal red blood cell morphology.

DIC, disseminated intravascular coagulation; TTP, thrombotic thrombocytopenic purpura; HUS, hemolytic uremic syndrome; HELLP, hemolysis, elevated liver function tests, low platelets.

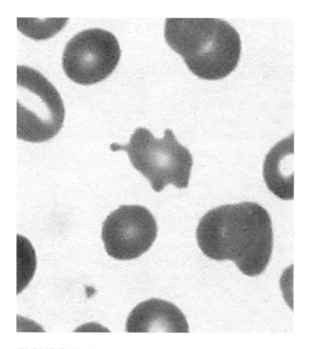

FIGURE 10–5 Peripheral blood smear with acanthocytes.

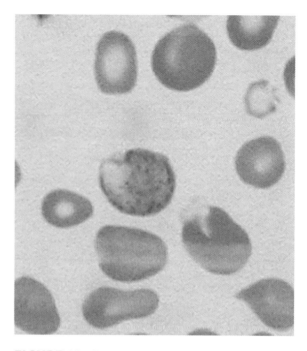

FIGURE 10–6 Peripheral blood smear with basophilic stippling.

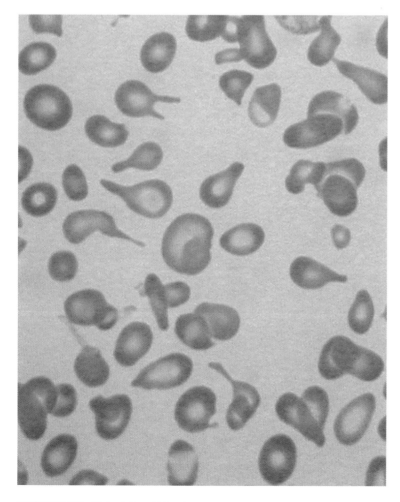

FIGURE 10–7 Peripheral blood smear with dacrocytes.

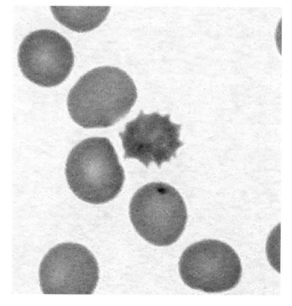

FIGURE 10–8 Peripheral blood smear with echinocyte.

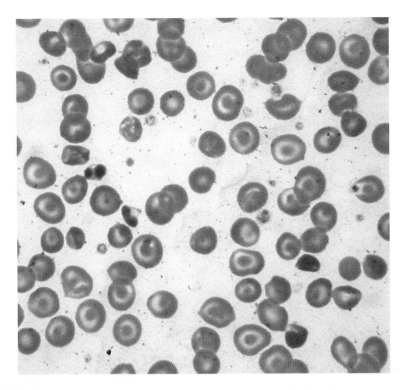

FIGURE 10–9 Peripheral blood smear from a patient with hemoglobin C disease.

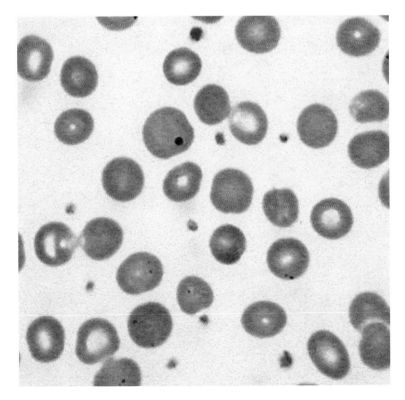

FIGURE 10–10 Peripheral blood smear showing a Howell-Jolly body.

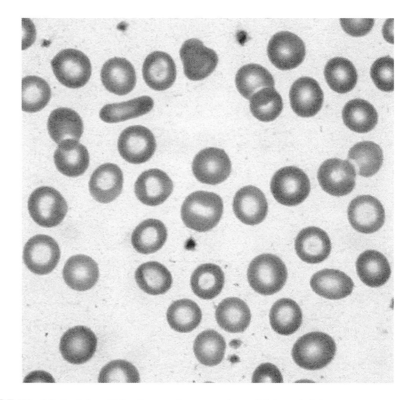

FIGURE 10–11 Peripheral blood smear from a patient with iron deficiency.

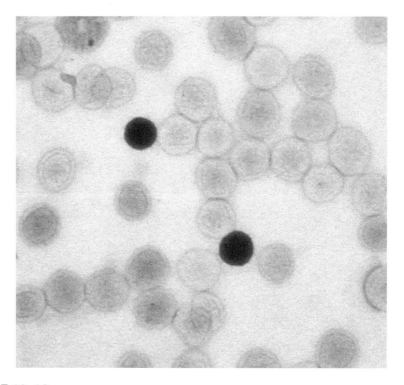

FIGURE 10–12 Slide showing the results of a Kleihauer–Betke test.

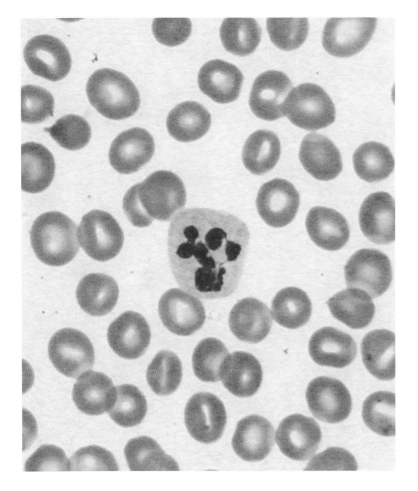

FIGURE 10–13 Peripheral blood smear from a patient with megaloblastic anemia and hypersegmented neutrophils.

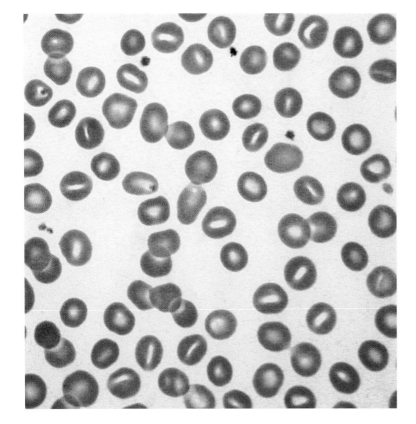

FIGURE 10–14 Peripheral blood smear from a patient with megaloblastic anemia and macroovalocytes.

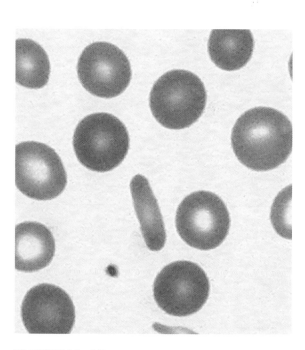

FIGURE 10–15 Peripheral blood smear showing an elliptocyte.

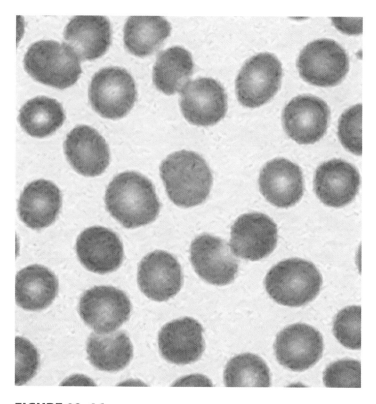

FIGURE 10–16 A peripheral blood smear stained with Wright's stain showing a reticulocyte.

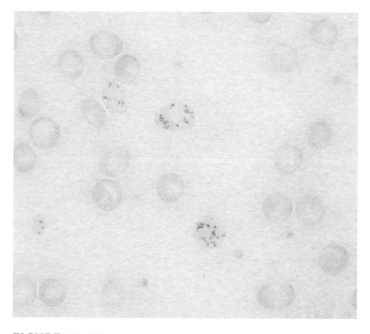

FIGURE 10–17 Four reticulocytes revealed by supravital staining.

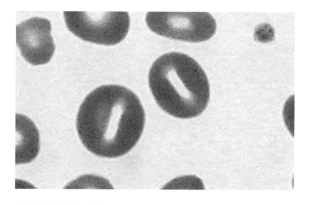

FIGURE 10–18 A peripheral blood smear from a patient with stomatocytes.

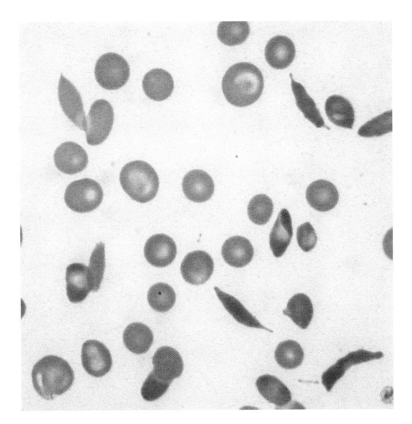

FIGURE 10–19 Peripheral blood smear with sickle cells.

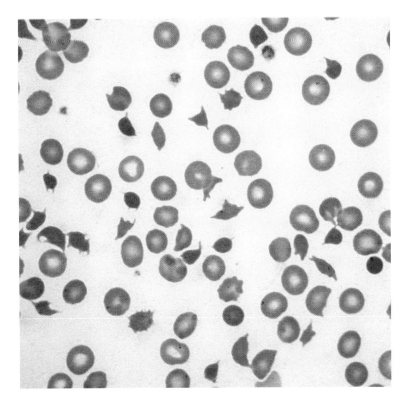

FIGURE 10–20 Peripheral blood smear with schistocytes.

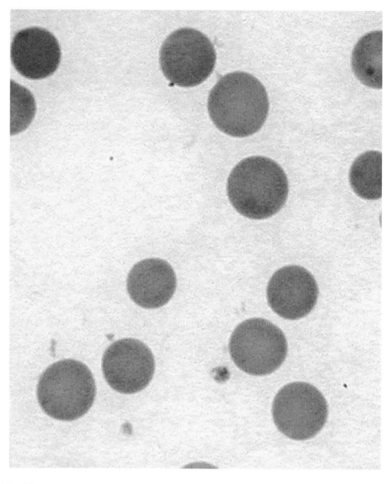

FIGURE 10–21 Peripheral blood smear with spherocytes.

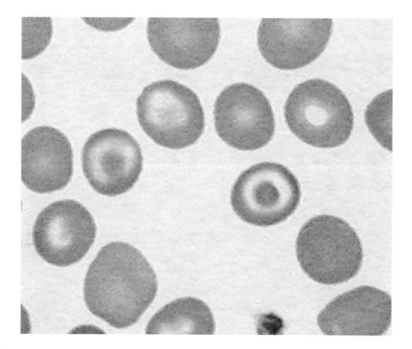

FIGURE 10–22 Peripheral blood smear with target cells.

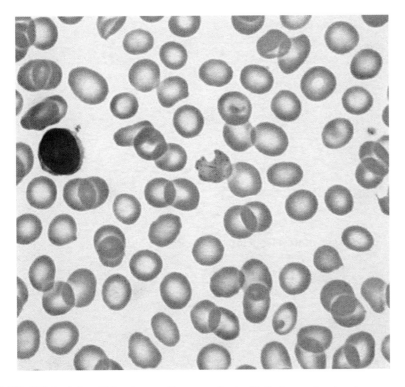

FIGURE 10–23 Peripheral blood smear from a patient with thalassemia, showing microcytic red cells, target cells, and basophilic stippling.

TABLE 10–5   Laboratory Distinction of Intravascular and Extravascular Hemolysis

Intravascular Hemolysis	Extravascular Hemolysis
Schistocytes	Microspherocytes
↑ LDH	↑ LDH
↓ Haptoglobin	Normal to ↓ haptoglobin
↑ Free Hb, ↑ urine Hb	↑ Indirect bilirubin
Hemosiderinuria	↑ Urine and fecal urobilinogen

Hb, hemoglobin; LDH, lactate dehydrogenase.

TABLE 10–6   Nonhemorrhagic Causes of Acute Severe Anemia

Acute Intravascular Hemolysis	Acute Exacerbation of Chronic Hemolysis
Microangiopathic hemolytic anemia	Parvovirus B19 bone marrow infection (aplastic crisis)
Mechanical hemolysis (e.g., heart valve)	Splenic sequestration crisis
Toxins (e.g., venoms)	Hyperhemolytic crisis
Infections (e.g., malaria, *Clostridium*)	
Oxidant stress (especially in glucose-6-phosphate dehydrogenase deficiency)	
Hemolytic transfusion reaction (ABO incompatibility)	
Paroxysmal nocturnal hemoglobinuria	
Paroxysmal cold hemoglobinuria	

TABLE 10–7   Causes of Iron Deficiency

Mechanisms	Examples
Iron-poor diet	Strict vegetarians
Iron malabsorption	Celiac sprue Small bowel resection Achlorhydria Hookworm infection
Chronic blood (iron) loss	Menses Colorectal cancer Idiopathic pulmonary hemosiderosis

TABLE 10–8   Stages of Iron Deficiency

Stage	Laboratory Findings	Clinical Findings
Iron store depletion	↓ Serum ferritin, ↓ Stainable marrow iron	None
Impaired erythropoiesis	All of the above plus ↑ TIBC, ↓ serum iron, and ↑ RDW	None
Iron deficiency anemia	All of the above plus microcytic, hypochromic anemia	Fatigue, pallor

TIBC, total iron binding capacity; RDW, red blood cell distribution width.

Diagnosis

The history and physical examination are the keys to arriving at the correct diagnosis. In perplexing situations, it may be necessary to exclude hemolysis. The main laboratory findings are a normocytic anemia with a marked reticulocytosis. The peripheral smear may be notable only for neutrophilia, a result of mobilization of granulocytes from marginal pools (demargination), which is a physiologic stress response. Somewhat later, there may be reactive thrombocytosis.

Iron Deficiency Anemia

Description

Within the cytoplasm of the marrow erythroblast, the predominant activity is the production of Hb molecules into which iron must be incorporated. Iron from the diet is absorbed principally in the duodenum. It is carried by transferrin to the marrow, where it is internalized into erythroblasts and incorporated into protoporphyrin to yield heme. Iron not utilized in this way is stored bound to ferritin. When there is inadequate iron intake or excessive iron loss (**Table 10–7**), the ferritin–iron stores of the reticuloendothelial system become progressively depleted. Red cells are produced that contain an inadequate concentration of Hb, giving rise to the appearance of small, hypochromic red cells that are poorly equipped for the carriage of oxygen. Fewer mature red cells are subsequently produced, lowering the Hct (**Table 10–8**). The clinical manifestations include those directly attributable to anemia (fatigue and pallor), in addition to pica (a desire to ingest solids such as rock, dirt, or ice), atrophic glossitis, koilonychias, and esophageal webs. The coexistence of esophageal webs in iron deficiency has been called Plummer–Vinson syndrome. These latter manifestations are not commonly seen and follow prolonged, untreated iron deficiency.

Iron deficiency is the most common cause of anemia. Worldwide, the most common cause of iron deficiency is a dietary lack of iron. In the United States, iron intake is not usually problematic, although supply can lag demand in some populations, such as toddlers and pregnant women. The finding of iron deficiency produces an obligation to identify and treat the underlying cause. In American adults, this underlying cause is usually found within the gastrointestinal tract. Iron deficiency often is the first sign of an occult gastrointestinal malignancy.

> Iron deficiency is the most common cause of anemia. The finding of iron deficiency produces an obligation to identify and treat the underlying cause.

Diagnosis

In many cases, the CBC and peripheral blood findings are highly characteristic: low RBC count, low MCV, low mean corpuscular hemoglobin concentration (MCHC), and high red cell distribution width (RDW). The platelet count is often elevated. The peripheral blood shows hypochromic, microcytic red cells with scattered elliptocytes This is in contrast to the most commonly entertained other diagnostic consideration, thalassemia, in which the RBC count is high, the RDW tends to be lower, elliptocytes are not seen, and target cells and basophilic stippling are more frequent.

To confirm the diagnosis of iron deficiency, the best single test is the serum ferritin. A ferritin above 15 μg/L essentially excludes iron deficiency, and the serum ferritin in iron deficiency is often below 10 μg/L. Lowered ferritin is the earliest finding in iron deficiency and persists throughout the course of the illness. The diagnostic difficulty with the use of ferritin is that it is an acute-phase reactant, an analyte that increases in response to inflammation. It may also be spuriously elevated in hepatic insufficiency, due to impaired clearance. Thus, other assays may occasionally be needed to make a diagnosis of iron deficiency anemia.

In established iron deficiency, the serum iron is typically low, the total iron binding capacity (TIBC) is elevated, and the percent transferrin saturation is low. These findings are somewhat in contrast to those seen in ACD (see below). Serum soluble transferrin receptor is elevated whenever there are cells depleted of iron; thus, it is elevated in iron deficiency anemia and in erythroid hyperplasia (hemolytic anemia, polycythemia). Lastly, the zinc protoporphyrin (ZPP) and free erythrocyte protoporphyrin (FEP) are elevated in iron deficiency but also elevated in lead poisoning and ACD. As a last resort, marrow iron stores can be examined directly under the microscope if an adequate bone marrow aspirate is obtained.

Anemia of Chronic Disease

Definition

Sustained systemic inflammation alters iron utilization in the marrow, suppresses hematopoiesis, and blunts the response of EPO to anemia. This combination of factors leads to a mild, refractory, hyporegenerative anemia that is usually normocytic and normochromic, but is microcytic in up to one third of cases. Although iron deficiency is the most common cause of anemia worldwide, ACD is the most common cause of anemia in both hospitalized and ambulatory hospital patients in the United States. The vast majority of cases are due to rheumatoid arthritis, collagen vascular disease, such as lupus, chronic infection, and malignancy.

The means by which chronic inflammatory diseases cause anemia are still being elucidated. Marrow biopsies in patients with ACD display bountiful iron stores in the face of decreased iron uptake by erythroid precursors. Decreased transferrin receptors have been demonstrated on erythroblasts in ACD. In addition, patients with ACD have decreased production of EPO in response to anemia. Cytokines, including IFNγ, TNFα, IL-1, and hepcidin, have been shown to produce the conditions of ACD when injected into laboratory animals.

Diagnosis

The diagnosis of ACD is made difficult by the presence of numerous comorbid factors, in patients who, by definition, are ill. In such patients, ACD may be coincident with iron deficiency, folate deficiency, renal insufficiency, and/or frequent phlebotomy. Furthermore, in up to 30% of those with iron indices characteristic of ACD, no chronic illness can be identified.

The laboratory diagnosis of ACD depends on demonstrating a hypoproliferative (low reticulocyte count) normocytic or microcytic anemia in the presence of characteristic iron studies. The iron studies should document increased iron stores (normal to high serum ferritin or increased stainable iron in a bone marrow biopsy) and a low serum iron, low transferrin, and low TIBC.

A normal or elevated ferritin level is crucial for distinguishing ACD from iron deficiency. However, interpretation of the results for ferritin can be problematic because ferritin is an acute-phase reactant. Thus, while a low ferritin is essentially diagnostic of iron deficiency, a normal ferritin does not entirely exclude it. In confusing situations, the soluble serum transferrin receptor assay may be helpful. This analyte is increased in iron deficiency anemia and normal in ACD.

> Anemia of chronic disease is the most common cause of anemia in both hospitalized and ambulatory hospital patients in the United States. The vast majority of cases are due to rheumatoid arthritis, collagen vascular disease, such as lupus, chronic infection, and malignancy.

Thalassemia

Description

Mutations in the genes that encode globin chains may result in 2 broad categories of disease. Some mutations lead to the production of a structurally abnormal globin chain, resulting in a *hemoglobinopathy* such as hemoglobin S (sickle cell disease and sickle cell trait). Other mutations lead to reduced production of a structurally normal globin chain, resulting in *thalassemia*.

A Hb molecule is composed of 4 polypeptide chains. The major adult Hb, hemoglobin A (HbA), is composed of 2 alpha chains and 2 beta chains. The minor adult hemoglobin (HbA2) is composed of 2 alpha chains and 2 delta chains. The major fetal hemoglobin (HbF) is composed of 2 alpha chains and 2 gamma chains. The one constant feature of all Hbs is the alpha chain. The alpha chain genes are located on chromosome 16. Each chromosome 16 contains 2 separate alpha chain genes, for a total of 4 genes per normal cell, each transcriptionally active. Thus, to render an individual completely deficient of alpha chains, inheritance of 4 mutated genes is required. The beta, gamma, and delta chain genes are located on chromosome 11. Each chromosome 11 contains 1 beta, 1 gamma, and 1 delta gene. Should a mutation occur in the beta chain, there can be a degree of compensation by increasing the production of gamma, delta, or both. There is no such substitute for the alpha chain.

With decreased alpha chain production, α-thalassemia arises. Harm comes to the red cell, however, not from a deficiency of alpha chain, but from an excess of nonalpha chains (e.g., beta). The excess chains form precipitates in the cell, leading to ineffective erythropoiesis, microcytosis, and enhanced splenic red cell destruction. Likewise, decreased beta chain production (β-thalassemia) leads to precipitation of excess alpha chains and subsequent red cell destruction. Disease severity reflects the genotype (**Table 10–9**).

Diagnosis

Since alpha chains are present in utero, α-thalassemia can be diagnosed at birth. The diagnosis of β-thalassemia is somewhat delayed, since beta chains are not produced to adult levels until 3 to 6 months of age. The CBC is notable for microcytosis, usually in the presence of a normal or high RBC count. The peripheral smear often displays target cells and may display basophilic stippling. When there are microcytosis, "thalassemic" indices, and normal iron studies, the diagnosis of thalassemia is essentially assured. In the case of β-thalassemia, an Hb electrophoresis displays increased HbA2 and sometimes HbF (**see description of Hb electrophoresis later in this chapter and in Chapter 2**). In α-thalassemia (recall that the alpha chain is needed for all Hb types), the proportion of Hbs appears normal. These findings are usually sufficient for the diagnosis. If further definition is required, molecular genetic testing is available.

Folate Deficiency

Description

Folate and vitamin B_{12} deficiency (described next) are the classic causes of megaloblastic anemia. The term *megaloblastic* refers to the appearance of hematopoietic precursor cells in the marrow. Their nuclei appear abnormally large and immature, resulting from nuclear maturation that lags cytoplasmic maturation. This megaloblastic change affects not only erythroblasts, but other rapidly dividing cells as well, including maturing granulocytes, megakaryocytes, and enterocytes. It results from impairment of DNA synthesis and has more than just morphologic consequences.

Erythropoiesis becomes ineffective, resulting in a hypercellular marrow. Many erythroblasts are destroyed while still in the marrow. Thus, megaloblastic anemia is in part a hemolytic anemia; indeed, intramedullary destruction of maturing erythrocytes leads to increased LDH and bilirubin, as one would associate with hemolytic anemia. The red cells that do proceed to maturity are macrocytic, with the MCV in fully developed megaloblastic anemia exceeding 115 fL.

Folate deficiency does not cause the same neurologic defect that vitamin B_{12} deficiency causes. However, supplementation of folate in early pregnancy is known to reduce the incidence of neural tube defects. No clear mechanism for this effect has been established.

Dietary factors are a major cause of folate deficiency. Folate is found in leafy green vegetables, fruits, and legumes. Dietary folate is absorbed in the duodenum, and the body stores

TABLE 10-9   Thalassemia Syndromes

Category	Syndrome	Genotype	Manifestations
Normal	Normal	αα/αα β/β	None
α-Thalassemia syndromes	α-Thalassemia (silent) carrier	αα/α■ β/β	None
	α-Thalassemia minor	αα/■■ β/β α■/α■ β/β	Mild
	Hemoglobin H	α■/■■ β/β	Moderate to severe
	Hemoglobin Barts	■■/■■ β/β	Fatal
β-Thalassemia syndromes	β-Thalassemia minor	αα/αα β/β⁺ αα/αα β/β°	Mild to moderate
	β-Thalassemia major	αα/αα β/β° αα/αα β⁺/β⁺ αα/αα β⁺/β°	Moderate to severe

Notation: α, normal α gene; ■, severely suppressed α gene; β, normal β gene; β⁺, moderately suppressed β gene; β°, severely suppressed β gene.

TABLE 10-10   Causes of Folate Deficiency

Inadequate intake	Malnutrition, chronic alcoholism
Malabsorption	Celiac sprue, small bowel resection
Increased demand	Pregnancy, chronic hemolysis
Renal loss	Dialysis

about a 4- to 5-month supply of it. Thus, within a relatively short time, poor diet, malabsorption, or excessive utilization can lead to folate deficiency (**Table 10–10**).

Diagnosis

The blood smear shows the classic features of megaloblastic anemia: marked oval macrocytosis, hypersegmented neutrophils, and large platelets. The diagnosis can be confirmed by measuring the serum or RBC folate. However, there are several confounding factors in the use of these tests. Several balanced meals can quickly normalize the serum folate, but the RBC folate reflects folate status better over time. Vitamin B_{12} deficiency can produce a falsely low RBC folate, but it does not affect the serum folate.

TABLE 10–11   Causes of Vitamin B$_{12}$ Deficiency

Inadequate intake	Strict vegetarians
Malabsorption	Pernicious anemia, achlorhydria, gastrectomy, ileal disease or resection, *D. latum* infestation
Increased demand	Pregnancy, chronic hemolysis
Impaired transport	Trancobalamin deficiency

Vitamin B$_{12}$ Deficiency

Description

Like folate deficiency, vitamin B$_{12}$ deficiency leads to megaloblastic anemia. The main difference between the 2 conditions is that B$_{12}$ deficiency may also produce a degenerative neurologic syndrome, the manifestations of which are attributable to demyelination of and loss of nerve fibers within the dorsal columns. The neurologic symptoms include paresthesia, weakness, and an unsteady gait. It is critical to make the diagnosis of B$_{12}$ deficiency and treat it appropriately, because these neurologic changes are not reversible.

Malabsorption is the major cause of vitamin B$_{12}$ deficiency (**Table 10–11**), most commonly from pernicious anemia. Pernicious anemia is a deficiency in gastric intrinsic factor (IF) due to an autoimmune assault on the gastric mucosa. Unlike folate deficiency, B$_{12}$ deficiency is rarely due to a poor diet. This is because 1) B$_{12}$ is abundant in a wide range of dietary sources and 2) the body stores several years worth of vitamin B$_{12}$. Dietary deficiency thus requires multiple years of a highly restrictive vegetarian diet.

Diagnosis

The blood smear shows the classic features of megaloblastic anemia: marked oval macrocytosis, hypersegmented neutrophils, and large platelets. The diagnosis can be confirmed by measuring serum B$_{12}$ levels.

Identifying the cause of the deficiency is the next step in the evaluation. The Schilling test is designed for this purpose. The patient is given a parenteral dose of unlabeled B$_{12}$ followed by an oral dose of radiolabeled vitamin B$_{12}$. The purpose of the unlabeled dose is to fully saturate the body with B$_{12}$ so that the radiolabeled dose will be quickly excreted in the urine. A 24-hour urine sample is then collected. A low level of urinary radioactivity confirms B$_{12}$ malabsorption, but it does not identify the specific gastrointestinal defect. The second part of the Schilling test is then undertaken. The patient is given another oral dose of radiolabeled B$_{12}$ in addition to oral IF. Patients with pernicious anemia will demonstrate enhanced absorption (increased urinary radioactivity) in this second part of the test.

Lead Poisoning (Plumbism)

Description

Lead toxicity affects RBC, renal epithelium, and the nervous system. It generally presents insidiously, with nonspecific features such as abdominal pain and cognitive impairment. However, it may present abruptly with vomiting, seizures, and altered mental status. In addition, lead poisoning may present as a microcytic, hypochromic anemia. Exposure to lead occurs through environmental sources, such as lead-based household paint, contaminated soil, lead plumbing, and manufacturing facilities.

Lead exerts its hematologic effects in 2 ways: inhibition of heme synthesis in the maturing erythrocyte and decreased survival of mature erythrocytes. Lead has a strong affinity for certain amino acids, particularly the sulfhydryl group of cysteine, and certain organelles, particularly mitochondria. Since heme synthesis takes place within mitochondria, and 2 enzymes instrumental in this process, delta-aminolevulinic acid dehydratase (δ-ALA) and ferrochelatase, are rich in the sulfhydryl groups, this process is exquisitely sensitive to lead. Ferrochelatase catalyzes the insertion

Like folate deficiency, vitamin B$_{12}$ deficiency leads to megaloblastic anemia. The main difference between the 2 conditions is that B$_{12}$ deficiency may also produce a degenerative neurologic syndrome.

TABLE 10-12   Common Hemoglobinopathies

Hemoglobin Gene Defects	Definition
Hemoglobin S	Change in 6th amino acid of the beta chain from glutamate to valine (β_6 glu → val)
Hemoglobin E	Change in 26th amino acid of beta chain from glutamate to lysine (β_{26} glu → lys)
Hemoglobin C	Change in 6th amino acid of beta chain from glutamate to lysine (β_6 glu → lys)
Hemoglobin D	Change in 121st amino acid of beta chain from glutamate to glutamine (β_{121} glu → gln)
Hemoglobin G	Change in 68th amino acid of alpha chain from asparagine to lysine (α_{68} asn → lys)

of iron into the protoporphyrin ring. Its inhibition leads to the accumulation of FEP (iron-free), much of which binds nonenzymatically to zinc to form ZPP. Separate from its effects on heme synthesis, lead inhibits ATPase-driven sodium channels, leading to increased osmotic fragility and hemolysis. Lead also inhibits the enzyme 5'-nucleotidase, leading to basophilic stippling.

Despite all these vulnerabilities, anemia does not develop until blood lead levels are above 50 μg/dL. A blood lead level >10 μg/dL is considered elevated. Iron deficiency enhances the effects of lead toxicity in 2 ways. The absence of iron enhances the blockage of the ferrochelatase step in heme synthesis, and in an effort to absorb more iron, the gastrointestinal absorption of lead increases.

Diagnosis

Basophilic stippling is noted in the peripheral blood smear and in maturing erythroblasts in the marrow. The Centers for Disease Control has defined lead poisoning as a blood lead level >10 μg/dL. Elevations in FEP and ZPP do not occur until blood lead levels exceed 35 μg/dL; thus, these assays are not sufficiently sensitive to screen for lead poisoning.

The advantage of FEP measurement, however, is that it can be performed reliably on small finger- or heel-prick samples. Furthermore, this assay can easily identify patients grossly intoxicated with lead. Elevated FEP and ZPP are not specific for lead poisoning and may also be seen in iron deficiency.

Sickle Cell Anemia and Other Hemoglobinopathies

Description

A hemoglobinopathy is a structural defect in Hb, usually resulting from a germline single-nucleotide point mutation in 1 of the Hb genes. There are examples of post-synthetic modifications in normally formed Hb, such as carboxyhemoglobin from carbon monoxide poisoning. The common hemoglobinopathies are listed in **Table 10-12**. In the United States, hemoglobin S is the most common abnormal Hb, followed by hemoglobin C, and hemoglobin E. Worldwide, hemoglobin S remains most common, but is followed closely by hemoglobin E (which is very common in Southeast Asia), followed by hemoglobin C, D, and G. In all, several hundred structurally abnormal Hbs have been described.

Homozygous sickle cell anemia (genotype SS, sickle cell disease) is associated with abnormal polymerization of Hb in red cells, leading to a cell with an altered shape that is rapidly cleared from the circulation. Polymerization of hemoglobin S is enhanced in hypoxic conditions. While normal red cells have a lifespan of about 120 days, the red cells in SS have an average lifespan less than 30 days. Hb electrophoresis shows that the red cells contain mostly hemoglobin S, with small quantities of hemoglobin F and hemoglobin A2. The clinical course in hemoglobin SS patients is one of chronic hemolysis punctuated by a wide range of complicating events (often called crises). Chronic hemolysis leads to a chronic anemia with growth retardation, delayed puberty, impaired exercise tolerance, jaundice, and cholelithiasis (due to

In the United States, hemoglobin S is the most common abnormal Hb, followed by hemoglobin C, and hemoglobin E. Worldwide, hemoglobin S remains most common, but is followed closely by hemoglobin E (which is very common in Southeast Asia), followed by hemoglobin C, D, and G.

the formation of pigmented gallstones). The patients are usually in need of intermittent transfusions. Episodic complications include vaso-occlusive events (e.g., stroke, avascular necrosis of bone, and splenic autoinfarction), splenic sequestration crises, aplastic crises (due most often to marrow infection with parvovirus B19), bacterial sepsis, and hyperhemolytic crises. The risk of bacterial infection is related to an underlying functional asplenia that affects most sickle cell patients by late childhood. This confers a particular susceptibility to infection by encapsulated bacterial organisms such as *Haemophilus influenzae and Streptococcus pneumoniae*. The most common cause of death in sickle cell disease is infection, followed by stroke and other thromboembolic events.

Heterozygotes (genotype SA, sickle cell trait) are essentially asymptomatic and have normal red cell indices. The presence of sickle Hb can be detected by Hb electrophoresis, where it is found to represent about 35% to 45% of total Hb. When exposed to hypoxic conditions such as high altitude, these patients are at risk for splenic infarcts. Interestingly, patients who are double heterozygotes for hemoglobin S and β-thalassemia are more severely affected than heterozygous SA, having red cells that contain >50% hemoglobin S. Conversely, double heterozygotes for S-α-thalassemia manifest less hemoglobin S (<35%) and less severe symptoms.

Hemoglobin E is relatively benign clinically, in both heterozygous and homozygous forms. Patients with hemoglobin E have red cell indices, however, that closely resemble those of a thalassemic patient (microcytic with high RBC count). Hemoglobin E is prevalent in Southeast Asia. Double heterozygotes for S and E (SE disease) manifest moderate to severe hemolysis.

Hemoglobin C disease (genotype CC) is generally associated with mild hemolysis, and heterozygotes (CA) are clinically normal. In both, target cells tend to be numerous in the peripheral smear. Patients who are doubly heterozygous for S and C (SC disease) have manifestations intermediate between SS and SA. While manifestations are generally milder than SS, there is a greater incidence of avascular necrosis of bone and retinal damage in SC than in SS. The peripheral blood film shows both sickle cells and target cells.

Hemoglobins D and G are benign Hb variants. They can lead to confusion in interpreting an abnormal Hb electrophoresis, since they appear in the same location as hemoglobin S. However, these patients are clinically well.

Diagnosis

The identification of variant Hbs is usually performed with Hb electrophoresis. However, many laboratories now use high-performance liquid chromatography (HPLC). One limitation of both of these techniques is that several different variants can give similar results, though this is significantly less problematic in HPLC. Findings must be correlated with knowledge of the patient's clinical status and red cell indices before a definitive diagnosis can be rendered.

There are a number of screening tests for sickle Hb. These are based on the tendency of hemoglobin S to polymerize. A positive sickle screen is not specific for sickle cell disease, however, and can be present in sickle cell trait, SC disease, and hemoglobin C_{harlem}. Furthermore, a negative screening test does not entirely exclude hemoglobin S, particularly in infants who may still have significant quantities of hemoglobin F, which inhibits polymerization of hemoglobin S.

> There are a number of screening tests for sickle Hb. These are based on the tendency of hemoglobin S to polymerize. A positive sickle screen is not specific for sickle cell disease, however, and can be present in sickle cell trait, SC disease, and hemoglobin C_{harlem}.

Hereditary Spherocytosis

Description

HS was once known as hereditary hemolytic jaundice. Its cardinal features are chronic hemolysis, jaundice, and splenomegaly. It is a fairly common condition, particularly among people of Northern European descent, in whom it is the most common inherited red cell disorder. In the United States, the incidence is about 1 in 5,000. HS is usually transmitted as an autosomal dominant trait, but about 25% of affected families display autosomal recessive inheritance. This variation derives from the fact that HS can be caused by any 1 of several defects in RBC cytoskeletal proteins, including band 3, protein 4.2, spectrin, and ankyrin. A deficiency in any of these components leads to cytoskeletal instability. Subsequently, there is loss of the biconcave shape in favor of the stoichiometrically more attainable sphere.

The plurality of underlying molecular defects also contributes to clinical heterogeneity, with phenotypes ranging from mild to severe. HS may present early as neonatal jaundice, or it may present in late childhood with splenomegaly and mild anemia. While anemia in some cases is quite severe, in most cases the hemolytic anemia is mild and well compensated by the marrow. Some patients require splenectomy, which usually results in clinical remission. However, splenectomy carries with it an increased susceptibility to bacterial sepsis. As HS patients age, they are at risk for pigmented gallstones.

Diagnosis

The peripheral blood film shows numerous spherocytes. These appear as red cells that lack central pallor. Larger polychromatophilic cells are often numerous, reflective of an increased reticulocyte count. While spherocytes are typically smaller than normal red cells, the MCV may be low, normal, or high, owing to reticulocytosis. The MCHC is characteristically increased.

When numerous spherocytes are observed on a peripheral blood film, the 2 primary considerations are immune hemolysis and HS. Immune hemolysis can usually be excluded with a negative direct antiglobulin test (DAT, Coombs test).

The osmotic fragility test can be useful in supporting the diagnosis of HS. However, spherocytes from any cause will result in a positive test.

Hereditary Elliptocytosis (HE)

Description

This autosomal dominant disorder is due to defective tetramerization of cytoskeletal spectrin, resulting in elliptocytes, also called ovalocytes. There are several clinical variants. The common type of HE is seen primarily in African Americans and manifests as a mild lifelong hemolytic anemia. Hereditary pyropoikilocytosis is a variant of HE in which RBC are exquisitely sensitive to damage from heat. The peripheral blood smear is notable for a profound degree of poikilocytosis with red cells of every size and shape. This condition is usually most pronounced in infancy and tends to abate with age, giving way to a phenotype of common HE. A stomatocytic type of HE exists that is also called Southeast Asian ovalocytosis. This phenotype confers some protection against infection by *P. vivax* malaria.

Diagnosis

There is no specific laboratory test for HE. The diagnosis depends on finding elliptocytes in the peripheral blood. By definition, these cells are twice as long as they are wide, and in HE they comprise >25% of all red cells. Elliptocytes are not unique to HE and may be seen in iron deficiency anemia and thalassemia. The proportion of elliptocytes is usually much less than 25% in these other conditions, and they are easily excluded on other grounds. Once these are ruled out, the diagnosis is made of HE.

Autoimmune Hemolytic Anemia

Description

When an antibody attaches to a red cell, the consequences depend largely on the nature of the antibody. Some antibodies are capable of activating complement and producing brisk intravascular hemolysis. Others behave as opsonins, promoting red cell destruction in the spleen. Some antibodies react only in a cold environment, some only in warmth. Some coat the red cell and do nothing more. Most cases of immune hemolytic anemia are due to antibodies of either the IgG or IgM type. Antibodies against red cells may be the result of autoimmunity, alloimmunity, or the presence of a drug.

These disorders present with the typical manifestations of anemia, with variable rates of onset. Mild splenomegaly is common when hemolysis is extravascular. Dark urine, abdominal or back pain, and fever may accompany intravascular hemolysis. In severe IgM-induced cold autoimmune hemolytic anemia (CAIHA), the skin may have a livedo reticularis pattern, and there may be acrocyanosis on exposure to cold.

When an antibody attaches to a red cell, the consequences depend largely on the nature of the antibody. Some antibodies are capable of activating complement and producing brisk intravascular hemolysis. Others behave as opsonins, promoting red cell destruction in the spleen.

TABLE 10–13   Drug-induced Immune Hemolytic Anemia

Mechanism	Drug Absorption (Hapten)	Immune Complex	AIHA
Type of hemolysis	Extravascular	Intravascular	Extravascular
Implicated drugs	Penicillin Ampicillin Methicillin Carbenicillin Cephalothin	Quinidine Phenacetin Thiazides Rifampin Sulfonamides	Alpha-methyldopa Mefenamic acid L-DOPA Isoniazid Procainamide Hydralazine Ibuprofen

Warm autoimmune hemolytic anemia (WAIHA) is mediated by IgG autoantibodies that optimally bind RBC at body temperature (37°C). The red cell antigens most commonly the target in WAIHA are the Rh antigens. IgG molecules must form cross-links to activate complement, and the target red cell antigens in WAIHA are usually insufficiently dense on the red cell surface to permit this. A higher density antigen is involved in a condition known as PCH, described below. Thus, IgG antibodies opsonize the red cell in WAIHA, leading to membrane damage mediated by splenic macrophages with the formation of small, spherocytic cells (microspherocytes). In some cases, there is concomitant immune thrombocytopenia, and this association is known as Evans syndrome.

CAIHA, also called cold agglutinin disease, is mediated by IgM antibodies that bind RBC at lower temperature ranges. The target antigens are usually the red cell antigens I or i. Those binding over a limited thermal amplitude (e.g., 0 to 22°C) will obviously not produce clinical consequences. However, these antibodies may cause difficulty in the laboratory, where studies are routinely carried out at room temperature, which could be within this thermal amplitude. Antibodies with broader thermal amplitude may bind to red cells in the extremities, where temperature falls a bit below core body temperature, resulting in acrocyanosis. IgM antibodies are capable of activating complement. Most often, the clinical consequence is a result of opsonization by C3, leading to extravascular hemolysis similar to that seen in WAIHA. C3-mediated hemolysis is more of a hepatic process than a splenic one. Sometimes, however, the complete complement cascade is activated on the cell surface, resulting in intravascular hemolysis.

Both WAIHA and CAIHA are often idiopathic conditions. However, a significant number are secondary to another underlying condition, including lymphoid neoplasms (e.g., chronic lymphocytic leukemia), medication use, systemic autoimmune diseases (e.g., systemic lupus erythematosus), immunodeficiency (e.g., common variable immunodeficiency), and infection (infectious mononucleosis, HIV, and *Mycoplasma pneumoniae*).

PCH is caused by IgG antibodies that are directed at the red cell P antigen. The antibody responsible for PCH is called the Donath–Landsteiner antibody. This particular IgG antibody has peculiar tendencies, including the binding of red cells in colder temperatures (in the blood of the extremities) and the activation of complement, producing intravascular hemolysis. Originally described in association with syphilis, the antibody now is more often seen in children with viral infections. Mortality can be quite high, up to 30%.

Drug-induced immune hemolytic anemia arises through several pathophysiologic mechanisms (**Table 10-13**). An antibody may be raised against a drug that is capable of adhering nonspecifically to the red cell membrane (drug adsorption or hapten mechanism). Second, drug–antibody immune complexes may coat the red cell surface (immune complex mechanism). What distinguishes these first 2 mechanisms is that the antibody is directed against the drug, not a red cell antigen. Lastly, a drug may be responsible for eliciting a true autoimmune hemolytic anemia, with antibody against red cell antigens. This condition is clinicopathologically indistinguishable from AIHA, and it may or may not abate when the drug is discontinued.

Drug-induced immune hemolytic anemia arises through several pathophysiologic mechanisms.

Lastly, alloimmune hemolytic anemia is due to transfusion of red cells bearing an antigen foreign to the recipient. Most responsible antibodies arise as a result of prior sensitization, commonly prior transfusion or pregnancy, and most cause extravascular hemolysis of mild to moderate severity. In the case of ABO antigens, the antibodies are naturally occurring, and prior sensitization is not required for there to be a problem. Furthermore, ABO antibodies produce severe intravascular hemolysis, which can be fatal.

Diagnosis

The DAT, also known as the direct Coombs test, is pivotal for the diagnosis of immune hemolysis. This test is capable of demonstrating the presence of antibodies or complement on the surface of RBC.

Additional laboratory findings include anemia, reticulocytosis, indirect hyperbilirubinemia, decreased haptoglobin, and an increased LDH. The peripheral blood smear often demonstrates spherocytes, polychromasia, and, in severe cases, nucleated red cells. In cold agglutinin disease, red cell clumping is seen.

An important consequence of red cell antibodies is their tendency to interfere with pretransfusion testing.

Hemolytic Disease of the Newborn (HDN)

Description

If there is mingling of fetal and maternal blood (a fetomaternal hemorrhage), then the mother can become sensitized to antigens of the fetal blood cells. Some of these antigens are paternal in origin and may therefore be foreign to the mother, and a maternal antibody reaction may occur. If the antibody idiotype produced is one that can cross the placenta (most IgG subtypes can cross the placenta, IgM cannot), it can produce fetal hemolysis.

The severity of fetal hemolysis depends on several factors, including the identity of the immunizing antigen and the titer of maternal antibody. The pregnancy that creates sensitization is usually spared, as the initial reaction produces largely IgM that does not cross the placenta. In subsequent pregnancies, an IgG-mediated anamnestic response may be raised, producing HDN. Furthermore, pregnancy-induced maternal sensitization may complicate future transfusions.

When this syndrome was first recognized, it was most commonly associated with antibodies to the Rh antigen known as D. This D antigen is the basis for categorizing blood types as Rh+ or Rh−. However, prevention strategies have reduced the incidence of RhD HDN to about 0.1% of all pregnancies. The incidence of maternal anti-Kell antibody now exceeds that of anti-D antibodies in many centers.

If a pregnant woman does have antibodies against a fetal antigen, the fetus is at risk for HDN. Mild HDN may only manifest as compensated hemolysis in which fetal erythropoiesis is capable of keeping up with the rate of red cell destruction. Severe HDN manifests with fetal anemia, hyperbilirubinemia, and numerous circulating nucleated RBC (erythroblastosis fetalis). Hypoproteinemia may ensue, leading to decreased serum osmotic pressure, and severe edema (hydrops fetalis). A pregnancy in which there is known sensitization (maternal antibodies to fetal red cell antigens have been detected) must be monitored to determine the severity of fetal hemolysis.

RhD HDN is prevented by the administration of Rh immune globulin (RhIg) to Rh-negative women during pregnancy. The RhIg binds to and effectively conceals D antigenic sites, precluding an immune response. RhIg is given routinely at 28 weeks, at term, and whenever a fetomaternal hemorrhage is suspected (amniocentesis, trauma, abortion, abruption, etc.).

Diagnosis

Several laboratory tests support the diagnosis and treatment of HDN. First, there is blood typing to confirm the maternal, paternal, and neonatal Rh status.

Second, in Rh-negative women, a screening test for antibodies must be performed. This is a test in which maternal serum is incubated with a panel of red cells having known antigenic status. If an alloantibody is detected, its titer is determined by serially diluting the sample until reactivity is abolished. If a titer of >1:32 is present, the risk of HDN is considered sufficiently high to warrant fetal monitoring.

If there is mingling of fetal and maternal blood (a fetomaternal hemorrhage), then the mother can become sensitized to antigens of the fetal blood cells. Some of these antigens are paternal in origin and may therefore be foreign to the mother, and a maternal antibody reaction may occur.

In Rh-negative women with alloantibodies, the fetus must be monitored to determine the severity of hemolysis. Amniocentesis is performed to determine the quantity of amniotic fluid bilirubin. When low, monitoring is continued. When high, consideration is given to therapeutic intervention, including intrauterine transfusion and, when possible, delivery.

In Rh-negative women without antibodies, laboratory tests are available to confirm and quantify a fetomaternal hemorrhage. These include the Kleihauer–Betke test, the erythrocyte rosette test, and others. If positive, a dose of RhIg may be given.

Microangiopathic Hemolytic Anemias
Description

This group of disorders shares the ability to create a microvascular environment capable of shredding red cells. They do this usually by inducing endothelial injury and thrombosis, generating a jagged lattice of fibrin against which red cells are thrust with the pressure of arterial blood. The result is intravascular hemolysis and the appearance of schistocytes in the peripheral blood film. Often the creation of thrombi is so brisk that thrombocytopenia results. The disorders associated with MHA include disseminated intravascular coagulation (DIC), thrombotic thrombocytopenic purpura (TTP), hemolytic uremic syndrome (HUS), and the pregnancy-associated syndrome of hemolysis, elevated liver enzymes, and low platelets (HELLP). A similar clinical picture can be created by malignant hypertension and macrovascular red cell trauma caused by mechanical heart valves.

Diagnosis

The peripheral blood smear shows schistocytes and, usually, thrombocytopenia. The associated conditions are clinicopathologic diagnoses for which there is no single diagnostic test.

Glucose-6-phosphate Dehydrogenase (G6PD) Deficiency
Description

This is the most common red cell enzyme defect. Since red cells lack a nucleus, they lack the capacity to make new enzymes. Even normal red cells have greater enzymatic capacity when young than when old. However, if the activity of a critical enzyme significantly degrades before the average red cell lifespan (120 days), then the cell dies prematurely. Red cells rely on G6PD to produce glutathione that absorbs oxidant stress to protect Hb from oxidation. Oxidized Hb forms precipitate within the red cell, known as Heinz bodies, whose excision by splenic macrophages results in bite cells.

There are numerous defective forms (disease-causing alleles) of G6PD. Most abnormal alleles result in a functionally normal enzyme but have a shortened lifespan within the red cell. Uncommon alleles result in decreased G6PD production, and even young cells have low activity in these cases. In most forms of the disease, young red cells, especially reticulocytes, have normal G6PD activity, whereas, in other forms, enzyme activity is universally decreased. Furthermore, the magnitude of this decrease varies. This heterogeneity results in 3 classes of G6PD deficiency: class 1, in which there is chronic low-level hemolysis; class 2, in which there is profound intravascular hemolysis following oxidant stress; and class 3, in which there is mild to moderate intravascular hemolysis following oxidant stress.

Most G6PD-deficient persons are clinically well until exposed to excess oxidant (class 2 or 3). Such exposures arise in the form of ingestion (e.g., fava beans), medication use (e.g., nitrofurantoin, antimalarials, and sulfa drugs), or infection. In most individuals, there is preferential destruction of older red cells.

Diagnosis

The peripheral smear shows a combination of bite cells and Heinz bodies. The latter require special (supravital) staining in order to be visualized. Laboratory assays are available for measuring G6PD activity. G6PD activity may appear normal during an acute episode, because only nonhemolyzed, younger cells are available to be assayed. If a normal result is obtained, consider repeating the assay in 3 months.

Most G6PD-deficient persons are clinically well until exposed to excess oxidant. Such exposures arise in the form of ingestion (e.g., fava beans), medication use (e.g., nitrofurantoin, antimalarials, and sulfa drugs), or infection.

Pyruvate Kinase (PK) Deficiency

Description

A steady generation of ATP is needed to maintain the integrity of the red cell membrane. Red cells generate ATP principally via the glycolytic pathway, in which PK is an active enzyme. Deficient ATP production leads to progressive red cell dessication, causing predominantly extravascular hemolysis.

PK deficiency is usually a recessively inherited condition. The disease is worldwide in distribution but slightly more concentrated in particular populations, notably people of Northern Europe descent and the Pennsylvania Amish.

Diagnosis

Echinocytes are the classic peripheral smear finding, but these appear in large numbers only after splenectomy. An autohemolysis test is positive and corrects with the addition of ATP. A fluorescent spot test is performed in which red cells are incubated with NADH (which fluoresces) to check for conversion to NAD (which does not).

Paroxysmal Nocturnal Hemoglobinuria

Description

Complement activation occurs at a low level continuously in the blood, and formed C3b that does not bind to an available surface (bacterium, leukocyte, platelet, or RBC) is rapidly degraded. Bound C3b can proceed to induce lysis of the cell to which it is attached. Thus, blood cells must have a mechanism for regularly shedding C3b to avoid lysis.

PNH is due to an acquired (somatic) mutation in the PIG-A gene of a hematopoietic stem cell, the major consequence of which is decreased production of the glycosylphosphatidylinositol (GPI) anchor. This is a molecule that functions as a transmembrane anchor for several surface proteins, many of which are involved in protecting the cell from complement lysis. Affected cells have decreased expression of, among others, CD16 (the F(c) receptor type III), CD55 (decay-accelerating factor or DAF), and CD59 (membrane inhibitor of reactive lysis or MIRL). Since this defect is found within an early stem cell, all cell lines (red cells, white cells, and platelets) are affected.

PNH manifests as hemolysis, and its severity oscillates. Hemoglobinuria reflects the intravascular nature of the hemolysis. While hemolysis tends to be episodic (paroxysmal), many patients experience chronic hemolysis of uniform intensity. Furthermore, exacerbations are not usually nocturnal as implied in the original description. PNH is associated with a thrombotic tendency that can be the initial manifestation. Over time, the disease may evolve to or present as aplastic anemia.

Diagnosis

A sucrose hemolysis test or acidified serum (Ham's) test may be used to screen for PNH. In these assays, patient blood is exposed to an environment that promotes complement activation. Enhanced hemolysis in the patient sample as compared to a normal control is interpreted as a positive test. The diagnosis may also be made by flow cytometry, a modality that allows quantitation of the surface proteins known to be diminished in PNH.

A sucrose hemolysis test or acidified serum (Ham's) test may be used to screen for PNH. In these assays, patient blood is exposed to an environment that promotes complement activation. Enhanced hemolysis in the patient sample as compared to a normal control is interpreted as a positive test.

Sideroblastic Anemia

Description

In the developing erythrocyte, it is within mitochondria that iron is incorporated into porphyrin to make heme. Ringed sideroblasts are the morphologic expression of the abnormal sequestration of iron within mitochondria. With increased iron-laden mitochondria, the differential diagnosis includes myelodysplastic syndrome, alcohol abuse, copper deficiency (Wilson's disease), lead toxicity, medication effect (isoniazid and pyrazinamide), pyridoxine (vitamin B_6) deficiency, and hereditary sideroblastic anemia.

TABLE 10-14   Polycythemia Vera vs Secondary Erythrocytosis

Parameter	Polycythemia Vera	Secondary Erythrocytosis
RBC mass	↑	↑
PaO$_2$	Normal	Normal to ↓
Leukocytes and basophils	Normal to ↑	Normal
LAP score	↑	Normal
Serum vitamin B$_{12}$	↑	Normal
Serum EPO	↓	↑
Serum iron/stainable iron	↓	Normal

LAP, leukocyte alkaline phosphatase; EPO, erythropoietin.

Diagnosis

In the peripheral blood, one finds anemia with a dimorphic red cell population, that is, there are normocytic macrocytes and hypochromic microcytes. The diagnosis of sideroblastic anemia requires a bone marrow biopsy. Nonringed sideroblasts, defined as red cell precursors with 1 to 4 faint siderotic granules, are normal in the marrow. Ringed sideroblasts are defined as red cell precursors with at least 10 siderotic granules that surround at least one third of the nucleus. Though they may be seen in small number in some normal individuals and in a wide range of disorders, when they are found in >15% of all red cell precursors, the diagnosis of sideroblastic anemia is made.

Pure Red Cell Aplasia
Description

Aplastic anemia is a term that refers to the complete absence of hematopoiesis, affecting granulocytic precursors, erythroid precursors, and megakaryocytes. A proliferative disorder may be isolated to a single cell line, however, as is the case in pure red cell aplasia. This condition may be acquired or congenital. Acquired pure red cell aplasia may be due to thymoma, EPO therapy, or infection with parvovirus B19. Congenital pure red cell aplasia is called the Blackfan–Diamond Syndrome.

Parvovirus B19 may cause transient arrests of red cell production in healthy children and adults without serious consequences. Infection usually lasts about 2 weeks, and in those with a normal red cell life span of 120 days, this usually goes unnoticed. However, in those with chronic hemolytic anemia, a transient arrest of erythropoiesis may be catastrophic. The virus infects erythroid progenitor cells, causing a maturation arrest at the pronormoblast stage. Marrow examination finds numerous giant pronormoblasts, a reduction of the more mature forms, and viral nuclear inclusions.

Congenital pure red cell aplasia (Blackfan–Diamond Syndrome) is a rare, constitutional red cell aplasia, which usually becomes evident by the age of 5 years. Erythroid precursors in the marrow are typically low or absent. HbF is increased.

Aplastic anemia is a term that refers to the complete absence of hematopoiesis, affecting granulocytic precursors, erythroid precursors, and megakaryocytes. A proliferative disorder may be isolated to a single cell line, however, as is the case in pure red cell aplasia.

Diagnosis

The diagnosis is made in a patient with isolated anemia, that is usually normocytic, with reticulocytopenia. The bone marrow biopsy shows an isolated decrement in erythropoiesis.

ERYTHROCYTOSIS

Differential Diagnosis

The primary considerations are myeloproliferative disorders (MPDs; polycythemia vera [PV]), reactive (secondary) erythrocytosis, and spurious erythrocytosis due to dehydration (Gaisbock's syndrome) (**Table 10-14**). Secondary polycythemia is associated with low PaO$_2$ states (such as smoking and living at high altitudes), abnormal Hb variants, and certain neoplasms (renal cell carcinoma and cerebellar hemangioblastoma) in which there is elevated EPO.

TABLE 10–15 Criteria for PV: A1+A2+ Any Other A Criterion *or* A1+A2+ Any 2 B Criteria

A1	Increased RBC mass *or* Hb>18.5 g/dL (men), >16.5 g/dL (women)
A2	Erythrocytosis is primary—no familial erythrocytosis, hypoxemia (PaO_2<92%), high-affinity hemoglobin variant, truncated erythropoietin (EPO) receptor, or tumor that is producing EPO
A3	Splenomegaly
A4	Clonal cytogenetic abnormality other than Philadelphia chromosome
A5	Endogenous erythroid colony formation in vitro
B1	Thrombocytosis >400 × 10^6 μL^{-1}
B2	WBC>12 × 10^6 μL^{-1}
B3	Panmyelosis on bone marrow biopsy
B4	Low serum EPO

Polycythemia Vera

Description

PV is an MPD that is due to a clonal neoplastic proliferation of erythroid precursors. It presents at a mean age of 60 years, most commonly with hypertension, thrombosis, pruritus, erythromelalgia, or headache. The erythrocytosis is usually normocytic. Neutrophilia and basophilia are common, and sometimes thrombocytosis is present. The cause of death is most commonly thrombosis. Some patients, however, progress to acute leukemia.

> Polycythemia vera is an myeloproliferative disease that is due to a clonal neoplastic proliferation of erythroid precursors. It presents at a mean age of 60 years, most commonly with hypertension, thrombosis, pruritus, erythromelalgia, or headache.

Diagnosis

The diagnosis of PV is made according to strict criteria (**Table 10–15**). The RBC mass is measured using isotope dilution, in which a sample of patient red cells is labeled with a radioactive isotope and reinfused. The red cell mass can then be calculated from the degree of dilution of the labeled red cells. This direct measurement of the red cell mass distinguishes reduced plasma volume from a true absolute erythrocytosis.

Examination of the bone marrow shows a marked expansion of erythroid precursors. In PV, erythroid precursors are capable of spontaneous erythroid colony formation in vitro. In testing for endogenous erythroid colony formation, patient marrow is cultured. In PV, one can observe the spontaneous formation of erythroid colonies (without addition of EPO). In healthy patients or those with secondary erythrocytosis, erythroid colony formation requires exogenous EPO.

The janus kinase 2 (JAK-2) mutation has now been identified in >80% of PV cases. The JAK-2 mutation is a valine to phenylalanine substitution at codon 617 (Val617Phe) that appears to confer cytokine-independent growth to cells bearing it.

METHODS

Also see Chapter 2 on Methods for illustrations of several of the methods described below.

Red Cell Indices

Measurement of total Hb is carried out most commonly through a chemical reaction. In the cyanohemoglobin (hemiglobin cyanide [HiCN]) method, Hb is converted to HiCN whose concentration is measured by spectrophotometry. The absorbance of the solution at 540 nm reflects the amount of Hb originally present.

The Hct can be measured directly (manual technique), by centrifuging a tube of whole blood. The ratio of the packed red cell column height to the total height is the Hct. Note that the Hct is a unitless value (a percentage), as the units cancel out in its calculation.

Erythrocytes (as well as leukocytes and platelets) can be counted manually, through the use of a hemocytometer. This is a labor-intensive method that is still used when, for various reasons, the automated analyzer gives erroneous results. RBC counts may be given in terms of cells per cubic millimeter (e.g., 5.5×10^6 mm^{-3}), per microliter (conventional units), or per liter (SI units). When the Hct and RBC count are determined manually, the remaining red cell indices can be calculated. For example, MCV = Hct × 1,000/RBC. The MCV is stated in femtoliters (fL).

Automated techniques are widely used in clinical laboratories. On most instruments, the red cell count (RBC), MCV, and RDW are measured directly (as is the total Hb). The instrument then calculates the other indices, such as Hct. There are at least 3 different methods used by automated instruments to count cells: impedance (counts any particle of given size), optical methods (light scatter), or combination of impedance and light scatter.

In impedance counting, cells are suspended in a conductive diluent and passed one-by-one through an aperture across which a current is flowing. A cell within the aperture causes a momentary increase in electrical resistance (impedance). Voltage, a product of resistance and current ($V = I \times R$), increases when the resistance increases. The instrument interprets a momentary increase in voltage as a single cell. The amount of voltage change is proportional to the size of the cell. The instrument is programmed to count particles measuring between 36 and 360 fL as red cells. Of course leukocytes, which are within this size range, will be counted as erythrocytes, but their relative number is so small (usually) that their effect is typically negligible. RBC passing through the aperture come in a range of sizes (volumes), distributed in a roughly Gaussian curve. The mean of this distribution is taken as the MCV. The variance in the curve is the RDW. The rest of the red cell indices can be calculated as follows: Hct = MCV × RBC; MCHC = (Hb/Hct) × 100.

> Automated techniques are widely used in clinical laboratories. On most instruments, the red cell count (RBC), MCV, and RDW are measured directly (as is the total Hb). The instrument then calculates the other indices, such as Hct.

Reticulocyte Counting

Reticulocytes can be measured manually or by automation. In the manual method, a blood smear is stained with a supravital dye (e.g., new methylene blue) that highlights the endoplasmic reticulum that persists within reticulocytes. Red cells and reticulocytes are counted, and the result is given as a percentage (number of reticulocytes per 100 red cells).

Automated methods are more accurate, since many more cells can be counted. A blood sample is incubated with a supravital dye, and then passed through an automated counter in which they are exposed to a laser. Light scatter (which will be greatest in stained reticulocytes) is used to enumerate the reticulocytes.

Normally reticulocytes are <1.5% of all red cells. This proportion increases when red cells are lost or destroyed peripherally, reflecting a marrow response. A normal reticulocyte count in the face of anemia is indicative of an impaired marrow.

However, the reticulocyte percentage can be somewhat misleading in the presence of anemia. This is because anemia leads to increased EPO production, and EPO stimulates the proliferation of red cell precursors and the release of reticulocytes from the marrow. Even if the marrow capacity for proliferation is impaired, the latter effect can produce a transient appearance of reticulocytosis. Thus, to correct for this, one can calculate the reticulocyte index (RI): RI = reticulocyte percentage × (patient's HCT normal HCT). A normal RI is <3%.

Hemoglobin Electrophoresis

Electrophoresis is the separation of proteins through the application of voltage. Most proteins have a net charge, usually a net negative charge, and when placed into a semisolid medium (a gel) will move in response to a voltage. The distance that a protein moves depends on its size and the magnitude of its charge, so that different proteins can be separated from one another. The positively charged electrode attracts negatively charged proteins and is called the anode. Proteins that end up closest to the anode are called fast-migrating or anodal. Proteins that end up farthest from the anode are considered slow-migrating or cathodal.

If RBC are lysed, the predominant protein within the lysate is Hb. In the normal adult, this Hb is largely HbA, with about 2% to 3% HbA2. When this lysate is applied to a gel across which a voltage is applied, the result is a prominent band (HbA) near the anode (fast-migrating) and a dim band (HbA2) near the anode. Any deviation from this pattern is indicative of a hemoglobinopathy or thalassemia. Routine Hb electrophoresis is performed by placing a sample of lysed blood on a cellulose acetate gel at pH 8.6 (alkaline electrophoresis). The gel is subjected to electromotive force, fixed, and stained.

Thalassemia, being a quantitative defect in production of entirely normal Hbs, does not produce abnormal bands on the electrophoresis. Instead, β-thalassemia is diagnosed by the presence of "thalassemic indices" (low Hct, increased RBC count, and low MCV) and a quantitatively increased HbA2. α-Thalassemia has "thalassemic indices" and normal HbA2.

True hemoglobinopathies are due to production of a structurally abnormal Hb molecule that usually produces a distinct band on electrophoresis. The identity of most, but not all, abnormal Hbs can often be determined by routine electrophoresis, particularly when supplemented with some clinical information and CBC data. When there is uncertainty, electrophoresis on citrate agar at pH 6.2 (acid electrophoresis) produces a different set of electrophoretic positions that, in combination with the alkaline gel, can help identify an abnormal band.

Screening Tests for Sickle Hemoglobin

Rapid detection of sickling Hb, without having to perform electrophoresis, is possible with 1 of 2 types of assays. In the first, the Hb solubility (dithionate) test, one can detect insoluble forms of Hb within a lysate of blood. Red cells are lysed in sodium dithionate buffer with saponin. After several minutes, marked turbidity indicates a positive screen. Note that this test detects free Hb with altered solubility and may be positive in a number of different genotypes: SS, SA, SC, SD, and some types of HbC. This test may be negative when the concentration of HbS is too small, for example, in neonates.

The second type of screening test, the sickling (metabisulfite) test, detects red cells with sickling Hbs. In this test, whole blood is subjected to metabisulfite, which encourages cells containing HbS to sickle. A smear is then examined microscopically for sickling. Like the solubility test, this test does not give genotypic information and may be positive in SS, SA, SC, S-other, and some types of HbC. The test requires at least 10% HbS to be positive. Thus, it may not be positive in neonates or those very aggressively transfused.

Osmotic Fragility Test

All red cells expand and eventually undergo lysis in a hypotonic environment, and spherocytic red cells do so at a faster rate than normal biconcave red cells. This is the basis of the osmotic fragility test. Red cells are incubated in progressively more hypotonic solutions, parallel with normal controls. Enhanced lysis, as compared to controls, is a positive test. A positive osmotic fragility test is not diagnostic of HS, however, since red cells that are spherocytic from any cause will give a positive result. The most common acquired cause of red cell spherocytosis is autoimmune hemolytic anemia.

Direct Antiglobulin Test (Coombs Test)

The reagent used in this test is an antibody, obtained from rabbit or goat, that reacts with (binds to) human globulins (antihuman globulin—AHG). Specifically, these antibodies may have reactivity with IgG, complement protein C3, or both. Patient blood is mixed with AHG and then observed for agglutination (clumping). Depending on the reagent used, agglutination suggests that the patient's red cells are coated with IgG, C3, or both. Furthermore, since these were not added to the red cells in vitro, agglutination indicates that coating occurred in vivo.

In the usual case of WAIHA, the red cells agglutinate mainly with anti-IgG. There may or may not be reactive with anti-C3. In cold agglutinin disease, red cells agglutinate only with anti-C3. While the titer of a warm autoantibody provides little useful clinical information, the titer of a cold agglutinin can be helpful. The cold agglutinin titer is the highest dilution of patient serum that causes agglutination of normal RBC.

> Thalassemia, being a quantitative defect in production of entirely normal Hbs, does not produce abnormal bands on the electrophoresis. True hemoglobinopathies are due to production of a structurally abnormal Hb molecule that usually produces a distinct band on electrophoresis.

Kleihauer–Betke Test

The Kleihauer–Betke (acid elution) test is based on the observation that a weak acid is capable of eluting normal HbA out of red cells. In contrast, HbF is resistant to acid elution and remains within red cells. Thus, if blood is subjected to a weak acid, and then smeared and stained, the cells containing HbA will appear as pale "ghosts," whereas cells containing HbF appear bright red. In a pregnant woman, the presence of red cells with HbF is indicative of a fetomaternal hemorrhage.

REFERENCES

Annibale B, et al. Gastrointestinal causes of refractory iron deficiency anemia in patients without gastrointestinal symptoms. *Am J Med.* 2001;111:439–445.

Beutler E. The common anemias. *JAMA.* 1988;259:2433.

Beutler E, Waalen J. The definition of anemia: what is the lower limit of normal of the blood hemoglobin concentration? *Blood.* 2006;107:1747–1750.

Bilgrami S, Greenberg BR. Polycythemia rubra vera. *Semin Oncol.* 1995;22:307.

Bowie LJ, et al. Alpha thalassemia and its impact on other clinical conditions. *Clin Lab Med.* 1997;17:97.

Cash JM, Sears DA. The anemia of chronic disease: spectrum of associated diseases in a series of unselected hospitalized patients. *Am J Med.* 1989;87:638–644.

Fitzsimons EJ, et al. Erythroblast iron metabolism and serum soluble transferrin receptor values in the anemia of rheumatoid arthritis. *Arthritis Rheum.* 2002;47:166–171.

Gehrs BC, Friedberg RC. Autoimmune hemolytic anemia. *Am J Hematol.* 2002;69:258–271.

Geifman-Holtzman O, et al. Female alloimmunization with antibodies known to cause hemolytic disease. *Obstet Gynecol.* 1997;89:272–275.

Goddard AF, et al. Guidelines for the management of iron deficiency anaemia. British Society of Gastroenterology. *Gut.* 2000;46(suppl 3–4):IV1–IV5.

Harkness UF, Spinnato JA. Prevention and management of RhD isoimmunization. *Clin Perinatol.* 2004;722(31):721–742.

Kettaneh A, et al. Pica and food craving in patients with iron-deficiency anemia: a case–control study in France. *Am J Med.* 2005;118:185–188.

Lane PA. Sickle cell disease. *Pediatr Clin North Am.* 1996;43:639.

Manci EA, et al. Causes of death in sickle cell disease: an autopsy study. *Br J Haematol.* 2003;123(2):359–365.

Marchand A, et al. The predictive value of serum haptoglobin in hemolytic disease. *JAMA.* 1980;243:1909–1911.

Nilsson-Ehle H, et al. Blood haemoglobin values in the elderly: implications for reverence intervals from age 70 to 88. *Eur J Haematol.* 2000;65:297–305.

Nissenson AR. Prevalence and outcomes of anemia in rheumatoid arthritis: a systematic review of the literature. *Am J Med.* 2004;116:50S–57S.

Perrotta PL, Snyder EL. Non-infectious complications of transfusion therapy. *Blood Rev.* 2001;15:69–83.

Rivera S, et al. Hepcidin excess induces the sequestration of iron and exacerbates tumor-associated anemia. *Blood.* 2005;105(4):1797–1802.

Rosse WF, Ware RE. The molecular basis of paroxysmal nocturnal hemoglobinuria. *Blood.* 1995;86:3277.

Wilson A, et al. Prevalence and outcomes of anemia in inflammatory bowel disease: a systematic review of the literature. *Am J Med.* 2004;116:44S–49S.

Wolf AW, et al. Effects of iron therapy on infant blood lead levels. *J Pediatr.* 2003;143:789–795.

11

Bleeding and Thrombotic Disorders

Elizabeth M. Van Cott and Michael Laposata

LEARNING OBJECTIVES

1. Learn the basic molecular events in clot formation and fibrinolysis.

2. Understand the basic classification of disorders in hemostasis.

3. Identify the appropriate laboratory tests for evaluation of the bleeding patient and the thrombotic patient.

4. Learn the prominent clinical and laboratory features of the individual disorders of hemostasis.

CHAPTER OUTLINE

The coagulopathies are grouped into disorders of bleeding and thrombosis. The hemorrhagic diseases are further subdivided into the 2 major categories of coagulation factor disorders and platelet disorders. To understand the diseases with abnormal coagulation that follow, a brief introduction to normal hemostasis precedes the discussions of the diseases.

INTRODUCTION TO HEMOSTASIS

Normal hemostasis is the controlled activation of coagulation factors and platelets leading to clot formation, with subsequent clot lysis, in a process that stops hemorrhage without excess clotting (thrombosis). Effective hemostasis is a rapid and localized response to an interruption in vascular integrity (vessel wall injury), such that clots are formed only when and where they are needed.

Clot Formation

Clot formation involves platelet activation and the subsequent generation of fibrin via the coagulation cascade. The 2 processes are discussed separately in the sections that follow.

Platelet Plug Formation

Platelet plug formation is initiated in vivo by exposure of platelets to vascular subendothelium when a vessel is injured. The platelets adhere to the subendothelium, spread out along the surface, and release substances that promote the aggregation of other platelets at that site. The platelets also accelerate fibrin clot formation by providing a reactive surface for several steps in the coagulation cascade.

Adhesion of platelets to the subendothelial surface is facilitated by a plasma protein, von Willebrand factor (vWF), especially in vessels with high shear forces. vWF binds to a specific receptor on the platelet surface. Deficiency of vWF results in poor adherence of platelets to subendothelium. The severity of bleeding in von Willebrand disease (vWD) varies widely among patients. Another related platelet adhesion defect occurs in patients whose platelets lack the receptor for vWF. This bleeding disorder, known as Bernard–Soulier disease, results from an inability of platelets to bind vWF.

Platelet activation occurs from interaction of platelet agonists, most of which are soluble, with specific receptors on the platelet membrane. Physiologically important agonists include adenosine diphosphate (ADP), thrombin, epinephrine, collagen, and thromboxane A_2, which is derived from arachidonic acid. A sequence of membrane and cytoplasmic events is initiated by the agonist–receptor interaction, involving an increase in cytoplasmic calcium ion concentration and a platelet shape change from a disc to a spiny sphere. The change in cytoplasmic calcium concentration leads to contractile events in the platelet, causing alpha and delta granules (also known as dense bodies) to fuse with the platelet plasma membrane and release their granule contents into the extracellular space. Successful granule release requires the formation of thromboxane A_2 from endogenous arachidonate via the enzyme cyclooxygenase. This enzyme is inhibited irreversibly by aspirin and inhibited reversibly by a number of other anti-inflammatory agents. Treatment with aspirin can cause a platelet secretion defect (reduced release of granule contents) that is often clinically significant in patients with underlying coagulopathies. Alpha granules contain vWF, fibrinogen, Factor V, 2 platelet-specific proteins—platelet factor 4 (PF4) and beta-thromboglobulin—as well as a number of other proteins. Delta granules contain serotonin, adenosine triphosphate (ATP), ADP, pyrophosphate, and calcium. The release of some of these substances, in particular ADP, activates unstimulated platelets nearby. Absence or deficiency of alpha or delta granules occurs as a feature of several congenital and acquired platelet function disorders, collectively known as storage pool disorders. Individuals whose platelets possess appropriate numbers of intact granules that cannot be released on appropriate stimulation have a platelet release defect, and on that basis also may have a bleeding tendency. Aspirin is a common cause of a platelet release defect, because it impairs thromboxane production.

Release of platelet granule contents is followed by platelet aggregation, that is, the binding of platelets to one another to form the platelet plug. Normal aggregation requires fibrinogen binding to platelets via the fibrinogen receptor, which is the glycoprotein IIb/IIIa complex (GP IIb/IIIa), on the platelet surface. Congenital absence of GP IIb/IIIa results in a bleeding diathesis known as Glanzmann thrombasthenia (GT).

The platelet surface serves as a site for certain coagulation pathway enzyme reactions (see below). For example, the platelet membrane can bind the Factor Xa/Factor Va complex that activates prothrombin to thrombin. Thus, platelet activation and fibrin formation via the coagulation cascade are interactive biological processes.

Clot formation involves platelet activation and the subsequent generation of fibrin via the coagulation cascade.

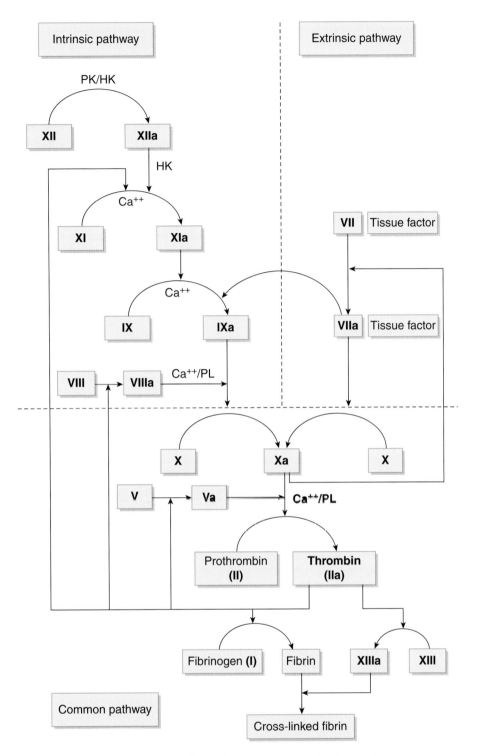

FIGURE 11–1 **The coagulation cascade. (Redrawn with permission from Roberts HR, Lozier JN. New perspectives on the coagulation cascade.** *Hosp Prac.* **1992;27:98.) PK, prekallikrein; HK, high-molecular-weight kininogen; PL, phospholipid.**

Fibrin Clot Formation

The coagulation factor pathway is an enzymatic cascade with sequential conversion of proenzymes (zymogens) to fully activated enzymes, which then convert other zymogens to their activated forms (**Figure 11–1**). The final steps directly preceding fibrin formation can be activated through both the intrinsic and extrinsic pathways; hence, this part of the pathway is called the common pathway. Numerous positive and negative feedback mechanisms exist in the coagulation pathways so that the cascades do not proceed in an uncontrolled fashion. The pathways are now known to be extremely complex, with multiple interactions between factors in the intrinsic, extrinsic, and common pathways. The following description is a version of coagulation factor interactions that highlights the fundamental reactions.

The coagulation cascade is activated by the appearance of tissue factor (also known as Factor III), which is not normally exposed. Tissue factor is presented when a blood vessel is injured. It binds with Factor VII and small amounts of circulating Factor VIIa, resulting in a complex of Factor VII or VIIa and tissue factor. The Factor VII in the complex can be autoconverted to Factor VIIa, resulting in a greater number of Factor VIIa–tissue factor complexes. This complex activates Factor IX to Factor IXa in the intrinsic pathway, with some activation of Factor X to Factor Xa in the common pathway. Factor IXa, with support from Factor VIII as a cofactor (or Factor VIIIa which is a much more effective cofactor), activates Factor X to Factor Xa. Factor Xa with the assistance of Factor V or, more effectively Factor Va, converts prothrombin to thrombin. At this point, the coagulation cascade is markedly amplified because thrombin activates Factor VIII to Factor VIIIa, a more effective cofactor, and activates Factor V to its more effective Factor Va form. In addition, thrombin activates Factor XI to Factor XIa, which, like Factor VIIa and tissue factor, activates Factor IX to Factor IXa. Thrombin catalyzes the conversion of fibrinogen to fibrin, which is then cross-linked by Factor XIII to create a stabilized form of fibrin. Factor XIII is also activated to Factor XIIIa by thrombin.

Factor XII, prekallikrein (PK), and high-molecular-weight kininogen (HMWK) are not required for the generation of fibrin in vivo because even when they are completely absent, there is no increased risk for bleeding. This cascade, as it is currently understood and described above, explains 2 longstanding clinical observations. First, it explains the significant bleeding tendency associated with Factors VIII and IX deficiencies because these factors are important in the early stages of cascade amplification. Factor VIIa and tissue factor activate Factor IX to Factor IXa, and Factor IXa requires Factor VIII to convert Factor X to Factor Xa. Second, this scheme provides an explanation for the clinical observation that deficiencies of Factor XII, PK, and HMWK are not associated with an increased risk for bleeding.

Two of the coagulation cascade reactions occur on the platelet surface. The first of these is the activation of Factor X to Factor Xa, which is produced by platelet-bound Factor IXa and platelet-bound Factor VIIIa. In the second, platelet-bound Factor Xa and platelet-bound Factor Va convert prothrombin (Factor II) to thrombin (Factor IIa) in a subsequent step in the coagulation sequence. As noted below, single factor deficiency states, most of which are congenital, exist for all of the factors, but multiple factor deficiencies, which are usually not congenital, are much more commonly encountered. Inhibitors, as antibodies directed against a specific coagulation factor, can arise to any of the individual factors to create deficiency states. With some exceptions, most factor inhibitors are rare.

There are 2 major regulatory pathways that determine the rate at which the cascade is amplified. One of these is the protein C–protein S anticoagulant pathway (**Figure 11–2**). As shown in the figure, excess thrombin, which is generated through the activation of the coagulation sequence, provides the signal to shut off the coagulation cascade by binding to a protein on the endothelial surface known as thrombomodulin. The thrombin/thrombomodulin complex converts protein C into its activated form. The activated protein C then binds free protein S as a cofactor. Protein S may be bound to C4b binding protein and to a limited number of other proteins, in which case protein S becomes inactive because it is unable to bind to activated protein C. Once free (unbound) protein S binds to activated protein C, the activated protein C/protein S complex then proteolytically degrades Factors Va and VIIIa, reducing the flux through the coagulation sequence by removing these 2 activated cofactors. A mutation in the Factor V molecule, known as the Factor V Leiden mutation, makes Factor V resistant to proteolytic degradation by the activated protein C/protein S complex. This condition is known as activated protein C resistance. This permits the prothrombotic action of Factor Va to persist and contribute to a hypercoagulable state.

An additional mechanism for control of the coagulation cascade involves the inhibitory action of antithrombin (formerly known as antithrombin III) (**Figure 11–3**). Antithrombin has a limited anticoagulant effect of its own, but in the presence of heparin or selected other negatively

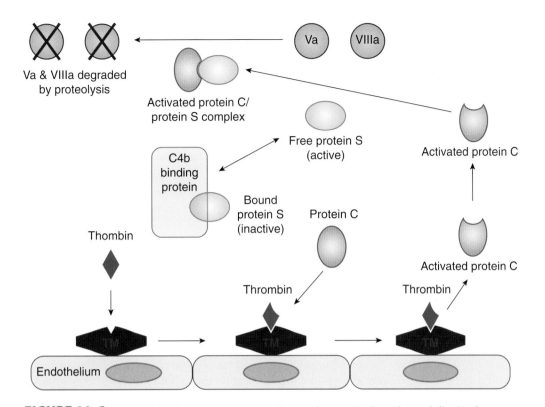

FIGURE 11–2 The protein C–protein S anticoagulant pathway. TM, thrombomodulin. (Redrawn with permission from Van Cott EM, Laposata M. Laboratory evaluation of hypercoagulable states. *Hematol Oncol Clin North Am*. 1998;12:1141–1166.)

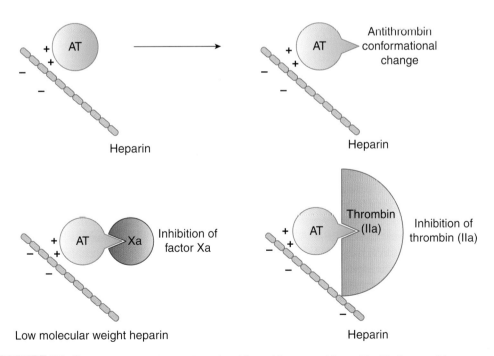

FIGURE 11–3 The anticoagulant action of antithrombin. AT, antithrombin. (Redrawn with permission from Kabakibi A, et al. The hypercoagulable state. In *Turnaround Times* [a newsletter for physicians at the Massachusetts General Hospital, Boston]. 1994;3:1:1.)

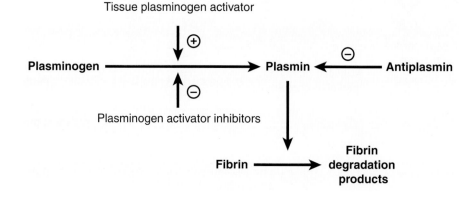

FIGURE 11–4 The fibrinolytic pathway. A plus sign indicates that tissue plasminogen activator converts plasminogen into plasmin. A minus sign indicates inhibitory action. (Redrawn with permission from Kabakibi, A et al. The hypercoagulable state. In *Turnaround Times* [a newsletter for physicians at the Massachusetts General Hospital, Boston]. 1994;3:1:1.)

charged heparin-like molecules, antithrombin adopts a new conformation that permits it to inhibit most of the activated coagulation factors in complexes where both antithrombin and heparin bind to the activated coagulation factor. Inhibition of Factor Xa, however, does not require the direct binding of the activated coagulation factor by heparin. Factor Xa can be neutralized when it is bound only to antithrombin (after antithrombin has been activated by heparin or related molecule). The antithrombotic action of short chains of heparin, notably low-molecular-weight heparin and fondaparinux, is directed primarily against Factor Xa because short heparin chains inhibit predominantly only Factor Xa (longer chains are required for Factor IIa inhibition). It should be noted that all of the coagulation factors in the coagulation cascade are synthesized in the liver, and that the activity of Factors II, VII, IX, and X is vitamin K-dependent. Tissue factor is constitutively expressed on some cell types, and in other cell types, such as endothelial cells, it becomes exposed in the initiation of the clotting reaction. There is little (if any) tissue factor in the circulating plasma under normal conditions. It is not exclusively synthesized in the liver. The half-lives of the coagulation factors in the plasma vary markedly, with Factor VII showing the shortest half-life of 5 hours and Factor XIII having the longest half-life of more than 120 hours. There is also a wide range of plasma concentrations for the coagulation factors. Factor VII is in the lowest concentration of the circulating coagulation factors at 500 ng/mL. The highest concentration is found for fibrinogen at 200 to 400 mg/dL.

Fibrinolysis

Fibrinolysis is the controlled dissolution of the formed clot. It occurs when the injured vessel begins to heal, and is initiated to a limited extent when clot formation begins. In this way, fibrinolysis serves as a regulatory mechanism to limit excess clot formation.

Fibrinolysis is the controlled dissolution of the formed clot. It occurs when the injured vessel begins to heal, and is initiated to a limited extent when clot formation begins. In this way, fibrinolysis serves as a regulatory mechanism to limit excess clot formation.

The principal enzyme involved in fibrinolysis is plasmin, which exists in a zymogen form known as plasminogen (**Figure 11–4**). Pharmacologic agents that produce thrombolysis, by converting plasminogen into plasmin, include streptokinase, urokinase, and derivatives of these compounds. Urokinase is a physiologic plasminogen activator. Another physiologic plasminogen activator is tissue plasminogen activator (TPA), which in its recombinant form is also used as a thrombolytic agent. Clinically effective derivatives of TPA from genetic manipulation are also used for thrombolysis. TPA is released by endothelial cells, and its secretion into the plasma is increased by thrombin. Plasminogen activator inhibitors are secreted by platelets and endothelial cells, particularly when they are activated. Plasminogen activator inhibitors stabilize a newly formed clot by blocking the action of TPA, thereby preventing premature dissolution of the clot. Plasmin degrades fibrin polymers, and to a limited degree, fibrinogen as well, by specific and sequential proteolytic cleavages, generating fibrin degradation products (FDP). These FDP (fragments X, Y, D, D-dimer, and E) may be detected in the plasma of patients experiencing fibrinolysis. Deficiency of plasminogen predisposes to thrombosis, and deficiency of plasminogen activator inhibitor may increase the risk for bleeding. Antiplasmin inhibits plasmin, but only when it is circulating and not when it is clot-bound. This prevents the circulation of a proteolytically active form of plasmin, while permitting clot lysis to proceed by plasmin within the clot. Deficiency of antiplasmin may result in a hemorrhagic tendency.

BLEEDING DISORDERS

Figure 11–5 provides a classification of coagulation disorders. The major division in the classification is between disorders associated with bleeding and disorders associated with thrombosis. There are 2 major subdivisions of bleeding disorders—those associated with coagulation factor and fibrinolytic pathway factor deficiencies, and those associated with an abnormal platelet count or impaired platelet function. Isolated factor deficiencies are usually congenital, although occasionally an isolated acquired factor deficiency develops. An example of an acquired isolated coagulation factor deficiency is the Factor X deficiency associated with amyloidosis. The deficiency of antiplasmin is listed in this section because its absence permits increased plasmin activity and overactive clot dissolution, resulting in a bleeding tendency. Another major category of coagulation factor abnormalities is multiple coagulation factor deficiencies. There are several commonly encountered situations associated with multiple factor deficiencies. These include vitamin K deficiency or warfarin intake (which results in a reduced amount of functional Factors II, VII, IX, and X as well as protein C and protein S); disseminated intravascular coagulation (DIC), which results in the consumption of multiple coagulation factors; and liver disease that results in decreased synthesis of coagulation factors. Several activated coagulation factors are inhibited by heparin. Heparin administration results in inactivation of most of the activated coagulation factors.

The group of disorders associated with platelets is divided first into quantitative platelet disorders and qualitative platelet disorders. *Quantitative platelet disorders* include thrombocytopenia and thrombocytosis. Thrombocytopenia can be produced as a result of increased platelet destruction, from a variety of immune or nonimmune causes, or decreased platelet production. Common causes of decreased platelet production include tumor infiltration of bone marrow from metastases or a hematologic malignancy, and drug-induced thrombocytopenia as occurs with chemotherapy. Thrombocytopenia can also occur as a result of increased sequestration of platelets in the spleen, usually in patients with splenomegaly. Thrombocytosis is much less common than thrombocytopenia. Thrombocytosis can be divided into reactive thrombocytosis, in which there is a transiently increased number of platelets from a stimulus to increase platelet production, or neoplastic thrombocytosis, as seen in myeloproliferative disease and, less commonly, myelodysplastic disorders.

Qualitative platelet disorders are characterized by abnormal platelet function in the presence of a normal platelet count. vWD is a disorder in which there is defective platelet function, but from a defect originating outside the platelet, since vWF is generated primarily in endothelial cells. vWF coats the surface of the activated platelet to allow it to adhere to the cut surface and initiate platelet plug formation.

Other causes of defective platelet function result from abnormalities within the platelet. These disorders may be congenital or acquired. The congenital ones are extremely rare, and the acquired ones are very frequently encountered. Congenital platelet abnormalities associated with defective function include GT, Bernard–Soulier disease, and storage pool disease (SPD). The much more common acquired qualitative platelet disorders include drug-induced platelet dysfunction, as produced by aspirin and clopidigrel (Plavix), and uremia-induced platelet dysfunction, which occurs in patients with impaired renal function.

Quantitative platelet disorders include thrombocytopenia and thrombocytosis. *Qualitative platelet disorders* are characterized by abnormal platelet function in the presence of a normal platelet count.

Fibrinogen Deficiencies

Description

Fibrinogen is produced in the liver by hepatocytes. Abnormalities of fibrinogen production may be congenital or acquired and, in general, involve either decreased production of a normal

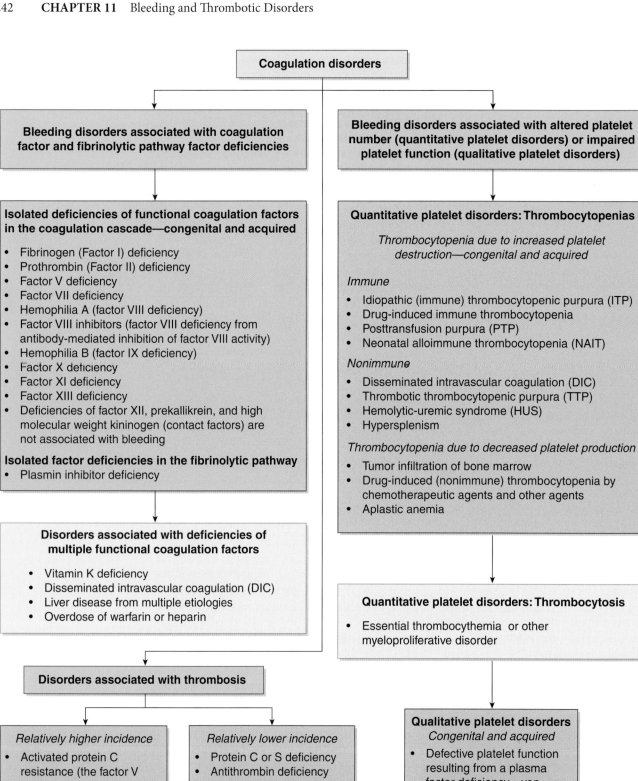

FIGURE 11–5 A classification of coagulation disorders.

TABLE 11–1   Laboratory Evaluation for Fibrinogen Deficiencies

Laboratory Test	Results/Comments			
	Quantitative Deficiencies		Dysfibrinogenemia (Qualitative Deficiencies)	
	Afibrinogenemia	Hypofibrinogenemia	Homozygous	Heterozygous
PT	Markedly prolonged	Normal to slightly prolonged	Markedly prolonged	Slightly prolonged to normal
PTT	Markedly prolonged	Normal to slightly prolonged	Markedly prolonged	Slightly prolonged to normal
Functional fibrinogen	Low	Slightly low to normal	Low	Slightly low to normal
Immunologic fibrinogen	Low	Slightly low to normal	Normal	Normal
Thrombin time	Prolonged	Normal to prolonged	Prolonged	Prolonged
Reptilase time	Prolonged	Normal to prolonged	Prolonged	Prolonged

PT, prothrombin time; PTT, partial thromboplastin time.

molecule (afibrinogenemia and hypofibrinogenemia) or production of an abnormal molecule (dysfibrinogenemia) (see **Table 11–1**).

In *congenital afibrinogenemia and hypofibrinogenemia*, there is a reduced (hypofibrinogenemia) or absent (afibrinogenemia) production of a normal fibrinogen molecule. In general, the homozygous deficiency results in afibrinogenemia, and the heterozygous state results in hypofibrinogenemia. Both disorders are rare. Homozygotes suffer a mild to moderate spontaneous bleeding tendency. Manifestations include umbilical stump hemorrhage and bleeding from mucous membranes, among many other possible signs and symptoms related to blood loss. Severe bleeding may occur with trauma or surgery. Hypofibrinogenemic patients are usually asymptomatic, but may bleed significantly with surgery or trauma.

Congenital dysfibrinogenemia is a result of inheritance of a gene for an abnormal fibrinogen molecule, which is produced in normal or near-normal quantities. All the fibrinogen produced by a homozygote for dysfibrinogenemia is abnormal, and approximately half of the fibrinogen in a heterozygote is abnormal. Hundreds of abnormal fibrinogens have been described. The true incidence of dysfibrinogenemia is not known because many forms of the disorder are asymptomatic. Homozygotes may have a mild bleeding tendency, perhaps because the fibrinogen molecule is cleaved too slowly to form fibrin monomers or because abnormal fibrin monomers polymerize too slowly. The bleeding tendency is characterized by easy or spontaneous bruising, menorrhagia, and prolonged or severe bleeding with surgery or trauma. Heterozygotes are usually asymptomatic, but may show excessive bleeding with surgery or trauma. Several types of dysfibrinogenemia (approximately 10% to 15% of cases) are associated with an increased risk of thrombosis rather than bleeding. A few types of congenital dysfibrinogenemia are associated with both bleeding and thrombosis.

Acquired hypofibrinogenemia is observed predominantly in patients with advanced liver disease, in patients with a consumptive coagulation disorder such as DIC, and in those treated with thrombolytic therapy.

Acquired dysfibrinogenemia represents the acquired production of an abnormal fibrinogen molecule in normal or near-normal quantities, most often in patients with acute or chronic liver disease, especially those with primary or metastatic hepatic malignancies. The patient may or may not be symptomatic, depending on 1) whether there is simultaneous production of normal fibrinogen in amounts sufficient to allow normal hemostasis and 2) whether the abnormal fibrinogen can polymerize like a normal fibrinogen molecule (see the section "Hemostatic Abnormalities in Liver Disease").

Acquired hypofibrinogenemia is observed predominantly in patients with advanced liver disease, in patients with a consumptive coagulation disorder such as DIC, and in those treated with thrombolytic therapy.

Diagnosis

See **Table 11–1** for the laboratory evaluation of the patient with a fibrinogen deficiency.

Prothrombin (Factor II) Deficiency

Description

Prothrombin (Factor II) is the precursor to thrombin (Factor IIa), which converts fibrinogen into fibrin in the common pathway of the coagulation cascade. Deficiency of prothrombin, either inherited or acquired, may result in a hemorrhagic diathesis. Inherited abnormalities of prothrombin are rare. As with fibrinogen, abnormalities occur in 2 major forms. The first is reduced or absent production of a normal prothrombin molecule. The second is production of normal amounts of an abnormal prothrombin molecule with decreased activity (dysfunctional form or dysprothrombinemia). Heterozygotes usually have approximately 50% of normal activity and may be asymptomatic or have a bleeding tendency. In 1 study, 83% of a small cohort of heterozygotes had bleeding, with Factor II levels ranging from 21% to 35%. Homozygotes usually have 1% to 25% of normal activity and have a mild to severe hemorrhagic tendency. Acquired hypoprothrombinemia occurs most often along with deficiencies of Factors VII, IX, and X in vitamin K deficiency and with warfarin (Coumadin) therapy; with deficiencies of multiple coagulation factors in liver disease or DIC; as an isolated coagulation factor deficiency in some patients with lupus anticoagulant (LA); and in patients exposed to topical bovine thrombin who develop antibodies to prothrombin (and not uncommonly to Factor V also). Bleeding manifestations depend on the level of prothrombin activity; usually no bleeding occurs with a prothrombin level >50% of normal.

> Abnormalities occur in 2 major forms. The first is reduced or absent production of a normal prothrombin molecule. The second is production of normal amounts of an abnormal prothrombin molecule with decreased activity (dysfunctional form or dysprothrombinemia).

Diagnosis

See **Table 11–2** for the laboratory evaluation of the patient with a prothrombin (Factor II) deficiency.

Factor V Deficiency

Description

Factor V is a high-molecular-weight protein (approximately 300,000 Da) that acts as an accelerating cofactor for the enzymatic conversion of prothrombin to thrombin by Factor Xa. When Factor V is cleaved to Factor Va by thrombin, its cofactor activity is significantly increased. Factors Va and VIIIa are degraded by activated protein C. An isolated deficiency of Factor V is a rare cause of bleeding.

Apparent heterozygous and homozygous deficient states have been observed. Heterozygotes usually have levels of approximately 50% of normal and can experience bleeding or may be asymptomatic. In a cohort of 19 heterozygous patients, 50% had bleeding, with Factor V levels ranging from 21% to 55%. Homozygotes have variable levels below 50%; they are most likely to be symptomatic if the level is 10% or less.

As with the other coagulation factors, 2 major forms of the inherited deficiency are described: reduced or absent production of a normal Factor V molecule (absence form) and production of an abnormal molecule with reduced activity in normal amounts (dysfunctional form). A rare combined deficiency of Factors V and VIII is due to a genetic defect in intracellular transport of Factors V and VIII. Acquired deficiencies of Factor V occur with liver dysfunction or DIC.

Diagnosis

See **Table 11–2** for the laboratory evaluation of the patient with a Factor V deficiency.

Factor VII Deficiency

Description

Factor VII is a vitamin K-dependent coagulation factor precursor that, when activated by thrombin, Factor Xa, or Factor IXa, is converted to Factor VIIa. This activated factor then converts phospholipid-bound Factor X into Factor Xa in the presence of calcium and tissue factor. It also converts Factor IX to Factor IXa. Factor VII deficiency is rare and may occur as an inherited or acquired disorder.

TABLE 11–2   Laboratory Evaluation for Coagulation Factor Deficiencies

Deficient Factor(s)	PT Prolonged if Deficient?	PTT Prolonged if Deficient?	Other Tests Useful in Diagnosis/Comments
Fibrinogen—see **Table 11–1**			
Prothrombin (Factor II)	Yes	Yes (usually less prominent than the PT prolongation)	Factor II assay; selected other factor assays to determine if Factor II is low along with other factors, especially VII, IX, and X—this often establishes the cause of a low Factor II level A lupus anticoagulant test to determine if a low Factor II level is associated with a lupus anticoagulant
Factor V	Yes	Yes (usually less prominent than the PT prolongation)	Factor V assay; selected other factor assays to determine if a low Factor V level is accompanied by other factor deficiencies
Factor VII	Yes	No	Factor VII assay; selected other factor assays to determine if Factor VII is low along with other factors, especially II, IX, and X
Factor VIII	No	Yes	Factors VIII and IX assays, as these 2 deficiency states are clinically indistinguishable von Willebrand factor antigen and ristocetin cofactor to determine if a low Factor VIII level represents hemophilia A or von Willebrand disease
Factor IX	No	Yes	Factors VIII and IX assays as these 2 deficiency states are clinically indistinguishable; selected other factor assays to determine if Factor IX is low along with other factors, especially II, VII, and X
Factor X	Yes	Yes (usually less prominent than the PT prolongation)	Factor X assay; selected other factor assays to determine if Factor X is low along with other factors, especially II, VII, and IX
Factor XI	No	Yes	Factor XI assay
Factor XII	No	Yes	Factor XII assay
Prekallikrein	No	Yes	Prekallikrein assay
High-molecular-weight kininogen	No	Yes	High-molecular-weight kininogen assay
Factor XIII	No	No	The screening test for Factor XIII deficiency assesses the solubility of the patient's clot in urea—clots from patients with Factor XIII levels <2% dissolve; a quantitative assay not involving clot solubility is also available and can detect mild deficiencies of Factor XIII

PT, prothrombin time; PTT, partial thromboplastin time.

The rare inherited deficiency state may be present as reduced or absent production of a normal molecule (absence form) or production of an abnormal molecule with decreased activity in normal amounts (dysfunctional form). An inherited isolated deficiency of Factor VII in heterozygotes is usually associated with a Factor VII activity level of approximately 50%. In a cohort of 88 heterozygous patients, 36% had a bleeding tendency, with Factor VII levels ranging from 21% to 69%. In homozygotes, there are variable Factor VII activity levels below 50%. The bleeding risk is difficult to predict in these patients because the factor activity level correlates poorly with the patient's tendency to hemorrhage. A large proportion of patients with less than 2% Factor VII do not bleed. Acquired Factor VII deficiency occurs in vitamin K deficiency and with warfarin therapy along with deficiencies of Factors II, IX, and X; and in DIC or severe liver disease along with multiple other coagulation factor deficiencies.

Intracranial hemorrhage has been reported in Factor VII-deficient patients, most often occurring in infants <1 year of age. Elevated Factor VII levels have been associated with an increased risk of cardiovascular disease.

> The bleeding risk is difficult to predict because the factor activity level correlates poorly with the patient's tendency to hemorrhage. A large proportion of patients with less than 2% Factor VII do not bleed.

Diagnosis

See **Table 11–2** for the laboratory evaluation of the patient with a Factor VII deficiency.

Hemophilia A (Factor VIII Deficiency)

Description

Hemophilia A is a bleeding disorder resulting from a deficiency of Factor VIII procoagulant activity. Factor VIII circulates in the plasma bound to vWF. Approximately 90% of patients with hemophilia A synthesize low amounts of normal Factor VIII molecules, and 10% of patients with hemophilia A synthesize normal amounts of an abnormal (nonfunctional) Factor VIII. Hemophilia A is inherited as an X-linked trait, and 65% to 75% of patients have a positive family history. Disease prevalence in the United States is 1 in 10,000 males; the carrier state in females is rarely symptomatic. Hemophilia A and hemophilia B (Factor IX deficiency, see below) are clinically indistinguishable. The likelihood of hemorrhage depends on the amount of Factor VIII present; the majority of patients (approximately 50% to 70% of hemophilia A patients) have severe disease. The severity of disease is categorized as follows:

- In mild disease: the VIII level is 6% to 20% of normal, with rare spontaneous bleeding.
- In moderate disease: the VIII level is 1% to 5% of normal, with occasional spontaneous bleeding.
- In severe disease: the VIII level is <1% of normal, with frequent spontaneous bleeding.

All hemophilia patients (A and B) may experience severe hemorrhage following trauma or surgery if there is no prior treatment to elevate the factor level. Bleeding that is characteristic of hemophilia (A and B) includes intra-articular (joint), intracranial, and intramuscular hemorrhage. The latter can produce a compartment compression syndrome. Easy bruising and prolonged bleeding after minor cuts and abrasions are also characteristic. The onset of hemorrhage is typically delayed following injury, and pathologic bleeding may occur hours after injury. Primary hemostasis (dependent on platelet plug formation) is intact, but secondary hemostasis (dependent on the fibrin clot generated by the coagulation cascade) is defective. Up to 15% of hemophilia A patients develop an inhibitor to Factor VIII at some time during the course of their disease. The inhibitor develops only in those transfused with Factor VIII-containing products, and most often in patients with <1% Factor VIII. Factor VIII inhibitors may also spontaneously occur in nonhemophiliacs (see the section "Factor VIII Inhibitors").

> Hemophilia A is a bleeding disorder resulting from a deficiency of Factor VIII procoagulant activity. Factor VIII inhibitors are antibodies, usually IgG, that bind to Factor VIII and inhibit its coagulant activity.

Diagnosis

See **Table 11–2** for information regarding the laboratory evaluation for Factor VIII deficiency.

Factor VIII Inhibitors

Description

Factor VIII inhibitors are antibodies, usually IgG, that bind to Factor VIII and inhibit its coagulant activity.

Factor VIII inhibitors have been found in several clinical situations.

- Inhibitors are diagnosed most commonly in patients with hemophilia A. Inhibitors occur in 10% to 15% of these patients and make the treatment of hemorrhage much more difficult. The vast majority of cases of Factor VIII inhibitors in hemophilia A patients occur in those with severe hemophilia A (<1% Factor VIII activity). Inhibitor formation is related to transfusion of exogenous Factor VIII, and usually develops before 100 treatment days if it appears. Two immune response patterns have been observed in hemophilia A patients. The first is a high response pattern. Inhibitors rise to a high titer in response to exposure to Factor VIII. The titer may not decline for months to years, even without further exposure to Factor VIII. Rapid anamnestic responses are often seen within 3 to 7 days of re-exposure in these patients. In the second pattern, there is a low response. In addition, inhibitors usually remain at a low titer despite re-exposure. They may occasionally disappear and reappear spontaneously. Little, if any, anamnestic response is likely in a low responder.

TABLE 11-3   Laboratory Evaluation for Factor VIII Inhibitor

Laboratory Test	Results/Comments
PT	Normal
PTT	Prolonged; normalizes in a 1:1 PTT mixing study of patient plasma and normal plasma with a 0-minute incubation (i.e., PTT performed immediately after mixing), but becomes prolonged with a longer incubation of the mixed plasma (60 or 120 minutes) at 37°C; the PTT of the mixed plasma at 60–120 minutes incubation with a clinically significant inhibitor is typically at least 8 seconds longer than the PTT of the mixed plasma at 0-minute incubation
Factor VIII activity	Decreased
Factor VIII inhibitor assay	Used for quantitation of inhibitor; inhibitor levels are expressed in Bethesda units (BU); 1 BU/mL is the amount of inhibitor that produces a 50% reduction in Factor VIII activity

PT, prothrombin time; PTT, partial thromboplastin time.

- Spontaneous inhibitors to Factor VIII can occur in the postpartum patient. Usually they are recognized 2 to 5 months after the birth of the first child and disappear spontaneously after 12 to 18 months. However, the course is variable, and there are reports of death from hemorrhage in some patients. Antigenic differences between mother and fetus do not sufficiently explain the development of a Factor VIII inhibitor, and its cause remains unknown.
- Inhibitors may occur in those with allergic and enhanced immunologic reactions, including patients with:
  - (a) rheumatoid arthritis
  - (b) systemic lupus erythematosus
  - (c) reactions to drugs, such as penicillin, chloramphenicol, sulfonamides, and phenytoin
  - (d) malignancy
  - (e) asthma
  - (f) Crohn disease
  - (g) ulcerative colitis
  - (h) pemphigus
  - (i) multiple myeloma
- Inhibitors may appear in patients without any obvious underlying disorder. These are usually older individuals, and the inhibitor may remit in several months, persist for years, or disappear with immunosuppressive therapy.

In a hemophilia A patient, a poor response to treatment with Factor VIII concentrate may be the first indication that an inhibitor is present, or there may be an increased frequency of bleeding episodes. In nonhemophiliacs, development of a new hemorrhagic tendency is usually the presenting feature of a spontaneous Factor VIII inhibitor. The most favorable prognoses are for patients with low titer inhibitors, peripartum women, and patients without an underlying disorder.

Hemophilia B is an inherited hemorrhagic disorder resulting from a lack of procoagulant activity of Factor IX.

Diagnosis

See **Table 11-3** for information regarding the laboratory evaluation for a Factor VIII inhibitor.

Hemophilia B (Factor IX Deficiency)

Description

Hemophilia B is an inherited hemorrhagic disorder resulting from a lack of procoagulant activity of Factor IX. Factor IX is a vitamin K-dependent factor that, in its active form (Factor IXa), is a serine protease of the intrinsic pathway of the coagulation cascade. Approximately 70% to 90% of hemophilia B patients have a deficiency of a normal coagulant protein, and 10%

to 30% produce an abnormal Factor IX that is nonfunctional. Inheritance is sex-linked, with affected male and female carriers. Of hemophilia B patients, 60% to 70% have a positive family history for bleeding. The prevalence of hemophilia B is much less than that of hemophilia A. Approximately 1 in 50,000 males in the United States has hemophilia B versus 1 in 10,000 males with hemophilia A. The hemophilia B carrier state in the female is usually asymptomatic, as is the case with hemophilia A. Acquired Factor IX deficiency may occur along with deficiencies of Factors II, VII, and X in patients with vitamin K deficiency or those receiving warfarin therapy, and with deficiencies of other coagulation factors in patients with liver disease, DIC, or nephrotic syndrome.

As previously noted, hemophilia B is clinically indistinguishable from hemophilia A. The severity of hemorrhage depends on the amount of Factor IX activity present:

- In mild disease: 6% to20% of normal IX activity is present, with rare spontaneous bleeding.
- In moderate disease: 1% to 5% of normal IX activity is present, with occasional spontaneous bleeding.
- In severe disease: <1% of normal activity is present, with frequent spontaneous bleeding.

Profuse bleeding may occur in any hemophilia B patient with trauma or surgery if there is no prior treatment to elevate the factor level. Bleeding in hemophilia B resembles that found in hemophilia A and includes: deep tissue bleeding, intra-articular bleeding (hemarthrosis), intracranial bleeding (which may be lethal), and intramuscular bleeding with potential compartment compression syndrome. Severe mucosal membrane bleeding can occur in hemophilia, particularly after dental surgery.

Inhibitors develop to Factor IX in 1% to 5% of hemophilia B cases. These antibodies often occur in high titer and frequently present a major bleeding problem despite treatment.

Diagnosis

See **Table 11–2** for information regarding the laboratory evaluation for patients with hemophilia B.

Factor X Deficiency
Description

An inherited isolated deficiency of Factor X is a rare disorder. Homozygotes and heterozygotes have been identified. Homozygotes usually possess <2% of normal activity. Heterozygotes usually possess 40% to 70% of normal activity. In a cohort of 15 heterozygous patients, 33% had a bleeding tendency, with Factor X levels ranging from 23% to 47%. Inherited Factor X deficiency, like the other factor deficiency states, occurs in 2 major forms: reduced or absent synthesis of a normal molecule (absence form) and synthesis of an abnormal molecule in normal amounts (dysfunctional form).

Acquired Factor X deficiency may result from warfarin or vitamin K deficiency (in the presence of deficiencies of Factors II, VII, and IX), from liver disease (with deficiencies of other factors synthesized in the liver), with DIC, or as an isolated deficiency in cases of amyloidosis. In amyloidosis, Factor X becomes irreversibly bound to amyloid fibrils in the extracellular space, and is thereby removed from the circulation.

Diagnosis

See **Table 11–2** for information regarding the laboratory evaluation of patients with Factor X deficiency.

Factor XI Deficiency
Description

Factor XI deficiency is a commonly encountered disorder. Homozygotes typically have less than 20% of normal Factor XI activity. Heterozygotes have 20% to 70% of normal Factor XI activity. The deficiency in almost all cases appears to be a reduced or absent production of a normal molecule, rather than production of an abnormal or dysfunctional molecule.

The vast majority of the cases of Factor XI deficiency are in people of Jewish descent, particularly those of Ashkenazi origin. The frequency of the homozygous deficient state is 0.2% to 0.3% in the Ashkenazi population, and the frequency of the heterozygous state is extremely high, at approximately 5.5% to 11.0%.

The hemorrhagic tendency is variable for both heterozygotes and homozygotes. Bleeding does not correlate well with the level of Factor XI activity. Some homozygotes have an abnormal partial thromboplastin time (PTT), a very low Factor XI level of less than 10%, and no bleeding, even with surgery. The bleeding tendency of a particular individual is more closely related to the bleeding tendency of the patient's kindred than to the measured Factor XI level. The explanation, which is true for all mutations affecting coagulation factors, is that certain mutations produce a low level of Factor XI and a prolonged PTT but are not clinically significant in vivo. This is because they only affect the activity of the factor in the in vitro clotting factor assays, which are not exact replicas of clot formation in vivo. Acquired decreases in Factor XI can occur with pregnancy, proteinuria, liver dysfunction, and DIC.

Diagnosis

See **Table 11–2** for information regarding the laboratory evaluation of patients with Factor XI deficiency.

Deficiencies of the Contact Factors

Description

The contact coagulation factors (so named because they were originally thought to activate the coagulation cascade by contacting the cut surface) include Factor XII, PK, and HMWK. A deficiency of any of the contact factors prolongs the PTT because the PTT assay is constructed to involve these factors, even though the coagulation cascade in vivo does not depend on these factors. Bleeding diatheses have not been reported in patients with deficiencies at any level of Factor XII, PK, or HMWK. Factor XII deficiency is fairly common, with many thousands affected, especially individuals of Asian descent and children with tonsillitis. HMWK deficiency and PK deficiency are rare.

> A deficiency of any of the contact factors prolongs the PTT because the PTT assay is constructed to involve these factors, even though the coagulation cascade in vivo does not depend on these factors. Bleeding diatheses have not been reported in patients with deficiencies at any level of Factor XII, PK, or HMWK.

Diagnosis

See **Table 11–2** for information regarding the laboratory evaluation for contact factor abnormalities.

Factor XIII Deficiency

Description

Factor XIII circulates in plasma as a zymogen and is converted to its active form (Factor XIIIa) by thrombin. Factor XIIIa catalyzes the formation of covalent bonds between chains of adjacent fibrin monomers. This stabilizes the fibrin clot, making it rigid and more resistant to the action of plasmin. Congenital deficiency of Factor XIII is rare. A bleeding tendency is observed in homozygotes, but is unlikely in heterozygotes. The hemorrhagic tendency is characterized by umbilical stump bleeding in newborns (>90% of patients with clinically significant Factor XIII deficiency have this finding) and posttraumatic hematomas, with bleeding often delayed hours to days after the trauma.

Diagnosis

See **Table 11–2** for information regarding the laboratory evaluation for Factor XIII deficiency.

Antiplasmin Deficiency

Description

Antiplasmin or plasmin inhibitor (formerly known as alpha-2 antiplasmin) is a glycoprotein that serves as a regulator of fibrinolysis in several ways (see **Figure 11–4**). It blocks the

TABLE 11-4   Laboratory Evaluation for Antiplasmin Deficiency

Laboratory Test	Results/Comments
PT	Normal
PTT	Normal
Antiplasmin	Decreased

PT, prothrombin time; PTT, partial thromboplastin time.

enzymatic activity of plasmin (the major fibrinolytic enzyme) and other serine proteases, some of which are coagulation factors, and it inhibits the binding of plasminogen to fibrin. A bleeding diathesis is associated with the congenital deficiency of plasmin inhibitor. It is an extremely rare disorder and only homozygotes with <10% of normal plasmin inhibitor activity appear to be clinically affected. Those who do bleed may experience mucosal membrane bleeding (particularly in the genitourinary tract), subcutaneous hematomas, spontaneous bruising, and severe bleeding with trauma. Most heterozygotes are asymptomatic, but those few who are symptomatic have only a mild bleeding tendency. Acquired deficiency of plasmin inhibitor can occur in liver disease, nephrotic syndrome, amyloidosis, DIC, and, most notably, following thrombolytic therapy. In thrombolytic therapy, plasminogen is purposefully converted to plasmin, which results in the formation of plasmin–antiplasmin complexes, thereby reducing the amount of available antiplasmin.

Diagnosis

See **Table 11-4** for information for the laboratory evaluation of plasmin inhibitor deficiency.

Vitamin K Deficiency
Description

In adults, vitamin K deficiency most often occurs secondary to disease or drug therapy; it rarely occurs as a dietary deficiency. Causes of vitamin K deficiency include:

- warfarin therapy (reduces the amount of active vitamin K);
- antibiotic therapy (capable of suppressing bowel flora which synthesize vitamin K);
- malabsorption syndromes: cystic fibrosis, sprue, ulcerative colitis, Crohn disease, parasitic infections, short-bowel syndrome, and ileojejunostomy (for morbid obesity);
- dietary restriction with incidental decrease in vitamin K intake;
- long-term total parenteral nutrition;
- biliary obstruction.

Vitamin K depletion can occur in as little as 2 weeks if both intake (enteral and parenteral) and endogenous production of vitamin K are eliminated. In early deficiency, Factor VII only, or Factors VII and IX only, may be decreased due to their shorter half-lives. Vitamin K deficiency may present as an asymptomatic prolongation of the PT in mild cases or as a major spontaneous hemorrhage in severe deficiencies. The degree of prolongation of the PT does not accurately predict the risk of hemorrhage.

Most antibiotics destroy bacterial flora and must be considered as a possible cause of vitamin K deficiency in the bleeding patient. However, certain cephalosporins produce vitamin K deficiency much more rapidly than other antibiotics. Cephalosporins with an *N*-methylthiotetrazole (MTT) group in position 3 directly inhibit the vitamin K-dependent carboxylase that is responsible for converting Factors II, VII, IX, and X to their active form. Cephalosporins in the MTT group include cefamandole, cefoperazone, cefotetan, moxalactam, cefmetazole, and cefmenoxime. Weekly prophylaxis with vitamin K has been recommended when MTT-cephalosporins are given to patients at high risk for vitamin K deficiency.

In adults, vitamin K deficiency most often occurs secondary to disease or drug therapy; it rarely occurs as a dietary deficiency.

TABLE 11–5   Laboratory Evaluation for Vitamin K Deficiency

Laboratory Test	Results/Comments
PT	Always prolonged
PTT	May be prolonged, depending on severity
Factors II, VII, IX, and X, protein C, and protein S	The combined deficiencies of Factors II, VII, IX, and X, protein C, and protein S are diagnostic of vitamin K deficiency or ingestion of a vitamin K antagonist, such as warfarin, especially if a non-vitamin K-dependent coagulation factor (e.g., Factor V) level is normal; Factor VII and protein C decrease before the others because they have the shortest half-lives in the plasma

PT, prothrombin time; PTT, partial thromboplastin time.

Diagnosis

See **Table 11–5** for information on the laboratory evaluation for vitamin K deficiency.

Disseminated Intravascular Coagulation

Description

DIC is a common acquired coagulation disorder that occurs secondary to a variety of underlying disorders. The most common cause is infection; 10% to 20% of patients with gram-negative sepsis develop DIC. Other causes of DIC include obstetrical complications (retained dead fetus, placental abruption, amniotic fluid embolism, hypertonic saline-induced abortion, and septic abortion), extensive tissue injury (including trauma, ischemia, infarction, and burns), liver disease, transfusion of ABO-incompatible blood, and adult respiratory distress syndrome. The clinical presentation varies from an asymptomatic condition, detectable only by laboratory abnormalities, to a severe coagulopathy with a mortality of up to 80%.

The major events in acute DIC, independent of the cause, are microvascular thrombosis with consumption of platelets and coagulation factors, and then hemorrhage as a result of low levels of platelets and coagulation factors and overactivation of the fibrinolytic system to remove the thrombi. Infrequently patients will develop macrovascular (large vessel) thrombosis as well, most likely as a deep vein thrombosis. Hemorrhagic symptoms can include any of the following—petechiae, ecchymoses, mucosal oozing, hematuria, gastrointestinal tract bleeding, bleeding into surgical wounds, and prolonged bleeding at venous access sites. Severe bleeding may contribute to hypotensive shock.

DIC may present as a more chronic condition in patients with malignancy, including those with solid tumors or leukemias, especially acute promyelocytic leukemia.

The prolongations of the PT and the PTT reflect a decrease in fibrinogen and other coagulation factors that are consumed by clotting. In addition, fibrinogen is degraded by excess plasmin activation in the fibrinolytic system. Platelets are also consumed, and therefore, the platelet count is typically low. The presence of FDP, 1 of which is the D-dimer, indicates that fibrin clots have been formed and subsequently degraded. There is no single laboratory test that can diagnose or exclude DIC, and the diagnosis is made when the characteristic laboratory abnormalities are present along with a known stimulus for DIC. A practical approach to diagnosis of DIC is to perform the PT, the PTT, and a D-dimer assay, with serial measurements of fibrinogen and platelets. In severe acute DIC, most of the laboratory test results will be abnormal although fibrinogen may be normal or even elevated. In chronic DIC, the laboratory abnormalities may be less pronounced or even absent because the liver and bone marrow can increase production of coagulation factors and platelets, respectively, to offset the losses from consumption.

The major events in acute DIC, independent of the cause, are microvascular thrombosis with consumption of platelets and coagulation factors, and then hemorrhage as a result of low levels of platelets and coagulation factors and overactivation of the fibrinolytic system to remove the thrombi.

TABLE 11–6   Commonly Used Assays in the Laboratory Evaluation for Disseminated Intravascular Coagulation (DIC)

Laboratory Test	Results/Comments
FDP or D-dimer	Elevated in essentially all cases, both acute and chronic; elevated due to fibrinolysis of fibrin deposits in the microvasculature
PT	Prolonged in most cases of clinically significant DIC, due to a decrease in fibrinogen, prothrombin (Factor II), and multiple other coagulation factors
PTT	Prolonged less often than the PT in DIC, but increases along with severity of DIC due to a decrease in fibrinogen, Factor VIII, and multiple other coagulation factors
Platelet count	Decreased in most cases of acute DIC due to consumption of platelets
Fibrinogen	Low or decreasing with serial samples in <50% of acute DIC cases, due to the conversion of fibrinogen into fibrin; the fibrinogen level can be normal or even elevated in DIC by a variety of mechanisms, 1 of which is increased fibrinogen synthesis in the liver as part of the acute phase response to infection or other stimulus
Schistocytes	Present in the peripheral blood smear in approximately 50% of acute DIC cases; results from microangiopathic hemolysis of RBCs as they traverse through vessels that are partially occluded by fibrin strands

FDP, fibrin degradation products; PT, prothrombin time; PTT, partial thromboplastin time.

Diagnosis

See **Table 11–6** for information on the laboratory evaluation for DIC.

Hemostatic Abnormalities in Liver Disease
Description

Patients with acute and chronic liver disease often have laboratory evidence of a hemostatic abnormality. These patients may be asymptomatic or have only mild bleeding problems, but those with advanced liver disease may experience a severe hemorrhage.

Hemorrhage in patients with liver disease may be due to 1 or more of the following:

- Coagulation factor abnormalities: This is caused by decreased hepatic synthesis of vitamin K-dependent factors (II, VII, IX, and X) and non-vitamin K-dependent factors. Decreased fibrinogen is usually found only in patients with severe hepatic failure; in fact, patients with acute hepatitis without hepatic failure usually have an increased fibrinogen level. The Factor VIII level is usually normal or elevated in liver disease because not all the Factor VIII is synthesized in the liver.
- Thrombocytopenia: This frequently occurs as a consequence of sequestration in the spleen, impaired platelet production, or increased platelet destruction. It is not usually a severe decrease in platelet number.
- Platelet dysfunction: The dysfunction is usually mild and its clinical significance is uncertain; platelet dysfunction may be clinically important only in liver disease patients with severe thrombocytopenia or severe renal failure, which can result in uremia-induced platelet dysfunction.
- DIC or a DIC-like syndrome: There is no general agreement as to whether the coagulation abnormalities that occur in patients with liver disease are due to DIC, liver disease alone, or to a combination of these and other mechanisms. A DIC-like syndrome occurs frequently in patients with acute hepatic failure. Laboratory abnormalities in these cases include hypofibrinogenemia, thrombocytopenia, increased FDP such as D-dimer, and decreased levels of Factors V and VIII.
- Acquired dysfibrinogenemia (in patients with selected liver diseases [see the section "Fibrinogen Deficiencies"]): Impaired fibrin polymerization may result and thereby predispose the patient to bleeding.

Patients with acute and chronic liver disease often have laboratory evidence of a hemostatic abnormality. These patients may be asymptomatic or have only mild bleeding problems, but those with advanced liver disease may experience a severe hemorrhage.

TABLE 11-7   Laboratory Evaluation for Hemostatic Defects in Liver Disease

Laboratory Test	Results/Comments
PT and PTT	Both will be prolonged, but the PT prolongation is usually greater than the PTT prolongation
D-dimer or FDP	Elevated due to decreased clearance by the liver
Fibrinogen	Most often slightly low or normal; can be elevated if underlying illness causes acute phase reaction
Platelet count	Most often slightly low or normal
Coagulation factor assays	Used to investigate the extent of coagulation factor deficiencies; in the absence of a concomitant DIC, Factor VIII is usually normal or elevated in liver disease as it can also be synthesized extrahepatically

DIC, disseminated intravascular coagulation; FDP, fibrin degradation products; PT, prothrombin time; PTT, partial thromboplastin time.

- Increased fibrinolysis: Hemostatic abnormalities in patients with cirrhosis may be due to increased fibrinolysis. This may occur as a result of decreased hepatic clearance of plasminogen activators and decreased synthesis of inhibitors of fibrinolysis (see **Figure 11-4**).

Diagnosis

The laboratory evaluation for hemostatic defects from liver disease is shown in **Table 11-7**.

Idiopathic or Immune Thrombocytopenic Purpura (ITP)

Description

ITP (where the I can stand for either idiopathic or immune) exists in both an acute and a chronic form. The disorder is one in which accelerated platelet destruction occurs in the absence of other causes such as DIC, thrombotic thrombocytopenic purpura (TTP), drug-induced thrombocytopenia, and neonatal thrombocytopenia.

The destruction of platelets in ITP is antibody mediated. The amount of platelet associated IgG is increased in the majority of patients with acute and chronic ITP. Many patients with chronic ITP have increased levels of antiplatelet antibodies in the serum, as well as on the platelet surface. It should be noted that there are a host of disorders unrelated to immune thrombocytopenias, which are associated with increased IgG on the platelet surface. *Helicobacter pylori* infection has been associated with ITP.

In acute ITP, the platelet may be an innocent target of an antipathogen antibody that cross-reacts with an epitope on the platelet membrane. Chronic ITP appears to be more of a classic auto-immune illness in which the target antigens for platelet autoantibodies are platelet glycoproteins. Sequestration and destruction of antibody-coated platelets occur predominantly in the spleen.

Acute ITP usually presents as a childhood illness with peak incidence between 2 and 9 years. It is heralded by a prodromal illness, such as a viral respiratory infection, in 60% to 80% of cases. The infection occurs 2 to 21 days prior to onset of thrombocytopenia. The risk of hemorrhage is greatest during the first 1 to 2 weeks after the onset of acute ITP. Intracranial hemorrhage is the most feared complication of ITP. The majority of patients experience a spontaneous resolution of acute ITP 3 weeks to 3 months after onset. A small percentage of patients do not recover fully after 12 months, and advance to a diagnosis of chronic ITP.

Chronic ITP occurs most commonly between the ages of 20 and 50 years, and in females more often than males (ratio of 2:1 to 3:1). Chronic ITP is characterized by the absence of a prodromal illness and the presence of mild bleeding that may continue for months before medical attention is sought. Manifestations include scattered petechiae or purpura, mostly on distal extremities, mild mucosal bleeding, easy bruising, epistaxis, and menorrhagia. ITP is often discovered in an asymptomatic patient found to have a low platelet count as part of a complete blood count (CBC). The diagnosis of ITP is made only after ruling out other causes for an isolated thrombocytopenia by history, physical examination, and laboratory studies.

Acute ITP usually presents as a childhood illness with peak incidence between 2 and 9 years. Chronic ITP occurs most commonly between the ages of 20 and 50 years, and in females more often than males.

TABLE 11-8   **Laboratory Evaluation for Idiopathic or Immune Thrombocytopenic Purpura (ITP)**

Laboratory Test	Results/Comments
Platelet count	In acute ITP, most cases have <20,000 platelets/μL; in chronic ITP, counts range from 5,000 to 75,000 μL^{-1} commonly, and, on average, are higher than platelet counts in patients with acute ITP
Platelet morphology	Large platelets are often seen on peripheral smear
PT and PTT	Normal
Hemoglobin and hematocrit	May be low if an accompanying blood loss is severe or longstanding; if there is no evidence of blood loss but there is an anemia, the possibility of a concomitant autoimmune hemolytic anemia and thrombocytopenia (Evans syndrome) should be considered
Antiplatelet antibodies	A test for antiplatelet antibodies is not required for diagnosis of ITP; it is generally neither sensitive nor specific for ITP; most patients with acute or chronic ITP will have increased immunoglobulin on the platelet surface; however, many disorders have increased levels of platelet-associated antibodies, including sepsis, drug-induced thrombocytopenia, lymphoproliferative disorders, disseminated intravascular coagulation, and autoimmune diseases; the test for antiplatelet antibodies, using various methodologies, detects small quantities of antibody on the platelet surface (much less antibody than is found on RBCs in patients with a positive direct antiglobulin test result)
Bone marrow aspirate	The bone marrow shows normal RBC and WBC precursors, and a normal or increased number of megakaryocytes; bone marrow platelet production may be increased greatly in an attempt to compensate for rapid platelet destruction

PT, prothrombin time; PTT, partial thromboplastin time.

Diagnosis

See **Table 11–8** for information on the laboratory evaluation for ITP.

Drug-induced Immunologic Thrombocytopenia
Description

Many drugs have been implicated in drug-induced immune thrombocytopenia. However, most cases can be attributed to relatively few drugs, notably heparin, quinidine/quinine, gold salts, and sulfonamides. Exposure to most of these compounds is readily ascertained. However, when obtaining the patient's history, one should include inquiries regarding consumption of over-the-counter medications and topical medications, as well as soft drinks, mixers, and aperitifs to rule out exposure to quinine. The pathogenesis of thrombocytopenia for most drugs involves both the drug and IgG (as the predominant class of antibody involved). A plasma protein bound to the drug serves as the antigen; the antigen combines with a specific antibody, and this complex binds to the platelet membrane. This is known as an "innocent bystander" effect. The antibody-coated platelet is then sequestered and destroyed. Certain other drugs (e.g., protamine, bleomycin, and ristocetin) can cause destruction of platelets by a direct toxic effect that is nonimmune. In heparin-induced thrombocytopenia (HIT), a complex of heparin and a circulating protein derived from the platelet, known as PF4, acts as the antigen. The complex, along with bound antibody, binds to the platelet surface, causing platelet activation, and unlike other drug-induced thrombocytopenias, an increased risk for thrombosis.

The true incidence of drug-induced immunologic thrombocytopenia is not known. The incidence varies with the drug in question and the clinical condition or treatment of the patient. It may be as high as 1% to 3% of people exposed to the drug, as is the case with unfractionated (standard) heparin. Of quinidine users, approximately 1 in 1,000 develop symptomatic thrombocytopenia. Drug-induced immunologic thrombocytopenia occurs most commonly in patients more than 50 years old, but it also has been reported in infants less than 1 year old. It is not possible to predict that patients will develop thrombocytopenia from drug treatment.

Many drugs have been implicated in drug-induced immune thrombocytopenia. However, most cases can be attributed to relatively few drugs, notably heparin, quinidine/quinine, gold salts, and sulfonamides.

TABLE 11–9   Laboratory Evaluation for Drug-Induced Immunologic Thrombocytopenia

Laboratory Test	Results/Comments
Platelet count	Extremely low to slightly low
Tests for drug-dependent antibodies bound to the platelet and for drug-dependent antiplatelet antibodies in the serum unbound to platelets	Both test results are usually positive; however, they may be negative if the reaction is dependent on an in vivo drug metabolite, rather than the parent drug if only the parent drug is used in the laboratory test; an assay for platelet activation by the drug should be positive if the mechanism of thrombocytopenia, in the presence of the drug, includes activation of platelets by antigen–antibody complexes; an in vivo challenge with the suspected drug to confirm toxicity can be extremely dangerous and is rarely, if ever, indicated; there are a variety of methodologies for tests assessing drug-induced platelet activation, including flow cytometry and the measurement of serotonin released from activated platelets; an ELISA assay for HIT detects antibodies to heparin–platelet factor 4 complexes

Ingestion of a drug that induces thrombocytopenia may produce flushing, fever, headache, and chills prior to onset of thrombocytopenia. The onset of thrombocytopenia may be abrupt following drug exposure or, if it requires antibody generation to lower the platelet count, it may be delayed for 7 to 10 days. Anamnestic responses may occur and if they arise, the delay is shorter. Bleeding may occur as early as 6 to 12 hours after exposure to the drug in highly responsive patients. Bleeding manifestations may include 1 or more of the following: petechiae, purpura (usually the first symptom), mucosal hemorrhagic bullae, gastrointestinal or genitourinary hemorrhage, intrapulmonary hemorrhage, and lastly, intracranial hemorrhage, which is rare, but often lethal. HIT is unique in that bleeding is uncommon, and as noted above, HIT patients are at risk for thrombosis rather than bleeding.

> Heparin-induced thrombocytopenia is unique in that bleeding is uncommon, HIT patients are at risk for thrombosis rather than bleeding.

Diagnosis

See Table 11–9 for information on the laboratory evaluation for drug-induced immunologic thrombocytopenia. Laboratory tests for drug-induced thrombocytopenia are not routinely available, with the exception of testing for HIT. If HIT is considered, a platelet count should be performed first. If the platelet count decreases to 50% or less of its apparent baseline value, a test for antibodies to the heparin–PF4 complex or a functional test that shows platelet activation in the presence of heparin and the patient's plasma should be performed.

Posttransfusion Purpura

Description

Posttransfusion purpura (PTP) is a syndrome characterized by the sudden onset of thrombocytopenia 7 to 10 days following transfusion of blood or blood products containing platelets or platelet material. The thrombocytopenia appears to be due to antibody-mediated destruction of autologous as well as transfused platelets. The disorder is rare. In over 90% of cases, the antibody that develops in the affected individuals is directed against the antigen HPA-1a, formerly known as Pl^{A1}, on platelet membrane glycoprotein IIIa. In these cases, the recipient's own platelets are HPA-1a negative. It is not known why there is destruction of the patient's own HPA-1a-negative platelets following platelet transfusion with HPA-1a-positive platelets. Only 2% to 3% of the population in the United States lacks this antigen. Antibodies against other platelet-specific antigens have been reported in PTP, but they are much less commonly encountered. In almost all cases, the development of anti-HPA-1a antibody is thought to be an anamnestic response, with prior sensitization occurring through previous transfusion or pregnancy.

PTP occurs predominantly in females, perhaps due to the likelihood of sensitization through pregnancy. The interval between the first exposure to the HPA-1a antigen and the transfusion

TABLE 11–10   Laboratory Evaluation for Posttransfusion Purpura

Laboratory Test	Results/Comments
PT and PTT	Normal
Platelet count	Usually decreased to <10,000 μL^{-1}
Tests for antiplatelet antibodies in the serum	Positive (see below)
Test for HPA-1a antigen on platelets in cases involving the HPA-1a antigen	The HPA-1a antigen is absent from the patient's platelets; anti-HPA-1a antibody is present in the patient's serum in the majority of cases and an attempt should be made to demonstrate the specificity of this antibody to HPA-1a

PT, prothrombin time; PTT, partial thromboplastin time.

that incites the thrombocytopenia is greater than 3 years in most cases in which the information has been reported. The onset of thrombocytopenia is fulminant in most cases, with the platelet count decreasing to <10,000 μL^{-1}. Hemorrhage usually begins with purpura and mucocutaneous bleeding, and may progress to gastrointestinal and genitourinary bleeding, epistaxis, oozing from intravenous access sites, and intracranial hemorrhage. In severely affected patients sustained with supportive therapy of red blood cells and/or platelets, the thrombocytopenia usually begins to resolve in 14 days (mean value with a range 1 to 35 days). Cases with less severe thrombocytopenia apparently require a longer recovery period (24 days average, range 6 to 70 days). The outcome is fatal in approximately 10% of cases, usually due to hemorrhage. The risk of fatal hemorrhage appears to be greatest at the onset of the disease. Recurrent PTP has been documented, with the recurrence appearing no sooner than 3 years after the first episode, even though antibody may persist in the patient's blood during the intervening time and there may be repeated challenges with exogenous platelets.

Diagnosis

See **Table 11–10** for information on the laboratory evaluation for PTP.

Neonatal Alloimmune Thrombocytopenia (NAIT)

Description

NAIT is a disorder in which there is destruction of platelets in the fetus and newborn. The destruction occurs following transplacental passage of maternal IgG antibodies directed against a platelet-specific antigen present on fetal platelets and absent from the mother's platelets. The antibody-coated platelets are removed from the circulation by the neonate's reticuloendothelial system around the time of birth. The estimated incidence ranges from 1 in 5,000 to 1 in 2,000 births, with an increasingly higher incidence in recent years attributed to improved surveillance and serologic testing for the disorder. The platelet-specific antigen implicated in 80% to 90% of all cases (and 95% of symptomatic cases) of NAIT is HPA-1a. As previously noted, this antigen is present on the platelets of 97% to 98% of the general population. In approximately 50% of cases, NAIT occurs during the first pregnancy; when it does occur, there is a 97% chance that the next pregnancy will be affected.

Affected newborns are usually the product of an otherwise uncomplicated pregnancy and delivery. Within hours after birth, petechiae and ecchymoses appear in a generalized distribution. Other clinical signs include neurologic abnormalities if intracranial hemorrhage occurs, and pallor from anemia, if the bleeding is severe. Intracranial hemorrhage is the leading cause of death in NAIT, with a 50% mortality. Overall mortality from NAIT is approximately 5% to 10%. Thrombocytopenia usually persists for approximately 2 weeks in untreated cases (range of 1 week to 2 months), and 1 week in treated cases.

Diagnosis

See **Table 11–11** for information on the laboratory evaluation for NAIT.

Neonatal alloimmune thrombocytopenic purpura is a disorder in which there is destruction of platelets in the fetus and newborn. The destruction occurs following transplacental passage of maternal IgG antibodies directed against a platelet-specific antigen present on fetal platelets and absent from the mother's platelets.

TABLE 11-11   Laboratory Evaluation for Neonatal Alloimmune Thrombocytopenia (NAIT)

Laboratory Test	Results/Comments
PT and PTT	Normal
Platelet count (in infants)	Normal to slightly decreased at birth, continues to increase after birth with gradual decline beginning several hours after birth; many cases show only mild thrombocytopenia, but most symptomatic cases have <30,000 platelets/μL; approximately 50% have <20,000 platelets/μL; returns to normal within 2–3 weeks
Hemoglobin/hematocrit	May be decreased with hemorrhage
Anti-HPA-1a antibodies (in HPA-1a-related cases)	A mother with HPA-1a-negative platelets is positive for the anti-HPA-1 antibody in serum

PT, prothrombin time; PTT, partial thromboplastin time.

Discussions of TTP and hemolytic–uremic syndrome (HUS), which are thrombocytopenias associated with thrombosis, are presented among the thrombotic disorders.

Essential Thrombocythemia

Description

Essential thrombocythemia is a chronic myeloproliferative disorder, characterized by thrombocytosis arising from the clonal proliferation of a neoplastic multipotent stem cell. Life expectancy can be essentially normal with a median survival of 10 to 15 years, but the disease course is frequently complicated by both hemorrhage and thrombosis. A small percentage (<5%) of patients progress to acute leukemia, predominantly those patients previously treated with radioactive phosphorus or alkylating agents to reduce their platelet counts. At the time of diagnosis using older criteria, mild splenomegaly occurs in 30% to 50% of patients, and hepatomegaly in 15% to 20%. Using 2008 WHO diagnostic criteria, splenomegaly is present in only a minority of patients at diagnosis. The incidence of the disorder is higher in older age groups.

The principal diagnostic feature of essential thrombocythemia is a persistently elevated platelet count with bone marrow megakaryocyte hyperplasia. Patients with this disorder can progress to a "spent" phase, characterized by myelofibrosis and a low platelet count. The purpose of the laboratory testing is to eliminate other possible etiologies for the thrombocytosis. Other entities in the differential diagnosis of an elevated platelet count include reactive thrombocytosis and other myeloproliferative disorders—myelofibrosis, polycythemia vera, and chronic myelogenous leukemia.

Diagnosis

See **Table 11-12** for information on the laboratory evaluation for essential thrombocythemia.

von Willebrand Disease

Description

vWD is caused by a quantitative deficiency of normal vWF in the majority of cases and a qualitatively abnormal vWF in the remainder of cases. vWF normally polymerizes to form multimers, which are aggregates of a single vWF polypeptide; in normal plasma, the multimers have a range of sizes. vWF has 2 major roles:

- Platelet adhesion: Large multimers of vWF (i.e., those with many units of the single polypeptide) effectively promote platelet adhesion to the subendothelium in injured vessels; if only small multimers are present, platelet plugs form poorly.
- Binding of Factor VIII: vWF circulates in the plasma with Factor VIII, the coagulant protein that is lacking in hemophilia A. vWF prolongs the half-life of Factor VIII by protecting it from rapid degradation. If vWF is reduced, Factor VIII coagulant activity is often reduced as well.

von Willebrand disease is caused by a quantitative deficiency of normal von Willebrand factor in the majority of cases and a qualitatively abnormal von Willebrand factor in the remainder of cases.

TABLE 11–12   Laboratory Evaluation for Essential Thrombocythemia (ET)

Laboratory Test	Results/Comments
Platelet count	[a]Sustained platelet count >450,000 μL^{-1}
Hemoglobin	[a]Lack of elevation in hemoglobin helps exclude polycythemia vera
DNA testing	[a]*JAK2* V617F or other clonal marker [a]Absence of *BCR-ABL* (to exclude chronic myelogenous leukemia)
Bone marrow biopsy	[a]Proliferation mainly of the megakaryocytic lineage with increased numbers of enlarged, mature megakaryocytes. No significant increase or left shift of neutrophil or red cell lineages. Absence of fibrosis helps exclude myelofibrosis
Platelet aggregation	Does not contribute to diagnosis, but platelets may be hypoaggregable or hyperaggregable
Acute phase reactants	Elevated acute phase reactants, such as C-reactive protein or fibrinogen, raise the possibility that the thrombocytosis is reactive rather than ET. Causes of reactive thrombocytosis include iron deficiency, splenectomy, surgery, infection, inflammation, connective tissue disease, malignancy, and other causes ([a]if *JAK2* V617F is absent, the diagnosis requires absence of evidence for reactive thrombocytosis; however, the presence of reactive thrombocytosis does not exclude ET if all of the other requirements are present)

[a]Required for diagnosis according to 2000 WHO guidelines.

TABLE 11–13   Classification of von Willebrand Disease (vWD)

Type (Newer Terminology) and Description of Defect	Type and Subtypes in Older Terminology
1: Partial quantitative deficiency of vWF	I
2: Qualitative defects in vWF	II
2A: Absence of high-molecular-weight multimers in plasma due to a defect in vWF	IIa
2B: Absence of high-molecular-weight multimers due to increased affinity of abnormal vWF for platelet glycoprotein Ib	IIb
2M: Decreased vWF function without the loss of high-molecular-weight multimers	Not previously designated
2N: Decreased affinity for Factor VIII ("autosomal hemophilia")	Normandy
3: Severe quantitative deficiency of vWF	III
Platelet-type vWD: Absence of high-molecular-weight multimers in plasma due to increased affinity of normal vWF by abnormal platelet vWF receptor	Platelet-type vWD
Acquired vWD: Reduction in plasma vWF associated with the presence of an underlying disease that leads to removal of vWF from the circulation	Acquired vWD

vWF, von Willebrand factor.

vWD prevalence estimates vary, with reported values as high as 1% of the general population. Unlike hemophilia A and B, vWD affects both men and women.

vWD prevalence estimates vary, with reported values as high as 1% of the general population. Unlike hemophilia A and B, vWD affects both men and women. It is likely to be the most common inherited bleeding disorder. There are 3 major types of vWD. The types were reorganized and renumbered with Arabic numerals in the 1990s (see **Table 11–13**). The most common type (type 1) is usually a mild bleeding disorder; it accounts for the majority of all cases of vWD. Type 2 vWD includes patients with qualitative vWF defects. Type 3 is rare and inherited as an autosomal recessive trait. It is associated with severe bleeding and very low to absent vWF levels. The types are distinguished from each other by laboratory testing.

TABLE 11-14 Laboratory Evaluation for von Willebrand Disease (vWD)

Laboratory Test	Results/Comments
Ristocetin cofactor activity (vWF:RCo)	A functional assay for vWF; assesses the ability of normal platelets to aggregate in the presence of ristocetin; normal aggregability to ristocetin requires large multimers of vWF
von Willebrand factor antigen (vWF:Ag)	An immunologic assay for vWF; assesses the quantity (not the function) of vWF
Factor VIII coagulant activity (Factor VIII)	Factor VIII becomes decreased secondary to the low vWF; if it is low enough, decreased Factor VIII coagulant activity is associated with a prolonged PTT
vWF multimer analysis	vWF multimer analysis assesses the size distribution of vWF multimers; an abnormal distribution of multimers occurs in type 2A and type 2B vWD

PTT, partial thromboplastin time; vWF, von Willebrand factor.

It should also be noted that the mean vWF levels vary with blood type as shown in the following table:

Blood group	Mean vWF (%)
O	75
A	106
B	117
AB	123

More than 65% of patients with vWD have type O, presumably because patients with this blood type start from a lower baseline value for vWF.

The severity of bleeding is highly variable among patients, even within the same subtype of vWD, and even within an individual patient over time. Typically, bleeding manifestations such as easy bruising or epistaxis begin in early childhood. Other manifestations include menorrhagia and mucous membrane bleeding (from the gingiva, oropharynx, and gastrointestinal and genitourinary tracts). Profuse hemorrhage may occur with a significant hemostatic challenge such as trauma or surgery.

Diagnosis

Laboratory test results vary with the type and subtype of vWD. Like the severity of bleeding, the laboratory values can also vary widely over time for an individual patient, and may sometimes be normal. Normal results from a single determination do not rule out the diagnosis. If the patient history strongly suggests vWD, and the test results are normal, the tests should be repeated at a later time because plasma levels for vWF are increased during pregnancy, stress, while receiving oral contraceptives, and during an acute illness or injury. Therefore, values obtained at these times may be unreliable for diagnosis. It is also not yet clear if the absolute level of vWF or the level relative to the mean vWF for the blood type of the patient is more important in establishing the diagnosis. Current guidelines note that the absolute level of vWF seems to be more important than the level relative to blood type.

See **Table 11-14** for information on the laboratory evaluation for vWD.

If the patient history strongly suggests vWD, and the test results are normal, the tests should be repeated at a later time because plasma levels for vWF are increased during pregnancy, stress, while receiving oral contraceptives, and during an acute illness or injury.

Selected von Willebrand Disease Types, Subtypes, and Their Expected Test Results

- Type 1: vWF multimers of all sizes are decreased due to a defect in synthesis or release of vWF from the endothelium, the site of most vWF synthesis. Functional (ristocetin cofactor or vWF:RCo) and antigenic (von Willebrand factor antigen or vWF:Ag) levels of vWF are usually proportionately decreased. Factor VIII activity might also be low. The vWF multimer pattern shows a normal distribution of multimers.

- Type 2A: Absence of large and intermediate-size vWF multimers from the plasma and platelet surface, due to a defect in the synthesis or polymerization of multimers, or from increased proteolysis of multimers. Functional activity (vWF:RCo) is decreased compared to antigenic levels (vWF:Ag). Therefore, vWF:RCo < vWF:Ag < Factor VIII is the most commonly observed pattern in type 2A. The vWF multimer pattern shows an abnormal distribution of multimers, with the absence of large and intermediate size multimers.
- Type 2B: Marked deficiency of large vWF multimers from plasma. Intermediate size multimers are present. Large multimers are present on the patient's platelets, due to increased affinity of the abnormal vWF molecule for the platelet surface. Functional and antigenic levels in plasma samples are similar to those in type 2A (vWF:RCo < vWF:Ag < Factor VIII). The vWF multimer pattern shows the absence of large multimers from plasma. The patient's platelets show increased aggregation at low concentrations of ristocetin that do not cause normal platelets to aggregate. The patient's platelets aggregate at low concentrations of ristocetin because they are coated with large vWF multimers.

Types 2M and 2N are uncommon and are briefly described in **Table 11–13**.

- Type 3: Severe deficiency of all vWF multimers, due to a marked defect in synthesis. Factor VIII activity is less severely affected than vWF activity. Both functional and antigenic vWF levels are markedly reduced. The vWF multimer pattern shows a virtual absence of all-size multimers.
- Platelet-type Willebrand disease: vWF is qualitatively normal, but abnormal platelets have an increased affinity for large multimers of vWF due to a defect in platelet glycoprotein Ib. The laboratory test values are similar to those in type 2B.
- Acquired vWD: This disorder has been found in patients with systemic lupus erythematosus, multiple myeloma, Waldenström macroglobulinemia, lymphoproliferative disorders, and other diseases. Patients have no congenital or familial history of bleeding. The decrease in circulating vWF can result from adsorption of large multimers onto cells (e.g., lymphocytes or tumor cells) or from the presence of neutralizing antibodies to vWF. Acquired vWD resolves when the underlying disorder is effectively treated.

Bernard–Soulier Disease and Glanzmann Thrombasthenia

Description

Bernard–Soulier **syndrome and Glanzmann Thrombasthenia are rare congenital hemorrhagic disorders that result from absent or defective specific platelet membrane glycoproteins, impairing platelet function.**

Bernard–Soulier syndrome (BS) and GT are rare congenital hemorrhagic disorders that result from absent or defective specific platelet membrane glycoproteins, impairing platelet function. BS is characterized by a decrease of functional glycoprotein 1b/IX/V, the platelet receptor for vWF. GT is characterized by a decrease of functional GP IIb/IIIa, the complex that binds fibrinogen to the platelet surface when platelets are activated.

GT often decreases in severity with age. Manifestations include easy bruising, epistaxis, mucous membrane bleeding—particularly in the gastrointestinal tract, and menorrhagia. The amount of hemorrhage is highly variable among affected patients.

Diagnosis

See **Table 11–15** for information on the laboratory evaluation for BS and GT.

Platelet Storage Pool Disease

Description

Platelet SPD represents a group of disorders in which there is a deficiency of platelet granules. Decreased secretion of platelet granular contents at the time of platelet activation makes the platelets less hemostatically effective. The congenital forms of SPD include:

- Delta SPD: platelets have a decreased number of delta (dense) granules; these secretory granules contain ADP, serotonin, and calcium.
- Alpha-delta or alpha-partial delta SPD: decreased number of delta granules with either a complete or partial deficiency of alpha granules; alpha granules contain many proteins including fibrinogen, PF4, platelet-derived growth factor, and beta-thromboglobulin.

TABLE 11–15 **Laboratory Evaluation for Bernard–Soulier Disease and Glanzmann Thrombasthenia**

Laboratory Test	Results/Comments
Platelet count	Slightly to moderately decreased in BS, occasionally normal; in GT, the platelet count is usually normal, but may be slightly decreased
Platelet morphology on peripheral smear	In BS, the platelets are very large (>80% of platelets are >2.5 mm in diameter) accounting for the synonym for this disorder as the "giant platelet syndrome"; in GT, platelets usually appear normal
PT and PTT	Normal
Platelet aggregation studies	In BS, there is decreased aggregation with ristocetin, but a normal response with epinephrine, ADP, arachidonic acid, and collagen; in GT, aggregation is absent (with nearly flat line tracings) with epinephrine, ADP, collagen, and arachidonic acid, but there is normal aggregation with ristocetin
Quantitative tests for platelet glycoproteins	BS patients have low amounts of glycoprotein Ib/IX; GT patients have low amounts of glycoprotein IIb/IIIa

ADP, adenosine diphosphate; BS; Bernard–Soulier disease; GT, Glanzmann thrombasthenia; PT, prothrombin time; PTT, partial thromboplastin time.

- Alpha SPD ("gray platelet syndrome"): decreased number of alpha granules, and a normal number of delta granules; platelets appear gray, large, and vacuolated on a peripheral blood smear.

SPD also may occur as an acquired abnormality, acutely in patients who have been supported on a cardiopulmonary bypass device and chronically in some cases of acute leukemia and myeloproliferative disorders. The molecular basis of most types of congenital SPD is unknown. It may result from abnormal granule morphogenesis or abnormal granule maturation in megakaryocytes. SPD may be a manifestation of a global defect in granule formation as in the Hermansky–Pudlak syndrome (see below). Hereditary SPD is the most common congenital qualitative platelet disorder, but it is still quite rare.

Most patients with SPD have mild bleeding symptoms. Bleeding manifestations of SPD include mild mucous membrane bleeding, easy bruising, menorrhagia, and excessive bleeding following dental or general surgery. SPD may also occur as a component of the following syndromes:

- Hermansky–Pudlak syndrome: Features include delta SPD, oculocutaneous albinism, pulmonary fibrosis, and the accumulation of ceroid-like material in cells of the reticuloendothelial system. One subtype is due to a defective gene (called HSP1) on chromosome 10.
- Chediak–Higashi syndrome: Features include delta SPD with giant platelet granules, photophobia, nystagmus, pseudoalbinism, lymphadenopathy, splenomegaly, and increased susceptibility to infection. It is attributed to defects in a gene called CHS1 on chromosome 1, affecting protein trafficking.
- Thrombocytopenia with absent radius: Features include alpha SPD and absence of the radius bone.
- Wiskott–Aldrich syndrome: Features of this X-linked recessive disorder include delta SPD with other metabolic platelet defects, recurrent infections, eczema, lymphocytopenia, multiple cellular and humoral immunologic defects, and thrombocytopenia with microplatelets (small platelets); the thrombocytopenia may resolve following splenectomy. It is attributed to a genetic defect in a gene called WASP on the X chromosome, affecting signal transduction and other functions.

Most patients with storage pool disease have mild bleeding symptoms. Bleeding manifestations of SPD include mild mucous membrane bleeding, easy bruising, menorrhagia, and excessive bleeding following dental or general surgery.

TABLE 11–16   Laboratory Evaluation for Storage Pool Deficiency

Laboratory Test	Results/Comments
PT and PTT	Normal
Platelet count	Variable
Peripheral blood smear	Shows thrombocytopenia with large, gray, vacuolated platelets in alpha SPD; giant granules in platelets, neutrophils, eosinophils, lymphocytes, and monocytes in Chediak–Higashi syndrome; microplatelets and thrombocytopenia in Wiskott–Aldrich syndrome
Platelet aggregation studies	Absent or extreme diminution of the secondary wave of aggregation with ADP and epinephrine
Platelet ATP/ADP ratio	Increase in delta granule deficiency due to low ADP in these platelets
Electron microscopy of circulating platelets	May reveal a decrease in alpha granules, delta granules, or both
Alpha granule quantitation	Alpha granule contents may be assayed by measuring the amount of platelet beta-thromboglobulin or platelet factor 4, both of which are normally present in alpha granules

ADP, adenosine diphosphate; ATP, adenosine triphosphate; PT, prothrombin time; PTT, partial thromboplastin time; SPD, storage pool deficiency.

TABLE 11–17   Laboratory Evaluation for Hemostatic Defects in Uremia

Laboratory Test	Results/Comments
PT and PTT	Normal
Platelet count	May be decreased, but it is rarely <80,000 µL^{-1}; hemodialysis can exacerbate the thrombocytopenia, but the function of the platelets may improve
Platelet aggregation studies	No typical pattern of responses to platelet agonists; decreased response to ADP, collagen, and epinephrine often observed

ADP, adenosine diphosphate; PT, prothrombin time; PTT, partial thromboplastin time.

Diagnosis

See **Table 11–16** for information on the laboratory evaluation for storage pool deficiency.

Hemostatic Defects in Uremia
Description

The bleeding tendency in uremia-induced hemorrhage is attributed to platelet dysfunction and endothelial cell dysfunction.

Bleeding manifestations may be mild or severe and can include petechiae, ecchymoses, epistaxis, and purpura. Paradoxically, chronic renal failure is also associated with an increased incidence of arterial and venous thrombosis, and, therefore, can influence hemostasis toward bleeding or clotting.

Diagnosis

See **Table 11–17** for information on the laboratory evaluation for hemostatic defects in uremia.

Drug-induced Qualitative Platelet Disorders
Description

Platelet dysfunction may occur on ingestion of a wide variety of drugs, particularly aspirin and clopidigrel (Plavix). Due to the ubiquity of aspirin in over-the-counter medications, many

> The bleeding tendency in uremia-induced hemorrhage is attributed to platelet dysfunction and endothelial cell dysfunction. Bleeding manifestations may be mild or severe and can include petechiae, ecchymoses, epistaxis, and purpura.

TABLE 11–18   Drug-induced Qualitative Platelet Disorders

Laboratory Test	Results/Comments
Platelet count	The platelet count is necessary to identify an underlying thrombocytopenia, if one exists, which is aggravated by a drug effect
PT and PTT, von Willebrand factor antigen, and ristocetin cofactor	Abnormal only if there is an underlying coagulation factor abnormality
Platelet aggregation studies	Abnormal platelet aggregation may be observed in patients exposed to certain drugs in vivo, especially to weak platelet agonists such as epinephrine; however, the presence of abnormal aggregation does not correlate well with the risk of bleeding

PT, prothrombin time; PTT, partial thromboplastin time.

medications are implicated in platelet dysfunction. Some patients consume multiple drugs, such as aspirin and clopidigrel, with different and additive antiplatelet effects and thereby inhibit platelet function by more than 1 mechanism. Drug-induced platelet dysfunction can present a high bleeding risk in patients with existing hemostatic defects, but typically does not result in clinically significant bleeding in normal individuals. When hemorrhage does occur, there is usually an underlying hemostatic disorder affecting either the platelets or coagulation factors, or an anatomic lesion, such as an ulcer, that predisposes the patient to bleeding.

Commonly encountered coagulopathies that place patients at risk for bleeding when there is a superimposed drug-induced platelet defect include vWD, thrombocytopenia of any cause, and anticoagulation therapy. Hemorrhagic manifestations can include petechiae and purpura, ecchymoses, mucosal membrane bleeding, hematuria, epistaxis, and oozing from intravenous access sites and surgical incisions.

Diagnosis

Laboratory tests are of little value in predicting the clinical significance of drug-induced platelet defects. They can confirm the presence of abnormal platelet function, but cannot assess the risk of bleeding. Furthermore, laboratory abnormalities in platelet function are not specific for a particular drug. See **Table 11–18** for information on the laboratory evaluation for drug-induced platelet defects.

THROMBOTIC DISORDERS

In this chapter, the disorders associated with thrombosis (**Figure 11–5**) are grouped into those with a relatively higher prevalence and those with a relatively lower prevalence. Among those with a higher prevalence is activated protein C resistance, which is produced by the Factor V Leiden mutation. This mutation is present in 3% to 5% of Caucasian populations. Other thrombotic disorders with a high prevalence are the prothrombin G20210A mutation, and the antiphospholipid antibody syndrome (an acquired disorder). The thrombotic disorders with a lower prevalence include protein C deficiency, protein S deficiency, and antithrombin deficiency. Markedly elevated plasma homocysteine levels may also increase the risk for thrombosis, but it is unlikely that modest elevations contribute to thrombotic risk. Plasminogen deficiency is also rare, and its association with thrombosis is controversial. Two other rare conditions, dysfibrinogenemia of certain types and essential thrombocythemia, can produce either thrombosis or bleeding. Also rare are TTP and HUS.

Hypercoagulable States

Description

Hypercoagulable states are associated with an increased risk for thrombosis (**Table 11–19**). There are both hereditary and acquired hypercoagulable states. Hereditary forms are characterized by a thrombotic tendency that may become manifest at any age. They may arise from a quantitative or qualitative deficiency of a regulatory anticoagulant protein, such as protein C, protein S, or

The disorders associated with thrombosis are grouped into those with a relatively higher prevalence and those with a relatively lower prevalence. Among those with a higher prevalence is activated protein C resistance, which is produced by the Factor V Leiden mutation, the prothrombin G20210A mutation, and the antiphospholipid antibody syndrome (an acquired disorder).

TABLE 11–19   Laboratory Evaluation for Hypercoagulable States

Hypercoagulable State	Incidence in General Population	Site of Thrombosis	Relevant Laboratory Test Results	Comments
Inherited				
Activated protein C resistance (nearly always associated with the presence of the Factor V Leiden mutation)	3%–5% in Caucasians	Venous (arterial thrombosis risk uncertain)	Positive activated protein C resistance test; DNA test positive for Factor V Leiden	Uncommon in those of African and Asian descent
Prothrombin G20210A mutation	1.5%–3% in Caucasians	Predominantly venous	DNA test positive for the prothrombin G20210A	Uncommon in those of African and Asian descent
Hyperhomocysteinemia (congenital forms with extremely high values)	Extremely rare	Venous and arterial; often with atherosclerosis	Markedly elevated homocysteine	It has not been shown that vitamins decrease thrombotic risk
Protein C deficiency[a] (congenital deficiency only)	0.2%–0.4%	Predominantly venous	Low functional and/or antigenic protein C	Risk of warfarin-induced skin necrosis if anticoagulation is initiated with warfarin in the absence of heparin
Protein S deficiency[a] (congenital deficiency only)	0.2%–0.4%	Predominantly venous	Low functional and/or antigenic protein S	Estrogen, pregnancy, and oral contraceptives cause acquired decreases, as do acute phase reactions
Antithrombin deficiency[a] (congenital deficiency only)	0.01%–0.02%	Predominantly venous	Low functional and/or antigenic antithrombin	Heparin use can cause an acquired deficiency
Acquired				
Antiphospholipid antibody (APA) (the presence of a lupus anticoagulant, an anticardiolipin antibody, and/or anti-beta 2 glycoprotein I antibody)	1%–5% in the general population; much higher incidence in groups with certain underlying conditions, especially systemic lupus erythematosus; higher incidence with age	Venous and arterial	Positive test results for lupus anticoagulant and/or anticardiolipin antibody, and/or anti-beta 2 glycoprotein I antibody	To make a diagnosis of antiphospholipid syndrome, test results for the lupus anticoagulant, anticardiolipin antibody, and/or anti-beta 2 glycoprotein I antibody must be positive on 2 separate occasions 12 weeks apart, in the setting of thrombosis, or specific pregnancy complications
Selected other acquired predisposing conditions for thrombosis				

For venous thromboembolism: postoperative state, immobility, trauma, obesity, congestive heart failure, pregnancy and postpartum state, estrogen and progesterone use, nephrotic syndrome, L-asparaginase therapy, infection, prolonged travel, dehydration, smoking, and malignancy

For arterial thromboembolism: atherosclerosis, damaged endothelium, bypass grafts, cardiac emboli (from atrial fibrillation, mitral stenosis, or mural thrombus following myocardial infarction), and arteritis

For both venous and arterial thromboembolism: disseminated intravascular coagulation, malignancy, myeloproliferative disorders, systemic lupus erythematosus, paroxysmal nocturnal hemoglobinuria, and heparin-induced thrombocytopenia

[a] If protein C and protein S are both decreased, vitamin K deficiency or warfarin intake should be considered, especially if the prothrombin time is prolonged; if protein C, protein S, and antithrombin are all decreased, decreased synthesis of these proteins from liver disease, or recent/active clotting with consumption of the factors, may be the explanation.

antithrombin (see **Figures 11–2** and **11–3**). Activated protein C resistance is caused by a mutation in the Factor V molecule (nearly always the Factor V Leiden mutation), which prevents activated protein C-mediated inactivation of Factor Va. The prothrombin G20210A mutation is prevalent in Caucasian populations, such as Factor V Leiden. Prothrombin G20210A is a mutation in the promoter of the prothrombin gene, causing increased synthesis of prothrombin (Factor II). Observational studies have shown that hyperhomocysteinemia, a disorder in which there is an abnormally high level of plasma homocysteine, can be hereditary or acquired. Hyperhomocysteinemic individuals are at increased risk for coronary artery disease and deep venous thrombosis. However, studies have not yet shown that reducing slightly or moderately elevated homocysteine with vitamin therapy reduces the thrombotic risk. A block in the pathway at any 1 of the several steps results in the accumulation of homocysteine. When the homocysteine level is manyfold higher than the upper limit of normal, this very high value may contribute to the damaging effects on the blood vessel wall. Acquired hypercoagulable states arise from a diverse array of clinical conditions. They include malignancy, immobilization, surgery, trauma, obesity, smoking, infection, prolonged travel, and the use of oral contraceptives, estrogen replacement therapy, and progesterone, among many others. An acquired hypercoagulable state for which specific coagulation testing is available is the antiphospholipid antibody syndrome.

The presence of 1 hypercoagulable condition alone is not usually sufficient to initiate thrombosis. The presence of a second (or more), superimposed hypercoagulable condition (often called a "second hit") appears to be required to provoke a thrombotic event. For example, a person with activated protein C resistance may not experience a thrombotic event until suffering major trauma as a "second hit."

Diagnosis

Laboratory testing for hypercoagulable states is most often performed for patients presenting with a personal or family history of thrombosis. The laboratory evaluation for hereditary hypercoagulable states is best performed as a panel of test results. The most common disorders are activated protein C resistance (caused nearly always by Factor V Leiden) and prothrombin G20210A, and the less common are deficiencies of protein C, protein S, and antithrombin. Frequently, antiphospholipid antibody testing is performed in conjunction with the tests for hereditary hypercoagulable disorders. If all of these tests are negative and the clinical suspicion for a congenital hypercoagulable state remains high, additional testing for the more rare hypercoagulable disorders can be performed. There are many acquired conditions or treatments that reduce the level of protein C, protein S, and antithrombin in the test panel for hypercoagulability, but despite this, the risk for thrombosis is not significantly increased on that basis. For example, warfarin reduces the levels of protein C and protein S but reduces thrombotic risk. Antithrombin is lowered by heparin therapy. Pregnancy, oral contraceptives, and estrogen therapy can all decrease the activity of protein S, although they can induce a hypercoagulable state by other mechanisms. Active clot formation, liver dysfunction, or DIC can lower protein C, protein S, and antithrombin. In situations where such a confounding variable exists that alters the level of protein C, protein S, or antithrombin, the tests should be repeated (if possible) when the variable is no longer present to obtain the patient's true baseline values. This should allow determination of whether a heritable deficiency of any of the following 3 proteins truly exists:

- Activated protein C resistance: Usually, the first assay performed is a functional assay for activated protein C resistance. If the result is abnormal, genetic analysis is performed, to confirm whether Factor V Leiden is present in the heterozygous state, present in the homozygous state, or absent.
- Prothrombin G20210A: This mutation is identified by genetic analysis that can specifically identify heterozygous and homozygous states.
- Hyperhomocysteinemia: Plasma homocysteine levels are measured by a variety of automated methods.
- Protein C, protein S, and antithrombin deficiencies: Individual functional assays to measure the activity of these endogenous anticoagulant proteins detect both qualitative (normal number of abnormally functioning molecules) and quantitative (low number of normally functioning molecules) deficiencies. In contrast, an antigenic (immunologic) assay, which measures only the quantity of protein present, can detect quantitative but not

qualitative deficiencies. Therefore, the first assay performed should be a functional assay. If the result is abnormal, an antigenic assay can be performed to determine if the cause of the decreased activity is a quantitative or qualitative deficiency of the protein.

- LA (an antiphospholipid antibody): A variety of tests can be used to detect a LA. This antibody interferes with the cofactor action of phospholipid in the coagulation cascade in laboratory assays only (see the section "Antiphospholipid Antibodies: The Lupus Anticoagulant, Anticardiolipin, and Beta-2 Glycoprotein I Antibodies"). Various phospholipid-dependent coagulation test times, especially PTT-based or dilute Russell viper venom time (DRVVT) assays, can be used. The DRVVT is the clotting time obtained using Russell viper venom, which contains a Factor X activator.
- Anticardiolipin antibody or beta-2 glycoprotein I antibody (antiphospholipid antibodies): These antiphospholipid antibodies may or may not be associated with the presence of a LA (see the section "Antiphospholipid Antibodies: The Lupus Anticoagulant, Anticardiolipin, and Beta-2 Glycoprotein I Antibodies"), and they are detected by enzyme-linked immunoassays.

See **Table 11–19** for characteristics of the hypercoagulable states.

Antiphospholipid Antibodies: The Lupus Anticoagulant, Anticardiolipin, and Beta-2 Glycoprotein I Antibodies
Description

Antiphospholipid antibodies recognize specific phospholipid–protein complexes rather than phospholipid alone. They can be immunoglobulin type IgG or IgM, or less commonly, IgA. The LA is an immunoglobulin that can interfere with phospholipid-dependent coagulation reactions in laboratory assays without inhibiting the activity of any specific coagulation factor. It targets phospholipids bound to prothrombin, beta-2 glycoprotein I, protein C, protein S, or other proteins bound to phospholipids. Anticardiolipin antibodies are another type of antiphospholipid antibody, which target beta-2-glycoprotein I bound to a particular phospholipid, cardiolipin; these can be detected by anticardiolipin antibody immunoassays. Anti-beta 2 glycoprotein I antibodies are another type of antiphospholipid antibody that target anti-beta 2 glycoprotein I in the presence or absence of phospholipid.

An antiphospholipid antibody may occur in apparently healthy individuals with no detectable illness. It also occurs in patients with a variety of clinical conditions or disorders including:

- systemic lupus erythematosus and other autoimmune disorders;
- malignancy;
- following ingestion of selected drugs (procainamide, quinidine, phenytoin, chlorpromazine, valproic acid, amoxicillin, augmentin, hydralazine, streptomycin, and propranolol have all been reported to induce an LA);
- infectious diseases—bacterial (including spirochetal and mycobacterial), viral, fungal, and protozoal infections;
- following vaccination.

A lupus anticoagulant is the most common cause of a prolonged PTT that remains prolonged in a PTT mixing study (a PTT performed on a sample of mixed patient and normal plasma).

Estimates of prevalence have been highly variable because results are completely dependent on the test(s) used for detection of antiphospholipid antibodies, and some methods are more sensitive than others. Approximately 2% of patients with a prolonged PTT will have an LA as the cause of the prolongation. LA is the most common cause of a prolonged PTT that remains prolonged in a PTT mixing study (a PTT performed on a sample of mixed patient and normal plasma). It is estimated that 1% to 5% of the general population has an antiphospholipid antibody. The frequency of antiphospholipid antibody in systemic lupus erythematosus patients is in the 30% to 40% range. Antiphospholipid antibodies due to infections are typically transient and asymptomatic.

Although the LA acts as an anticoagulant in vitro, it does not appear to be associated with hemorrhage, even with surgical challenge. Rare cases of bleeding in patients with the LA can almost always be attributed to specific abnormalities in hemostasis that happen to be present along with the LA. Decreased prothrombin (Factor II) is occasionally found with the LA. The LA can bind directly to prothrombin, but typically the LA does not neutralize the procoagulant activity of prothrombin even when it does bind to it. In an occasional patient, however, antibody binding does reduce the prothrombin concentration by accelerated clearance of prothrombin/antiprothrombin complexes, and these patients can have hemorrhagic complications. Concomitant thrombocytopenia is not infrequently found in patients with the LA, and this also may be a cause for hemorrhage.

Antiphospholipid antibodies are associated with an increased risk for venous or arterial thrombosis. The role of the antiphospholipid antibody in thrombosis is not clear, although several mechanisms for thrombosis have been proposed. The incidence of clinically apparent thromboembolism in patients with the LA, with or without systemic lupus erythematosus, is difficult to determine because of the variety of tests used to detect the LA. However, data suggest that the percentage of patients with the LA who will develop thrombosis is 1% per year if there is no history of thrombosis and 5.5% per year if there has been at least 1 prior thrombotic event. High titers of anticardiolipin or anti-beta 2 glycoprotein I antibodies present a higher risk for complications than low titers, and IgG is thought to be higher risk than IgM or IgA. There is a greater risk for thrombosis if more than 1 of the 3 antiphospholipid antibody tests (LA, anticardiolipin antibodies, and anti-beta 2 glycoprotein I antibodies) are abnormal.

Recurrent spontaneous abortion has been reported to be increased in patients with antiphospholipid antibodies. There is evidence suggesting that thrombosis and infarction in the placenta mediate antiphospholipid antibody-associated spontaneous abortion in a significant number of women experiencing recurrent fetal loss or premature birth.

Diagnosis

There are no "gold standard" tests that unequivocally establish the presence of antiphospholipid antibodies:

- *For the LA*: A prolonged PTT and a PTT mixing study that does not correct into the normal range are clues to the presence of the LA, although some PTT reagents are not sensitive to the LA. Therefore, it should be noted that the routine PTT is not an appropriate screening test for the LA. A PTT- or DRVVT-based test with a reduced amount of phospholipid can be used as a screening test for the LA. If it is prolonged, a 1:1 mixing study should be performed. In the presence of an LA, the PTT or DRVVT remains prolonged when equal portions of patient plasma and normal plasma are mixed. If the mix is positive (prolonged), the result should be confirmed by a test that is specific for a LA. The PT is not typically increased by the LA, unless the patient has an associated hypoprothrombinemia or the thromboplastin used in the PT is one that is particularly sensitive to inhibition by the LA.
- *For anticardiolipin or anti-beta 2 glycoprotein I antibodies*: An enzyme-linked immunosorbent assay (ELISA) is used that quantitates IgG and IgM antibody levels in arbitrary units. IgA is also measured in some kits.

Patients with antiphospholipid antibodies may have a false-positive serologic test result for syphilis (such as Venereal Disease Research Laboratories [VDRL] and rapid plasma reagin [RPR]).

See **Table 11–19** for information on the laboratory diagnosis of antiphospholipid antibodies.

Thrombotic Thrombocytopenic Purpura

Description

TTP is a clinical syndrome that is characterized by a triad (1 to 3 below, more commonly) or pentad (1 to 5 below, less commonly) of signs and symptoms:

1. thrombocytopenia with generalized purpura, and mucous membrane bleeding;
2. hemolytic anemia (microangiopathic) sufficient to cause jaundice or pallor;
3. neurologic abnormalities, which may include fluctuating weakness, dysphagia, headache, dementia/behavioral changes, obtundation, seizures, diplopia, paresthesias, and coma;
4. fever;
5. renal dysfunction, which may include hematuria, proteinuria, or renal insufficiency.

The characteristic, but not pathognomonic, pathology includes platelet and fibrin "hyaline" thrombi in the small arteries, arterioles, and capillaries in a widespread organ distribution. Organ ischemia and infarction that arise from these thrombi are thought to give rise to the observed fever and organ dysfunction. The etiology for TTP has been shown to be a deficiency of

Thrombotic thrombocytopenic purpura is a clinical syndrome that is characterized by a triad (more commonly) or pentad (less commonly) of signs and symptoms.

TABLE 11–20   **Laboratory Evaluation for Thrombotic Thrombocytopenic Purpura**

Laboratory Test	Results/Comments
Activity of von Willebrand factor-cleaving protease activity	A low value for this enzyme activity is the diagnostic hallmark for the disease, but the assay may not be available for rapid diagnosis of TTP
PT, PTT, and fibrinogen levels	Usually normal
Fibrin degradation products or D-dimer	Normal or slightly elevated
Hemoglobin/hematocrit	Mild to moderate decrease in most cases; hemorrhage and hemolysis can result in severe anemia in some patients
Haptoglobin	Low as a reflection of intravascular hemolysis
Platelet count	Decreased, often in the range of 10,000–50,000 μL^{-1}
Peripheral blood smear	Shows schistocytes, nucleated RBCs, and decreased platelet number
Direct and indirect antiglobulin tests	Negative, ruling out an immune hemolytic anemia
Indirect bilirubin	Mild to moderate elevation
Serum lactate dehydrogenase (LDH)	Elevated, correlating with the severity of hemolysis and possibly tissue damage from ischemia
WBC count and differential	Shows a mild leukocytosis with a left shift
Urinalysis	Characterized by mild to moderate proteinuria and hematuria (without casts)
BUN and creatinine	May or may not be elevated, depending on the presence of renal impairment

BUN, blood urea nitrogen; PT, prothrombin time; PTT, partial thromboplastin time.

vWF-cleaving protease. Nonfamilial cases of TTP are a result of an inhibitor to the vWF-cleaving protease; the familial form of TTP is apparently caused by a constitutional deficiency of the protease. The unusually large forms of vWF in the plasma of patients with TTP promote the aggregation of platelets in vivo, which accounts for most of the clinical findings.

TTP can occur at any age but is most common between the ages of 20 and 50 years. Peak incidence is in the third decade. There is a female to male ratio of 3:2. TTP usually occurs as an acute, fulminant disease, but may also occur in a chronic form or in an acute relapsing form. The acute and acute relapsing types are often preceded by a viral prodrome. Nonspecific signs such as malaise, weakness, fatigue, and anorexia may predominate at first, until the above triad or pentad develops in days to weeks. The chronic type usually pursues an indolent, low grade course, with ongoing disease activity for months.

Nonspecific manifestations in other organ systems resulting from ischemia may include:

- Cardiac: conduction defects, sudden death, and heart failure.
- Pulmonary: lung infiltrates and acute respiratory failure.
- Gastrointestinal: abdominal pain due to visceral ischemia, pancreatitis, and gastrointestinal mucosal hemorrhage.

Diagnosis

See **Table 11–20** for information on the laboratory evaluation for TTP.

Hemolytic–Uremic Syndrome

Description

Hemolytic uremic syndrome is a clinical syndrome with presentation and manifestations similar to TTP. Despite the clinical similarity, evidence has shown that the low levels of vWF-cleaving protease found in TTP are not found in HUS.

HUS is a clinical syndrome with presentation and manifestations similar to TTP. Despite the clinical similarity, evidence has shown that the low levels of vWF-cleaving protease found in TTP are not found in HUS. Thus, the pathogenesis of these 2 disorders is apparently completely

TABLE 11–21 Laboratory Evaluation for Hemolytic–Uremic Syndrome

Laboratory Test	Results/Comments
PT, PTT, and fibrinogen	Normal
Fibrin degradation products or D-dimer	Absent or minimally increased
Hemoglobin/hematocrit	Decreased with microangiopathic changes on the peripheral blood smear (nucleated RBCs, schistocytes)
Platelet count	Mild to moderate decrease
Urinalysis	Hematuria, proteinuria, and red cell casts
Creatinine	Elevated
Lactate dehydrogenase (LDH)	Elevated
Indirect bilirubin	Elevated
Haptoglobin	Low
Direct antiglobulin test (DAT)	Negative
E. coli O157:H7	Commonly positive

PT, prothrombin time; PTT, partial thromboplastin time.

different. HUS is characterized by fever, microangiopathic hemolytic anemia, thrombocytopenia, and renal dysfunction. HUS differs clinically from TTP in the following ways: neurologic symptoms are less pronounced or absent in HUS; renal function is usually more impaired in HUS than in TTP; HUS occurs in a younger population than TTP with a peak incidence between 6 months and 4 years, with males and females equally affected; HUS is a more common entity than TTP; as with TTP, hyaline thrombi may be found, but in most cases they tend to be confined to the glomerular capillaries and afferent arterioles.

HUS occasionally occurs in adults, and is often distinguished from childhood HUS because of its strong association in adults with obstetrical complications such as eclampsia. The prognosis is worse in adults than in affected children, with an adult mortality as high as 60%.

Acute HUS occurs in nonfamilial and familial forms, which may have different causes. Nonfamilial forms are most often associated with a diarrheal illness caused by a Shiga-toxin-producing *E. coli* (in particular, *E. coli* O157:H7). Familial forms have been linked to abnormalities in complement factor H and factor I. The majority of childhood cases resolve without sequelae, if children with acute renal failure receive dialysis when necessary. The prognosis depends on the duration of renal failure and the severity of the neurologic disturbance. Renal function returns to normal in approximately 90% of childhood cases.

Diagnosis

See **Table 11–21** for information on the laboratory evaluation for HUS.

A portion of this chapter, primarily the material in the section "Introduction to Hemostasis," was adapted with permission with modifications from Laposata M, Connor AM, Hicks, DG, Phillips DK. The Clinical Hemostasis Handbook. Chicago: Year Book Medical Publishers; 1989.

REFERENCES

Acharya SS, et al. Rare bleeding disorder registry: deficiencies of factors II, V, VII, X, XIII, fibrinogen and dysfibrinogenemias. *J Thromb Haemost.* 2004;2:248.

Boyce T, et al. *Escherichia coli* O157:H7 and the hemolytic–uremic syndrome. *N Engl J Med.* 1995;333:364.

Bussell JB, et al. Fetal alloimmune thrombocytopenia. *New Engl J Med.* 1997; 337:22–26.

Cines DB, Bussel JB. How I treat idiopathic thrombocytopenic purpura (ITP). *Blood.* 2005;106:2244–2251.

Dahlback B. Advances in understanding pathogenic mechanisms of thrombophilic disorders. *Blood.* 2008;112:19.

Feinstein DI. Immune coagulation disorders. In: Colman, W, et al., eds. *Hemostasis and Thrombosis: Basic Principles of Clinical Practice*. 4th ed. Philadelphia, PA: Lippincott Williams & Wilkins; 2001:1003.

Feinstein DI, Marder VJ, Colman RW. Consumptive thrombohemorrhagic disorders. In: Colman W, et al., eds. *Hemostasis and Thrombosis: Basic Principles of Clinical Practice*. 4th ed. Philadelphia, PA: Lippincott Williams & Wilkins; 2001:1197.

Finazzi T, et al. Natural history and risk factors for thrombosis in 360 patients with antiphospholipid antibodies: a four-year prospective study from the Italian registry. *Am J Med*. 1996;100:530.

Furlan M, et al. Von Willebrand factor-cleaving protease in thrombotic thrombocytopenic purpura and the hemolytic–uremic syndrome. *N Engl J Med*. 1998;339:1578.

George JN. Thrombotic thrombocytopenic purpura. *N Engl J Med*. 2006;354:1927–1935.

George JN, et al. Chronic idiopathic thrombocytopenic purpura. *N Engl J Med*. 1994;331:1207.

George JN, et al. Idiopathic thrombocytopenic purpura: a practice guideline developed by explicit methods for the American Society of Hematology. *Blood*. 1996;88:3.

Gill JC, et al. The effect of ABO blood group on the diagnosis of von Willebrand's disease. *Blood*. 1987;69:1691–1695.

Gillis S. The thrombocytopenic purpuras: recognition and management. *Drugs*. 1996;51:942.

Hoyer L. Hemophilia A. *N Engl J Med*. 1994:330:38

Joist JH, George JN. Hemostatic abnormalities in liver and renal disease. In: Colman W, et al., eds. *Hemostasis and Thrombosis: Basic Principles of Clinical Practice*. 4th ed. Philadelphia, PA: Lippincott Williams & Wilkins; 2001:839.

Kempton CL, White GC Jr. How we treat a hemophilia A patient with a factor VIII inhibitor. *Blood*. 2009,113.11–17.

Kottke-Marchant K. Platelet disorders. In: Kottke-Marchant K, ed. An algorithmic approach to hemostasis testing. Northfield, IL: College of American Pathologists Press; 2008:185–216.

Kurtzberg J, Stockman JA. Idiopathic autoimmune thrombocytopenic purpura. *Adv Pediatr*. 1994;41:111.

Laposata M, et al. *The Clinical Hemostasis Handbook*. St. Louis, MO: The CV Mosby Company; 1989.

Miyakis S, et al. International consensus statement on an update of the classification criteria for definite antiphospholipid syndrome (APS). *J Thromb Haemost*. 2006;4:295–306.

Nichols WL, et al. *Diagnosis, Evaluation, and Management of von Willebrand Disease*. National Heart, Lung, Blood Institute (NHLBI); 2007 (NIH publication number 08-5832).

Roberts HR, White GC Jr. Inherited disorders of prothrombin conversion. In: Colman W, et al., eds. *Hemostasis and Thrombosis: Basic Principles of Clinical Practice*. 4th ed. Philadelphia, PA: Lippincott Williams & Wilkins; 2001:839.

Rodeghiero F, et al. Standardization of terminology, definitions and outcome criteria in immune thrombocytopenic purpura of adults and children: report from an international working group. *Blood*. 2009;113(11):2386–2393.

Rothenberger SS, McCarthy LJ. Neonatal alloimmune thrombocytopenia: from prediction to prevention. *Lab Med*. 1997;28:592.

Siegler RL. The hemolytic uremic syndrome. *Pediatr Clin North Am*. 1995;42:1505.

Seitz R, et al. ETRO Working Party on Factor XIII questionnaire on congenital Factor XIII deficiency in Europe: status and perspectives. *Semin Thromb Hemostasis*. 1996;22:415.

Seligsohn U, et al. Inherited deficiencies of coagulation factors II, V, VII, X, XI and XIII and combined deficiencies of factors V and VIII and of the vitamin K-dependent factors. In: Lichtman MA, et al., eds. *Hematology*. 7th ed. New York, NY: McGraw-Hill; 2006:1887.

Souid A, Sadowitz PD. Acute childhood immune thrombocytopenic purpura: diagnosis and treatment. *Clin Pediatr*. 1995;34:487.

Swerdlow SH, et al. *WHO Classification of Tumours of Haematopoietic and Lymphoid Tissues*. Lyon: IARC; 2008:32.

Taaning E, Svejgaard A. Post-transfusion purpura: a survey of 12 Danish cases with special reference to immunoglobulin G subclasses of the platelet antibodies. *Transfus Med*. 1994;4:1.

Tarr PI, Gordon CA, Chandler WA. Shiga-toxin-producing *Escherichia coli* and haemolytic uraemic syndrome. *Lancet*. 2005;365:1073–1086.

Tsai H-M, Lian EC-Y. Antibodies to von Willebrand factor-cleaving protease in acute thrombotic thrombocytopenic purpura. *N Engl J Med*. 1998;339:1585.

Van Cott EM, Laposata M. Laboratory evaluation of hypercoagulable states. *Hematol Oncol Clin North Am*. 1998;12:1141.

Verhovsik M, et al. Laboratory testing for fibrinogen abnormalities. *Am J Hematol*. 2008; 83:928–931.

Waters AH. Autoimmune thrombocytopenia: clinical aspects. *Semin Hematol*. 1992;29:18.

Zhang B, et al. Genotype–phenotype correlation in combined deficiency of factor V and factor VIII. *Blood*. 2008; 111: 5592–5600.

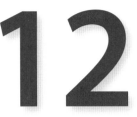

Transfusion Medicine

Christopher P. Stowell and Jacqueline J. Haas

LEARNING OBJECTIVES

1. Understand the process of blood collection and the preparation of blood components and plasma derivatives.

2. Learn which tests must be performed to assure safe transfusion.

3. Learn the specific indications for transfusion of individual blood components and alternatives to allogeneic transfusion.

4. Understand the clinical complications that may arise after transfusion of blood components.

5. Learn about the collection and use of hematopoietic progenitor cells.

6. Learn the process of apheresis and its clinical indications.

CHAPTER OUTLINE

Transfusion medicine is the field of medicine that encompasses blood banking (the collection, storage, and testing of blood components and derivatives) as well as the therapeutic uses of blood components, plasma derivatives, and apheresis technology. It also includes the collection, storage, and use of hematopoietic and other blood-derived cells. An overview of the steps from collection of the blood to transfusion of its components is shown in **Figure 12–1**. Briefly (with more complete descriptions to follow), blood is collected as whole blood or by apheresis from screened, volunteer donors, and samples of the blood are tested

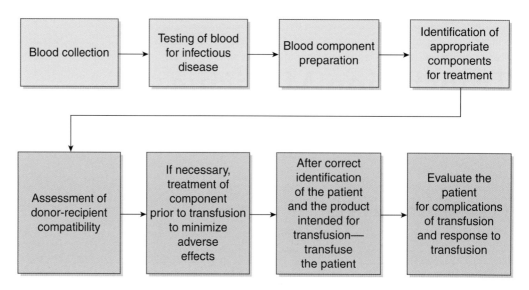

FIGURE 12–1 An overview of blood collection, processing, and transfusion.

for infectious diseases and to determine the blood type. Whole blood may be fractionated into packed red blood cells (RBCs), platelets, and a plasma product. Alternatively, all 3 components can be collected by apheresis. Plasma can be further processed to provide albumin, clotting factor concentrates, and immunoglobulin preparations. The transfusion of blood components requires testing to be done to establish compatibility between the product and the intended recipient. Blood components may also be treated to reduce complications of transfusion (e.g., remove leukocytes to prevent febrile reactions). As complex, biologically derived therapeutic agents, blood components and derivatives are responsible for a variety of potential untoward effects that must be evaluated and managed. The entire process, from blood collection to transfusion and post-transfusion evaluation, is described in this chapter (see **Figure 12–1**).

> Whole blood may be fractionated into packed red blood cells (RBCs), platelets, and a plasma product.

COLLECTION OF BLOOD AND PREPARATION OF BLOOD COMPONENTS

Blood Collection

The cornerstone of a safe blood supply is the volunteer blood donor who is motivated by altruism. In the past, the use of paid donors was associated with increased levels of transfusion-transmitted hepatitis. Concerns remain about the impact of significant financial incentives on the frank disclosure of health problems or high-risk behaviors that might disqualify a potential blood donor. In the United States, virtually all of the blood is collected from volunteer donors. Regional blood centers collect and distribute more than 90% of the US blood supply while hospital blood banks collect the remainder. The Food and Drug Administration (FDA) Center for Biologics Evaluation and Research regulates all aspects of blood collection and processing, but most blood banks and donor centers are also accredited, on a voluntary basis, by the American Association of Blood Banks (AABB). Blood donors are screened for behaviors or medical conditions that might make blood donation unsafe for them (e.g., anemia, coronary artery insufficiency) or the donated blood hazardous for the transfusion recipient (e.g., exposure to viral hepatitis, use of a teratogenic medication). The AABB has developed, and the FDA has sanctioned, a Uniform Donor Health Questionnaire that is in wide use in the United States and reflects the consistency of donor criteria throughout the country. To qualify for blood donation, the prospective donor must also pass a basic physical screening that includes temperature, blood pressure, pulse, and examination of the arms for signs of intravenous drug use, and have a hemoglobin level of at least 12.5 g/dL from a fingerstick or venous blood sample. The collecting agency must check its records to be sure that the donor has not previously been disqualified from donating.

In the process of blood collection, the venipuncture site is disinfected and a needle, which is connected to a collecting set, is inserted into a vein in the arm. The collecting set includes a primary collection bag and several integrally connected satellite bags that are used to make components. The primary collection bag contains a solution that includes an anticoagulant (citrate) and a variety of substances, such as phosphate, adenine, and dextrose, which improve the recovery of the RBCs when transfused and permit their storage in the refrigerator for 35 to 42 days. The typical donation is approximately 450 to 500 mL of whole blood, but may not exceed 10.5 mL/kg, and must be collected in no more than 10 minutes if a unit of platelets is to be made. This volume of blood represents approximately 10% of the total blood volume of a donor weighing 70 kg, and its loss is well tolerated by healthy individuals. Samples of blood for serologic and infectious disease testing are also obtained at the time of donation, often by collecting the first 15 to 25 mL of blood drawn, which has the advantage of diverting blood most likely to be contaminated with skin bacteria away from the collection bag. Once the collection is complete, the needle is withdrawn from the donor's arm, and the tubing connecting the needle to the primary collection bag is heat-sealed off.

> The typical donation is approximately 450 to 500 mL of whole blood. This volume of blood represents approximately 10% of the total blood volume of a donor weighing 70 kg, and its loss is well tolerated by healthy individuals.

Component Preparation

Almost all of the whole blood collected is separated into its components—RBCs, platelets, and plasma—in order to be able to store each under optimal conditions. This separation process entails 2 centrifugation steps and relies on the system of integrally connected satellite bags to carry out all of the preparation steps in a closed, aseptic environment (see **Table 12–1** for a description of blood components, and Chapter 2 for a diagram of blood component preparation). In the procedure used in the United States, RBCs are separated from platelet-rich plasma by the first, relatively low *g* force, centrifugation step. The platelet-rich plasma is expressed from the primary collection bag into 1 of the satellite bags that is heat-sealed off from the packed RBCs in the primary collection bag. The packed RBCs remaining in the primary collection bag may be stored for up to 35 days at 1°C to 6°C (CPDA-1 RBCs). In some collection systems, additional additive–preservative solution from another satellite bag may be added to the packed RBC, creating a product with a lower hematocrit (but identical RBC mass) and an additional week of storage (42 days).

The platelet-rich plasma, which was expressed off the packed RBC after the first spin, is then separated into platelets and plasma by a second, higher *g* force, centrifugation step. The platelet-poor plasma is expressed into another satellite bag after this second centrifugation step and is usually frozen within 8 hours of collection (as fresh frozen plasma or FFP) or within 24 hours of collection (24-hour plasma). The platelet pellet that remains is suspended in 40 to 60 mL of plasma and is called a platelet concentrate or whole blood-derived platelets. Platelets are stored at 20°C to 24°C for up to 5 days, whereas the various plasma-derived components are stored frozen (≤−18°C for 1 year; ≤−65°C for 7 years).

FFP can be used to prepare another useful component, called cryoprecipitated anti-hemophilic factor (or "cryoprecipitate"). When FFP is thawed at 1°C to 6°C, a precipitate forms. Most of the plasma can be expressed into a satellite bag, leaving behind this cryoprecipitate that is suspended in 10 to 20 mL of plasma, refrozen, and then stored (≤−18°C for 1 year). Cryoprecipitate contains about half of the factor VIII, von Willebrand factor, factor XIII, and fibrinogen that was present in the original unit of plasma, but in a much smaller volume. The plasma remaining after the cryoprecipitate has been removed may also be refrozen. "Plasma–cryoprecipitate reduced" (or cryo-poor plasma) may be used as the starting material (source plasma) for the preparation of plasma derivatives such as albumin and immunoglobulins, and occasionally for replacement during plasmapheresis for patients with thrombotic thrombocytopenic purpura (see **Table 12–2**). Thus, each unit of whole blood can be separated into a unit of packed RBCs, a platelet concentrate, and either FFP or cryoprecipitate plus a plasma product. The different plasma products (absent cryoprecipitate) may all be used as source plasma for the preparation of derivatives.

Blood components also may be donated by a procedure known as apheresis, in which whole blood is removed from the donor, the component of interest (plasma or platelets most commonly, but RBCs as well) is removed, and the remaining blood elements are returned to the

TABLE 12-1   Blood Component Descriptions and Indications

Category	Description of Product	Major Indications	Actions	Precautions
Packed RBCs	Packed RBCs are the product of a centrifugal separation of red cells from plasma; this component has a hematocrit of 55%–80%	Packed RBCs are used for treatment of a symptomatic anemia; this component may also be used for exchange transfusion when treating sickle cell crisis or hemolytic disease of the newborn	Packed RBCs provide RBC mass and increase oxygen-carrying capacity in the blood	RBCs must be ABO- and Rh-compatible, and crossmatched
RBCs, leukoreduced	Packed RBCs may be modified by removal of leukocytes by filtration or washing; washing RBCs is less effective at removing leukocytes than filtration techniques	The indications for this product are the same as for packed RBCs; leukoreduced RBCs are used for individuals who have experienced febrile reactions due to passenger WBCs in a blood component; they are also used to prevent alloimmunization in a patient who may require multiple platelet transfusions, or to prevent cytomegalovirus infection in a susceptible patient	Packed RBCs provide RBC mass and increase oxygen-carrying capacity in the blood	RBCs must be ABO- and Rh-compatible, and crossmatched
Fresh frozen plasma	Plasma that is separated from the cellular components and frozen within 8 hours of collection of whole blood is known as fresh frozen plasma (FFP)	Because fresh frozen plasma contains significant levels of all the plasma coagulation factors, including Factors V and VIII that are labile, it is useful to control bleeding in patients who have multiple coagulation factor deficiencies; fresh frozen plasma should not be used to correct a deficit of blood volume; other volume expanders that are less potentially infectious should be used	Fresh frozen plasma restores plasma proteins, particularly coagulation factors, and this may result in control of a bleeding episode	This component should be ABO-compatible with the recipient's RBCs, but crossmatching is not performed prior to transfusion; Rh type is not a consideration
Cryoprecipitate	Cryoprecipitate is generated by thawing fresh frozen plasma at 1°C–6°C; the precipitate is collected and refrozen; a typical bag of cryoprecipitate contains at least 80 units of Factor VIII and at least 150 mg of fibrinogen in a volume of less than 25 mL	This component is used for patients with a deficiency of fibrinogen (often from disseminated intravascular coagulation), or deficiency of Factor XIII	Transfusion of cryoprecipitate to raise fibrinogen levels to greater than 100 mg/dL may be useful to provide hemostasis for fibrinogen deficiency	Crossmatch testing is unnecessary; although ABO-compatible cryoprecipitate is preferred, it is not necessary; the Rh type is not a consideration
Platelet concentrates (whole blood-derived platelets)	Platelet concentrates are obtained from a single unit of whole blood, and contain at least 5.5×10^{10} platelets; suspended in 40–60 mL of plasma, which is stored at 20°C–24°C	Platelet transfusions are indicated for patients who are thrombocytopenic due to decreased platelet production or blood loss and for those patients who do not have an adequate number of functioning platelets; platelet transfusions are not usually effective in conditions associated with rapid platelet destruction; platelets may be useful in preventing a bleeding episode if given as a prophylactic measure to patients with very low platelet counts	The elevation of the platelet count in a thrombocytopenic patient or the transfusion of functionally active platelets into a patient with dysfunctional platelets can result in the cessation or prevention of bleeding	Although crossmatching is not necessary, platelet products that are ABO-compatible with the recipient are preferred to minimize the infusion of incompatible plasma

Continued next page—

TABLE 12–1 Blood Component Descriptions and Indications (continued)

Category	Description of Product	Major Indications	Actions	Precautions
Platelets collected by apheresis	Platelets obtained by apheresis contain at least 3×10^{11} platelets/unit; the product has a volume between 200 and 400 mL	Same as for platelet concentrates	Same as for platelet concentrates	Same as for platelet concentrates
Granulocytes collected by apheresis	Granulocytes are collected from a single donor by apheresis; the product, which contains other blood cells as well, is in a volume of 200–300 mL	Granulocytes may be indicated for the patient who has both neutropenia and a documented infection that is not responsive to therapy; this product should not be used for prophylaxis against infection; in general, it has been more effective in infants than in adults	The granulocytes may contribute to the eradication of infection in a neutropenic recipient	Crossmatching must be performed before transfusion because of the large number of RBCs in the product; in addition, the granulocytes are very labile, so this product should be transfused as soon as possible after collection

TABLE 12–2 Derivatives of Blood Components and Indications for Their Use

Derivative	Description and Indication
Factor VIII concentrate	Prepared for treatment of hemophilia A; Factor VIII can be purified from human plasma and treated to remove and inactivate infectious agents; a recombinant Factor VIII product is also available; some plasma-derived preparations contain significant amounts of von Willebrand factor and are suitable for treatment of this disease as well
Factor IX concentrate	Prepared using methods similar to those for Factor VIII; it is used for the treatment of patients with hemophilia B; recombinant factor IX is available; concentrates that contain Factors II, VII, and X along with Factor IX are also available, and are known as prothrombin complex concentrates; some of these concentrates are potentially thrombogenic and are therefore not the preferred product for treatment of hemophilia B
Albumin	Prepared from pooled donor plasma as a 5% or a 25% solution in a manner that removes infectious agents; albumin is used as replacement fluid for plasmapheresis, for hypoalbuminemic patients with acute lung injury, in conjunction with large-volume paracentesis, for diuresis in patients with ascites unresponsive to diuretics, in selected patients with subarachnoid hemorrhage to prevent vasospasm and in selected burn patients; it should not be used routinely for volume expansion when crystalloid or synthetic colloid volume expanders such as dextran and hyroxyethyl starch are available
Intravenous immunoglobulin (IV Ig)	The IgG fraction prepared from pooled donor plasma is processed to minimize IgG dimerization and remove or inactivate infectious agents; used as antibody replacement therapy in humoral immunodeficiency states (see Chapter 3) and in the treatment of selected autoimmune disorders such as idiopathic or immune thrombocytopenic purpura (ITP)
Rh immune globulin	The IgG fraction prepared from pooled plasma from donors with high-titer anti-D treated to remove or inactivate infectious agents; administered by intramuscular injection to Rh-negative women to prevent their alloimmunization by the Rh-positive RBCs of their offspring; Rh-negative women should receive this product at 28 weeks of gestation and again within 72 hours of the birth of an Rh-positive baby, or at the time of abortion, miscarriage, vaginal hemorrhage, ectopic pregnancy, abdominal trauma, or invasive procedure such as amniocentesis or chorionic villous sampling; an intravenous formulation of this product is used for treatment of ITP
Antithrombin concentrate	Prepared for treatment of patients with low amounts of circulating antithrombin who are susceptible to thrombosis; antithrombin is purified from pooled human plasma and treated to remove or inactivate infectious agents
Recombinant, activated factor VII	A recombinant version of activated Factor VII prepared for treatment of patients with acquired Factors VIII and IX inhibitors and for patients with congenital Factor VII deficiency; widespread off-label use in bleeding patients with complex coagulopathies is being tempered by poor outcomes in randomized trials; should be used with caution in patients with prothrombotic tendencies

donor (see Chapter 2 for a diagram of apheresis). This procedure may be done manually, but is now usually carried out using an automated device. Using an apheresis instrument, whole blood is drawn from the donor's vein as an anticoagulant solution (usually citrate) is added, and pumped into a centrifuge where it is separated into its components. The component of interest is drawn into a collection bag, and the rest of the blood is returned to the donor via the same or a different vein. This process may be discontinuous (fill the instrument, separate the components, return the residual blood, and repeat) or continuous. The entire extracorporeal circuit is sealed except at the points of contact with the donor's vein(s). Apheresis is commonly used to obtain plasma, usually for further processing into derivatives such as albumin, clotting factor concentrates and immunoglobulins, as well as platelets. A unit of apheresis platelets (commonly called "single donor platelets") contains more platelets than a unit derived from a whole blood donation. Transfusion of a unit of apheresis platelets, which must contain at least 3×10^{11} platelets, usually elevates an adult patient's platelet count by 30,000 to 50,000 platelets/µL. Since 1 unit of whole blood-derived platelets must only contain 5.5×10^{10} platelets, the usual adult dose is 4 to 10 units or 1 unit/10 kg. Whole blood-derived platelets are less expensive to prepare than apheresis platelets because they do not require special equipment for their isolation. However, apheresis platelets can easily be prepared in such a way that they contain very few residual white blood cells ("process leukoreduced"), which is an advantage for some patient groups. Apheresis platelets also lend themselves more readily to bacterial screening by culture than do the smaller units of whole blood-derived platelets.

Granulocytes also can be harvested by apheresis for transfusion to patients who are neutropenic and suffering from severe infection. Instruments designed to collect RBCs by apheresis (typically 2 units at a time if the donor meets the somewhat more stringent size and hematocrit requirements) or various combinations of RBCs, platelets, and plasma are also in use. Finally, apheresis is used to collect peripherally circulating hematopoietic progenitor cells (HPCs) for autologous and allogeneic HPC transplantation.

Testing of Donated Blood

Donated blood is held in quarantine following collection while a variety of laboratory tests are performed using blood specimens obtained from the donor. The ABO and Rh types are determined on an RBC sample obtained at each donation, and the donor serum or plasma is screened for the presence of unexpected RBC alloantibodies. The concern is that such alloantibodies could cause destruction of a transfusion recipient's RBCs if they express the target antigen. Plasma or platelets from a donor with an alloantibody are not used for transfusion, although RBCs are generally safe, particularly if they have been saline washed. Records from any previous donations, including the results of ABO and Rh typing, are also checked, to reduce the opportunity for donor or unit misidentification.

Infectious Disease Testing

Transmission of viruses, bacteria, and parasites by transfusion of blood components has been well documented. To minimize infectious disease transmission, blood donors are screened for evidence of infection and for participation in activities that may have exposed them to infectious agents. In addition, each blood donation is subjected to several tests for infectious agents before it is made available for transfusion. The tests required for each donation are shown in **Table 12–3**. Platelets, which are stored at 20°C to 24°C, must also be screened for evidence of bacterial contamination, which is currently responsible for the majority of transfusion-transmitted infections. A limited number of commercial blood culture systems have been licensed for the testing of leukoreduced platelets. Options are more limited for nonleukoreduced platelets and whole blood-derived platelets, but alternate screening methods (e.g., pH testing and Gram staining) have been deployed in the absence of suitable culture techniques. Donors who have resided in South or Central America, or whose birth mothers have done so, are screened for antibody to *Trypanosoma cruzi*, the organism that causes Chagas disease.

Transmission of viruses, bacteria, and parasites by transfusion of blood components has been well documented. To minimize infectious disease transmission, blood donors are screened for evidence of infection and for participation in activities that may have exposed them to infectious agents.

TABLE 12–3 Infectious Disease Testing of Donated Blood

Required	Optional
Serologic test for syphilis	Antibody to cytomegalovirus
Antibody to HIV-1 and HIV-2 HIV-1 RNA	Alanine aminotransferase activity for liver function abnormalities resulting from infection
Antibody to hepatitis C virus (HCV)	
HCV RNA	
Hepatitis B surface antigen	
Antibody to hepatitis B core antigen	
Antibody to HTLV-I and HTLV-II	
West Nile Virus RNA	
Antibody to *Trypanosoma cruzi*[a]	
Screen for bacteria (platelets only)	

HIV, human immunodeficiency virus; HCV, hepatitis C virus; HTLV, human T-cell lymphotropic virus.

[a]For donors who have lived in South or Central America, or whose birth mothers have done so.

COMPATIBILITY TESTING

Pretransfusion Testing to Assess Donor/Recipient Compatibility for Blood Components Containing RBCs

Prior to transfusion, the compatibility of donor RBCs with the intended transfusion recipient must be established (see **Tables 12–4** and **12–5** for RBC compatibility issues). Part of this process involves various serologic tests. But an equally important part of this process is the proper identification of the patient when the blood bank specimen is obtained, and again when the transfusion is initiated. Misidentification of patients and mislabeling of specimens are the most common serious errors encountered in transfusion. ABO mistransfusion as a result of this kind of error is far more frequent than the transmission of HIV and all of the hepatitis viruses, combined. Compatibility testing includes:

- The identification of patient and proper labeling of the specimen for compatibility testing. The blood bank specimen (tube of blood) must be labeled at the bedside using the patient's armband for identification. The label must include 2 patient identifiers (typically name and medical record number) and the date. There must also be some means of identifying the phlebotomist (commonly, but not necessarily, by signing or initialing the tube or requisition).
- The determination of the ABO and Rh type of the donor. The collecting facility determines the ABO group (by front- and back-typing as described below) and Rh type of the donated unit (and checks prior records). The hospital transfusion service must confirm the ABO group (front type only) and the Rh type of Rh(D)-negative units that have been received from the collecting facility.
- The determination of the ABO and Rh type of the patient on a current specimen, and a comparison to previous records, if any. The ABO group (front and back types) and Rh type are determined on a current specimen. The specimen must be <3 days old for any patient who has been transfused or pregnant within the past 3 months; however, many transfusion services require new specimens every 3 days to keep things simple.
- A screen of the recipient's serum/plasma for unexpected RBC alloantibodies. If unexpected antibodies (i.e., not anti-A or anti-B) are found, as described below, the antigen specificity of these antibodies must be identified to establish the risk of a hemolytic transfusion reaction (HTR) and to help identify potentially compatible donor RBCs that lack the target antigen. A record check for previously identified alloantibodies must also be made.

Misidentification of patients and mislabeling of specimens are the most common serious errors encountered in transfusion. ABO mistransfusion as a result of this kind of error is far more frequent than the transmission of HIV and all of the hepatitis viruses, combined.

TABLE 12–4　**RBC Compatibility**

ABO Group of Patient	Isoagglutinins Present	Compatible Donor RBC Units	Incompatible Donor RBC Units
A	Anti-B	A, O	B, AB
B	Anti-A	B, O	A, AB
AB	Neither	A, B, AB, O	None
O	Anti-A, anti-B, anti-AB	O	A, B, AB

RBC D Antigen	Acceptable Donor Units		Unacceptable Donor Units
Rh-Positive	Rh(D)-positive, Rh(D)-negative		None
Rh-negative	Rh(D)-negative		Rh(D)-positive

TABLE 12–5　**The Major RBC Antigens: Frequencies and Clinical Significance**

System	Antigen	Antigen Frequency in Caucasians	Antigen Frequency in Africans	Implicated in Hemolytic Disease of the Newborn	Implicated in Hemolytic Transfusion Reactions
Rh	D	0.85	0.92	Yes	Yes
	C	0.68	0.27	Yes	Yes
	c	0.80	0.96	Yes	Yes
	E	0.29	0.22	Yes	Yes
	e	0.98	0.99	Yes	Yes
Kell	K	0.09	0.02	Yes	Yes
	k	0.99	0.98	Yes	Yes
Duffy	Fy^a	0.66	0.10	Yes	Yes
	Fy^b	0.83	0.43	Yes	Yes
	$Fy^{(a-b-)}$	Rare	0.68	NA	NA
Kidd	Jk^a	0.77	0.91	Yes, mild case	Yes
	Jk^b	0.72	0.23	Yes, mild cases	Yes
MNSs	M	0.78	0.70	Yes, few cases	Yes, few cases
	N	0.72	0.74	Yes, rarely	No
	S	0.55	0.31	Yes	Yes
	s	0.89	0.97	Yes	Yes
Lewis	Le^{a*}	0.22	0.23	No	Yes, few cases
	Le^{b*}	0.72	0.55	No	No
	Le$^{(a-b-)}$	0.06	0.22	NA	NA

NA, not applicable.

*Not allelic pair.

- The performance of a crossmatch. Several techniques for performing the crossmatch are described below.
- The identification of the patient when the transfusion is initiated. The patient must once again be properly identified using the armband to be sure that the unit is intended for the patient. The armband is the only link between the patient, the specimen, and the blood component.

ABO Grouping

After the identification of the patient and the specimen for compatibility testing, the most important step in assuring the safety of an RBC transfusion is the determination of the ABO group of the donor unit and the intended recipient. The specificity of the A and B blood group antigens lies in the presence of carbohydrate structures that are borne by membrane-associated glycoproteins and glycolipids. During the first year of life, individuals begin to make antibodies to whichever A and B antigens they lack. Thus, a person with A antigen on his or her RBCs (group A) has naturally occurring anti-B antibodies in the plasma (see **Table 12–4**). It is the presence of these antibodies (called isoagglutinins because of their ability to agglutinate RBCs in vitro) that makes ABO mistransfusion so hazardous. The isoagglutinins are largely IgM and fix complement readily. Hence, they can cause intravascular hemolysis.

Because determining the ABO group is so critical, it is required not only to test for A and B antigens on the RBCs, but also to demonstrate the presence of the appropriate anti-A and anti-B isoagglutinins in the plasma or serum (see Chapter 2 for a diagram of ABO and Rh typing). The presence of A or B antigens on patient or donor RBCs is detected by combining them with reagent "anti-A" in 1 test tube and reagent "anti-B" in another test tube, and then assessing RBC agglutination. Agglutination with anti-A, for example, indicates the presence of A antigen on the RBCs. This test is called the "front" or "cell" typing. The plasma of a patient or donor is tested for the presence of anti-A or anti-B antibodies by combining the plasma with reagent RBCs known to be either group A or group B, and then assessing RBC agglutination. Agglutination of the reagent B cells indicates the presence of anti-B isoagglutinin in the plasma, which would be the expected finding in a person who is blood group A. This test is called the "back" or "serum" typing. The results of the front- and back-typing must be congruent.

Rh Typing

The second most important antigen system with respect to transfusion safety is the Rh system. Approximately 85% of Caucasians express the D (or Rh) antigen and are called D (or Rh)-positive (see **Table 12–4**). Rh-negative individuals, who lack the D antigen, are vulnerable to development of an alloantibody to the D antigen, the most immunogenic antigen on human RBCs, if they are exposed to D-positive RBCs by transfusion or, for a woman, by maternal–fetal hemorrhage. Anti-D is the most common cause of severe hemolytic disease of the newborn, although the frequency of this complication of pregnancy has been considerably decreased since the advent of Rh immune globulin. This product is an immunoglobulin fraction obtained by pooling the plasma of people with high-titer anti-D. When given by intramuscular injection to individuals who have been exposed to D-positive RBCs (e.g., women pregnant with a D-positive fetus), it reduces the chance of sensitization presumably by binding to D-positive fetal cells, leading to their rapid clearance from the maternal circulation before an immune response can be generated (see the section "Hemolytic Disease of the Newborn (HDN)" in Chapter 10).

The Rh type is determined by incubating the RBCs with a reagent antibody to the D antigen. Rh-positive cells expressing the D antigen are agglutinated by the reagent antibody. RBCs that do not agglutinate in the presence of the Rh antibody are incubated a second time, usually after the addition of an enhancer of agglutination. RBCs that do not agglutinate after this second step are considered to be Rh(D)-negative. A small number of people have RBCs that do not agglutinate in the first step but are agglutinated after the second, enhanced, incubation step. These individuals are considered to have the weak D (formerly D^u) phenotype. Donors, and usually patients as well, who are weak D are treated as if they are D-positive, since some weak D RBCs can elicit the formation of anti-D alloantibodies in D-negative individuals, or can be the target for anti-D alloantibodies.

The Antibody Screen and the Indirect Antiglobulin Assay Used to Detect Antibodies

To determine if the patient has an alloantibody to a RBC antigen, an antibody screen is performed. In this test, the patient's serum or plasma is combined with 2 or 3 reagent RBCs that are specifically chosen because they bear a number of the antigens to which clinically significant RBC alloantibodies are made. These cells are group O so that they will not be agglutinated by the anti-A or anti-B isoagglutinins that may be present. If the patient serum does not produce agglutination of the reagent screening cells, then no unexpected RBC alloantibodies are present.

Although the anti-A and anti-B isoagglutinins are predominantly IgM and readily produce agglutination in vitro, most of the other clinically significant RBC alloantibodies are IgG and do not. To detect IgG alloantibodies, an assay called the indirect antiglobulin test (formerly the indirect Coombs' test) is used in the antibody screen (see Chapter 2 for a diagram of the indirect antiglobulin test). In this technique, the patient's serum is combined with the reagent screening cells, often in the presence of an additive, such as low ionic strength saline or polyethylene glycol, which promotes binding of antibody to RBCs, and the mixture is incubated at 37°C. If an RBC alloantibody is present, it will bind to the screening cell with the target antigen. The cells are then washed with saline and the "antiglobulin reagent" is added. Antiglobulin reagent consists of a mixture of antibodies to IgG and/or complement. These antibodies bind to any IgG or complement attached to the screening cell. By binding to IgG or complement on adjacent target cells, the anti-IgG "crosslinks" the RBCs and produces RBC agglutination in vitro. It is called the indirect antiglobulin test because it requires first an incubation with the alloantibody (the serum sample) followed by a second step when the antiglobulin reagent is added. The antiglobulin test is commonly performed in a test tube, but has also been adapted to assays based on solid phase or gel column techniques.

If 1 or more of the screening cells is agglutinated by the patient's serum, indicating the presence of an RBC alloantibody, steps must be taken to identify its specificity by determining its target antigen. This is accomplished again using the indirect antiglobulin test and adding the patient's serum to a panel of group O RBCs (typically around 10) that have been chosen to express the target antigens of the most commonly encountered clinically significant alloantibodies. The pattern of which panel cells are agglutinated in the indirect antiglobulin test can be used to determine the antigen to which the patient's alloantibody is directed. Based on the accumulated clinical experience with alloantibodies of a given specificity, it is usually possible to predict the likelihood that a particular alloantibody will cause an HTR or hemolytic disease of the newborn (see **Table 12–5**). If the alloantibody has the potential of causing hemolysis, donor RBCs that lack the target antigen must be chosen for transfusion. The typing of RBCs for specific antigens is accomplished in a manner similar to that used for the determination of the ABO and Rh type using commercial antisera directed at specific antigens. Patients who have multiple alloantibodies, or alloantibodies directed at high-frequency antigens, may pose the challenge that very few donors will lack the target antigen(s). Under these circumstances, the blood bank may have to screen the red cell inventory for antigen-negative units, request their blood supplier to do the same, or in some instances, locate suitable units through a national rare blood registry.

The RBC Crossmatch

There are 3 crossmatch techniques in common use: the antiglobulin technique crossmatch, the immediate spin crossmatch, and the electronic crossmatch.

The antiglobulin crossmatch was the standard for years and still must be performed when a patient has an RBC alloantibody (see Chapter 2 for a diagram of the blood crossmatch). This crossmatch procedure is very similar to the antibody screen and is based on the indirect antiglobulin technique, except in this case the patient's serum is combined with RBCs from the donor unit. If the patient has an alloantibody to the donor RBCs, the antibody will become bound to the donor RBCs during the incubation step and the cells will be agglutinated by the antiglobulin reagent added in the final step. If agglutination occurs, the crossmatch is incompatible and the unit of RBCs should not be transfused to that patient. If the RBCs from this donor were mistakenly transfused, they would be destroyed prematurely, that is, an HTR would occur. If there is no agglutination, the patient does not have alloantibodies to the antigens present on this donor's RBCs and the crossmatch is compatible.

The immediate spin crossmatch is done by combining the patient's serum with a sample of the donor RBCs intended for transfusion, centrifuging them without incubation or the use of the antiglobulin reagent, and observing them immediately for agglutination. This technique detects ABO incompatibilities, but is not sensitive to the presence of other RBC alloantibodies. It may

There are 3 crossmatch techniques in common use: the antiglobulin technique crossmatch, the immediate spin crossmatch, and the electronic crossmatch.

only be used in patients who do not have unexpected alloantibodies (i.e., they have a negative antibody screen), in massive transfusion (transfusion of the equivalent of 1 entire blood volume), and in emergency circumstances when an abbreviated crossmatch procedure is imperative for providing blood rapidly.

In the electronic crossmatch, blood bank personnel rely on the computer to verify the ABO (and Rh) compatibility between donor RBCs and the patient. A number of requirements must be met by the information system and the bench procedures involved in the typing, and extensive validation must be performed. This technique is again only suitable for patients who do not have unexpected RBC alloantibodies, or in emergency situations.

Direct Antiglobulin Test (Formerly Direct Coombs' Test)

This test detects the presence of IgG or complement that is bound, in vivo, to the patient's RBCs, by using antiglobulin reagent specific for IgG or various complement components including C3b, C3d, and/or C4d. In this technique, the patient's RBCs are washed with saline, and the antiglobulin reagent is then added directly (hence the name of the test) (see Chapter 2 for a diagram of the direct antiglobulin test). The cells are observed for agglutination after incubation. The presence of RBC coated with immunoglobulin and/or complement is evidence of immune-mediated hemolysis. Disorders associated with a positive direct antiglobulin test include hemolytic disease of the newborn, autoimmune hemolytic anemia, and drug-induced hemolytic anemia. A positive direct antiglobulin test result is also observed in patients experiencing an HTR where donor RBCs are circulating coated with the recipient's alloantibody. Note that most patients with positive direct antiglobulin tests do not have hemolysis. A positive direct antiglobulin test is found in many patients with lymphoproliferative and autoimmune disorders, or who are taking various medications such as procainamide, vancomycin, and drugs in the penicillin and cephalosporin families.

Compatibility Testing for Other Blood Components That Do Not Contain RBCs

Compatibility testing for blood components without RBCs (i.e., platelets and plasma) is much less complex than it is for products with RBCs since no crossmatching must be done. ABO grouping of donor units and the patient must be performed to avoid the transfusion of plasma that is ABO-incompatible with the recipient's RBCs. The amount of anti-A and/or anti-B isoagglutinin in a unit of apheresis platelets or FFP (200 to 300 mL) could lead to destruction of some of the recipient's RBCs if there were an ABO mismatch. Rh-negative recipients may receive plasma products or apheresis platelets from a donor of any Rh type, since these components do not contain RBCs. Whole blood-derived platelets from Rh-negative donors may be preferentially selected for Rh-negative patients, particularly if there is visible RBC contamination of the platelet product, to avoid the possibility of alloimmunization to the D antigen.

INDICATIONS FOR TRANSFUSION

Table 12–6 is a list of indications for transfusion of RBCs, platelets, plasma, and cryoprecipitate.

Red Blood Cells

A National Institutes of Health (NIH) Consensus Conference established broad parameters for perioperative RBC transfusion. Although the conclusion of the conference was that "no single measure can replace good clinical judgment as the basis for decisions regarding perioperative transfusion," it was suggested that patients with hemoglobin levels exceeding 10 g/dL (100 g/L) rarely require transfusion, while those with hemoglobin levels less than 7 g/dL (70 g/L) frequently do. Several professional organizations have also established guidelines for RBC transfusion. There have been a small number of randomized trials comparing the clinical outcomes of liberal and stringent RBC transfusion triggers that have consistently failed to demonstrate any benefit of transfusing patients for hematocrits of 30% (10 g/dL) compared to triggers as low as 21% (7 g/dL).

> Hemoglobin levels exceeding 10 g/dL (100 g/L) rarely require transfusion, while those with hemoglobin levels less than 7 g/dL (70 g/L) frequently do.

TABLE 12–6   Indications for Transfusion

Packed RBCs
Hgb <7 g/dL or hematocrit <21% in a patient with uncompromised cardiovascular function
Hgb <10 g/dL or hematocrit <30% in a patient with cardiovascular disease, sepsis, or hemoglobinopathy

Platelets
Prophylactically for platelet count <10,000 μL^{-1} (adults), or <50,000 μL^{-1} (neonate)
<30,000 platelets/μL and bleeding or minor bedside procedure
<50,000 platelets/μL and intra- or postoperative bleeding
<100,000 platelets/μL and bleeding post cardiopulmonary bypass
Do not transfuse platelets in setting of thrombocytopenic thrombotic purpura, heparin-induced thrombocytopenia. Platelet transfusions are unlikely to be useful in idiopathic thrombocytopenic purpura or posttransfusion purpura

Fresh frozen plasma
Bleeding in patients with INR ≥2
Bedside procedure and INR ≥2
Prophylaxis (nonbleeding) with INR ≥6
FFP is not indicated for patients with INR <1.5
Thrombotic thrombocytopenic purpura

Cryoprecipitate
Bleeding in the setting of: • Dysfibrinogenemia • Fibrinogen <100 mg/dL • von Willebrand disease

Hgb, hemoglobin; INR, international normalized ratio.

Platelets

Indications for platelet transfusion have also been addressed by an NIH Consensus Conference and by professional organizations. Of particular interest in the last several years has been a reassessment of the use of prophylactic platelet transfusions in thrombocytopenic patients with marrow failure. In general, the traditional trigger level of 20,000 platelets/μL for prophylactic transfusion has been replaced with a level of 10,000 platelets/μL. There has even been a challenge to the utility of any prophylactic platelet transfusion, including before minor procedures such as line placement and lumbar puncture. This challenge suggests that platelets should only be administered in cases of actual bleeding. Appropriate uses of platelets in other settings are included in **Table 12–6**.

> In general, the traditional trigger level of 20,000 platelets/μL for prophylactic transfusion has been replaced with a level of 10,000 platelets/μL.

Fresh Frozen Plasma

Clinical situations in which FFP is likely to be useful also have been established by an NIH Consensus Conference and professional organizations. FFP has been used as replacement therapy for deficiencies of clotting factors and regulatory proteins, including protein C and protein S, for which specific concentrates or recombinant products are not available. The use of FFP to reverse patients with mild coagulation abnormalities is probably not warranted. The risk of bleeding appears to be very low when the prothrombin time (PT) and the international normalized ratio (INR) derived from it are only mildly elevated (<1.5 times the control) or the INR is ≤1.5. The same can be said for mild elevations of the partial thromboplastin time (PTT) associated with coagulation factor deficiencies. It is also unlikely to provide any benefit to patients with mild elevations in the PT or PTT who are undergoing minor procedures (e.g., line placement). On the other hand, FFP is effective in the treatment of thrombotic thrombocytopenic purpura, reversing the effects of warfarin in an emergency situation, the treatment of the bleeding patient with disseminated intravascular coagulation, and massive transfusion cases.

Cryoprecipitate

The practice of using cryoprecipitate as a source of fibrinogen and Factor XIII is well accepted. In addition, cryoprecipitate can be mixed with thrombin to form topical fibrin "glue," which is used to initiate anatomic connections and control bleeding over large surfaces; however, products with standardized amounts of fibrinogen that have undergone viral inactivation procedures are now commercially available and are generally preferable. The role of cryoprecipitate in the treatment of bleeding in uremic patients is controversial. Cryoprecipitate is no longer recommended for treatment of hemophilia A or von Willebrand disease because of the availability of other products.

COMPLICATIONS OF BLOOD TRANSFUSION

An adverse effect of blood transfusion occurs in an estimated 3.0% to 3.5% of transfusions in the United States. These complications of transfusion can be classified as immunologic, infectious, or due to the chemical or physical characteristics of blood components.

Immunologic Reactions
RBC Reactions

Hemolytic Transfusion Reactions
Although HTR are much discussed, they are fortunately quite uncommon, reflecting the efficacy of the serologic and procedural techniques in place to prevent their occurrence. Although HTR occur with less than 0.1% of the units transfused in the United States, they can be life-threatening complications. It bears noting that fatal, acute HTR due to ABO incompatibility is a more frequent adverse outcome of transfusion than infection with HIV or HCV, and it is more often the result of patient or sample misidentification than to serologic mishaps or exotic blood types.

HTR are mediated by antibodies directed against alloantigens present on transfused RBCs. Most alloantibodies to RBC antigens, other than the AB isoagglutinins, develop in response to exposure to allogeneic RBCs by transfusion or maternal–fetal hemorrhage. There are hundreds of RBC antigens comprising more than 50 systems. Fortunately, only a small proportion of these have clinical significance. In addition to the AB isoagglutinins, antibodies to antigens in the Rh, Kell, Duffy, Kidd, and MNSs systems are responsible for the preponderance of HTR. Identification of these alloantibodies, by the techniques discussed above, is important because the degree and severity of hemolysis differs among them.

HTR can either be acute, occurring within 24 hours of transfusion, or delayed, in a reaction that appears 5 to 7 days (range 3 to 21 days) after the transfusion is completed. Acute reactions are more severe than their delayed counterparts, and occur in patients who already have antibodies to RBC alloantigens when they are transfused with RBCs bearing those target antigens. The most severe acute HTRs are due to ABO incompatibility because the AB isoagglutinins are present at a substantial titer and fix complement efficiently, being largely IgM. The A and/or B antigen sites are also abundant on RBCs (typically 1 to 2×10^6 antigen sites per cell). Antibodies to antigens in the Kell, Kidd, and Duffy systems also have been responsible for acute HTR.

Acute HTR typically present with temperature elevation. Nausea, vomiting, hypotension, low back pain, and substernal pressure may also signal the occurrence of acute hemolysis. Hemolysis is generally intravascular in this setting. The hemoglobin released into the plasma from the lysed RBCs is apparent as hemoglobinemia (red plasma rather than yellow) and hemoglobinuria (red urine which remains red after centrifugation). Disseminated intravascular coagulation and systemic hemodynamic instability may be triggered by the hemolysis. Together with the direct toxic effects of cell-free hemoglobin on the tubular cells of the kidney, these conditions are responsible for the impaired kidney function that often accompanies acute intravascular hemolysis. Therapy is largely supportive but preservation of renal function is sought through the use of intravenous hydration and diuretics.

An adverse effect of blood transfusion occurs in an estimated 3.0% to 3.5% of transfusions in the United States. These complications of transfusion can be classified as immunologic, infectious, or due to the chemical or physical characteristics of blood components.

Delayed HTR occur in 2 situations. In 1, the patient is exposed to a foreign RBC alloantigen by a transfusion and mounts a primary immune response. As the amount of antibody increases, hemolysis may ensue. A delayed response may also occur when a patient is re-exposed to an alloantigen to which he or she was sensitized in the past by previous transfusion or pregnancy. Even if the alloantibody to this antigen is not detectable prior to the transfusion, exposure to the alloantigen can stimulate an anamnestic response. Antibodies to Kidd and Rh antigens are frequently responsible for such reactions. Hemolysis is typically extravascular in delayed HTR with the only clinical and laboratory signs being a decrease in the hemoglobin level, a rise in the bilirubin level, a low grade temperature, and a feeling of malaise. When no hemolysis can be detected in a delayed HTR, the reaction is called a delayed serologic (rather than hemolytic) transfusion reaction.

Reactions to Plasma Components

Hypersensitivity Reactions—Allergic and Anaphylactic Transfusion Reactions

Allergic reactions occur in 1% to 3% of patients receiving blood products containing plasma. In most cases, these hypersensitivity reactions are a host response to foreign plasma proteins in the donor blood components. The vast majority of these reactions consist of hives, pruritis, and erythema, and can be managed with antihistamines or steroids. More serious responses such as bronchospasm, laryngeal edema, gastrointestinal disturbance (nausea, vomiting, cramps, and diarrhea), and hypotension (anaphylactoid reaction) are much less frequent. IgA-deficient patients with anti-IgA antibodies in their plasma are at risk for serious reactions including frank anaphylaxis if exposed to IgA in a transfused blood component. If transfusion is required, these patients should be provided with components from IgA-deficient donors, or, in an elective situation, store their own components. Washing packed RBC can effectively remove IgA. Patients who are IgA deficient, but who do not have anti-IgA, do not require special preparations, but should be observed closely during transfusion.

White Blood Cell Reactions

Febrile-Nonhemolytic Transfusion Reactions (FNHTRs)

These reactions are among the most common transfusion-related complications and accompany 1% to 3% of transfusions of cellular components. They are more common in multiply transfused patients and with nonleukoreduced cellular components. An FNHTR usually presents with a temperature elevation of 1°C or more, during or shortly after a transfusion (usually within 1 to 2 hours), that is unlikely to be associated with the patient's underlying disease or therapy. The temperature elevation is often accompanied by chills, rigors, and generalized discomfort, and in some patients, nausea and vomiting as well. The majority of these reactions are mild and do not persist for more than 8 hours. Anti-pyretics may be administered, and occasionally meperidine may be required to treat severe rigors. These reactions have long been considered to be the product of anti-leukocyte antibodies present in the recipient's plasma, reacting with WBCs or WBC fragments in the transfused product. There may, however, be other etiologies for the FNHTRs, including the presence of cytokines released by lymphocytes in the donated unit during storage.

Transfusion-associated Graft Versus Host Disease (TA-GVHD)

Immunocompetent T lymphocytes present in cellular blood components may engraft in an immunoincompetent transfusion recipient, particularly if cellular immunity is compromised. The engrafted, allogeneic T cells mount an alloimmune response to cells in the skin and gastrointestinal tract, as in TA-GVHD, and to the cells in the bone marrow as well, making this complication of transfusion often lethal. Fortunately, T lymphocytes in cellular blood components can be inactivated by exposure to gamma irradiation, which effectively prevents this complication. Patients at risk for this rare complication include those undergoing HPC transplantation or who have hematologic malignancies. Low-birth-weight infants, infants born with hemolytic disease of the newborn, and fetuses receiving intrauterine transfusions are also at risk. Patients with congenital T-cell immunodeficiencies (e.g., Wiskott–Aldrich and diGeorge syndromes) have also developed this complication. Cellular components from blood relative donors are also routinely irradiated to prevent TA-GVHD that may occur in the circumstance when the donor is homozygous for an HLA haplotype shared with the transfusion recipient. In this situation, the transfused T cells

Febrile-nonhemolytic transfusion reactions are among the most common transfusion-related complications and accompany 1% to 3% of transfusions of cellular components.

remain immunologically invisible to the otherwise immunocompetent host and, rather than being cleared, engraft and attack the host, recognizing the mismatched host haplotype as foreign. Most of the reports of TA-GVHD in other patients with solid tumors or who were undergoing surgery pre-date the awareness of this 1-way haplotype match, which is the most likely explanation for the occurrence of this event in these immunocompetent patients.

Transfusion-related Acute Lung Injury (TRALI)

TRALI is characterized by the development of acute respiratory distress, hypoxia, and bilateral infiltrates on chest X-ray, often accompanied by fever and hypotension, during or within 6 hours of completion of a transfusion. To meet the current working definition of TRALI, there must be no pre-existing form of acute lung injury or other risk factors such as sepsis, aspiration, or pneumonia. Most patients recover completely with supportive care, which usually includes mechanical ventilation, and the pulmonary infiltrates usually resolve within 2 to 4 days without long term sequelae. However, there is a 5% mortality rate. This complication has been attributed to the presence of anti-leukocyte antibodies in the plasma of donor blood (often from females with a history of pregnancy) that react with the recipient's WBCs. This results in the formation of immune complexes that are trapped in the pulmonary vasculature and lead to alveolar edema. At present, various steps are being taken to reduce the incidence of TRALI such as not making FFP from female donors or donors with a history of pregnancy or transfusion, or by testing for HLA antibodies.

Platelet Reactions

Posttransfusion Purpura (see the section "Bleeding Disorders" in Chapter 11)

This rare complication occurs in patients who lack a common platelet antigen (often HPA-A1) and have developed an alloantibody by exposure through prior transfusion or pregnancy. When re-exposed to HPA-A1 by transfusion of a platelet product or an RBC product containing contaminating platelets, these patients appear to develop an anamnestic response and become severely thrombocytopenic 7 to 10 days later. Paradoxically, the patient's own platelets, which are HPA-A1 negative, are also cleared. Several explanations have been offered including the observation that there is an initial IgM response that reacts with GP IIb–IIIa (essentially a platelet autoantibody) but then "matures" with the production of an IgG with anti-HPA-A1 specificity. The reaction is self-limiting, but may be complicated by severe hemorrhage. Steroids and intravenous immunoglobulin have been used successfully to manage this immunologic reaction.

Refractoriness to Platelet Transfusions

Patients may become sensitized to leukocyte and platelet antigens through transfusion or pregnancy. Transfused platelets may be cleared rapidly when given to a patient who has preformed antibodies directed at foreign platelet antigens or HLA Class I molecules, which are also expressed on the platelet membrane. As a result, it may be extremely difficult to elevate the platelet count in such patients. A patient is considered to be refractory to platelet transfusion if the increment measured between 15 and 60 minutes after the platelet transfusion is lower than expected on 2 occasions. Note that counts done several hours afterward are not useful for determining which patients are immunologically refractory. The posttransfusion count may be corrected for the number of platelets administered and the patient's body surface area (the "corrected count increment") as follows:

$$\text{Corrected count increment} = \frac{\text{Platelet count increment} \times \text{Body surface area} \times 10^{11}}{\text{Number of platelets transfused}}$$

Here the default for number of platelets transfused is: 1 unit whole blood-derived platelets = 5.5×10^{10} platelets. 1 unit apheresis platelets = 3×10^{11} platelets.

A corrected count increment of <7,500 is a strong evidence of immunologic refractoriness. Note that other causes of refractoriness should be ruled out, among them: active bleeding, fever, sepsis, splenomegaly (splenic sequestration), disseminated intravascular coagulation, marrow transplantation, antibiotics (e.g., vancomycin), IV amphotericin B, thrombotic thrombocytopenic purpura, idiopathic or immune thrombocytopenic purpura, and heparin-induced thrombocytopenia.

Patients with immunologic refractoriness may respond well to platelets from donors who lack the HLA antigens corresponding to the patient's HLA alloantibodies (or to platelets which are HLA matched) or to platelets that have been chosen by platelet crossmatching.

Leukocytes in the transfused unit appear to be necessary for stimulating the immune response to both platelet and leukocyte antigens. Alloimmunization may be prevented by transfusion of cellular components from which leukocytes have been removed, usually by passage of the product through a filter that retains the leukocytes. Patients who are likely to need extensive platelet transfusion support (e.g., HPC transplants or hematologic malignancies) often receive leukoreduced cellular components to reduce the likelihood of alloimmunization.

Nonimmunologic Reactions

Complications Created by the Physical Characteristics of Blood

Hypothermia

Transfusion of small volumes of cold blood may be associated with minor discomfort. This complication can be averted by using blood warmers or blankets. In the setting of massive transfusion, however, the rapid transfusion of large amounts of blood that is at 1°C to 10°C contributes to hypothermia. Hemostasis is impaired when the circulating blood is below 37°C and in extreme situations, cardiac dysrhythmias and arrest may occur. In this setting, the use of high-throughput blood warmers is warranted.

Transfusion-associated Circulatory Overload (TACO)

Volume overload is a relatively common but often overlooked complication of transfusion. Patients with congestive heart failure or renal failure, the very young, and the very old are particularly at risk. It should be suspected in a patient who complains of dyspnea, orthopnea, cough, or chest pain, during or soon after transfusion, particularly if there are signs of hypoxia, rales, tachycardia, or hypertension. Supplemental oxygen and diuresis may be required. Future transfusions should be carried out slowly and perhaps with the aid of a diuretic.

Chemical Complications

> Volume overload is a relatively common but often overlooked complication of transfusion. Patients with congestive heart failure or renal failure, the very young, and the very old are particularly at risk.

Iron Overload

Each unit of packed RBC contains approximately 200 mg of iron. Chronic RBC transfusion can overwhelm the body's mechanisms for eliminating excess iron resulting in accumulation in various tissues. An individual who has received 100 or more units of RBCs (20 g of iron) is at risk to develop various complications of iron overload including cardiac dysrhythmias, pancreatic failure ("bronze diabetes"), and liver function abnormalities. Tissue iron can be mobilized and excreted using chelating agents such as desferroxamine or deferasirox. Chelation therapy is a slow process and is more effective if deployed well before tissue accumulation of iron is extensive.

Potassium Toxicity

Potassium leaks out of RBCs during storage as ATP levels decline and the ATPase-dependent Na^+/K^+ pump activity diminishes. Once the banked RBCs are transfused, they transport glucose, restore their ATP levels, and take up the K^+ that was lost during storage. In the short term, however, each unit of RBCs might contain as much as 6 mmol of extracellular K^+ at the time of outdate. There have been a handful of reports of neonates, or patients with renal failure receiving large volumes of banked blood, who have developed life-threatening cardiac dysrhythmias. Neonates usually receive RBC units that have been stored for less than 1 week and have not yet accumulated much extracellular K^+. Washing RBC is also an effective means of removing extracellular K^+, although it is very rarely required.

Citrate Toxicity

Citrate is the anticoagulant used in the collection of all blood products and is therefore transfused with the blood product into the patient. Citrate is present in the plasma. Hence, most of it ends up in platelet and plasma products while there is relatively little in RBC products. Citrate is metabolized by every nucleated cell of the body, but in circumstances where large volumes of banked blood are being infused rapidly, as in massive transfusion, the rapid influx of citrate may overwhelm the body's metabolic capacity, leading to an accumulation in the patient's plasma. Most patients can receive up to 1 unit of FFP every 6 minutes without evidence of citrate toxicity. Patients with liver failure metabolize citrate more slowly, however, and are particularly susceptible. The accumulating citrate chelates calcium, causing the ionized calcium levels to drop and producing perioral tingling and extremity paresthesias. In extreme circumstances, it may produce severe hypo(ionized)calcemia that can lead to cardiac dysrhythmias.

Depletion of 2,3-Diphosphoglycerate (2,3-DPG)

With increasing storage time of RBCs, the intracellular level of 2,3-DPG decreases, producing a left shift of the oxyhemoglobin dissociation curve. Once banked RBCs are transfused, they restore the levels of 2,3-DPG over a period of 24 to 48 hours. It has been suggested that the high oxygen affinity of the hemoglobin in the 2,3-DPG-deficient banked RBCs might impair oxygen delivery, particularly to neonates. As a result, it has become a general practice to transfuse neonates with RBCs that have been banked less than 1 week. However, most of the literature demonstrating unfavorable outcomes for neonates receiving older units was based on studies with RBC storage systems in which maintenance of 2,3-DPG levels was not as effective as it is using the current systems.

Infectious Complications (see the section "Infectious Disease Testing")

The Classic Pathogens

Transfusion transmission of the hepatitis viruses and the retroviruses has been substantially reduced through the interventions of donor education, screening on the basis of medical history and risk behaviors, and testing, including the use of highly sensitive techniques based on amplification of viral genetic nucleic acids. The residual risk of HIV or HCV infection through transfusion is in the range of 1 event per 1 to 2×10^6 units transfused. Viral transmission by pooled plasma products has also been largely eliminated by the use of robust viral inactivation techniques or replacement with recombinant proteins.

Transfusion transmission of the hepatitis viruses and the retroviruses has been substantially reduced through the interventions of donor education, screening on the basis of medical history and risk behaviors, and testing.

The Current Significant Pathogens

At the present time, bacterial contamination of blood components is the most significant infectious complication of transfusion in developed countries, in terms of both the number of transmitted infections and the number of fatalities. It has been estimated that in the United States, approximately 1 in 500,000 units of RBCs, or 1 in 10,000 to 20,000 units of platelets, is associated with transfusion-transmitted sepsis. The organisms most frequently associated with septic RBC transfusions are psychrophilic gram-negative bacteria such as *Yersinia enterocolitic* and *Pseudomonas* spp., as well as *Enterobacter* spp. and *Serratia* spp. Platelet units have been reported to transmit gram-positive cocci (*Streptococcus aureus, S. epidermidis,* and *Staphylococcus* spp.) as well as gram-negative organisms (*Klebsiella* spp., *Serratia* spp., *Salmonella* spp., and *Enterobacter* spp.). The sources of these bacteria are thought to be skin commensals picked up and introduced into the blood donation with the venipuncture, or less commonly, cryptic bacteremia in clinically healthy donors. Even if the inoculum is quite small, blood provides a superb culture medium, particularly when stored at room temperature, as is the case for platelets. Although donors are now questioned specifically about antibiotic use, the health history is neither a sensitive nor a specific screening tool. The implementation of tests to screen platelet products for evidence of bacterial contamination was discussed above.

Cytomegalovirus (CMV) is a ubiquitous member of the herpes virus family to which approximately 30% to 60% of adults in developed countries have been exposed. CMV can be transmitted by transfusion of blood components that contain leukocytes, such as packed RBCs and platelets. Although primary infection rarely produces serious disease in immunologically intact hosts, it is associated with systemic infection in immunocompromised patients who are CMV-seronegative. The following groups of patients have been shown to be susceptible to transfusion-transmitted CMV primary infection and disease and should receive CMV reduced-risk cellular blood components:

1. premature, low-birth-weight (<1,200 g) neonates;
2. CMV-seronegative pregnant women (including those undergoing intrauterine transfusions);
3. CMV-seronegative recipients of, or candidates for, hematopoietic or solid organ transplants;
4. CMV-seronegative, HIV-infected patients.

CMV reduced-risk blood components can be obtained by screening donors for CMV antibody (IgG) that indicates past exposure, or by removing the leukocytes that contain latent CMV by filtration with leukocyte reduction filters. These 2 approaches have been shown to be equally effective in preventing transfusion-transmitted CMV infection. Only cellular components need to be CMV reduced-risk, since intact mononuclear cells are required to transmit CMV.

Emerging Pathogens.

The blood supply will always be vulnerable to the introduction of new pathogens into the donor population. In some instances, the pathogen may truly be a new organism, or one that has recently acquired the ability to infect humans, such as the SARS virus, various strains of avian flu, and the bovine prion responsible for variant Creutzfeldt–Jakob disease. Population shifts in response to natural or man-made catastrophes, or simply travel for business or pleasure, spread pathogens from one part of the world to another, such as the West Nile Virus, *Plasmodium* spp., and *Trypanosoma* spp. In some circumstances, questioning donors about exposure to a pathogen or a history of a characteristic illness, or the rapid development of a screening test has been an effective means of interdicting transfusion transmission of a new infectious agent. However, an effective response is more difficult in the circumstance where the organism has not been identified, its biology is unique, the routes of transmission are not well understood, or the clinical effects are not well defined. As a result, work continues to develop pathogen inactivation technology that would be suitable for cellular blood components.

Transfusion Reaction Work-up

If a reaction is suspected, the transfusion must be stopped immediately while maintaining intravenous access, and the patient must be assessed. Emergent airway and hemodynamic issues should be dealt with immediately and appropriate measures taken to alleviate the patient's major symptoms and concerns. If the assessment reveals that the patient's only symptoms are cutaneous manifestations of hypersensitivity (flushing, pruritis, and urticaria), then the transfusion may be resumed under careful observation. In all other situations, the transfusion of that unit should be stopped and a clerical check should be performed to verify that the correct unit (i.e., one labeled for that patient) has been administered. A transfusion reaction form should be filled out and a new blood bank specimen should be drawn from the patient. The transfusion reaction form, the unit involved, and the new specimen should be returned to the blood bank for evaluation. A posttransfusion urine specimen should also be obtained and sent for urinalysis.

The blood bank will perform a clerical check, and compare the posttransfusion specimen with the pretransfusion specimen used for compatibility testing for the appearance of hemolysis or hyperbilirubinemia. The ABO and Rh type of the posttransfusion specimen will be done to confirm that the pretransfusion specimen was indeed from this patient and that the ABO and Rh type of the unit that was being transfused was appropriate. A direct antiglobulin test is also performed on the posttransfusion specimen looking for antibody-coated RBC (i.e., donor cells coated with recipient alloantibody) indicating an immune-based HTR. Any findings suggestive of an HTR trigger a more extensive investigation in the blood bank. If the work-up rules out a hemolytic reaction, transfusion may resume.

ALTERNATIVES TO ALLOGENEIC TRANSFUSION

The 1980s saw the considerable development of techniques to avoid allogeneic transfusion (transfusion with someone else's blood), particularly in elective surgery. The major driver was concern about the infectious complications of transfusion. Before the development of a screening test

If a reaction is suspected, the transfusion must be stopped immediately while maintaining intravenous access, and the patient must be assessed.

in 1985, HIV transmission rates may have been as high as 1 in 10,000 units transfused, while as many as 5% to 10% of transfusion recipients developed what was then called non-A, non-B hepatitis, and is now known to have been due primarily to HCV, which was only identified in 1989. Although demand for these blood-sparing techniques is not as great as it was 20 years ago, they are still in use and continue to be helpful for patients with unusual blood types or multiple alloantibodies for whom it is difficult to find compatible blood. In addition, the drive to avoid allogeneic blood exposure has reinforced common sense measures: treatment of medically correctable anemia, greater physician tolerance of asymptomatic anemia, meticulous surgical hemostasis, and the wider use of hemostatic medications. The licensing of recombinant erythropoietin also reduced the dependence of patients with renal failure, malignancies, and HIV infection on regular RBC transfusion.

Four techniques in particular were developed to reduce the dependence of surgical patients on banked RBC: preoperative autologous blood donation (PABD), acute normovolemic hemodilution (ANH), intraoperative blood recovery and reinfusion, and postoperative blood recovery and reinfusion.

PABD is suitable for patients undergoing elective surgical procedures for which RBC transfusion is commonly required, and in this setting can reduce allogeneic blood use. Since the blood may only be used by the donor/recipient, donor qualifications are simple and no testing (other than ABO/Rh typing) is required. Note that mistransfusion, bacterial contamination, and volume overload are just as likely to occur with an autologous unit as an allogeneic unit. Since the hazards averted (especially of infection) are very small, donors who might be put at even a small risk by donation (e.g., mild anemia and coronary artery insufficiency) should be discouraged from PABD.

ANH is a technique whereby several units of blood are removed from a patient in the operating room immediately before a procedure. The volume is replaced with crystalloid. The blood is returned if bleeding occurs, or at the end of the procedure. The practice is more common in Europe than in the United States. It has the advantage that little advance planning is necessary, but it is not very efficacious at reducing allogeneic RBC transfusions for patients with moderate anemia from whom few units can be withdrawn at the beginning of the procedure.

Blood recovered from the operative field can be collected, processed in some manner, and reinfused. Shed blood is collected by suction from a reservoir, usually with heparin or citrate, and then usually washed in a centrifugal device specially designed for this purpose. The washed RBCs are suspended in normal saline and pumped into a bag suitable for reinfusion to the patient. The washing procedure removes materials that might cause reactions such as cell debris, activated clotting factors, and complement. A similar process can be carried out manually. This technique is particularly helpful in procedures where large volumes of blood are lost. Although somewhat expensive, the recovery of 3 to 4 units of RBCs is usually adequate to recover the costs. This technique is suitable for elective as well as emergency procedures during which blood loss is extensive.

Devices are also available for collecting blood shed in the postoperative period. Many of them rely on filtration of the shed blood. The filtration technique is not adequate to remove materials that can provoke a reaction and is generally not worth risking for the small amounts of blood that can be recovered. A small, centrifugal device that washes the blood collected postoperatively is also available. Although it provides a much cleaner product, the small volumes of blood recovered in this manner do not make it very cost-effective.

CELLULAR THERAPIES

Cellular therapies encompass the collection, processing, storage, and therapeutic use of hematopoietic cells, most commonly HPCs. In addition, mononuclear cell fractions from HPC donors have been used to enhance the graft versus tumor effect of allogeneic transplantation, and dendritic cells sensitized to tumor antigens have been used to treat solid tumors. Allogeneic HPC have the advantage that they are free of malignancy and may have a significant graft versus tumor effect; they are preferred for most forms of leukemia, Hodgkin disease, and the myelodysplastic syndromes. Allogeneic transplantation has also occasionally been used to treat certain genetic disorders of the hematopoietic system, such as sickle cell disease and thalassemia. Autologous

> Cellular therapies encompass the collection, processing, storage, and therapeutic use of hematopoietic cells.

HPC transplants are not complicated by rejection and have a lower incidence of GVHD. They are performed in patients with some forms of non-Hodgkin lymphoma and multiple myeloma, and as rescue therapy after intensive chemotherapy for some solid tumors (e.g., testicular, breast, and ovarian cancer).

Potential allogeneic donors must in general meet the criteria for blood donation, including infectious disease testing, although some of these criteria may be waived if an alternate suitable donor cannot be found. Potential donors must be typed for HLA Class I and II antigens using molecular techniques. Class I mismatches are at increased risk for rejection and failure to engraft, whereas Class II mismatches are associated with increased incidence of GVHD. A single Class I or II mismatch usually has little impact on survival. Two Class I mismatches, or a Class I and a Class II mismatch, are usually associated with poorer outcomes. Haploidentical sibling donors have been used successfully. If a suitable family member donor cannot be found (and only 1 in 4 siblings is likely to be a 2 haplotype match), a donor may be sought through the National Marrow Donor Program, a registry of people who have been HLA typed and have expressed a willingness to donate HPCs. The search may take a few months and is less likely to be successful for patients with unusual phenotypes. There has been considerable effort in the past few years to register donors from previously under-represented minority populations. ABO or Rh matching is not necessary since the transplant recipient will convert to the donor type if engraftment is successful, although RBC engraftment may be delayed if donor RBCs are incompatible with the recipient's anti-A or anti-B isoagglutinins. Donor isoagglutinins may also cause hemolysis of residual recipient RBCs, or at least a positive direct antiglobulin test. The conversion from recipient to donor blood type does pose problems for the transfusion service that must provide blood that is compatible with donor and recipient until the recipient's original RBCs and isoagglutinins are undetectable.

HPCs may be collected from peripheral blood by apheresis, from bone marrow by aspiration, or from cord blood. Apheresis collection now accounts for 90% of autologous transplants, and 50% of allogeneic transplants, a fraction which is increasing. Bone marrow aspiration is performed with multiple punctures and aspirations of the posterior iliac crest and must be performed in the operating room with the donor under general anesthesia. The aspirates are anticoagulated (heparin or citrate), filtered, and pooled into a bag that is then usually stored frozen until the time of the transplant.

Collection by apheresis is less invasive and less likely to recover residual malignant cells. In addition, it has been shown to be associated with quicker engraftment, although chronic GVHD is somewhat more likely to occur than with marrow transplantation. The number of HPCs in the peripheral blood is ordinarily very low, so donors are prepared by the administration of granulocyte colony-stimulating factor or granulocyte–macrophage colony-stimulating factor at the point when their marrow is rebounding from a cycle of chemotherapy. Under these circumstances, the levels of HPCs (which can be determined by measuring the number of CD34-positive cells in the peripheral blood by flow cytometry) may be elevated 200- to 1,000-fold. The pheresis instrument is configured to collect the mononuclear cell fraction. Large volume collections (with 3 blood volumes processed) are typically performed, which reduces the number of procedures needed to collect the targeted number of CD34-positive cells (typically 2 to 4×10^6 per kg patient weight). Large volume collection may also have the effect of recruiting HPCs from the marrow during the collection.

The HPC product undergoes extensive quality control testing including: ABO and Rh type, RBC and WBC counts (and differential), CD34 cell count, an assay to enumerate colony-forming units in vitro, cell viability and testing for bacteria, fungi, and mycoplasma. Products are frozen (usually at a controlled rate) in the presence of 10% dimethylsulfoxide and 10% protein (plasma or albumin) as cryoprotectants, and stored in mechanical freezers or liquid nitrogen tanks. At the time of transplant, the units are thawed at 37°C, usually at the patient's bedside, and then administered intravenously, much like a conventional transfusion.

Umbilical cord blood contains high levels of circulating HPCs, and this observation has led to the development of cord blood banking. If a mother meets the criteria for allogeneic blood donation (except for hemoglobin level and recent pregnancy because she has just delivered) including the usual infectious disease testing, and there is no history of genetic diseases in the family of either parent, she may give consent for the blood to be drained from the placenta via the umbilical

TABLE 12-7 **Categories of Indications for Therapeutic Apheresis**

Category	Use of Therapeutic Apheresis	Evidence for Clinical Efficacy
Category I	Primary therapy or a first-line adjunct to other therapies	Randomized, controlled clinical trials or a broad base of published experience
Category II	Supportive therapy or a second-line adjunct to other therapies	Benefit from apheresis is well accepted, supported by randomized, controlled clinical trials, small series, or informative case studies
Category III	Experimental therapy indicated when conventional therapies have failed or as part of a research protocol	Insufficient evidence exists to establish the efficacy of apheresis or risk/benefit; trials with conflicting results or small number of case reports
Category IV	Lack of therapeutic efficacy of apheresis has been demonstrated	Controlled studies or case reports fail to show clinical benefit

Adapted with permission from Szczepiorkowski Z, Shaz BH, Bandarenko N, Winters JL. A new approach to assignment of AFSA categories—introduction to the fourth special issue: clinical applications of therapeutic apheresis. *J Clin Apheresis.* 2007;22:97.

cord (after it has been severed or clamped off from the neonate) and then stored frozen. In addition to the usual quality control testing of the cord blood, HLA Class I and II typing is performed as well as ABO/Rh typing.

Over 5,000 related and unrelated (but HLA matched) cord blood transplants have been performed since the technique was first developed in 1988. Cord blood HPCs home readily to the host bone marrow and do not seem to be as alloreactive to recipient antigen-presenting cells as HPCs from adults. In addition, the large numbers of HLA-typed cord blood samples may improve the chances of finding unrelated matches. Cord transplants are also less likely to be complicated by GVHD and infection with CMV. However, the total number of HPCs in each cord blood sample is small and engraftment is slower. This has led to the use of double cord transplants that accelerate engraftment, even though eventually 1 of the donor's HPCs dominates.

THERAPEUTIC APHERESIS

Therapeutic apheresis is the process of withdrawing blood from the body, selectively removing one particular element (i.e., plasma, leukocytes, platelets, or RBCs), and returning the remaining elements along with a replacement solution (crystalloid and/or colloid) to maintain isovolemia. There are several different therapeutic apheresis procedures that are designed to remove, or treat, specific components of the blood. These are described below.

Indications for Therapeutic Apheresis

Indications for therapeutic apheresis have been classified according to the quality of the evidence demonstrating efficacy or the lack thereof (**Table 12–7**). The specific disorders for which therapeutic apheresis has been evaluated as a treatment are shown in **Table 12–8**.

Therapeutic apheresis has been used as a treatment for numerous disorders. While it is clearly effective in some diseases, such as thrombotic thrombocytopenic purpura, the therapeutic benefit of apheresis in many other disorders is much less clear, because many of them are uncommon, and therefore it is extremely difficult to obtain information about efficacy based on large-scale, prospective, randomized clinical trials.

Plasmapheresis

In plasmapheresis (plasma exchange; see the figure in Chapter 2), blood is withdrawn from a patient and the plasma is separated from the cellular components by centrifugation or, less commonly, by filtration, in an apheresis instrument. The plasma is discarded and the cellular components are returned to the patient. Liters of abnormal plasma can be removed from the

TABLE 12–8　**Categories of Indications for Therapeutic Apheresis**

Disorders	Category I	Category II	Category III	Category IV
Solid organ transplantation and renal	Cryoglobulinemia (1)[a] Goodpasture syndrome (1)	Acute humoral rejection (renal allograft) (1) Cardiac allograft humoral rejection (2) Rapidly progressive glomerulonephritis with ANCA (1)	Cardiac allograft humoral rejection (1) Hemolytic–uremic syndrome (1)	Diarrhea-associated hemolytic–uremic syndrome (1)
Neurologic	Acute Guillain–Barré syndrome (1) CIDP (1) Myasthenia gravis (1) PANDAS (1) Paraproteinemic peripheral neuropathy—IgG, IgA (1) Sydenham's chorea (1)	Acute CNS multiple sclerosis (1) Lambert–Eaton myasthenic syndrome (1) Paraproteinemic peripheral neuropathy—IgM (1)	Paraneoplastic syndromes (1) Chronic, progressive multiple sclerosis (1)	
Metabolic	Familial hypercholesterolemia (5)	Familial hypercholesterolemia (1) Mushroom poisoning (1) Refsum disease (1)	Acute hepatic failure (1) Nonmushroom poisonings (1) Thyrotoxicosis (1) Sepsis (1)	
Hematologic and oncologic	Erythrodermic cutaneous lymphoma (2) Hyperviscosity/ paraproteinemia (1) Leukocytosis/ leukostasis (3) Sickle cell crisis (severe) (4)	ABO-incompatible marrow transplant (apheresis of recipient) (1) Babesiosis/malaria (severe) (4) Graft vs host disease (skin) (2) Maternal alloimmunization (1) Thrombocytosis (symptomatic) (3)	Aplastic anemia/red cell aplasia (1) Autoimmune hemolytic anemia (1) Coagulation factor inhibitors (1) Posttransfusion purpura (1)	Cutaneous lymphoma— nonerythrodermic (2) Immune thrombocytopenia (1)
Autoimmune	TTP (1)		Pemphigus vulgaris (1, 2) Progressive systemic scleroderma (1) SLE (nonrenal) (1)	Progressive systemic scleroderma (2) SLE nephritis (1)

Abbreviations: ANCA, anti-neutrophil cytoplasmic antibody ; CIDP, chronic inflammatory demyelinating polyneuropathy; CNS, central nervous system; PANDAS, pediatric autoimmune neuropsychiatric disorders associated with streptococcal infections; SLE, systemic lupus erythematosus; TTP, thrombotic thromocytopenic purpura. Adapted with permission from Szczepiorkowski Z, Shaz BH, Bandarenko N, Winters JL. A new approach to assignment of AFSA categories—introduction to the fourth special issue: clinical applications of therapeutic apheresis. *J Clin Apheresis*. 2007;22:101–103.

[a]Number in parentheses refers to specific apheresis procedure as follows: 1) therapeutic plasma exchange; 2) photopheresis; 3) cytapheresis; 4) red cell exchange; 5) selective column adsorption.

patient and replaced by saline, albumin, starch solutions, FFP, or combinations of these. This technique is used to remove autoantibodies, immune complexes, paraproteins, and protein-bound toxins.

Cytapheresis

Cytapheresis is the removal of one of the cellular elements of the blood. *Leukapheresis* is occasionally indicated for patients with acute myelogenous leukemia or chronic myelogenous leukemia in the accelerated phase with a high level of circulating blasts and evidence of leukostasis with pulmonary or CNS involvement. Myeloid blast forms adhere to the vascular endothelium and can impede blood flow in the lungs and the brain. The collection of peripheral HPCs and granulocytes are variations on leukapheresis.

Plateletpheresis may be indicated in patients with myeloproliferative disorders, such as essential thrombocytosis, who develop platelet counts that exceed 1×10^6 μL^{-1} and also show signs of hemorrhage or thrombosis.

Erythrocytapheresis (RBC Exchange)

Although most sickle crises are managed with hydration, pain medication, and supplemental oxygen, RBC exchange is occasionally performed for patients who are experiencing a severe infarctive crisis complicated by stroke, acute chest syndrome, retinal infarction, or priapism. Exchange is performed less commonly to prepare patients for surgery. In the exchange replacement of sickle RBCs with normal RBCs, the usual goals are to reduce the hemoglobin S concentration to less than 30% of total hemoglobin, and to increase the hematocrit to 30%. Red cells chosen for exchange are often screened for hemoglobin S (since donors with sickle trait may be unaware of it and have a normal hemoglobin level) and may be partially phenotype matched (e.g., for Kell and the Rh antigens) to prevent alloimmunization. Red cell exchange also has been used to treat patients with malaria or babesiosis who have a high percentage (e.g., >10%) of RBCs infected with organisms despite adequate medical therapy, and signs of decompensation such as marked hemolysis, pulmonary involvement, CNS involvement, renal failure, or disseminated intravascular coagulation. Patients who are immunosuppressed, asplenic, or elderly seem to be particularly at risk to develop complications from infection with *Babesia*.

Photopheresis

In this apheresis procedure, the patient's leukocytes are separated from whole blood and exposed to ultraviolet light, usually after the patient has ingested psoralen. The psoralen/ultraviolet light-treated leukocytes are then returned to the patient. Photopheresis has been used to treat cutaneous T-cell lymphoma and has been shown to increase patient survival when compared to conventional chemotherapy. Photopheresis has also been used to treat GVHD and cardiac allograft rejection.

A portion of this chapter related to complications of transfusion appeared previously in Clinical Laboratory Reviews (a newsletter for physicians at the Massachusetts General Hospital, Boston, 1995;4:2).

REFERENCES

American Association of Blood Banks. *Circular of Information for the Use of Human Blood and Blood Components.* Bethesda, MD: American Association of Blood Banks; 2006. http://www.aabb.org/Documents/About_Blood/Circulars_of_Information/coiwnv0809.pdf; Accessed 01.12.09.

Bowden RA, et al. A comparison of filtered leukocyte-reduced and cytomegalovirus (CMV) seronegative blood products for the prevention of transfusion-associated CMV infection after marrow transplant. *Blood.* 1995;86:3598–3603.

Szczepiorkowski, Z., ed. Clinical applications of therapeutic apheresis: an evidence based approach. 4th ed. *J Clin Apheresis.* 2007;22:95–186.

Davenport RD. Therapeutic apheresis. In: Roback JD, Combs MR, Grossman BJ, Hillyer CD, eds. *Technical Manual.* 16th ed. Bethesda, MD: AABB Press; 2008:697–714.

Downes KA, Shulman IA. Pretransfusion testing. In: Roback JD, Combs MR, Grossman BJ, Hillyer CD, eds. *Technical Manual.* 16th ed. Bethesda, MD: AABB Press; 2008:437–464.

Fresh-Frozen Plasma, Cryoprecipitate, and Platelets Administration Practice Guidelines Development Task Force of the College of American Pathologists: practice parameter for the use of fresh-frozen plasma, cryoprecipitate, and platelets. *JAMA.* 1994;271:777.

Goldman M, et al. TRALI Consensus Panel. Proceedings of a consensus conference: towards an understanding of TRALI. *Transfus Med Rev.* 2005;19:2–31.

Hébert PC, et al. A multicenter, randomized, controlled clinical trial of transfusion requirements in critical care. *N Engl J Med.* 1999;340:409.

Herman JH, Manno CS. *Pediatric Transfusion Therapy.* Bethesda, MD: AABB Press; 2002.

Kakaiya R, et al. Whole blood collection and component processing. In: Roback JD, Combs MR, Grossman BJ, Hillyer CD, eds. *Technical Manual.* 16th ed. Bethesda, MD: AABB Press; 2008:189–228.

Leger RM. The positive direct antiglobulin test and immune-mediated hemolysis. In: Roback JD, Combs MR, Grossman BJ, Hillyer CD, eds. *Technical Manual*. 16th ed. Bethesda, MD: AABB Press; 2008:499–524.

McLeod BC, ed. *Apheresis: Principles and Practice*. 2nd ed. Bethesda, MD: AABB Press; 2003.

Mintz PD, ed. *Transfusion Therapy: Clinical Principles and Practice*. 2nd ed. Bethesda, MD: American AABB Press; 2005.

Popovsky MA, ed. *Transfusion Reactions*. 3rd ed. Bethesda, MD: AABB Press; 2007.

Practice guidelines for blood component therapy: a report by the American Society of Anesthesiologists' Task Force on Blood Component Therapy. *Anesthesiology*. 1996;84:732–747.

Rebulla P, et al. The threshold for prophylactic platelet transfusion in adults with acute myeloid leukemia. *N Engl J Med*. 1997;337:1870–1875.

Reid ME, Lomas-Francis C. *The Blood Group Antigens. Factsbook*. 2nd ed. San Diego, CA: Academic Press; 2004.

Roback JD, Combs MR, Grossman BJ, Hillyer CD, eds. *Technical Manual*. 16th ed. Bethesda, MD: AABB Press; 2008.

Simon TL, Snyder EL, Solheim BG, Stowell CP, Strauss RG, Petrides M, eds. *Rossi's Principles of Transfusion Medicine*. 4th ed. Bethesda, MD: AABB Press/Wiley-Blackwell; 2009.

Smith JW, Burgstaler EA. Blood component collection by apheresis. In: Roback JD, Combs MR, Grossman BJ, Hillyer CD, eds. *Technical Manual*. 16th ed. Bethesda, MD: AABB Press; 2008:229–240.

Standards for Blood Banks and Transfusion Services. 25th ed. Bethesda, MD: AABB Press; 2008.

Trial to Reduce Alloimmunization to Platelets Study Group. Leukocyte reduction and ultraviolet B irradiation of platelets to prevent alloimmunization and refractoriness to platelet transfusions. *N Engl J Med*. 1997;337:1861–1869.

Uniform Donor Health Questionnaire. http://www.aabb.org/Content/Donate_Blood/Donor_History_Questionnaires/AABB_Blood_Donor_History_Questionnaire; Accessed 01.12.09.

Diseases of White Blood Cells, Lymph Nodes, and Spleen

Daniel E. Sabath

LEARNING OBJECTIVES

1. Learn the differential diagnosis of leukopenia.

2. Distinguish between neoplastic and nonneoplastic proliferations of white blood cells.

3. Learn the diagnostic criteria for the different types of lymphomas, leukemias, myelodysplastic syndromes, myeloproliferative disorders, and plasma cell dyscrasias.

4. Understand the genetic, biochemical, and/or cellular defects associated with the more commonly encountered disorders of WBC function.

CHAPTER OUTLINE

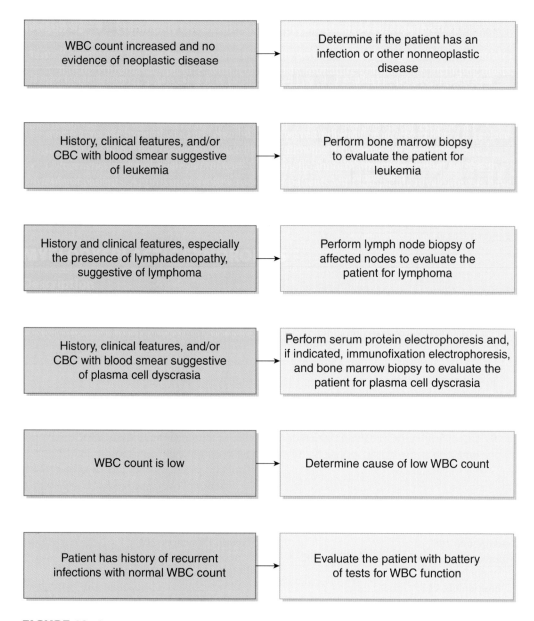

FIGURE 13–1 An approach to the patient with a white blood cell disorder.

bnormalities in white blood cells (WBCs) are nearly always quantitative (e.g., too many or too few WBCs). These disorders may be neoplastic, as found in leukemia, or nonneoplastic. A qualitative or functional disorder of WBCs may accompany the quantitative disorder. Qualitative defects in WBC function with a normal WBC count occur, but they are uncommon. The approach to diagnosis of WBC disorders is shown in **Figure 13–1**.

LEUKOPENIA

Description and Diagnosis

A low WBC count can occur because of a decreased number of lymphocytes, granulocytes, or both. A number of the immunodeficiency diseases are associated with a lymphocytopenia (see Chapter 3). Granulocytopenia primarily reflects a reduction in the number of neutrophils (neutropenia) in the peripheral blood. When the number of neutrophils decreases below about 1,000 neutrophils/μL, the neutropenic patient becomes susceptible to infections. These illnesses range from mild to severe, depending on the type of organism and the effectiveness of the antibiotics used to treat it. A classification of granulocytopenic disorders follows.

Defects in the production of granulocytes may be caused by:

- diseases associated with marrow failure, such as aplastic anemia;
- diseases in which the marrow is infiltrated by leukemic cells or by metastatic cancer cells originating from another site; the decreased neutrophil production in this setting is typically associated with defects in the production of other blood cells as well;
- suppression of granulocyte production by exposure to certain drugs; the list of drugs that can produce neutropenia is extensive; noteworthy examples are chemotherapeutic agents used in cancer treatment and certain nonsteroidal anti-inflammatory drugs (NSAIDs);
- vitamin B_{12} or folate deficiency; these disorders produce a megaloblastic anemia and defective DNA synthesis in granulocyte precursors;
- suppression of granulocyte production by neoplastic cells, for example, large granular lymphocytic leukemia.

Accelerated removal of granulocytes may be caused by:

- immunologically mediated injury to neutrophils following exposure to drugs, with the injury occurring from an immune response on the neutrophil surface;
- immunologically mediated injury to neutrophils as part of an autoimmune disorder; for example, Felty syndrome is a variant of rheumatoid arthritis with neutropenia, splenomegaly, leg ulcers, and the joint lesions found in rheumatoid arthritis; the neutropenia can dominate the clinical course in patients with Felty syndrome;
- immunologically mediated injury to neutrophils that is idiopathic and not associated with any identifiable abnormality;
- excessive destruction of granulocytes from splenic sequestration of the neutrophils in an enlarged spleen or from overwhelming infection.

NONNEOPLASTIC PROLIFERATION OF WBCs

Description and Diagnosis

An elevated peripheral WBC count is commonly found in patients with infections and other inflammatory states, such as those associated with autoimmune disorders.

An elevated peripheral WBC count is commonly found in patients with infections and other inflammatory states, such as those associated with autoimmune disorders.

Lymphocytes

Patients can develop a lymphocytosis in a variety of different conditions such as tuberculosis, acute bowel infections, and infectious mononucleosis and other viral infections.

Eosinophils

An increase in circulating eosinophils is most commonly found in patients with allergic disorders and those with asthma. An increase in circulating eosinophils is also found in patients with certain parasitic infections and in patients with dermatologic disorders such as eczema. Increases in eosinophils can also be caused by some drugs and some autoimmune disorders. Finally, increases in eosinophils can be seen in certain neoplastic conditions such as Hodgkin lymphoma and T-cell lymphomas.

Monocytes

The peripheral monocyte count is increased in a number of situations where the lymphocyte count is also increased, such as tuberculosis. Rheumatoid arthritis, systemic lupus erythematosus, and other connective tissue diseases also may be associated with a monocytosis.

Neutrophils

A mild increase in circulating neutrophils can occur without disease after strenuous exercise, during menstruation, and in the course of pregnancy. An increased neutrophil count is clinically significant when it is indicative of a bacterial infection, a neoplastic disorder, ischemia, an auto-immune disorder, or an effect of certain drugs, such as corticosteroids or epinephrine. The most frequently identified immature neutrophil in the blood when there is an increased WBC count is the neutrophilic band cell. The percentage of WBCs represented by band cells or more immature neutrophil precursors is a commonly used indicator of infection. However, band counts are poorly reproducible among medical technologists, so the current trend is to not report band counts. Other less mature neutrophil precursors can be seen in infections and other conditions where the bone marrow is attempting to produce granulocytes rapidly.

NEOPLASTIC PROLIFERATION OF WBCs

WBC neoplasms frequently involve the peripheral blood, and can result in leukocytosis. White cell neoplasms are broadly divided into 2 large categories, lymphoid (the lymphocyte lineage) and myeloid (the lineage including granulocytes, monocytes, megakaryocytes, and erythroid cells). Lymphoid disorders include acute lymphoblastic leukemias (ALL) and mature B-, T-, and NK-cell neoplasms. Myeloid disorders include acute myeloid leukemias, myeloproliferative disorders, and myelodysplastic syndromes.

LYMPHOID MALIGNANCIES

Description and Diagnosis

The lymphoid malignancies are caused by neoplastic transformation of lymphocytes or their precursors. Lymphoid cells can be found in the lymph nodes, blood, bone marrow, spleen, and extranodal sites such as the skin, mucosae, and respiratory and gastrointestinal tracts. Lymphoid neoplasms can occur at any of these sites. Neoplasms that primarily involve the bone marrow and peripheral blood are referred to as leukemias, and those involving tissue sites are called lymphomas. However, many lymphoid malignancies can involve both tissues and the blood/bone marrow, so the leukemia/lymphoma distinction is somewhat arbitrary. The World Health Organization (WHO) classification system for lymphoid malignancies is shown in **Table 13–1**.

Lymphoid leukemias can correspond to precursor B or T cells or mature lymphoid cells. Precursor lymphoid malignances are also called lymphoblastic leukemias/lymphomas. Relatively common B- and T-cell malignancies that frequently present in a leukemic phase include chronic lymphocytic leukemia (CLL)/small lymphocytic lymphoma, hairy cell leukemia, mantle cell lymphoma, Burkitt lymphoma/leukemia, T-cell prolymphocytic leukemia, T-cell large granular lymphocytic leukemia, and Sézary syndrome. Lymphoid leukemias generally present with elevated white counts (specifically lymphocytosis), and depending on the degree of bone marrow involvement, there can be decreased numbers of normal white cells, red cells, and/or platelets. Processes that involve the marrow extensively can result in the presence of myeloid and erythroid precursor cells in the peripheral blood. Leukemias are diagnosed by examination of the peripheral blood smear and bone marrow aspirates and biopsies. Additional studies such as immunophenotyping by flow cytometry, molecular diagnostic techniques, and cytogenetics are frequently used to establish a diagnosis.

When lymphoid malignancies are mostly tissue-based, they are referred to as lymphomas. Lymphomas are monoclonal, neoplastic proliferations of B, T, or NK cells. Most lymphomas are malignancies of mature lymphocytes, but precursor lymphocytic malignances can involve tissues, and thus be classified as lymphomas. Lymphomas are divided into 2 major groups, Hodgkin lymphoma and a much larger variety of lymphomas known generically as non-Hodgkin lymphomas. The patient with lymphoma often presents with an isolated, enlarged superficial lymph node, which may be discovered accidentally on physical exam. Alternatively, the patient may have generalized lymphadenopathy. If the enlarged lymph node develops in a site where it can produce signs and symptoms, it is more likely to be discovered early in the course of disease. An example is the enlargement of lymph nodes in the mediastinum, which can impair blood flow through the large vessels in the chest and produce symptoms on that basis. In some cases, organ involvement may be the first manifestation of a lymphoma. Non-Hodgkin lymphomas, for example, may become symptomatic when there is cellular proliferation in the orbit, the gastrointestinal tract, or the skin. Involvement of the bone marrow and peripheral blood also may be an initial indicator of the presence of a lymphoma.

White cell neoplasms are broadly divided into 2 large categories, lymphoid (the lymphocyte lineage) and myeloid (the lineage including granulocytes, monocytes, megakaryocytes, and erythroid cells).

TABLE 13-1   2008 World Health Organization Classification of Lymphoid Neoplasms

B-cell neoplasms

Precursor B-cell neoplasms
B-cell lymphoblastic leukemia/lymphoma, unspecified
B lymphoblastic leukemia/lymphoma with specific cytogenetic abnormalities

Mature B-cell neoplasms
Chronic lymphocytic leukemia/small lymphocytic lymphoma
B-cell prolymphocytic leukemia
Splenic marginal zone lymphoma
Hairy cell leukemia
Lymphoplasmacytic lymphoma/Waldenström macroglobulinemia
Heavy chain diseases (alpha, gamma, mu)
Plasma cell myeloma
Plasmacytoma (of bone or extraosseous)
Extranodal marginal zone lymphoma of mucosa-associated lymphoid tissue (MALT)
Nodal marginal zone B-cell lymphoma
Follicular lymphoma
Mantle cell lymphoma
Diffuse large B-cell lymphoma
Mediastinal (thymic) large B-cell lymphoma
Intravascular large B-cell lymphoma
ALK-positive large B-cell lymphoma
Plasmablastic lymphoma
Primary effusion lymphoma
Burkitt lymphoma/leukemia

T- and NK-cell neoplasms

Precursor T-cell neoplasms
Precursor T lymphoblastic leukemia/lymphoma
Blastic NK-cell lymphoma

Mature T- and NK-cell neoplasms
T-cell prolymphocytic leukemia
T-cell large granular lymphocytic leukemia
Aggressive NK-cell leukemia
Systemic EBV positive T-cell lymphoproliferative disease of childhood
Hydroa vacciniforme-like lymphoma
Adult T-cell leukemia/lymphoma
Extranodal NK/T-cell lymphoma, nasal type
Enteropathy-associated T-cell lymphoma
Hepatosplenic T-cell lymphoma
Subcutaneous panniculitis-like T-cell lymphoma
Mycosis fungoides
Sézary syndrome
Primary cutaneous anaplastic large cell lymphoma
Primary cutaneous gamma-delta T-cell lymphoma
Peripheral T-cell lymphoma, unspecified
Angioimmunoblastic T-cell lymphoma
Anaplastic large cell lymphoma

Hodgkin lymphoma

Nodular lymphocyte-predominant Hodgkin lymphoma
Classical Hodgkin lymphoma
Nodular sclerosis
Lymphocyte-rich
Mixed cellularity
Lymphocyte-depleted

Data from Swerdlow SH, Campo E, Harris NL, et al., eds. *WHO Classification of Tumours of Haematopoietic and Lymphoid Tissues.* Lyon: IARC; 2008.

Lymph node biopsy is the preferred method for diagnosis of lymphoma, since it allows the pathologist to determine the overall tissue architecture and get a large sample of the cells present. Because the lymphoma may not be distributed evenly in all lymph nodes, it may be necessary to biopsy several lymph nodes to establish the diagnosis. In recent years, fine needle aspiration and biopsy have been used more commonly to make diagnoses of lymphoma. Although this procedure does not allow optimal evaluation of tissue architecture, diagnostic procedures such as flow cytometry and/or molecular techniques can be used to render a diagnosis on minimal amounts of material.

Principal differentiating factors between Hodgkin and non-Hodgkin lymphomas are:

- Hodgkin lymphoma:
  - (a) proliferation of cells is typically localized to a single group of nodes such as the cervical or mediastinal nodes;
  - (b) proliferating cells spread by contiguity;
  - (c) mesenteric lymph nodes are rarely involved.
- Non-Hodgkin lymphomas:
  - (a) frequent involvement of multiple groups of nodes;
  - (b) proliferating cells spread widely and noncontiguously;
  - (c) mesenteric lymph nodes are commonly involved.

The Hodgkin and non-Hodgkin lymphomas are classified into clinical stages based on the distribution of the disease. These stages, with increased clinical severity associated with higher stage numbers, are as follows:

- Stage I—involvement of 1 group of lymph nodes or 2 contiguous lymph node clusters on the same side of the diaphragm.
- Stage II—involvement of 2 or more noncontiguous lymph node groups on the same side of the diaphragm.
- Stage III—lymph node involvement above and below the diaphragm; if there is involvement of the spleen, the lymphoma is classified as III(s); and if there is visceral involvement by direct extension, it is known as stage III(e).
- Stage IV—widespread disease, often involving the liver, bone marrow, lungs, bones, and skin.

In addition to the above staging scheme, the designation "B" is added for patients who have constitutional symptoms such as fever, night sweats, and weight loss. For example, a patient with involvement of 2 groups of lymph nodes on the same side of the diaphragm with fevers and night sweats would be considered stage IIB. In general, the presence of these "B symptoms" portends a more advanced stage of disease with worse prognosis. In addition, the designation "E" is used to designate lymphomas involving extranodal sites only (e.g., the gastrointestinal tract).

Lymphoma

Historically the diagnosis of Hodgkin and non-Hodgkin lymphoma was primarily based on the histological appearance of the lymph nodes. For Hodgkin lymphoma, the Rye classification system was used for decades and has now been incorporated with relatively few changes into the current WHO classification system for hematologic malignancies. Classification of non-Hodgkin lymphomas has been more problematic. Non-Hodgkin lymphomas were organized in the Rappaport classification in 1966, the Lukes–Collins classification in 1973–1974, and in 1982 they were reclassified according to the Working Formulation of Clinical Usage by an international panel of experts.

By the early 1990s, significant progress was made in understanding the biology of lymphomas, so newer classification systems were developed based on typing lymphomas with antibodies specific for cytoplasmic and cell surface proteins (immunohistochemistry and flow cytometry) and by detecting specific molecular lesions. In 1994, the REAL classification was introduced by the International Lymphoma Study Group. The goal of the new classification was to use morphological, immunologic, and genetic information to better define the disease entities. The REAL classification system was modified somewhat to form the basis for the current WHO classification system (**Table 13–1**).

The WHO classification system, like the REAL classification system preceding it, attempts to classify non-Hodgkin lymphomas according to the normal cell equivalent of the neoplastic cells. First, neoplastic cells are classified based on whether they are of B- or T-cell/NK-cell origin. Next, the cells are classified by the stage of differentiation to which they correspond. Most B- and T-cell neoplasms correspond to mature B and T cells.

In the end, lymphoma classification is determined by the architectural features observed under the microscope (e.g., follicular versus diffuse growth pattern and the microscopic appearance of the malignant cells), the spectrum of proteins expressed on the surfaces and in the cytoplasm of the malignant cells (e.g., T- or B-cell markers and proteins not expressed in normal lymphocytes), the presence of clonal rearrangements of the immunoglobulin or T-cell receptor genes, and in some cases, by the presence of specific genetic lesions in the malignant cells. The techniques used for lymphoma diagnosis include light microscopy, immunohistochemistry, flow cytometry, and molecular techniques including cytogenetics, fluorescence in situ hybridization (FISH), polymerase chain reaction (PCR), and newer techniques such as microarrays.

Since it is beyond the scope of this chapter to discuss all the lymphoid malignancies in detail, the more common disorders have been selected for inclusion.

Precursor B- and T-cell Neoplasms

Neoplasms of immature B and T cells most commonly present as leukemias, with extensive blood and bone marrow involvement, but they can also involve the lymphoid tissues as lymphomas. For example, precursor T-cell leukemia/lymphoma often presents with a mediastinal mass and may not demonstrate blood or bone marrow involvement. ALL accounts for almost one third of all childhood cancers and represents 75% of all pediatric leukemias. The median age at diagnosis is 10 years with a slight male predominance of 1.4:1. Pediatric leukemias are almost always (80% to 85%) of a precursor B-cell lineage, with the remainder being T-cell lineage.

Diagnosis

- *Morphology*—Morphologically, the involved tissues show monomorphic collections of medium sized cells with fine chromatin, high nuclear cytoplasmic ratios, and inconspicuous nucleoli.
- *Immunophenotyping*—Depending on lineage, the cells will express B- or T-cell surface proteins. Both B- and T-cell precursor cells contain the enzyme terminal deoxynucleotidyl transferase.
- *Cytogenetics*—There are a number of recurrent chromosomal translocations associated with ALL. Hyperdiploidy with 50 or more chromosomes is a favorable prognostic finding. The presence of the Philadelphia chromosome, t(9;22)(q43;q11), is an adverse prognostic finding.

Chronic Lymphocytic Leukemia
Description

CLL is the most common of the non-Hodgkin lymphomas. The median age at diagnosis is 70 years with a slight male predominance of 1.7:1. The neoplastic cells in CLL are mature B cells. CLL is an indolent disease with a highly variable life expectancy. Transformation to aggressive disease occurs in 5% to 10% of cases at any time during the course of the illness, and is usually a terminal event.

Diagnosis

- *Morphology*—The lymphocytes in CLL are usually small and well differentiated. They are sometimes difficult to distinguish from normal lymphocytes, but they can be identified by their somewhat larger size, coarsely clumped chromatin, and tendency to break apart on peripheral blood smears, forming "smudge cells." CLL can transform into a high-grade B-cell lymphoma known as Richter syndrome in approximately 3% of B-cell CLL cases. Another type of transformation is to the prolymphocytoid form, where patients can have a very high white count of characteristic prolymphocytes with prominent nucleoli.

Chronic lymphocytic leukemia is an indolent disease with a highly variable life expectancy. Transformation to aggressive disease occurs in 5% to 10% of cases at any time during the course of the illness, and is usually a terminal event.

- *Immunophenotyping*—The CLL tumor cells express low levels of surface IgM and IgD in the majority of cases, surface IgM only in approximately 25% of the cases, and surface IgD, other immunoglobulin isotypes, or no surface immunoglobulin in a small percentage of cases. A characteristic finding in CLL is expression of CD5, which is normally a pan-T-cell antigen, but is expressed on a minor normal subset of B cells. CLL cells also express the B-cell antigens CD19, CD20 (low level), and CD23. Immunophenotyping can also be used for prognosis: high-level expression of CD38 and ZAP-70 is associated with worse prognosis.
- *Cytogenetics*—Chromosomal abnormalities in CLL have prognostic significance. Trisomy 12 and 11q and 17p abnormalities are associated with significantly shorter survival.

Hairy Cell Leukemia

Description

Hairy cell leukemia is an uncommon form of non-Hodgkin lymphoma. This disease generally occurs in men with a median age at diagnosis of 50 years. The male to female ratio is approximately 4:1. The clinical manifestations are primarily the result of infiltration of the tumor cells into the bone marrow, liver, and spleen. A significant clinical finding on physical examination is the often massive splenomegaly. The liver is also enlarged, but to a much lesser degree than the spleen. Marrow failure is common in this disease, resulting in pancytopenia and its associated complications. Patients generally present with splenomegaly, leukopenia with a relative decrease in monocytes, and an inaspirable bone marrow.

Diagnosis

- *Morphology*—The diagnosis of hairy cell leukemia is supported by the identification of lymphocytes with bean-shaped nuclei and fairly abundant gray cytoplasm, giving the cells a somewhat monocytic appearance. Fine cytoplasmic projections that have a hair-like appearance on Wright–Giemsa-stained smears give this entity its name.
- *Cytochemistry*—The cells in hairy cell leukemia stain positively for acid phosphatase that is partially or completely resistant to removal on the addition of tartrate. This is known as TRAP, for **t**artrate-**r**esistant **a**cid **p**hosphatase. TRAP-positive lymphocytes with fine cytoplasmic projections are highly consistent with a diagnosis of hairy cell leukemia.
- *Immunophenotyping*—The hairy cells have a B-cell phenotype, with surface immunoglobulin, CD19 (increased), and CD20 (increased). Antigens that are relatively specific for hairy cell leukemia include the interleukin 2 receptor alpha, CD25, as well as surface CD11c and CD103. Immunohistochemistry performed on bone marrow biopsies or spleen can be used to detect DBA44, which is relatively selective, although not specific, for hairy cell leukemia. These results are all consistent with the identification of hairy cell leukemia as a B-cell disorder.

Plasma Cell Dyscrasias

The plasma cell dyscrasias are disorders in which there is an expansion of a single clone of immunoglobulin-secreting cells. This results in the appearance of high levels of complete or incomplete immunoglobulin molecules in the serum or urine. The monoclonal immunoglobulin in the serum is known as an M-component because it is found in the prototype disorder in this group of diseases, *multiple myeloma*. Incomplete immunoglobulins containing only light chains or only heavy chains may be produced in certain plasma cell dyscrasias. The free light chains, which are known as Bence-Jones proteins, may be excreted into the urine. The 5 disorders included in this grouping of plasma cell dyscrasias are: plasma cell myeloma, Waldenström macroglobulinemia, heavy chain disease, primary amyloidosis, and monoclonal gammopathy of unknown significance (MGUS). Amyloidosis was discussed in Chapter 3, and the other entities are described as follows.

Plasma Cell Myeloma

Description

Plasma cell myeloma, also known as multiple myeloma, is a disorder resulting from proliferation of a single plasma cell clone that produces a monoclonal immunoglobulin. The median age

> The monoclonal immunoglobulin in the serum is known as an M-component because it is found in the prototype disorder in this group of diseases, *multiple myeloma*.

TABLE 13-2   Diagnostic Criteria for Plasma Cell Myeloma

Plasma cell myeloma is divided between symptomatic and asymptomatic forms, depending on evidence of end-organ damage
Symptomatic plasma cell myeloma: • M-protein in serum >30 g/L or urine • Plasmacytoma or clonal plasma cells in bone marrow • Evidence of end-organ damage including hypercalcemia, renal insufficiency, anemia, or bone lesions
Asymptomatic (also known as smoldering) myeloma: No evidence of end-organ damage or myeloma symptoms with: • M-protein in serum >30 g/L • 10% of more clonal plasma cells in the bone marrow

for presentation is 62 years. The most frequent presenting symptom is bone pain resulting from osteolytic lesions produced by clusters of plasma cells infiltrating the bone. The bones most often affected are the skull, the ribs, the vertebrae, and the long bones of the extremities. Because patients with multiple myeloma are often anemic, fatigue and weakness are common presenting symptoms. Patients may also experience recurrent bacterial infections as a result of the leukopenia that occurs later in the disease. In addition, the passage of free light chains into the urine may result in "myeloma kidney" and lead to renal failure.

Diagnosis

The diagnosis of myeloma depends on the presence of a monoclonal protein in the serum or urine, and then the type of myeloma is further classified based on the severity of the disease (**Table 13–2**). The evaluation of a patient for multiple myeloma begins with protein electrophoresis of serum and urine to identify any monoclonal proteins (see Chapter 2 for protein electrophoresis and immunofixation). An M-component on an electrophoretic gel is a dense band of protein that is not usually present. It most often migrates in the gamma region of the gel, but occasionally appears in the beta or alpha-2 region. To increase the likelihood of M-component detection in the urine, the samples evaluated for M-components must be concentrated prior to electrophoresis. Confirmation that a band identified on serum or urine protein electrophoresis represents an M-component involves further analysis by immunofixation electrophoresis (see Chapter 2) or, much less frequently now, by immunoelectrophoresis. Both of these tests permit identification of the specific heavy chain and light chain of the M-component, if both are present. It is also necessary to quantify serum immunoglobulins to determine if the concentration of the M-component is greater than 35 g/L. Beta-2 microglobulin is the light chain of a class 1 major histocompatibility complex protein, and is present on the surface of all nucleated cells. Increased levels of the unbound beta-2 microglobulin in the plasma are found in multiple myeloma and are considered a reflection of tumor burden. Other tests used to evaluate myeloma include measurement of serum calcium, evaluation of renal function, and a skeletal survey to look for bone lesions.

Waldenström Macroglobulinemia

Description

Waldenström macroglobulinemia is the clinical syndrome associated with lymphoplasmacytic lymphoma in the WHO classification. There is a diffuse infiltration of the bone marrow by small lymphocytes and plasma cells that synthesize an IgM immunoglobulin, which is referred to as a macroglobulin. It is similar to plasma cell myeloma in that both have an M-component. However, the M-component in Waldenström macroglobulinemia is always an IgM molecule, and unlike the relatively rare IgM myeloma patient, individuals with Waldenström macroglobulinemia do not have lytic bone lesions. The mean age for presentation is 63 years, with a slight male predominance. Patients frequently present with fatigue, weight loss, weakness, and bleeding from anemia and thrombocytopenia. When present in sufficient concentration, the large circulating IgM protein produces a hyperviscosity syndrome in the plasma and tissue deposition of IgM. Most patients with Waldenström macroglobulinemia have an elevated serum viscosity, but only 15% to 20% are symptomatic. The most common symptoms associated with slow blood flow from hyperviscosity are blurred vision, mucosal bleeding, dizziness, and, on funduscopic examination of the eye, papilledema, hemorrhage, and distention of the retinal veins.

Diagnosis

The diagnosis of Waldenström macroglobulinemia requires demonstration of an IgM serum protein concentration greater than 30 g/L. As with multiple myeloma, Waldenström macroglobulinemia must be differentiated from an IgM MGUS.

Heavy Chain Disease

Description

The heavy chain diseases are a group of lymphoproliferative disorders in which there is production of monoclonal immunoglobulins with only heavy chains. Each type of heavy chain disease is named for the abnormal heavy chain produced, resulting in:

- alpha chain disease—a high serum concentration of the heavy chain present in IgA;
- gamma chain disease—a high serum concentration of the heavy chain present in IgG;
- mu chain disease—a high serum concentration of the heavy chain present in IgM.

All the heavy chain diseases are rare, with alpha chain disease having the highest incidence of the related disorders. In all 3 disorders, the monoclonal heavy chain is defective with internal deletions of most of the variable region of the protein and some portion of the first constant region domain. Common clinical findings in patients with heavy chain disease are splenomegaly, hepatomegaly, and lymphadenopathy. Almost all cases of mu chain disease have been associated with CLL. Gamma chain disease has been found in the presence of a variety of autoimmune disorders and in lymphoplasmacytic lymphoma. Alpha chain disease is associated with extranodal marginal zone lymphoma of the MALT type, which usually involves the gastrointestinal tract.

Diagnosis

The diagnosis of heavy chain disease is made primarily by demonstration of a monoclonal heavy chain by protein electrophoresis of serum, concentrated urine, or both. The diagnosis of heavy chain disease should prompt an investigation into the presence of lymphoma if that diagnosis has not already been made.

Monoclonal Gammopathies of Unknown Significance

Description

> Patients with MGUS are asymptomatic but have a monoclonal protein in their serum and/or urine. It is essential to differentiate patients who have MGUS from those who have plasma cell myeloma or Waldenström macroglobulinemia.

Patients with MGUS are asymptomatic but have a monoclonal protein in their serum and/or urine. There is an increasing incidence of MGUS with aging. Because the incidence of malignant monoclonal gammopathies also increases with age, it is essential to differentiate patients who have MGUS from those who have plasma cell myeloma or Waldenström macroglobulinemia. Most patients with MGUS remain clinically stable without therapy for many years. However, as many as 15% to 20% develop myeloma, macroglobulinemia, amyloidosis, or lymphoma. Indolent myeloma and smoldering myeloma, disorders with many features of multiple myeloma and Waldenström macroglobulinemia that do not meet the criteria for diagnosis, can be differentiated from MGUS because MGUS has a lower amount of immunoglobulin in the serum and a lower percentage of plasma cells in the bone marrow.

Diagnosis

MGUS is diagnosed by the presence of a monoclonal serum or urine immunoglobulin at a concentration less than that required for a myeloma diagnosis, less than 10% plasma cells in the bone marrow, no lytic bone lesions, and no symptoms suggestive of multiple myeloma.

Hodgkin Lymphoma

Description and Diagnosis

Hodgkin lymphoma is distinguished from non-Hodgkin lymphoma by the presence of a neoplastic giant cell known as a Reed–Sternberg cell in the lymph node. For many years the lineage of the Reed–Sternberg cell was controversial, but the best information now indicates that the Reed–Sternberg cell is an abnormal malignant B cell. Hodgkin disease is a common form of malignancy in young adults with a second peak incidence in older individuals. Unlike the multiple classification schemes for non-Hodgkin lymphomas, a classification of Hodgkin disease known as the Rye classification was accepted for decades. This classification system has now been incorporated into the WHO classification system for hematologic malignancies. Hodgkin lymphoma is divided into 2 broad categories, classical Hodgkin lymphoma and nodular lymphocyte-predominant Hodgkin lymphoma. Classical Hodgkin lymphoma is characterized by infrequent Reed–Sternberg cells in a background of normal lymphocytes, plasma cells, eosinophils, and granulocytes. The Reed–Sternberg cells lack expression of the pan-hematopoietic marker CD45; they occasionally express the B-cell marker CD20; and they characteristically express CD30 and CD15. The different subtypes of classical Hodgkin lymphoma in the WHO classification are characterized primarily by differences in tissue architecture and the composition of the cellular background.

Nodular lymphocyte-predominant Hodgkin lymphoma also shows scattered large abnormal cells, but these do not have the appearance of Reed–Sternberg cells. The abnormal cells in nodular lymphocyte-predominant Hodgkin lymphoma have convoluted nuclei, leading to the term "popcorn cells." These abnormal cells express the pan-hematopoietic marker CD45 and the B-cell marker CD20; they variably express CD30 and do not express CD15. The abnormal cells are frequently ringed by normal T cells. Nodular lymphocyte-predominant Hodgkin lymphoma is best thought of as a low-grade B-cell lymphoma.

> Hodgkin lymphoma is distinguished from non-Hodgkin lymphoma by the presence of a neoplastic giant cell known as a Reed–Sternberg cell in the lymph node.

MYELOID DISORDERS

Acute Myeloid Leukemias

Acute leukemias are hematologic malignancies that primarily involve the peripheral blood and bone marrow. An acute leukemia is a neoplasm of a hematopoietic stem cell that has lost its capacity to differentiate and regulate its own proliferation. The outcome of the expansion of the leukemic clone is an accumulation of poorly differentiated WBC precursors known as blasts in the bone marrow. These limit the production of normal blood cells. The blasts commonly appear in the peripheral blood and permit identification of an acute leukemia from review of the peripheral blood smear. A diagnosis of acute leukemia requires that 20% or more of the bone marrow cells be blasts. These disorders are usually rapidly progressive, and patients can die within days to weeks without therapeutic intervention. In the WHO classification, leukemias are not considered an independent group of diseases. Instead, they are classified according to their cell of origin. Acute leukemias of lymphoid cells are included in the B- and T-cell malignancy classification scheme. In this section, we will consider the acute myeloid leukemias, which are malignancies of myeloid stem and precursor cells.

Morphological examination of leukemias can be difficult. In particular, it is frequently not possible to distinguish leukemias of myeloid lineage from leukemias of B- or T-cell precursors. Special cytochemical stains can sometimes help identify the lineage of the leukemic cells, but definitive classification is best done by immunophenotyping using flow cytometry. It is also important to perform cytogenetic and/or molecular analysis of leukemias, to obtain both prognostic information and, in some cases, information that can be used to design specific therapy. The description and diagnosis for several acute leukemias are presented in the sections that follow.

A uniform classification for the acute leukemias was developed in 1976 by the French–American–British (FAB) cooperative group. The classification from the FAB cooperative group ultimately divided AML into 7 types, M1 to M7. These types were based primarily on the morphology of the leukemic blasts and in some cases on cytochemical staining. In 1990, guidelines were established by the National Cancer Institute for an M0 type of AML that is not within the M1 to M7 classification. It was also clarified at that time that AML was different from myelodysplastic syndromes (see the section "Myelodysplastic Syndromes"). The FAB system has long been a means to classify acute leukemias, particularly AML. However, the FAB system has several drawbacks. First, the different categories of the FAB classification do not correspond to distinct biological entities. For example, the translocation t(8;21) can be found in several different FAB types. Similarly, FAB type M5, monocytic leukemia, has a predilection to involve the skin and mucous membranes, but other leukemias can infiltrate extramedullary sites. The 1 exception is FAB type M3, acute promyelocytic leukemia. This leukemia reproducibly has a translocation t(15;17), and is unique among the myeloid leukemias in its response to treatment by all-*trans* retinoic acid.

The WHO classification system recognizes some of the drawbacks of the FAB system. New features of the WHO system include defining specific leukemias by their molecular pathology for those with recurrent chromosomal abnormalities, and creating categories for leukemias evolving from previous myelodysplastic syndromes and from patients treated with leukemogenic chemotherapy for prior malignancies that do not fit neatly into the FAB categories (see **Table 13–3**). For the remaining myeloid leukemias, classification is similar to the FAB system (see **Table 13–4**).

> The FAB system has long been a means to classify acute leukemias, particularly AML. The WHO classification system recognizes some of the drawbacks of the FAB system.

TABLE 13–3   2008 World Health Organization Classification of Myeloid Neoplasms

Acute myeloid leukemias
Acute myeloid leukemias with recurrent cytogenetic abnormalities AML with t(8;21)(q22;q22), *RUNX1/RUNX1T1* AML with inv(16) or t(16;16)(p13;q22), *CBFβ/MYH11* Acute promyelocytic leukemia (AML with t(15;17)(q22;q12), *PML/RARα* and variants AML with t(9;11)(p22;q23), *MLLT3/MLL* AML with t(6;9)(p32;q34), *DEK/NUP214* AML with inv(3)(q21;q26.2) or t(3;3)(q21;q26.2), *RPN1/EVI1* AML (megakaryoblastic) with t(1;22)(p13;q13), *RBM15/MKL1*
Acute myeloid leukemia with myelodysplasia-related changes *Acute myeloid leukemia, therapy-related* *Acute myeloid leukemia, not otherwise characterized* AML minimally differentiated AML without maturation AML with maturation Acute myelomonocytic leukemia Acute monoblastic and monocytic leukemia Acute erythroid leukemia Acute megakaryoblastic leukemia Acute leukemias of ambiguous lineage
Myeloproliferative neoplasms
Chronic myeloid leukemia *Chronic neutrophilic leukemia* *Polycythemia vera* *Primary myelofibrosis* *Essential thrombocythemia* *Chronic eosinophilic leukemia* *Mastocytosis* *Myeloid and lymphoid neoplasms with eosinophilia and abnormalities of PDGFRA, PDGFRB, or FGFR1* *Myelodysplastic/myeloproliferative neoplasms* Chronic myelomonocytic leukemia Atypical chronic myeloid leukemia Juvenile myelomonocytic leukemia
Myelodysplastic syndromes Refractory cytopenia with unilineage dysplasia (anemia, neutropenia, or thrombocytopenia) Refractory anemia with ringed sideroblasts Refractory cytopenia with multilineage dysplasia Refractory anemia with excess blasts MDS with isolated del(5q) chromosome abnormality

Data from Swerdlow SH, Campo E, Harris NL, et al., eds. *WHO Classification of Tumours of Haematopoietic and Lymphoid Tissues.* Lyon: IARC; 2008.

TABLE 13–4   Classification of Acute Myeloid Leukemias, Not Otherwise Specified

	Blast Percentage	Cytochemistry	Immunophenotype	Genetics	Other	Corresponds to FAB Type
AML minimally differentiated	≥20%	MPO and NSE negative	CD13, CD33, CD117, usually CD34, CD38, HLA-DR; may have low expression of lymphoid markers TdT, CD7, CD2, CD19, no monocytic markers	27% with RUNX/AML1 mutations; 16%–22% with FLT3 mutations		M0
AML without maturation	≥90%	MPO positive >3%, NSE negative	CD13, CD33, CD117, MPO, frequently CD34 and HLA-DR, generally negative for monocytic and lymphoid markers	No specific abnormalities		M1
AML with maturation	20%–89%	MPO positive, NSE negative	CD13, CD33, CD15, may express CD117, CD34, HLA-DR, 20%–30% with CD7	No specific abnormalities	Less than 20% monocytes in marrow	M2
Acute myelomonocytic leukemia	20%–89%	MPO and NSE positive	CD13, CD15, CD33, HLA-DR, positive for some monocytic antigens (including CD14, CD4, CD11b, CD11c, CD64, CD36, lysozyme), 30% have CD7, subset may have CD34, CD117	No specific abnormalities	Greater than or equal to 20% monocytes in marrow, may have peripheral monocytosis	M4
Acute monoblastic/ monocytic leukemia	20%–89%	MPO negative, NSE positive	CD13, CD33 (bright), HLA-DR, monocyte markers (including CD14, CD4, CD11b, CD11c, CD64, CD36, lysozyme), frequently have CD7, CD56	No specific abnormalities; occasional t(8;16)	Greater than 80% monoblasts or monocytes in marrow: if monoblasts, then acute monoblastic leukemia; if promonocytes, then acute monocytic leukemia	M5a (monoblastic), M5b (monocytic)
Acute erythroid leukemia (erythroleukemia and pure erythroid leukemia)	Erythroleukemia has ≥50% total marrow erythroid cells, ≥20% of nonerythroid cells are blasts; pure erythroid leukemia has ≥80% immature erythroid cells	MPO, NSE negative; PAS positive	CD13, CD33, CD117, may have MPO, CD34, HLA-DR, erythroid cells express glycophorin A, hemoglobin	Complex cytogenetics, no specific abnormalities		M6
Acute megakaryoblastic leukemia	20%–89%	MPO, NSE negative	Platelet markers: CD41, CD61, less CD42, some with CD13, CD33, CD36, often negative for CD34, CD45, HLA-DR	Complex cytogenetics, no specific abnormalities	Abnormal megakaryocytes in marrow, frequent marrow fibrosis	M7

Leukemias with Recurrent Genetic Abnormalities

Certain common chromosomal translocations are found in acute myeloid leukemia. These translocations usually result in the generation of an abnormal transcription factor that alters gene expression, leading to leukemia. The most common recurrent translocation is the t(8;21)(q22;q22). It is seen in several FAB types of AML and is associated with a relatively good prognosis. The inv(16) translocation is associated with a type of myelomonocytic leukemia that has increased eosinophils in the bone marrow (FAB type AML M4-Eo). It is also associated with a relatively good prognosis. The t(15;17) translocation is uniquely associated with acute promyelocytic leukemia (FAB type M3). This translocation results in an abnormal form of the retinoic acid receptor α. Interestingly, acute promyelocytic leukemia can be treated with all-*trans* retinoic acid in addition to standard leukemia chemotherapy, and many patients have a good outcome. The all-*trans* retinoic acid presumably interacts with the abnormal product of the t(15;17) fusion gene and interferes with its leukemogenic function. This was the first leukemic therapy described that was directed at the molecular pathology of the leukemia. A final recurrent chromosomal abnormality associated with AML is a set of translocations involving the *MLL* gene at chromosome 11q23. This gene forms fusion genes with many different partner genes. It is found more commonly in pediatric AML and is associated with a somewhat worse clinical outcome.

> Certain common chromosomal translocations are found in acute myeloid leukemia. The most common recurrent translocation is the t(8;21)(q22;q22).

Secondary Acute Myeloid Leukemia

Unlike the leukemias with recurrent chromosomal abnormalities, which are thought to represent de novo events, there is a group of leukemias that evolve out of previously existing conditions. One set consists of the leukemias that develop from patients with stem cell disorders such as the myelodysplastic syndromes (see below). These leukemias are associated with morphological abnormalities in all hematopoietic lineages. The other secondary leukemias develop in patients who have had previous chemotherapy for other malignancies. These leukemias occur in patients who were treated with alkylating agents such as cyclophosphamide or nitrogen mustard or with topoisomerase inhibitors such as the epipodophyllotoxins or anthracyclines. Both sets of leukemias are associated with complex cytogenetic abnormalities and have poor prognoses.

Other Acute Myeloid Leukemias

Leukemias that do not have characteristic cytogenetic abnormalities or documented previous stem cell disorders or therapy are characterized by their putative lineage as determined by immunophenotyping, morphology, and cytochemical staining. Their classification is most similar to the FAB system used prior to the WHO classification. The diagnostic criteria for these leukemias are shown in **Table 13–4**.

- *Cytochemistry*—Two cytochemical stains are widely used in the diagnostic evaluation of an acute leukemia. These are myeloperoxidase (MPO) and nonspecific esterase (NSE). MPO identifies cells of myeloid lineage, which usually stain intensely positive for MPO. Monoblasts and promonocytes, which appear in acute myelomonocytic leukemia, can also react with MPO. NSE is confined mostly to cells of monocytic lineage, which predominate in acute monoblastic/monocytic leukemia.
- *Immunophenotyping*—With the development of monoclonal antibodies that can be fluorochrome-conjugated to bind to and identify cell antigens, flow cytometry has become a useful tool in distinguishing AML from ALL, and identifying the individual subtypes of AML. Immunophenotyping is particularly important in the identification of blasts that show no morphological features to indicate their lineage, as found in the minimally differentiated subtype of AML. Markers such as CD14 and CD64 can be useful in identification of monocytic cells in AML. The detection of hemoglobin or glycophorin A aids in the diagnosis of erythroleukemia. Identification of platelet glycoprotein antigens supports a diagnosis of acute megakaryoblastic leukemia.
- *Molecular genetics*—Molecular genetic tests are also used to provide diagnostic and/ or prognostic information not available from morphological analysis. For example,

PCR gene amplification and FISH can be used to detect the recurrent cytogenetic translocations of AML. Molecular analysis can also be used to detect mutations in specific genes such as *FLT3* and *NPM1*, which frequently occur in AML with otherwise normal cytogenetics. Finally, PCR to detect translocation-specific fusion RNAs can sensitively detect residual leukemic cells after chemotherapy or transplantation and thereby permit earlier intervention.

Biphenotypic and Mixed Lineage Leukemias

There is a subset of acute leukemias that express both myeloid and lymphoid markers at the same time on the same blasts. These are called mixed lineage leukemias. These leukemias may reflect a lack of marker specificity or aberrant gene expression by a malignant hematopoietic stem cell. Biphenotypic leukemias have separate subpopulations of leukemic blasts with different immunophenotypes (e.g., myeloid on 1 set and lymphoid on another). Both types of leukemias generally have a relatively poor prognosis.

MYELOPROLIFERATIVE DISORDERS

Disorders in which there is a clonal neoplastic proliferation of a multipotent myeloid stem cell are grouped together in the myeloproliferative disorders. The major disorders in this grouping include:

- chronic myeloid leukemia, with cell proliferation in the granulocytic series;
- polycythemia vera, in which erythrocytic precursors dominate the picture (see the section "Erythrocytosis" in Chapter 10);
- essential thrombocythemia in which megakaryocytes are the primary cytological feature (see the section "Bleeding Disorders" in Chapter 11);
- primary myelofibrosis (see the following), a disorder in which the bone marrow is initially hypercellular in multiple cell lineages and then gradually becomes markedly hypocellular with the development of marrow fibrosis.

The myeloproliferative disorders have a fair amount of overlap in their clinical and hematologic findings, including increased numbers of red cells, platelets, and/or white cells, the presence of circulating immature cells, and the presence of marrow fibrosis. The fibrosis is a reactive response to the neoplastic elements of the bone marrow. Myeloproliferative disorders are differentiated from the myelodysplastic diseases because in the myeloproliferative disorders, there are few, if any, dysplastic changes in the blood cell precursors in the marrow. The prognosis of the myeloproliferative disorders varies depending on the diagnosis. Polycythemia vera and essential thrombocythemia tend to have very long survival and a low incidence of transformation to acute leukemia. Chronic myeloid leukemia and primary myelofibrosis have worse prognoses.

> Chronic myeloid leukemia is distinct from the other myeloproliferative disorders in that it contains a specific chromosomal translocation, t(9;22) (q34;q11), also known as the Philadelphia chromosome.

Chronic myeloid leukemia is distinct from the other myeloproliferative disorders in that it contains a specific chromosomal translocation, t(9;22)(q34;q11), also known as the Philadelphia chromosome. This will be discussed in detail below.

The other myeloproliferative disorders commonly contain a mutation in the *JAK2* tyrosine kinase gene. JAK2 is a tyrosine kinase involved in transmitting growth signals for several different hematopoietic growth factors. In approximately 80% to 90% of polycythemia and in approximately 40% to 50% of essential thrombocythemia and primary myelofibrosis, the valine at amino acid 617 is mutated to a phenylalanine (designated V617F). This mutation inactivates a domain of the JAK2 protein that normally inhibits its tyrosine kinase activity. The result is that the kinase becomes activated without growth factor stimulation, and this leads to uncontrolled proliferation of the cells. Molecular testing for the V617F mutation has become standard practice for patients suspected of having 1 of these myeloproliferative disorders.

Chronic Myeloid Leukemia

Description

CML represents approximately 15% of all leukemias in the United States. The median age at diagnosis is 65 years, and there is a slight male predominance, with a male to female ratio of 1.7:1. In CML, the disease begins with a chronic phase that usually lasts for 3 to 4 years after diagnosis. The chronic phase evolves into a more aggressive accelerated phase of the disease. This phase persists for 1 to 2 years in most cases. At least 25% of patients with CML die in this phase of the disease. The remainder progress to an acute leukemia, which is known as blast crisis. The blast crisis typically leads to death within 6 months because it is highly resistant to chemotherapy. Approximately 25% of the patients with CML advance rapidly from chronic phase to blast crisis, without a significant intervening period of acceleration.

CML is characterized by a characteristic chromosomal translocation, t(9;22), also known as the Philadelphia chromosome. Discovered in 1960, this was the first genetic lesion associated with a human cancer. When molecular cloning techniques became available, the t(9;22) was found to produce an abnormal RNA and protein product, BCR-ABL. BCR-ABL is a tyrosine kinase that is constitutively active and leads to uncontrolled proliferation of myeloid cells. In 1996, a drug, imatinib mesylate, was discovered that inhibits the tyrosine kinase activity of BCR-ABL, and this has led to a revolution in the treatment of CML, which previously relied primarily on interferon-alpha and bone marrow transplantation. Long-term treatment with imatinib leads to drug resistance however, and new BCR-ABL inhibitors are in development to overcome this problem. The only curative treatment for CML is still bone marrow transplantation.

> In Chronic myeloid leukemia, the disease begins with a chronic phase that usually lasts for 3 to 4 years after diagnosis. The chronic phase evolves into a more aggressive accelerated phase of the disease.

Diagnosis

The diagnosis of CML is based on the morphological appearance of the bone marrow, peripheral blood cell morphology, and cytogenetic and molecular genetic studies. Cytochemistry and immunophenotyping are not particularly valuable in the diagnosis of CML in its chronic phase. This is the stage of the disease in which most CML patients first present.

- *Chronic-phase CML*—A significant hematologic finding in this phase of CML is a moderate to significant elevation of the neutrophil count, often with all stages of neutrophil maturation detectable in the peripheral blood smear. An increase in basophils is important to recognize, as modest basophilia is an early indication of CML. Approximately 50% of CML patients also have an elevation in their platelet count. The appearance of the bone marrow is hypercellular as the disease progresses in the chronic phase of CML, with an increase in the myeloid/erythroid ratio from 2:1–4:1 to 10:1–30:1. There is complete maturation of the granulocytes in CML.
- *Accelerated-phase CML*—There is no widely accepted definition for the accelerated phase of CML. The characteristic features of this phase of the disease include splenomegaly, an increase in the proportion of myeloblasts (10% to 19%) and promyelocytes in the bone marrow over that found in the chronic phase, basophilia to >20% of the total WBC count, and anemia or thrombocytopenia.
- *CML in blast crisis*—By definition, when the percentage of blasts is 20% or more in the blood or bone marrow, blast transformation of CML has occurred. The blasts can be of either myeloid or lymphoid lineage; this determination is made by flow cytometry immunophenotyping. Approximately 70% of blast crises are myeloid. CML transforms into ALL in approximately 30% of cases of blast crisis. The immunophenotype is most commonly precursor B-cell ALL.
- *Cytogenetics*—The Philadelphia chromosome is present in essentially 100% of CML cases; if the Philadelphia chromosome cannot be demonstrated by cytogenetics, FISH, or molecular studies, another diagnosis should be considered. Blast crisis is usually accompanied by additional cytogenetic abnormalities that appear with clonal evolution.
- *Molecular genetics*—The diagnosis of CML is still possible in cases that are Philadelphia chromosome negative by using FISH or reverse transcriptase PCR to detect the *BCR-ABL* fusion RNA. PCR can also be used to detect minimal residual disease in patients being treated for CML. Newer techniques are now available to quantify BCR-ABL RNA in the peripheral blood or bone marrow. These are being used to assess clinical responses to imatinib and to detect early evidence of imatinib resistance.

Polycythemia Vera
Description
Polycythemia vera is diagnosed by an increase in red cell mass with no apparent cause such as chronic oxygen deprivation (living at high altitude or heavy smoker). Transformation to acute myeloid leukemia is rare, but patients with polycythemia vera are at increased risk for the development of leukemia (see Chapter 10 for additional information on polycythemia vera).

Diagnosis

- *Cell counts and the peripheral blood smear*—By definition, the hemoglobin, hematocrit, and red cell count are all elevated. Patients often present with microcytosis and a normal hematocrit due to the iron deficiency that develops due to excessive red cell production. Because of this, these patients are sometimes initially thought to have thalassemia trait. The WBC count and platelet count are also often moderately elevated.
- *Bone marrow morphology*—The bone marrow can appear normal, but is often hypercellular with an increase in red cell precursors. With progressive disease, the bone marrow can become fibrotic.
- *Cytogenetics and molecular pathology*—Cytogenetic findings are usually normal. Definitive diagnosis is made by demonstrating a point mutation in the JAK2 gene.

Polycythemia vera is diagnosed by an increase in red cell mass with no apparent cause such as chronic oxygen deprivation (living at high altitude or heavy smoker).

Essential Thrombocythemia
Description
Essential thrombocythemia is diagnosed by an increase in platelet count with no other explanation. Platelet counts can frequently exceed 1 million/μL. Patients with essential thrombocythemia can manifest abnormal bleeding or blood clotting, although these complications are not very common. Transformation to acute myeloid leukemia is rare (see Chapter 11 for additional information on essential thrombocythemia).

Diagnosis

- *Cell counts and the peripheral blood smear*—Diagnosis is made by demonstrating a chronically elevated platelet count. The WBC count and hematocrit may also be moderately elevated.
- *Bone marrow morphology*—The bone marrow demonstrates an increase in megakaryocytes and an overall increase in cellularity. With progressive disease, the bone marrow can become fibrotic.
- *Cytogenetics and molecular pathology*—Cytogenetic findings are usually normal. Definitive diagnosis is made by demonstrating a point mutation in the JAK2 gene, which occurs in about 50% of cases. Mutations in the thrombopoietin receptor, Mpl, have also been described.

Primary Myelofibrosis
Description
Patients with primary myelofibrosis typically present with marked splenomegaly and some degree of hepatomegaly. The disease affects primarily older individuals. As the marrow becomes fibrotic and cytopenias in the peripheral blood develop, the complications associated with the cytopenias appear. Bleeding from low platelet counts and infections from low WBC counts may be lethal. A minority of patients with primary myelofibrosis (less than 10%) progress to acute leukemia, with a higher incidence in those who are treated with radioactive phosphorus or alkylating agents in the highly proliferative phase of their disease.

Diagnosis

- *Cell counts and the peripheral blood smear*—The peripheral blood frequently demonstrates a "leukoerythroblastic" picture, with leukocytosis, immature granulocytes including blasts, thrombocytosis, and the presence of immature erythroid cells including reticulocytes and nucleated red cells. The cell counts decline with disease progression.
- *Bone marrow morphology*—Initially, the bone marrow shows trilineage hypercellularity with megakaryocyte hyperplasia and reticulin fibrosis. With disease progression, there is replacement of the bone marrow by extensive fibrosis allowing little space for hematopoiesis.
- *Cytogenetics and molecular pathology*—Cytogenetic abnormalities are present in 30% to 60% of patients. Approximately 40% to 50% of patients with idiopathic myelofibrosis have the *JAK2* V617F mutation.

MYELODYSPLASTIC SYNDROMES

Description

Myelodysplastic syndromes include a group of bone marrow disorders with dysplastic (not normal, but not neoplastic) changes of the cells of the myeloid series. In myelodysplasia, the myeloblasts in the bone marrow must represent less than 20% of all nucleated marrow cells, because if there are 20% or more blasts, a diagnosis of acute myeloid leukemia is made. Because the myelodysplastic cells originate from an abnormal stem cell clone that is genetically unstable, there is a tendency for myelodysplasia to evolve into acute leukemia.

Myelodysplastic syndrome can occur as a primary disease or as a secondary disorder following exposure to chemotherapeutic agents or radiotherapy. Most cases of primary myelodysplastic syndrome are found in individuals over the age of 50 years. Many names have been applied to what is now called myelodysplastic syndrome, including preleukemia, refractory anemia (RA), and smoldering leukemia.

Myelodysplastic syndromes include a group of bone marrow disorders with dysplastic (not normal, but not neoplastic) changes of the cells of the myeloid series.

Diagnosis

Peripheral blood cytopenias are a hallmark of the myelodysplastic syndrome. As a result of ineffective hematopoiesis, myelodysplasia patients present with the complications of reduced blood cell counts in 1 or more cell lines. The complications include infections from low WBC counts, hemorrhage from low platelet counts, and weakness from anemia. In all forms of myelodysplastic syndrome, the bone marrow biopsy reveals hypercellularity.

A cytogenetic abnormality is found in 40% to 80% of the cases of primary myelodysplasia and 90% to 97% of patients with secondary myelodysplasia. These abnormalities may be useful as prognostic indicators. The most common changes are an interstitial deletion of the long arm of chromosome 5 (5q–) and deletions of chromosome 7 (–7, 7p–, or 7q–).

WHO Classification of the Myelodysplastic Syndrome

The myelodysplastic syndromes include a heterogeneous, but definable group of disorders. A brief description of each the disorders in the myelodysplastic syndrome is provided as follows:

- *RA*—This is defined as an anemia refractory to therapy. Dysplastic changes are only seen in the erythroid lineage. There are less than 5% bone marrow blasts, and ringed sideroblasts are less than 15% of the erythroid precursors.
- *Refractory anemia with ringed sideroblasts (RARS)*—This disorder is like RA except that 15% or more of the nucleated RBCs in the marrow are ringed sideroblasts. A ringed sideroblast, as noted in the section "Sideroblastic Anemia" (Chapter 10), is a cell in which at least 30% of the circumference of the nuclear membrane is covered by mitochondria containing iron granules.
- *Refractory cytopenias with multilineage dysplasia (RCMD)*—This disorder is like RA except that dysplasia is present in 2 or more lineages (lineages being myeloid, erythroid, and megakaryocytic). Auer rods (abnormal inclusions in myeloid blasts) are absent.

- *Refractory cytopenias with multilineage dysplasia and ringed sideroblasts (RCMD-RS)*—This disorder is like RCMD except that 15% or more of the nucleated RBCs in the marrow are ringed sideroblasts.
- *Refractory anemia with excess blasts-1 (RAEB-1)*—The major criterion for RAEB-1 is the presence of 5% to 9% of total nucleated cells in the bone marrow as blasts. There can be unilineage or multilineage dysplasia. In addition, the percentage of WBC blasts in the peripheral blood must be less than 5% of nucleated cells. Auer rods are absent.
- *Refractory anemia with excess blasts-2 (RAEB-2)*—This disease is present if there are 10% to 19% blasts in the bone marrow, 5% to 19% blasts in the blood, or Auer rods in myeloblasts or other neutrophilic precursors. There can be unilineage or multilineage dysplasia.
- *Myelodysplastic syndrome, unclassified (MDS-U)*—This disease is similar to RA except that dysplasia is present in 1 lineage other than the erythroid lineage. There are less than 5% blasts, and there are no Auer rods.
- *MDS associated with del(5q)*—Also known as "5q-syndrome," there are normal to increased megakaryocytes with hypolobated nuclei, less than 5% blasts, no Auer rods, and the sole cytogenetic abnormality of del(5q).

MYELODYSPLASTIC/MYELOPROLIFERATIVE NEOPLASMS

The myelodysplastic/myeloproliferative neoplasm category was created for the WHO classification. This category is for clonal stem cell disorders that do not fit well into either the myelodysplastic or myeloproliferative disorders. The most common of these disorders is chronic myelomonocytic leukemia (CMML). Other rare disorders in this category include atypical chronic myeloid leukemia, juvenile myelomonocytic leukemia, and an unclassifiable category.

- *CMML*—This disorder is a chronic leukemia with dysplastic changes in the bone marrow that are indicative of an increased risk for transformation into acute myeloblastic leukemia. Patients with CMML have an absolute peripheral monocytosis greater than 1,000 monocytes/µL, less than 20% blasts in the bone marrow, and dysplasia of 1 or more myeloid lineages.

DISORDERS ASSOCIATED WITH IMPAIRED WBC FUNCTION

WBC functional abnormalities may be clinically significant and predispose to life-threatening infections.

WBCs must be present in appropriate numbers and also function normally. The disorders previously discussed in this chapter are associated with alterations in WBC number, and in some cases, impaired function as well. The 3 disorders presented in the following sections represent examples of WBC functional disorders with no alteration in WBC number. It is for this reason that they are also known as qualitative (as opposed to quantitative) WBC disorders. Many WBC qualitative disorders result in functional impairment and no increased risk for infections. However, other WBC functional abnormalities may be clinically significant and predispose to life-threatening infections.

Chediak–Higashi Syndrome
Description
This disorder is due to a mutation in a lysosomal trafficking regulator. The disorder is characterized by functional defects associated with azurophilic granules in the cells that have these granules. They are particularly prominent in neutrophils and melanocytes. Most patients with Chediak–Higashi syndrome are subject to recurrent infections. Chediak–Higashi patients also have partial albinism because they have defective melanosomes (which provide skin coloration). The platelets from these patients have a defect in storage granules. This platelet granule deficiency may produce a bleeding tendency because release of the granule contents is necessary for the platelets to aggregate and form platelet plugs.

Diagnosis
A personal and family history consistent with Chediak–Higashi syndrome, along with abnormal granules in all granulated hematopoietic cells and lymphocytes, strongly suggests the diagnosis.

Chronic Granulomatous Disease

Description

Chronic granulomatous disease (CGD) comprises a heterogeneous group of disorders in which recurrent bacterial infections can lead to an early death. The WBCs in CGD do not exhibit obvious morphological differences from normal WBCs. However, there are multiple biochemical defects in neutrophil function in CGD that limit their ability to produce peroxide and superoxides that destroy bacteria.

Diagnosis

Patients with CGD have a negative nitroblue tetrazolium (NBT) dye test. In this assay, a yellow dye is oxidized by the oxidative enzymes in the normal granules of neutrophils to form an insoluble blue-black compound detectable by light microscopy.

Myeloperoxidase Deficiency

Description

This disorder results from a defect in the pathway required for generation of free radicals, which are important in the destruction of invading microorganisms, similar to CGD. Although individuals with MPO deficiency may experience recurrent infections, the disorder is benign in most cases. The absence of MPO may be congenital or acquired.

Diagnosis

In patients with MPO deficiency, MPO staining of freshly prepared blood smears will produce only faint staining of the granules in neutrophils.

> There are multiple biochemical defects in neutrophil function in chronic granulomatous disease that limit their ability to produce peroxide and superoxides that destroy bacteria.

REFERENCES

Bain BJ. The relationship between the myelodysplastic syndromes and the myeloproliferative disorders. *Leuk Lymphoma*. 1999;34:443.

Baird SM. Plasma cell neoplasms: general considerations. In: Beutler E, et al., eds. *Williams Hematology*. 5th ed. New York, NY: McGraw-Hill; 1995:1097.

Barolgie B, et al. Plasma cell dyscrasias. *JAMA*. 1992;268:2946.

Bataille R, Harousseau J. Multiple myeloma. *N Engl J Med*. 1997;336:1657.

Bennett JM, et al. Proposals for the classification of the acute leukemias. *Br J Haematol*. 1976;33:451.

Bennett JM, et al. The morphological classification of acute lymphoblastic leukemia: concordance among observers and clinical correlations. *Br J Haematol*. 1981;47:553.

Bennett JM, et al. Proposed revised criteria for the classification of acute myeloid leukemia. *Ann Intern Med*. 1985;103:620.

Bennet JM, et al. Criteria for the diagnosis of acute leukemia of megakaryocyte lineage (M7). *Ann Intern Med*. 1985;103:460.

Boccadoro M, Pileri A. Diagnosis, prognosis and standard treatment of multiple myeloma. *Hematol Oncol Clin North Am*. 1997;11:111.

Brunning RD. Acute leukemias. In: Rosai J, ed. *Tumors of the Bone Marrow. Atlas of Tumor Pathology*. Washington, DC: Armed Forces Institute of Pathology; 1994:19. Series 3, Fascicle 9.

Brunning RD, McKenna RW. Myelodysplastic syndromes. In: *Atlas of Tumor Pathology: Tumors of the Bone Marrow*. Washington, DC: Armed Forces Institute of Pathology; 1994:143. Series 3, Fascicle 9.

Campana D, Pui CH. Detection of minimal residual disease in acute leukemia: methodological advances and clinical significance. *Blood*. 1995;85:1416.

Cheson BD, et al. National Cancer Institute-sponsored working group guidelines for chronic lymphocytic leukemia: revised guidelines for diagnosis and treatment. *Blood*. 1996;87:4990.

Cortes JE, et al. Chronic myelogenous leukemia: a review. *Am J Med*. 1996;100:555.

Devine SM, Larson RA. Acute leukemia in adults: recent developments in diagnosis and treatment. *CA Cancer J Clin*. 1994;44:326.

Dickstein JI, Vardiman JW. Hematopathologic findings in the myeloproliferative disorders. *Semin Oncol*. 1995;22:355.

Dimopoulos MA, Alexanian R. Waldenström's macroglobulinemia. *Blood*. 1994;83:1452.

Durie BGM. Staging and kinetics of multiple myeloma. *Semin Oncol*. 1986;13:300.

Faderl S, et al. The biology of chronic myeloid leukemia. *N Engl J Med*. 1999;341:164.

Ferry JA, Harris NL. *Atlas of Lymphoid Hyperplasia and Lymphoma*. Philadelphia, PA: WB Saunders; 1997.

Foucar K. Myelodysplasia. In: *Bone Marrow Pathology*. Chicago, IL: ASCP Press; 1994:159.

Harris NL, et al. A revised European–American classification of lymphoid neoplasms: a proposal from the International Lymphoma Study Group. *Blood*. 1994;84:1361.

Heaney ML, Golde DW. Myelodysplasia. *N Engl J Med*. 1999;340:1649.

Janckila AJ, et al. Hairy cell identification by immunohistochemistry of tartrate-resistant acid phosphatase. *Blood*. 1995;85:2839.

Keating MJ. Chronic lymphocytic leukemia. *Semin Oncol*. 1999;26(suppl 14):107.

Kipps TJ. Chronic lymphocytic leukemia and related diseases. In: Beutler E, et al., eds. *Williams Hematology*. 5th ed. New York, NY: McGraw-Hill; 1995:1017.

Kjeldsberg C, et al. *Practical Diagnosis of Hematologic Disorders*. 2nd ed. Chicago, IL: ASCP Press; 1995

Rowley JD. Recurring chromosome abnormalities in leukemia and lymphoma. *Semin Hematol*. 1990;27:122.

Kyle RA. The monoclonal gammopathies. *Clin Chem*. 1994;40:2154.

Kyle RA, et al. The diverse picture of gamma heavy-chain disease: report of seven cases and review of literature. *Mayo Clin Proc*. 1981;56:439.

Lichtman MA. Chronic myelogenous leukemia and related disorders. In: Beutler E, et al., eds. *Williams Hematology*. 5th ed. New York, NY: McGraw-Hill; 1995:298.

Melnick SJ. Acute lymphoblastic leukemia. *Clin Lab Med*. 1999;19:169.

Morrison VA. Chronic leukemias. *CA Cancer J Clin*. 1994;44:353.

Rajkumar SV, Greipp PR. Prognostic factors in multiple myeloma. *Hematol Oncol Clin North Am*. 1999:13:1295.

Rowley JD. The role of chromosome translocations in leukemogenesis. *Semin Hematol*. 1999;36(suppl 7):59.

Rubnitz JE, Pui CH. Molecular diagnostics in the treatment of leukemia. *Curr Opin Hematol*. 1999;6:229.

Seligmann M, et al. Heavy chain diseases: current findings and concepts. *Immunol Rev*. 1979;48:145.

Swerdlow SH, Campo E, Harris NL, et al., eds. World Health *Organization Classification of Tumours of Haematopoietic and Lymphoid Tissues*. Lyon, France: IARC Press; 2008.

Teffari A, et al. Agnogenic myeloid metaplasia. *Semin Oncol*. 1995;22:327.

Wood B. 9-Color and 10-color flow cytometry in the clinical laboratory. *Arch Pathol Lab Med*. 2006;130:680.

The Respiratory System

Alison Woodworth

LEARNING OBJECTIVES

1. Learn the role of blood gases in the evaluation of the patient with pulmonary disease.
2. Understand how pleural fluid analysis is used in the diagnosis of pulmonary disorders.
3. Understand how bronchoalveolar lavage can aid in the diagnosis of respiratory disease.
4. Recognize the different laboratory tests used for assessing fetal lung maturity.

CHAPTER OUTLINE

APPROACH TO THE PATIENT WITH PULMONARY DISEASE

Impaired exchange of gases is the unifying theme of respiratory disorders (**Figure 14–1**). Although they do not play a significant role in the diagnosis of specific pulmonary diseases, blood gas and electrolyte measurements (see Chapter 2 for blood gas determinations) are commonly used to assess the severity of different pulmonary diseases. The analysis of fluid located in the pleural space, which collects with certain diseases, constitutes another battery of tests often useful in the evaluation of pulmonary diseases. Careful analysis of respiratory secretions along with accompanying white blood cells, immune mediators, and foreign pathogens through bronchoalveolar lavage (BAL) aids in the diagnosis and management of lung disease. Infections in the respiratory tract are a major category of pulmonary disorders. These are nearly always diagnosed using clinical laboratory tests (respiratory infections are discussed in Chapter 5). Respiratory distress syndrome (RDS) is among the most common lung diseases in infants and neonates and is directly correlated with incomplete lung maturation. Fetal lung maturity (FLM) can be assessed in a number of ways in the clinical laboratory. This chapter is organized by laboratory tests, rather than by diseases. The major sections of this chapter are discussions of blood gases, FLM testing, pleural fluid, and BAL analyses. There is also a disease-based section in this chapter, in which selected respiratory diseases are listed with their associated laboratory test abnormalities.

Pulmonary disorders other than infections and tumors can be classified into 3 major groups. One group of disorders includes emphysema, bronchitis, asthma, and RDS. These are airway-based

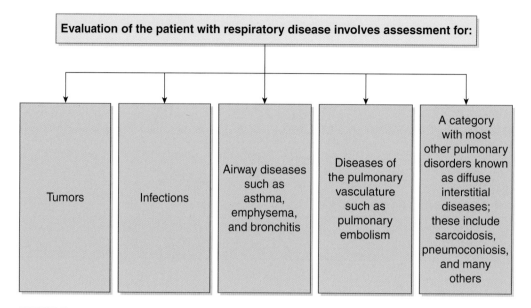

FIGURE 14–1 An overview of the evaluation of the patient for respiratory disease.

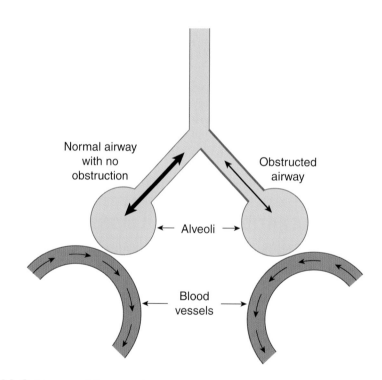

FIGURE 14–2 Diagram of diseases of the airway resulting in impaired ventilation.

diseases. Diseases of the airway result in impaired ventilation of alveoli (**Figure 14–2**). Another group of disorders affects the blood vessels, and, thereby, blood flow in the lung. Pulmonary diseases associated with reduced blood flow result in nonuniform perfusion of the lungs (**Figure 14–3**). The third major category of pulmonary diseases includes the diffuse interstitial, also known as infiltrative or restrictive, lung diseases. The disorders within this third group are heterogeneous and not uniformly classified. Such diseases are associated with a thickened interface between alveoli and adjacent capillaries resulting in impaired diffusion of gases (**Figure 14–4**).

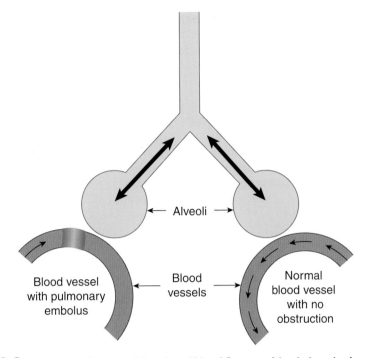

FIGURE 14–3 Diagram of diseases with reduced blood flow, resulting in impaired perfusion of the lung.

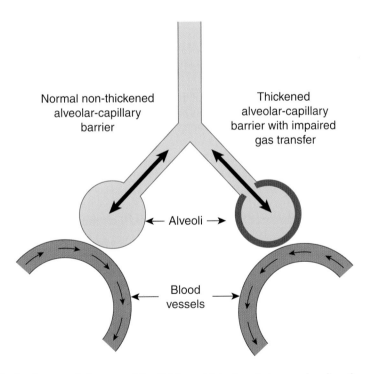

FIGURE 14–4 Diagram of diseases with a thickened interface between alveoli and adjacent capillaries, resulting in impaired diffusion of gases.

Clinical progression of pulmonary disease can lead to life-threatening respiratory failure. Acute RDS is a rapid onset disease associated with severe breathing problems resulting from multiple insults to the lung. It is distinct from "end-stage lung," which is the result of a chronic pulmonary disorder.

BLOOD GASES AND BLOOD pH

Many disorders are associated with abnormalities in arterial blood pO_2, pCO_2, and pH. While these tests are not themselves diagnostic, they are valuable in assessment of the severity of respiratory diseases. The blood gas test panel includes:

- pO_2 or partial pressure of oxygen
- pCO_2 or partial pressure of carbon dioxide
- pH

The functional abnormalities most commonly detected with this battery of tests are:

- low pO_2 (hypoxemia or low O_2 in blood, as opposed to hypoxia, which is reduced O_2 in tissues);
- high pCO_2 (hypercapnia);
- low arterial blood pH with a primary respiratory cause (respiratory acidosis from an increased arterial pCO_2);
- low arterial blood pH with a primary metabolic cause (metabolic acidosis, usually from increased acid production and/or impaired renal H^+ elimination, resulting in a decreased arterial HCO_3^-);
- high arterial blood pH with a primary respiratory cause (respiratory alkalosis from a decreased arterial pCO_2);
- high arterial blood pH with a primary metabolic cause (metabolic alkalosis from an increased arterial HCO_3^-).

The lungs respond within minutes to acid–base disturbances by 1) eliminating CO_2 (hyperventilation) to increase blood pH or 2) retaining CO_2 (hypoventilation) to decrease the pH. The kidney has the ability to 1) excrete H^+ and retain HCO_3^- to increase pH or 2) retain H^+ and excrete HCO_3^- to lower blood pH. However, renal compensation is slow and occurs over hours to days. **Table 14–1** lists selected respiratory and nonrespiratory disorders associated with hypoxemia, and **Table 14–2** presents selected respiratory and nonrespiratory disorders that can result in acid–base abnormalities.

The lungs respond within minutes to acid–base disturbances by 1) eliminating CO_2 (hyperventilation) to increase blood pH or 2) retaining CO_2 (hypoventilation) to decrease the pH.

TABLE 14–1   Selected Disorders Associated with Hypoxemia

Disorder	Basis of Abnormality
Chronic bronchitis	Impaired ventilation of lung
Emphysema	Impaired ventilation of lung
Asthma	Impaired ventilation of lung
Pneumoconioses	Impaired ventilation of lung
Central or peripheral neuromuscular disorders	Impaired ventilation of lung
Right-to-left shunts of great vessels	Impaired perfusion of blood into lungs
Pulmonary embolism and pulmonary infarction	Impaired perfusion of blood into lungs
Sarcoidosis	Impaired diffusion of gases into blood
Selected lung cancers	Impaired diffusion of gases into blood

TABLE 14–2   Selected Disorders Associated with Acid–Base Abnormalities[a]

Disorder	Metabolic Alterations
Selected causes of metabolic acidosis: Arterial pH decreased with arterial HCO_3^- decreased (often from increased acid production associated with an elevated anion gap or impaired renal elimination) as a primary change and arterial pCO_2 decreased as a compensatory change	
Uncontrolled diabetes	Increased ketoacids, increased anion gap
Methanol intoxication	Increased formic acid, increased anion gap
Tissue hypoxia	Increased lactic acid, increased anion gap
Renal failure from a variety of causes	Impaired H^+ excretion and/or HCO_3^- absorption
Gastrointestinal HCO_3^- loss from diarrhea	Decrease in HCO_3^- results in a relative increase in acidity
Selected causes of respiratory acidosis: Arterial pH decreased with arterial pCO_2 increased as a primary change and arterial HCO_3^- increased as a compensatory change	
Neuromuscular disorders that decrease breathing such as brain stem injury, myasthenia gravis, and poliomyelitis	Decreased pCO_2 excretion results in increased carbonic acid (H_2CO_3)
Severe pulmonary embolisms, infections, lung cancers, asthma, bronchitis, emphysema, and respiratory distress syndrome with impaired ventilation, perfusion, and/or diffusion	Decreased pCO_2 excretion results in increased carbonic acid (H_2CO_3)
Selected causes of metabolic alkalosis: Arterial pH increased with arterial HCO_3^- increased as a primary change and arterial pCO_2 increased as a compensatory change	
Vomiting or nasogastric suction	Loss of stomach acids (HCl)
Diuretic (ab)use	Increase in HCO_3^- due to renal acid loss often as a result of impaired renal function
Cushing syndrome and hyperaldosteronism	Impaired ion exchange in the kidney can result in a relative reduction in acidity
Selected causes of respiratory alkalosis: Arterial pH increased with arterial pCO_2 decreased as a primary change and arterial HCO_3^- decreased as a compensatory change	
Hyperventilation in response to hypoxemia from a variety of causes	Increased pCO_2 excretion results in decreased carbonic acid (H_2CO_3)
Hyperventilation without hypoxemia as a stimulus, as in anxiety and central nervous system disorders that increase the respiratory rate	Increased pCO2 excretion results in decreased carbonic acid (H_2CO_3)

[a]Blood pH = 6.1 + [log(arterial HCO_3^- concentration)/(0.03 × pCO_2)] is the equation that associates the measured parameters in this table.

ELECTROLYTES AND ANION GAP

Electrolytes are defined as either positively (cations) or negatively (anions) charged ions in the blood. Four freely circulating electrolytes are typically considered when evaluating acid–base disturbances (Na^+, K^+, Cl^-, and HCO_3^-). Blood gas and pH results are most important when investigating acid–base disruptions, and electrolytes play an important role in identifying the nature of the problem. Modern blood gas analyzers have expanded test menus to include electrolytes, facilitating their use in the evaluation of patients with suspected respiratory and/or metabolic disorders.

TABLE 14–3   Selected Disorders with Transudate or Exudate Formation

Disorders Associated with Transudate Formation	Basis of Abnormality
Congestive heart failure	An increased systemic venous pressure and pulmonary capillary pressure, due to the decreased effectiveness of the heart as a pump, results in leakage of fluid into the pleural space
Hypoalbuminemia	Decreased albumin results in a low vascular osmotic pressure and fluid accumulation in body tissues and cavities, including the pleural space
Disorders Associated with Exudate Formation	
Pulmonary embolism and pulmonary infarction	Blockage of blood vessels results in tissue damage and leakage of fluid, or in some cases whole blood, into the pleural space
Pulmonary infections	Tissue damage results in leakage of fluid into the pleural space
Lung tumors	Tissue damage results in leakage of fluid into the pleural space
Autoimmune diseases with pulmonary involvement	Tissue damage results in leakage of fluid into the pleural space
Trauma to the lung or chest wall	Tissue damage results in leakage of fluid into the pleural space

The anion gap refers to the difference between the major free cations (Na^+ and K^+) and free anions (Cl^- and HCO_3^-). The calculation of the anion gap from measured electrolyte concentrations is critical for evaluation of acidosis. An elevated anion gap occurs when acid anions (such as lactate or ketones) are present. The amount of the increase in anion gap is equal to the amount of acid present because an increase in acid results in a proportional decrease in bicarbonate. **Table 14–2** presents selected metabolic acidoses associated with an elevated anion gap.

> The anion gap refers to the difference between the major free cations (Na^+ and K^+) and free anions (Cl^- and HCO_3^-). The calculation of the anion gap from measured electrolyte concentrations is critical for evaluation of acidosis.

PLEURAL FLUID ANALYSIS

There are a number of disorders associated with the accumulation of fluid in the pleural space (**Table 14–3**). Pleural fluid can be collected by a pleural tap, also known as thoracentesis. An initial evaluation of color, physical characteristics, and odor of the fluid may help identify the source. Next, the fluid is identified as an exudate or a transudate to limit the differential diagnosis and help identify the cause of the fluid accumulation. Exudates and transudates are defined by the following criteria:

- Exudate—A filtrate of plasma out of the blood vessel, resulting from capillary damage or lymphatic obstruction (i.e., significant loss of the blood/tissue barrier), with a relatively high concentration of protein (>3.0 g/dL) and:

  (a) $\dfrac{\text{Pleural fluid total protein}}{\text{Serum total protein}} > 0.5$

  (b) Pleural fluid lactate dehydrogenase (LDH) > 20 IU/dL

  (c) $\dfrac{\text{Pleural fluid LDH}}{\text{Serum LDH}} > 0.6$

- Transudate—An ultrafiltrate of plasma with a relatively low protein concentration (<3.0 g/dL) and values for [(pleural fluid total protein)/(serum total protein)], pleural fluid LDH, and [(pleural fluid LDH)/(serum LDH)] below what is required to define the fluid as an exudate.

  (a) $\dfrac{\text{Pleural fluid total protein}}{\text{Serum total protein}} < 0.5$

  (b) $\dfrac{\text{Pleural fluid LDH}}{\text{Serum LDH}} < 0.6$

Other laboratory testing on pleural fluid, while not diagnostic, may provide useful information in identifying the source of the fluid accumulation. These include: total nucleated cell counts, WBC differential, Gram stain, pH, glucose, amylase, lipids, and tumor markers. The section "Infections of the Lung and Pleurae" in Chapter 5 contains information on pleural fluid testing that is specific for infections.

BRONCHOALVEOLAR LAVAGE FLUID ANALYSIS

Analysis of the components of BAL fluid is an important diagnostic tool in assessment of diffuse lung diseases. BAL analysis is most helpful when used in conjunction with clinical data and imaging results to aid in the diagnosis of pulmonary infections, particularly ventilator-acquired pneumonia, interstitial lung diseases, and lung cancers, and for monitoring of the allograft postlung transplant. Several aliquots of warmed saline are instilled in different areas of the lungs. At least 30% of the instilled fluid is carefully aspirated. BAL fluid is collected with the aid of a bronchoscope.

Bacterial cultures of the pooled fluid sample help identify an infectious cause of respiratory disease. Analysis of physical characteristics of the BAL collections also aids in the differentiation of disease. Bloody BAL fluid may indicate a diffuse alveolar hemorrhage, while cloudy BAL fluid suggests **a** diagnosis of pulmonary alveolar proteinosis. BAL fluid can also be processed to allow analysis of soluble biomarkers and cells. Studies of the BAL cell pellet include bacterial cultures, WBC count and differential, and Gram stain.

ASSESSMENT OF FETAL LUNG MATURITY

Respiratory Distress Syndrome

RDS of the newborn is most commonly associated with incomplete development of the fetal lungs. The pulmonary system is one of the last to completely develop, and as a result, RDS is a common cause of morbidity and mortality in preterm infants. Symptoms of RDS begin within a few hours of birth due to a deficiency of pulmonary surfactant. Surfactant, a mixture of phospholipids and proteins, coats the alveolar surfaces and separates alveolar airspace from liquid-coated lung epithelial cells, preventing lung collapse during exhalation. RDS patients suffer both lung collapse and hyperextension of alveoli leading to fibrosis, or hyaline membrane disease. The alveoli in an RDS lung are perfused, but not ventilated, resulting in hypoxia, hypercapnia, and respiratory acidosis.

RDS can be addressed by preventing preterm births or by administration of corticosteroids at least 48 hours prior to a premature birth. Corticosteroids induce surfactant production, significantly reducing neonatal morbidity and mortality due to RDS. Assessment of FLM status is essential for clinical decisions for women with symptoms of preterm labor and for those whose labor is induced prior to 39 weeks gestation.

Selected Laboratory Tests for Assessment of Fetal Lung Maturity

FLM is most commonly assessed by testing the amount of surfactant in the amniotic fluid in women after 30 weeks gestation. The diagnostic test most commonly used to assess FLM is the surfactant–albumin (S/A) ratio. The S/A ratio increases throughout gestation proportionally with lung maturity. The commercially available S/A ratio assay is called the TDX-FLM II where a result >55 mg surfactant/g albumin is consistent with lung maturity. Surfactant is packaged into

> Respiratory distress syndrome of the newborn is most commonly associated with incomplete development of the fetal lungs. The pulmonary system is one of the last to completely develop, and as a result, RDS is a common cause of morbidity and mortality in preterm infants.

TABLE 14–4   Selected Respiratory Diseases and Laboratory Tests Useful in Their Diagnosis or Management

Disorder	Results/Comment
Asthma	Demonstration of an elevated total IgE helps predict patients who will benefit from anti-IgE therapy; antigen-specific IgE testing is useful in young children and patients with a contraindication to skin testing
Sarcoidosis	Elevated serum angiotensin-converting enzyme is found in 30%–80% of sarcoidosis cases and may be a surrogate marker of disease burden
Pulmonary embolism	A diagnostic algorithm based on a clinical significance score combined with radiography and laboratory testing is most accurate in predicting an embolism. A negative test result for D-dimer (a fibrin degradation product) in a patient with low to moderate clinical probability effectively rules out PE. A pulmonary embolism is confirmed with a multidetector CT pulmonary angiogram in patients with a high clinical probability or a positive D-dimer test (see Chapter 8 for a related discussion in the section "Deep Vein Thrombosis"); thrombosis is also reviewed in Chapter 11
Lung cancer	Detection of EGFR mutations can aid in prediction of patients who will respond to tyrosine kinase inhibitor therapy in nonsmall cell lung carcinoma (NSCLC); CYFRA 21-1 may be used to monitor disease and response to therapy in NSCLC; neuron-specific enolase may be useful in monitoring tumor recurrence in SCLC
Emphysema in nonsmokers	Identification of an allelic variant in the alpha-1-antitrypsin gene correlating to reduced alpha-1-protease inhibition is critical in patients with clinical and radiologic indications of AAT deficiency; see Chapter 16 for a discussion of alpha-1-antitrypsin deficiency
Goodpasture syndrome	Increased concentrations of serum glomerular basement membrane (GBM) antibodies are found in Goodpasture syndrome; ANCA antibody testing helps classify disease and rule out other syndromes; blood cell counts are important to monitor anemia; and renal function tests are useful for detection of renal failure
Pulmonary vasculidites	Discussed in the section "Vasculitis" of Chapter 8 on blood vessels (such as Wegner granulomatosis and Churg–Strauss syndrome)
Cystic fibrosis	Discussed in Chapter 7
Autoimmune-related	Discussed in Chapter 3

Fetal lung maturity can also be predicted by measuring the lecithin–sphingomyelin ratio. An L/S ratio >2.0 indicates lung maturity.

storage granules called lamellar bodies that pass into amniotic fluid in the third trimester of pregnancy. Lamellar body counts (LBC) >50,000 µL^{-1} suggest maturity. Lamellar bodies are similar in size to platelets and can be counted on a standard whole blood counter.

Surfactant-based phospholipids, particularly lecithin (phosphatidylcholine) and phosphatidylglycerol (PG), increase in the amniotic fluid during fetal lung maturation, while lipids not originating from the lung, such as sphingomyelin, remain fairly constant throughout gestation. Because of this, FLM can also be predicted by measuring the lecithin–sphingomyelin ratio. An L/S ratio >2.0 indicates lung maturity. Qualitative detection of PG in amniotic fluid is a rapid and sensitive alternative for predicting FLM in late pregnancy. PG measurements are particularly useful in blood and meconium-contaminated amniotic fluid specimens as all other tests described above are affected by these contaminants.

LABORATORY TESTS USEFUL IN THE DIAGNOSIS OR MANAGEMENT OF SELECTED PULMONARY DISEASES

There are a number of pulmonary diseases for which laboratory tests (other than blood gases, BAL, and those for FLM and exudate/transudate determination discussed above) are useful in establishing a diagnosis. These disorders are listed in **Table 14–4** with their accompanying clinical laboratory test results. The infectious diseases of the respiratory tract and pleurae are presented in Chapter 5. Pulmonary function tests provide information on airflow and lung volumes. These tests quantitate the volume of air moved in different inspiratory and expiratory maneuvers, and the rate at which the air is moved. In addition, the uptake of a gas can be measured as an indicator of an impaired alveolar–capillary interface. These tests on airflow and gas exchange often do not identify a specific respiratory disorder, but they can suggest a category of diseases that may account for the airflow abnormalities. Because pulmonary function tests are performed outside the clinical laboratory, they are not discussed further in this text.

Radiologic studies, particularly plain chest radiographs, computed tomographic scans, magnetic resonance imaging, positron emission tomography (PET) scans, and nuclear medicine studies such as ventilation/perfusion scanning, play a prominent role in the diagnosis of pulmonary disorders.

REFERENCES

ACOG Educational Bulletin. Assessment of fetal lung maturity. Number 230, November 1996. Committee on Educational Bulletins of the American College of Obstetricians and Gynecologists. *Int J Gynaecol Obstet.* 1997;56:191–198.

Anderson DR, Wells PS. Improvements in the diagnostic approach for patients with suspected deep vein thrombosis or pulmonary embolism. *Thromb Haemost.* 1999;82:878–886.

Ball JA, Young KR Jr. Pulmonary manifestations of Goodpasture's syndrome. Antiglomerular basement membrane disease and related disorders. *Clin Chest Med.* 1998;19:777–791, ix.

Beane J, Kadar A, DeLisi C, et al. Diagnostic and prognostic impact of high-throughput genomic and proteomic technologies in the post-genomic era. In: McPherson RA, Pincus MR, eds. *Henry's Clinical Diagnosis and Management by Laboratory Methods.* Saunders Elsevier Philadelphia, PA; 2007:1381–1394.

Dufour DR. Evaluation of renal function, water, electrolytes, acid–base balance, and blood gases. In: Henry JB, ed. *Clinical Diagnosis and Management by Laboratory Methods.* WB Saunders Philadelphia, PA; 2001:159–179.

Froudarakis ME. Diagnostic work-up of pleural effusions. *Respiration.* 2008;75:4–13.

Gal AA, Staton GW Jr. Current concepts in the classification of interstitial lung disease. *Am J Clin Pathol.* 2005;123(suppl):S67–S81.

Greenberg AK, Lee MS. Biomarkers for lung cancer: clinical uses. *Curr Opin Pulm Med.* 2007;13:249–255.

Grenache DG, Gronowski AM. Fetal lung maturity. *Clin Biochem.* 2006;39:1–10.

Gupta R, et al. The predictive value of epidermal growth factor receptor tests in patients with pulmonary adenocarcinoma: review of current "best evidence" with meta-analysis. *Hum Pathol.* 2009;40:356–365.

Herbst RS, et al. Lung cancer. *N Engl J Med.* 2008;359:1367–1380.

Homburger HA. Allergic diseases. In: McPherson RA, Pincus MR, eds. *Henry's Clinical Diagnosis and Management by Laboratory Methods.* Saunders Elsevier Philadelphia, PA; 2007:961–971.

Hughes JM. Assessing gas exchange. *Chron Respir Dis.* 2007;4:205–214.

Janata-Schwatczek K, et al. Pulmonary embolism. II. Diagnosis and treatment. *Semin Thromb Hemost.* 1996;22:33–52.

Kardon EM. Acute asthma. *Emerg Med Clin North Am.* 1996;14:93–114.

Kohnlein T, Welte T. Alpha-1 antitrypsin deficiency: pathogenesis, clinical presentation, diagnosis, and treatment. *Am J Med.* 2008;121:3–9.

Konstantinides S. Clinical practice. Acute pulmonary embolism. *N Engl J Med.* 2008;359:2804–2813.

Lynch JP 3rd, Ma YL, Koss MN, et al. Pulmonary sarcoidosis. *Semin Respir Crit Care Med.* 2007;28:53–74.

Marshall WJ. Hydrogen ion homeostatis and blood gases. In: *Clinical Chemistry.* Mosby Philadelphia, PA; 2008:45–68.

Meyer KC. Bronchoalveolar lavage as a diagnostic tool. *Semin Respir Crit Care Med.* 2007;28:546–560.

Newman LS. Occupational asthma. Diagnosis, management, and prevention. *Clin Chest Med.* 1995;16:621–636.

Sahn SA. The value of pleural fluid analysis. *Am J Med Sci.* 2008;335:7–15.

Trape J, et al. Biological variation of tumor markers and its application in the detection of disease progression in patients with non-small cell lung cancer. *Clin Chem.* 2005;51:219–222.

The Gastrointestinal Tract

D. Robert Dufour

LEARNING OBJECTIVES

1. Understand the relative contributions of clinical laboratory tests and other diagnostic studies in the evaluation of the patient for a disorder of the gastrointestinal tract.

2. Learn the appropriate selection of diagnostic tests required to establish a diagnosis of ulcer disease from *Helicobacter pylori* infection.

3. Select the most appropriate tests for evaluation of suspected celiac disease, and learn the situations where results may be misleading.

4. Describe the recommended approaches to screening for colon cancer, and the benefits and limitations of laboratory tests for this purpose.

CHAPTER OUTLINE

Most diseases of the gastrointestinal tract can be directly visualized by endoscopy or from a histopathologic review of a biopsy obtained during the endoscopic procedure. In addition, many gastrointestinal tract disorders can be identified with various imaging studies. This accessibility of lesions for direct examination and biopsy has limited the need for clinical laboratory tests in identifying most gastrointestinal disorders. However, because imaging studies are often expensive, and endoscopic procedures are both expensive and invasive, there is a clinical need for laboratory tests to aid in the diagnosis and management of persons with a number of gastrointestinal disorders. Infectious diseases involving the gastrointestinal tract are numerous, and are discussed in Chapter 5. The clinical laboratory plays an important role in identifying pathogenic microorganisms of the gastrointestinal tract.

The clinical laboratory also plays a role in the evaluation of dyspepsia (abdominal discomfort caused by acid), and/or ulcer disease, particularly that induced by *Helicobacter pylori* infection; in the recognition and monitoring of celiac sprue; and in the detection of colon cancer. Laboratory tests for these disorders are presented in this chapter.

DYSPEPSIA, ULCER DISEASE, AND *H. PYLORI*

Description

According to the American Gastroenterological Association (AGA), dyspepsia is defined as chronic or recurrent pain or discomfort centered in the upper abdomen. Other conditions (particularly reflux of acid into the esophagus, referred to as gastroesophageal reflux disease or GERD) can also cause abdominal discomfort, and it is often difficult to specifically characterize the type and location of discomfort. About 10% of those with upper abdominal symptoms are

TABLE 15–1   Commonly Used Laboratory Tests for *Helicobacter pylori*

Test	Advantages	Disadvantages
H. pylori IgG antibodies (serology)	Less expensive Widely available Simple to collect	Not very sensitive or specific; does not reflect response to treatment
Urea breath test	Most reliable non-invasive test Reflects response to treatment in about 4–6 weeks Relatively expensive	Requires special test meal and special testing equipment; not widely available Falsely negative with effective acid suppression
Stool *H. pylori* antigen	Reliable non-invasive test Simple to perform Not affected by acid suppression Reflects response to treatment	Requires special handling of stool Not widely available Requires 6–12 weeks to reflect treatment response
CLO test	Simplest test to perform Widely available Reliable test Reflects response to treatment in 4–6 weeks	Requires endoscopy and biopsy Falsely negative with acid suppression

found to have peptic ulcers. Other causes include gastritis related to use of non-steroidal anti-inflammatory agents, and "functional dyspepsia," in which no obvious pathology is present in the stomach.

The major cause of peptic ulcer disease is infection with *H. pylori*. The infection is most likely to occur in childhood, especially if the children are living in low socioeconomic conditions. In developed countries, *H. pylori* infection prevalence increases with age. Not all patients with *H. pylori* infection develop ulcer disease, as many suffer from dyspepsia without ulcers. Up to 10% of infected individuals in the United States develop peptic ulcers, most often in the duodenum, and *H. pylori* infection is usually the cause. The infection initially produces an acute gastritis that lasts 1 to 4 weeks. Once infected, however, chronic active gastritis occurs in the majority of individuals and may lead to more serious outcomes. Especially when infected in early childhood, individuals are at risk for the development of multifocal atrophic gastritis and over time, subsequently, have an increased risk for gastric adenocarcinoma.

> The major cause of peptic ulcer disease is infection with *H. pylori*. Not all patients with *H. pylori* infection develop ulcer disease, as many suffer from dyspepsia without ulcers.

Diagnosis

The evaluation of individuals with dyspepsia depends on age and the severity of symptoms. According to AGA guidelines, direct visualization of the upper gastrointestinal tract by endoscopy is the preferred initial step in persons over age 55 years, or in younger patients who have a family history of gastric cancer or who also have more worrisome symptoms such as weight loss, difficulty swallowing food, recurrent vomiting, or gastrointestinal bleeding. In younger patients without these symptoms, the recommended approach is to test for the presence of active *H. pylori* infection and treat infected individuals. Those without evidence of infection are treated with drugs that inhibit acid production. Persons who do not respond to these treatments should then have an endoscopy.

Laboratory tests for *H. pylori* can be separated into those that identify exposure and those that detect active infection (**Table 15–1**). Serologic tests for IgG antibodies to *H. pylori* indicate past or current infection. They have a sensitivity and a specificity of only about 85% to 90%, and have largely been replaced by tests that directly identify the organism. Accepted guidelines recommend 1 of the 2 tests for detection of current infection. *H. pylori* has a unique surface antigen that can be detected in the stool of infected individuals, but not in those with inactive infection. While stool antigen testing (with kits using monoclonal antibodies to the antigen) is sensitive and specific, it is not widely available. In addition, stool samples require special handling to prevent loss of the antigen. Because *H. pylori* is able to split urea (it is a urease-positive organism), its presence can be detected by ability of the individual to metabolize urea.

The urea breath test involves ingestion of a food product containing urea labeled with a small amount of radioactive carbon. If urease activity is present, the urea will be split into ammonia and carbon dioxide, and the amount of radioactive carbon dioxide in the breath correlates with urease activity. Use of drugs that suppress acid production may cause falsely negative urea breath tests. Either of these tests can also be used to evaluate the success of antibiotic treatment for *H. pylori*. Successful treatment should lead to loss of stool antigen (after several weeks) and the loss of urease activity in the stomach. Unlike the antigen and urease tests, serologic tests remain positive for years after successful treatment, and are thus of no use to monitor the effects of treatment.

If endoscopy is performed, direct tests can be done on either the gastric fluid or biopsy samples to detect *H. pylori*. While culture and DNA detection methods using polymerase chain reaction are available, biopsies are more commonly assessed for urease activity. The CLOtest™ involves incubating a piece of a gastric biopsy in the presence of a pH indicator, which changes color as urea is split. Once *H. pylori* infection is diagnosed, treatment success can be evaluated using either a stool antigen test or the urea breath test.

CELIAC SPRUE

Description

Celiac sprue is an immunologic disease caused by immune reactions triggered by gluten and related proteins, that are components of wheat, barley, and rye (and to a more limited extent, oat) grain products. Antibodies reactive against gliadin, an antigenic component of gluten, and tissue transglutaminase (TTG), an enzyme involved in antigen processing, are present along with T-cells reactive to the same antigens. This leads to damage to the mucosa of the small intestine, and patients present with a variety of symptoms and complications. Dermatitis herpetiformis, an immunologic skin disease associated with blisters and itching, is a cutaneous manifestation of gluten sensitivity.

> Celiac sprue is an immunologic disease caused by immune reactions triggered by gluten and related proteins, that are components of wheat, barley, and rye (and to a more limited extent, oat) grain products.

The diagnosis of celiac sprue currently requires endoscopy with biopsy of the duodenum. In severe cases, there is atrophy of villi and flattening of the mucosa, but milder cases may show only lymphocytes infiltrating the mucosa.

Although long thought to be an uncommon childhood disease with serious clinical consequences such as failure to gain weight, diarrhea due to malabsorption of nutrients, and vomiting, it is now recognized that celiac sprue can initially present in adulthood and with much milder clinical manifestations. As many as 1 in 250 adults have evidence of immune reactions to gliadin. Mildly affected individuals may have symptoms such as bloating, irregular bowel movements, and cramps (often referred to as irritable bowel syndrome, most cases of which are not caused by celiac sprue). Celiac sprue patients may present with malabsorption of certain essential nutrients, including iron. About 5% of iron deficiency in adults is thought to be due to celiac sprue. Malabsorption of folate and vitamin D, which may present clinically as osteoporosis, can also occur.

Diagnosis

Laboratory testing for celiac disease is summarized in **Table 15–2**. Testing for antibodies associated with the disease has become the primary means to detect individuals with milder forms of the disease. The most widely used test currently involves the detection of IgA antibodies to TTG. This test has a sensitivity and a specificity over 98%, especially now that human TTG is used in the test as a reagent. As many as 3% of those with classic celiac sprue have a deficiency of IgA, which would result in a falsely negative test result. In a person with a high suspicion for celiac sprue and a negative anti-TTG result, measurement of IgA is recommended. Tests for antibodies to gliadin are less sensitive and less specific in adults for diagnosis of celiac sprue, but they are more sensitive than anti-TTG assays in children. Antibody tests to gliadin are less likely to be positive in milder cases, and often become negative when gluten is eliminated from the diet. Some patients may be monitored with antibody levels to gliadin to monitor compliance with treatment. Recently, tests that detect an antibody to a modified form of gliadin have been shown to have significantly improved sensitivity and specificity, and these are now available for clinical use.

TABLE 15-2   Commonly Used Diagnostic Tests for Celiac Disease

Test	Advantages	Disadvantages
Tissue transglutaminase (TTG) IgA antibodies	Most reliable non-invasive test Inexpensive Widely available Easy sample collection High sensitivity and specificity	Falsely negative with IgA deficiency (3% of patients with celiac disease) May be negative if on low gluten diet
Gliadin antibodies (IgG and IgA)	Inexpensive Widely available Easy sample collection Positive in IgA deficiency May be more sensitive in children	Not as sensitive or specific as TTG IgA antibodies May be negative if on low gluten diet
Deamidated gliadin antibodies (IgG and IgA)	Widely available Easy sample collection Positive in IgA deficiency High sensitivity and specificity	Not as widely available as first 2 tests above More expensive than anti-gliadin antibody test
Small bowel biopsy	Reliable test, considered gold standard Reflects response to treatment	Requires endoscopy and biopsy Very expensive

SCREENING FOR COLORECTAL CANCER

Because colorectal cancer is the second most common cause of cancer death in both men and women, and because early detection is associated with better survival, there is widespread acceptance of the benefits of screening those over age 50 years for colorectal cancer. Screening may also detect adenomas of the colon, which have been recognized to be the precursors of most cases of invasive cancer. The most sensitive screening test for colorectal cancer is colonoscopy. Not only can colonoscopy detect colorectal cancer, but it can also detect most adenomas. Removal of adenomas that are detected reduces the risk of subsequent development of cancer.

Because colonoscopy is an invasive and expensive procedure with risks involved, other approaches to screening are also approved. These include virtual colonoscopy using CT scanning, but the most widely used screening procedure involves testing stool for the presence of blood, termed fecal occult blood testing (FOBT). The testing is done by having an individual take 2 samples from 3 consecutive bowel movements, and smearing these small samples onto cards that are sent to a site where they can be tested. FOBT can be detected using 2 slightly different methods. The older test uses guaiac, a reagent that reacts with hemoglobin and a number of other substances to produce a blue color when blood is present. Guaiac tests react with animal hemoglobin as well, so restrictions on meat intake are required for several days before samples are collected. Iron and certain plants also can cause a blue color with guaiac, and their intake should also be restricted. More recently, tests using antibodies to human hemoglobin have been introduced. These tests are generally slightly more expensive, but do not require restriction of diet before testing. Both types of tests for hemoglobin are approved in AGA guidelines.

Colonoscopy needs to be repeated infrequently, every 10 years if no adenomas are found, although more frequently in those with adenomas or with a strong family history of colon cancer. FOBT testing, on the other hand, should be performed every year. Any abnormal results should be followed up by colonoscopy.

Colorectal cancer, like most cancers, is associated with a number of mutations in genes related to cell growth and regulation. Recently, it has become possible to identify DNA from shed cells in stool. Preliminary results have shown that testing for multiple mutations in genes associated with colon cancer has a higher sensitivity than FOBT testing, although not as high as colonoscopy. The DNA test requires special handling, with collection of stool into a container that has been stored frozen, and rapid delivery after collection to the testing laboratory. It is similar in expense to colonoscopy at present. The newest guidelines from the Joint Task Force on Colorectal

Colonoscopy needs to be repeated infrequently, every 10 years if no adenomas are found, although more frequently in those with adenomas or with a strong family history of colon cancer.

TABLE 15–3   Screening Tests for Colorectal Cancer

Test	Advantages	Disadvantages
Colonoscopy	Most reliable screening modality Detects and permits removal of pre-cancerous polyps Only needs to be done every 10 years (if initially negative) High sensitivity and specificity	Expensive Requires unpleasant bowel preparation Has low, but present, risk of complications
Virtual colonoscopy (CT)	Non-invasive, no complications Detects pre-cancerous polyps (if >1 cm), which represent highest cancer risk Only needs to be done every 5 years (if initially negative) High sensitivity and specificity	Expensive Requires unpleasant bowel preparation Needs to be followed by colonoscopy if lesions detected
Fecal DNA testing	Non-invasive No dietary preparation Relatively simple to collect Fairly high sensitivity and specificity Detects pre-cancerous polyps	Expensive Not widely available More difficult to collect sample than it is for fecal occult blood tests No information on optimal frequency Needs to be followed by colonoscopy if abnormal
Fecal occult blood testing by guaiac	Non-invasive Simple to collect Inexpensive	Must be done yearly Dietary preparation needed (no meat, peroxidase-containing vegetables) Needs to be followed by colonoscopy if abnormal
Fecal occult blood testing by anti-human hemoglobin antibodies	Non-invasive No dietary preparation Simple to collect Inexpensive	Must be done yearly Needs to be followed by colonoscopy if abnormal

Cancer support the use of fecal DNA testing as an acceptable initial screening modality, but have not made recommendations on the frequency of testing. Laboratory testing to screen patients for colorectal cancer is summarized in **Table 15–3**.

REFERENCES

Dyspepsia and *Helicobacter pylori*

Talley NJ, American Gastroenterological Association medical position statement: evaluation of dyspepsia. *Gastroenterology*. 2005;129:1753–1755.

Gisbert JP, et al. Accuracy of monoclonal stool antigen test for the diagnosis of *H. pylori* infection: a systematic review and meta-analysis. *Am J Gastroenterol*. 2005;101:1921–1930.

Goodwin CS. *Helicobacter pylori* gastritis, peptic ulcer, and gastric cancer: clinical and molecular aspects. *Clin Infect Dis*. 1997;25:1017.

Hirschl AM, Makristhathis A. Non-invasive *Helicobacter pylori* diagnosis: stool or breath tests? *Dig Liv Dis*. 2005;37:732–734.

McCallion WA, et al. *Helicobacter pylori* infection in children: relation with current household living conditions. *Gut*. 1996;39:18.

NIH Consensus Development Panel on *Helicobacter pylori* in Peptic Ulcer Disease. *Helicobacter pylori* in peptic ulcer disease. *JAMA*. 1994;272:65.

Parsonnet J. *Helicobacter pylori* in the stomach: a paradox unmasked. *N Engl J Med*. 1996;335:278.

Ricci C, et al. Diagnosis of *Helicobacter pylori*: invasive and non-invasive tests. *Best Pract Res Clin Gastroenterol*. 2007;21:299–313.

Vilaichone R, et al. *Helicobacter pylori* diagnosis and management. *Gastroenterol Clin North Am*. 2005;35:229–247.

Celiac Sprue

Agardh D. Antibodies against synthetic deamidated gliadin peptides and tissue transglutaminase for the identification of childhood celiac disease. *Clin Gastroenterol Hepatol.* 2007;5:1276–1281.

Green P, Cellier C. Celiac disease. *N Engl J Med.* 2007;357:1731–1743.

Rostom A, et al. The diagnostic accuracy of serologic tests for celiac disease: a systematic review. *Gastroenterology.* 2005;128:S38–S46.

Rostom A, et al. American Gastroenterological Association (AGA) Institute technical review on the diagnosis and management of celiac disease. *Gastroenterology.* 2006;131:1981–2002.

Colon Cancer

Levin B, et al. Screening and surveillance for the early detection of colorectal cancer and adenomatous polyps, 2008: a joint guideline from the American Cancer Society, the US Multi-Society Task Force on Colorectal Cancer, and the American College of Radiology. *CA Cancer J Clin.* 2008;58:161–179.

Sinatra MA, et al. Interference of plant peroxidases with guaiac-based fecal occult blood tests is avoidable. *Clin Chem.* 1999;45:125–126.

Traverso G, et al. Detection of APC mutations in fecal DNA from patients with colorectal tumors. *N Engl J Med.* 2002;346:311–320.

Young GP, et al. Choice of fecal occult blood tests for colorectal cancer screening: recommendations based on performance characteristics in population studies. A WHO and OMED report. *Am J Gastroenterol.* 2002;97:2499–2597.

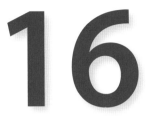
The Liver and Biliary Tract

William E. Winter

CHAPTER OUTLINE

INTRODUCTION

Laboratory evaluation of the hepatobiliary system centers on measurements of: 1) hepatocyte plasma membrane integrity, 2) measurements of the detoxifying and excretory functions of the hepatobiliary system, and 3) measurements of the synthetic capacity of hepatocytes.

TABLE 16–1   Enzymes Indicative of Liver Plasma Membrane Integrity

Indicative of hepatocellular disease
Alanine aminotransferase (ALT)
Aspartate aminotransferase (AST)
Lactate dehydrogenase (LDH)
Indicative of biliary tract disease
Alkaline phosphatase (ALP)
Gamma glutamyl transferase (GGT)
5′-Nucleotidase (5′-NT)

PLASMA MEMBRANE INTEGRITY AND DISORDERS PREDOMINANTLY ASSOCIATED WITH ELEVATED CONCENTRATIONS OF LIVER-DERIVED ENZYMES IN THE BLOOD

With hepatocyte or biliary tract disease, many cellular enzymes are released that enter the circulation. Enzymes indicative of hepatocyte disease are alanine aminotransferase (ALT) and aspartate aminotransferase (AST). Alkaline phosphatase (ALP) elevations relate to biliary tract disease (**Table 16–1**).

Enzyme concentrations are usually measured by determining the enzyme activity in serum or plasma. Such measurements are reported as units per liter (U/L) or international units per liter (IU/L), where the unit is an activity measurement (e.g., the rate of appearance of product or disappearance of substrate per unit time).

Normally, the healthy plasma membrane and various organelles contain (e.g., "hold") enzymes within the cell. An elevated enzyme level in the blood suggests organ dysfunction because of a functional or anatomic disruption in the plasma membrane. One way to assess the degree of elevation of an enzyme is to calculate the ratio of the patient's enzyme concentration relative to the upper limit of the reference interval. For example, if the upper limit of the reference interval for ALT were 40 U/L and the patient's ALT was 120 U/L, the patient's ALT would be said to be "3 times above the upper limit of normal."

While not specific for hepatocytes, elevations of ALT and AST are characteristic of hepatocellular disease. The major sources of ALT include the liver and the kidney. Lesser amounts are released from skeletal and cardiac muscle. AST is also found in these organs. ALT is exclusively localized in the cell cytoplasm. AST is located in the cytoplasm and mitochondria. However, AST derived from the cytoplasm and mitochondria cannot be distinguished through clinical laboratory testing. ALT is more specific for the liver than AST. Usually ALT and AST rise in tandem in liver disease states.

One condition where AST is elevated to a greater extent that ALT is in chronic liver disease resulting from chronic alcohol abuse. Alcoholics are not uncommonly pyridoxine deficient. While both AST and ALT are pyridoxine dependent for their activity, ALT is more dependent on pyridoxine than AST. Thus, a rise in the measured ALT may not be as great as the rise in measured AST because ALT activity suffers more from pyridoxine deficiency than does AST. If the AST to ALT ratio is greater than 2 in the setting of chronic liver disease, alcoholic liver disease is strongly suggested. With cirrhosis of any etiology, enzyme elevations may be modest, or their concentrations may be normal, reflecting a marked loss in hepatocyte mass and, thereby, a loss of enzymes within the liver.

In the past, lactate dehydrogenase (LDH) was also regularly employed as a marker of hepatocellular disease. However, LDH is not favored for routine evaluation of the hepatocyte integrity currently because LDH is released upon injury of many different tissues. Both ALT and AST are more specific for liver than LDH.

Enzymes indicative of hepatocyte disease are alanine aminotransferase (ALT) and aspartate aminotransferase (AST). Alkaline phosphatase (ALP) elevations relate to biliary tract disease.

TABLE 16–2 **Lactate Dehydrogenase (LDH) Isoenzymes: Subunit Composition and Distribution**

Isoenzyme	Subunits	Distribution
LD1	H4	Heart, red blood cell, renal cortex
LD2	H3M	Heart, red blood cell, renal cortex
LD3	H2M2	Pancreas, lung, lymphocyte, platelet
LD4	HM3	No specific distribution
LD5	M4	Hepatocyte, skeletal muscle, prostate

H, the heart subunit; M, the muscle subunit.

Measurement of LDH isoenzymes is possible, but there are more informative tests that can be ordered to evaluate specific organ dysfunction. LDH is composed of 4 subunits. The subunits are H (for heart) and M (for muscle). If required, LDH isoenzymes can be determined by electrophoresis. The subunit composition and major sources of each of the 5 isoenzymes are listed in **Table 16–2**. The LD4 isoenzyme provides no clinically useful information.

If the total LDH is increased in a patient with suspected liver disease, who lacks skeletal muscle and prostate disease, it is expected that LD5 will be elevated. The enzyme marker of choice for the evaluation of skeletal muscle injury or disease is creatine kinase (CK). If the CK is normal in the setting of an elevated LD5, skeletal muscle is not likely to be the source of the elevated LD5.

Biliary tract disease produces relatively greater increases in ALP than increases in ALT, AST, or LDH. ALP is associated with the plasma membrane of hepatocytes adjacent to the biliary canaliculus. Obstruction or inflammation of the biliary tract results in an increased concentration of the ALP in the circulation. Similar to ALT and AST, ALP is not specific for biliary tract disease. ALP is released by osteoblasts, the ileum, and the placenta. ALP is elevated: 1) in children 2- to 3-fold over adults because the child skeleton is growing, 2) with bone disease involving osteoblasts (e.g., metastatic cancer or following a fracture), 3) in cases of ileal disease, and 4) during the third trimester of pregnancy because the placental isoenzyme is elevated.

When the etiology of the elevated ALP is unclear, in the past ALP isoenzymes were determined. However, there are many technical problems with these assays. Today it has proven more pragmatic to measure other biliary tract enzyme markers such as gamma glutamyl transpeptidase (GGT) or 5'-nucleotidase (5'-NT). GGT is more commonly measured than 5'-NT because GGT testing is widely available on a variety of laboratory instruments. GGT is typically not elevated with bone disease. Combined elevations of ALP and GGT are compatible with biliary tract disease. However, if the ALP is elevated to a far greater extent than the GGT (or the GGT is normal), ALP sources other than the biliary tract, such as bone, must be investigated. GGT elevations occur in response to alcohol use and anticonvulsants as GGT is induced by such agents. While there is no specific biochemical test to prove that a patient suffers from alcohol abuse, carbohydrate-deficient transferrin levels can be elevated in patients suffering from alcoholism.

Using the information presented, we can develop an algorithm for the interpretation of liver enzyme elevations in patients with suspected liver disease. If the relative increase in ALT or AST over the upper limit of normal exceeds the relative increase in ALP over the upper limit of normal, the liver disease is predominantly hepatocellular.

Causes of acute hepatocellular disease include (**Table 16–3**): viral hepatitis (e.g., hepatitis A, B, or C), alcoholic hepatitis, toxic injury (e.g., acetaminophen poisoning), and ischemic injury (e.g., hypotension). In cases of ischemic injury or toxic injury following an acute toxic ingestion, the ALT and AST levels can rise and peak within 24 hours of the precipitating event. Less common causes of acute liver disease include hepatitis due to hepatitis D, hepatitis E, cytomegalovirus (CMV), Epstein–Barr virus (EBV), and herpes virus; autoimmune hepatitis (marked by positivity for antinuclear antibodies [ANA], smooth muscle autoantibodies [ASMA], and/or liver–kidney microsome autoantibodies [anti-LKM₁ autoantibodies] and negative antimitochondrial autoantibodies [AMA]); Wilson disease, and liver disease of pregnancy. Three forms of liver

Biliary tract disease produces relatively greater increases in ALP than increases in ALT, AST, or LDH. ALP is associated with the plasma membrane of hepatocytes adjacent to the biliary canaliculus.

TABLE 16–3   Causes of Hepatocellular Disease[a]

Acute: present for less than 6 months
Common Viral hepatitis (hepatitis A, B, or C) Alcoholic hepatitis Toxic injury Ischemic injury
Less common Viral hepatitis which is not hepatitis A, B, or C (includes hepatitis D, hepatitis E,   cytomegalovirus [CMV], Epstein–Barr virus [EBV], and herpes virus) Autoimmune hepatitis Wilson disease Liver disease of pregnancy
Chronic: present for more than 6 months
Viral hepatitis (hepatitis B or C) Drug toxicity Alcoholic liver disease Nonalcoholic fatty liver (NAFL) Inborn errors (includes hemochromatosis, alpha-1-antitrypsin deficiency, Wilson disease,   glycogen storage disease, and Gaucher disease) Autoimmune hepatitis

[a]The relative elevations in ALT and AST exceed the relative elevation in ALP.

disease in pregnancy include fatty liver, intrahepatic cholestasis, and hepatic dysfunction associated with toxemia (e.g., part of the HELLP syndrome: *h*emolysis, *e*levated *L*FTs [e.g., enzymes], and *l*ow *p*latelets).

Chronic hepatocellular disease is diagnosed when liver disease is present for more than 6 months (**Table 16–3**). Causes of chronic hepatocellular disease include: hepatitis B or C, drug toxicity (e.g., statins, sulfonamides, or INH), alcoholic liver disease, nonalcoholic fatty liver (NAFL), inborn errors, and autoimmune hepatitis. NAFL is one of the most common causes of nonviral and nonalcoholic liver disease. NAFL can progress to nonalcoholic steatohepatitis (NASH), cirrhosis, liver failure, and even hepatocellular carcinoma in some cases. Inborn errors causing chronic liver disease encompass hemochromatosis, alpha-1-antitrypsin deficiency, Wilson disease, glycogen storage disease (GSD), and Gaucher disease.

> Bilirubin is predominantly derived from hemoglobin in the normal turnover of red blood cells, and to a lesser extent, from myoglobin in muscle.

The AST to ALT ratio can be used to suggest alcoholic liver disease. One can argue that excluding the setting of alcoholism, hepatocellular disease can be adequately assessed with the measurement of ALT alone. However, it is common medical practice to measure both enzymes, and the enzyme measurements are rapidly available and can be performed at low cost in modern automated laboratories.

If the relative increase in ALP over the upper limit of normal exceeds the relative increase in ALT or AST over the upper limit of normal, the liver disease predominantly involves the biliary tract (**Table 16–4**). A major manifestation of obstructive biliary tract disease is an elevated bilirubin concentration. Clinical jaundice results when the total bilirubin exceeds 2 to 3 mg/dL.

DETOXIFYING AND EXCRETORY FUNCTIONS OF THE HEPATOBILIARY SYSTEM AND DISORDERS ASSOCIATED PREDOMINANTLY WITH AN ELEVATED BILIRUBIN CONCENTRATION

A major biochemical responsibility of the liver is to metabolize toxins, drugs, and biologic endproducts and excrete many of the resulting metabolites into the bile. The easiest endogenous endproduct to assess is bilirubin. Bilirubin is predominantly derived from hemoglobin in the normal turnover of red blood cells, and to a lesser extent, from myoglobin in muscle. Red blood

TABLE 16–4 Causes of Biliary Tract Disease[a]

Failure of formation of the bile ducts
Biliary atresia

Obstruction or obliteration of the bile ducts
Cholelithiasis   Cholangitis   Primary biliary cirrhosis   Primary sclerosing cholangitis   Post-surgical strictures   Parasitic infection

Compression of the bile ducts outside the liver
Pancreatic cancer   Pancreatitis   Hepatic cancers

[a]The relative elevation in ALP exceeds the relative elevations in ALT and AST.

cells normally circulate for approximately 120 days. Red blood cell senescence and destruction in monocytes/macrophages, primarily in the spleen, releases hemoglobin from red blood cells. Hemoglobin is then metabolized to biliverdin and finally to bilirubin. The bilirubin then enters the circulation. This form of bilirubin (i.e., "unconjugated" bilirubin) is relatively insoluble in water and is transported to the hepatocyte bound to albumin. It is not excreted in the urine. Unconjugated bilirubin is normally taken up into hepatocytes via a transport system. Inside the hepatocyte via the action of UDP-glucuronyl transferase, either 1 or 2 glucuronide molecules are conjugated to bilirubin, making the bilirubin water soluble. Conjugated bilirubin is bilirubin monoglucuronide or bilirubin diglucuronide. Conjugated bilirubin is then transported across the plasma membrane into the bile canaliculi along with bile via multiple drug resistance (MDR) transporter proteins. If the concentration of either conjugated or unconjugated bilirubin rises pathologically, the skin and sclera can develop a yellowish color, termed jaundice. With marked elevations in bilirubin, patients may acquire a green hue. Pathologic elevations in water-soluble bilirubin (e.g., conjugated bilirubin) can lead to bilirubin excretion in the urine (bilirubinuria), causing the urine to develop a yellow-brown or green-brown color.

Bilirubin is most often measured by reacting the patient's serum or plasma with Ehrlich's reagent that includes a diazo compound. The conjugated fraction reacts most rapidly with the reagent because the conjugated fraction is water soluble. This is termed "direct acting," or more commonly, "direct" bilirubin. To measure total bilirubin, solubilizing agents must be added to the serum or plasma to enhance the reaction of the water-insoluble bilirubin (i.e., unconjugated bilirubin) with the reagents. Caffeine or benzoate can be used for this purpose. Because only direct and total bilirubin can be measured, indirect (unconjugated bilirubin) is calculated as the difference between the total and the direct bilirubin. While this is the measurement scheme in the majority of automated chemistry analyzers, it is necessary to review how bilirubin is measured using dry slide technology that was originally developed by Kodak. The unique feature of dry slide technology (as provided in the Vitros series of analyzers) is the ability to spectrophotometrically determine the unconjugated (BU: bilirubin unconjugated) and conjugated bilirubin (BC: bilirubin conjugated) fractions. The difference between the sum of the BU and BC and the total bilirubin measured via the Ehrlich's reaction is the delta bilirubin. Delta bilirubin is bilirubin that is covalently bound to albumin. Elevated levels of delta bilirubin are consistent with chronic elevations in bilirubin. However, only 1 analytical system is able to estimate delta bilirubin (i.e., dry slide technology) and the calculation of the delta bilirubin has not yet been shown to be clinically informative.

In most cases involving hepatocellular dysfunction (notably, acute viral hepatitis), the major increase in bilirubin is an increased conjugated bilirubin fraction because transport of conjugated bilirubin into the bile canaliculus is typically the rate-limiting step in bilirubin excretion. With the failure of transport of conjugated bilirubin into the bile canaliculus, the conjugated bilirubin

If the concentration of either conjugated or unconjugated bilirubin rises pathologically, the skin and sclera can develop a yellowish color, termed jaundice.

TABLE 16–5   Unconjugated Hyperbilirubinemia with Hemolysis

	Comment
Schistocytes present	
Microangiopathic hemolytic anemia	Rule out DIC, TTP, and HUS
Artificial heart valve	History of valve replacemen
Autoimmune hemolytic anemia	Perform Coombs testing
Schistocytes absent	
Intramarrow hemolysis	Rule out vitamin B$_{12}$ deficiency
Red blood cell membrane defects	Review peripheral smear for spherocytes, elliptocytes
Red blood cell enzyme defects	Review peripheral smear for bite cells, measure G6PDH
Hemoglobinopathies	Perform hemoglobin electrophoresis

DIC, disseminated intravascular coagulation; TTP, thrombotic thrombocytopenic purpura; HUS, hemolytic uremic syndrome; G6PDH, glucose-6-phosphate dehydrogenase.

TABLE 16–6   Unconjugated Hyperbilirubinemia without Hemolysis

Newborn
Mild to moderate and transient unconjugated hyperbilirubinemia Physiological jaundice Breast milk jaundice
Persistent unconjugated hyperbilirubinemia Crigler–Najjar syndrome types I (severe) and II (mild)
Child or adult
Gilbert syndrome

It is useful to classify hyperbilirubinemia as predominantly unconjugated or conjugated. When the ratio of conjugated to total bilirubin is 0.4 or greater, predominantly a conjugated hyperbilirubinemia is present.

refluxes into the systemic circulation. However, with severe hepatocellular dysfunction, as might occur in cases of end-stage liver disease, there can be defective conjugation in addition to defective canalicular transport.

It is useful to classify hyperbilirubinemia as predominantly unconjugated or conjugated. This assists in the development of an appropriate differential diagnosis. If the ratio of the conjugated bilirubin to total bilirubin is less than 0.4, an unconjugated hyperbilirubinemia is present. When the ratio of conjugated to total bilirubin is 0.4 or greater, predominantly a conjugated hyperbilirubinemia is present. In neonates, the cutoff ratio is 0.2 because unconjugated bilirubin is normally much higher in neonates than in children or adults.

Causes of unconjugated hyperbilirubinemia involve 3 basic mechanisms: 1) increased red blood cell destruction ("prehepatic"), 2) defects in the transport of unconjugated bilirubin into the hepatocyte, and 3) defective conjugation. Major causes of increased red blood cell destruction include intramarrow hemolysis (e.g., vitamin B$_{12}$ deficiency causing ineffective erythropoiesis), intravascular or extravascular hemolysis (e.g., microangiopathic hemolytic anemia, hemolysis from an artificial heart valve, and autoimmune hemolytic anemia ["warm," IgG-mediated and "cold," IgM-mediated]), intrinsic membrane defects in red blood cells (e.g., congenital spherocytosis or elliptocytosis), red blood cell enzyme defects (e.g., glucose-6-phosphate dehydrogenase deficiency), and hemoglobinopathies (e.g., sickle cell anemia) (**Table 16–5**).

A variety of nonhemolytic conditions can cause an unconjugated hyperbilirubinemia (**Table 16–6**). Gilbert syndrome is an autosomal dominant disorder in which there is a mild defect in the uptake of bilirubin by the hepatocyte, combined with a mild defect in conjugation.

Clinical jaundice does not usually occur in the absence of concurrent disease (e.g., gastroenteritis or other mild conditions). Liver enzyme concentrations and hepatic synthetic ability are normal, and, therefore, Gilbert syndrome is best considered a variation of normal and not a disease. On the other hand, a congenital deficiency of UDP-glucuronyl transferase is a serious condition. Absolute deficiency of UDP-glucuronyl transferase, which results in Crigler–Najjar syndrome type I, will cause marked elevations in unconjugated bilirubin that will cause kernicterus if untreated. The treatment of this disease is liver transplantation. A milder deficiency of UDP-glucuronyl transferase, Crigler–Najjar syndrome type II, may be treated with barbiturates to stimulate production of the deficient enzyme. A transient, mild, self-limited deficiency of UDP-glucuronyl transferase activity is common in newborns (e.g., neonatal jaundice; a.k.a., icterus neonatorum). However, if the unconjugated bilirubin rises above ~15 to 20 mg/dL in a neonate, phototherapy is used to reduce the bilirubin concentration. An unconjugated, transient hyperbilirubinemia occurs in 2–10% of breast-fed infants (i.e., breast milk jaundice). In these infants, it is believed that a constituent in the breast milk interferes with bilirubin conjugation, thereby elevating unconjugated bilirubin.

The etiologies of conjugated hyperbilirubinemia involve 2 basic mechanisms: 1) hepatocellular disorders with decreased transport of conjugated bilirubin into the bile canaliculus (**Table 16–3**) or 2) biliary tract obstruction (**Table 16–4**). Moderate to severe acute or chronic hepatocellular disease can produce a conjugated hyperbilirubinemia. Hepatocellular disorders associated with impaired plasma membrane integrity and release of enzymes into the circulation were discussed earlier.

Of note are 2 disorders in which there is a conjugated hyperbilirubinemia with otherwise normal hepatic function. These are Dubin–Johnson syndrome and Rotor syndrome. Dubin–Johnson syndrome results from dysfunction of the multidrug resistance protein 2 (MRP2) that is a canalicular multispecific organic anion transporter (cMOAT) the gene product of *ABCC2*. The liver is stained black in this condition. Rotor syndrome is a consequence of decreased hepatic glutathione-*S*-transferase levels (hGSTA1-1). In the absence of a liver biopsy, Dubin–Johnson and Rotor syndromes have been distinguished by urine testing for coproporphyrins and coproporphyrin I. DNA testing is used progressively more often to distinguish these disorders.

> Biliary tract obstruction can be intrahepatic or extrahepatic. The most common cause of extrahepatic biliary tract obstruction after the neonatal period is cholelithiasis.

Biliary tract obstruction can be intrahepatic or extrahepatic. Infants with a persistent conjugated hyperbilirubinemia most commonly suffer from biliary atresia or neonatal hepatitis. The most common cause of extrahepatic biliary tract obstruction after the neonatal period is cholelithiasis. This can be accompanied by inflammation of the gall bladder, i.e., cholecystitis. Rupture of the gall bladder will produce peritonitis that can be life-threatening. Other causes of biliary tract obstruction include inflammation (e.g., cholangitis or pancreatitis), neoplasia (e.g., pancreatic adenocarcinoma or a hepatic cancer with compression of the bile duct), post-surgical strictures, autoimmunity (e.g., primary sclerosing cholangitis [PSC]), and parasites (e.g., helminths or their ova).

Compared to the timing of elevations in the enzymes of hepatic origin following a liver insult, elevations in bilirubin occur later. Also, while the degree of increase in the concentration of the hepatic enzymes correlates poorly with the degree of liver injury or disease, greater elevations in the level of conjugated bilirubin do correlate with more severe degrees of liver disease. In end-stage liver disease as found in alcoholic cirrhosis, for example, ALT and AST may only be modestly elevated, yet the patient may exhibit intense jaundice. In such cases, portal hypertension is frequent with ascites and esophageal varices, hemorrhoids, and splenomegaly.

SYNTHETIC FUNCTION OF THE LIVER AND DISORDERS ASSOCIATED WITH LOW CIRCULATING CONCENTRATIONS OF ALBUMIN, TRANSTHYRETIN, RETINOL-BINDING PROTEIN, AND COAGULATION FACTORS

Excluding immunoglobulins, which are the products of B cells and plasma cells, the liver is the major source of circulating proteins. On a strictly quantitative basis, albumin is a better measure of synthetic ability than total protein. A substantial degree of hypoalbuminemia can exist, yet the total protein may be normal or elevated because of a coexistent polyclonal or monoclonal hypergammaglobulinemia. Besides liver disease, there are several other causes of hypoalbuminemia

TABLE 16–7   Acute Phase Reactants Synthesized in the Liver

Positive acute phase reactants (concentrations increase with acute inflammation)
Immune-related Complement (C′) Mannose-binding lectin (MBL) C-reactive protein (CRP) Orosomucoid (alpha-1 acid glycoprotein)
Antiproteases (anti-enzymes) Alpha-1 antitrypsin (A1-AT) Alpha-2 macroglobulin (A2M)
Anti-oxidants Ceruloplasmin
Coagulation factors Fibrinogen Factor VIII
Others Haptoglobin Serum amyloid A (SAA) Plasma fibronectin Lipopolysaccharide binding protein (LBP) Ferritin
Negative acute phase reactants (concentrations decrease with acute inflammation)
Retinol-binding protein (RBP) Transthyretin (TBPA) Albumin Transferrin

including malnutrition and malabsorption (insufficient nutritional substrate for albumin synthesis), acute inflammation where protein synthesis is redirected from albumin to acute phase reactants (e.g., complement proteins, C-reactive protein, mannose-binding lectin, and serum amyloid A; **Table 16–7**), and protein loss from nephrosis or protein-losing enteropathy.

In nutritionally deficient patients, nutritional replenishment can be assessed by measurement of retinol-binding protein, or, more commonly, transthyretin (thyroxine-binding prealbumin). While transthyretin is commonly referred to as "prealbumin," strictly speaking, prealbumin is a region on a serum protein electrophoresis gel that precedes albumin. In contrast to albumin, transthyretin and retinol-binding protein are not usually measured as indices of hepatic dysfunction.

Assessment of clotting factor proteins through measurement of clotting factor activity tests (such as the prothrombin time [PT]) is a useful assessment of liver synthetic function. An increase in the PT, or the international normalized ratio (INR) derived from it, is a sign of serious liver dysfunction. Because the half-life of many clotting factors is much shorter than the half-life of albumin, in cases of acute liver dysfunction, measurement of the PT can provide a more sensitive index of decreased liver protein synthesis than albumin. The PT involves factors VII, X, V, II (prothrombin), and I (fibrinogen). The half-life of factor VII is the shortest of any clotting factor and is only 4 to 5 hours.

Moderate to serious liver disease can lead to bleeding for many reasons. Vitamin K malabsorption, decreased clotting factor concentrations and activity (the vitamin-K-dependent factors are II, VII, IX, and X), and impaired clearance of fibrin-split products can all occur with liver dysfunction. Fragments of fibrin can interfere with the formation of a stable and firm clot. With cirrhosis, increased portal pressure can produce esophageal varices that are easily traumatized, resulting in bleeding. Increased portal pressure can produce splenomegaly, leading to platelet sequestration. Thrombocytopenia is not uncommon in severe liver disease. Thrombopoietin is produced by the liver.

An increase in the prothrombin time (PT), or the international normalized ratio (INR) derived from it, is a sign of serious liver dysfunction.

TABLE 16–8   **Tests for Viral Hepatitis and Selected Liver Disorders**

	Importance in liver disease
HAV total antibody	Positivity indicates present or past infection with HAV or immunization against HAV infection
HAV IgM antibody	Positivity indicates acute infection with HAV
HBV surface antigen	Positivity indicates acute or chronic HBV infection
HBV e antigen	Positivity indicates acute or chronic HBV infection and increased infectivity
HBV core IgM antibody	Positivity indicates acute infection with HBV
HBV core total antibody	Positivity indicates present or past infection with HBV
HBV e antibody	Positivity indicates chronic or past infection with HBV
HBV surface antibody	Positivity indicates chronic or past infection with HBV or immunization against HBV infection
HCV antibody	Positivity indicates present or past infection with HCV
HDV IgM antibody	Positivity indicates acute infection with HDV
HDV antibody	Positivity indicates present or past infection with HDV
Antinuclear autoantibodies	Can be positive in autoimmune hepatitis
Antismooth muscle autoantibodies	Can be positive in autoimmune hepatitis
Anti-LKM1 autoantibodies	Can be positive in autoimmune hepatitis
Antimitochondrial autoantibodies	Can be positive in primary biliary cirrhosis
Alpha-fetoprotein	Marker of hepatocellular carcinoma
Ammonia	Can be elevated in cases of end-stage liver disease
Serum bile acids	Can be elevated in many forms of hepatocellular disease; sometimes ordered to support the diagnosis of cholestasis of pregnancy

THE DIAGNOSIS OF VIRAL HEPATITIS

Hepatitis serologic tests are used to diagnose viral hepatitis or recognize past exposure or immunization to a virus that can cause hepatitis. The hepatitis A virus (HAV) is an RNA virus that commonly causes acute hepatitis and is transmitted through the fecal–oral route. Fulminant hepatic necrosis is possible but very rare, and chronic liver disease does not result from HAV infection. Total antibody to HAV can be measured, and when it is positive, there are elevations of IgM and/or IgG antibodies to HAV. Positivity for the IgM antibody to HAV indicates acute or recent infection. Positivity for the HAV total antibody test does not distinguish patients with acute infection from those with a past infection who have recovered or from immunized individuals (**Table 16–8**).

Acute hepatitis B virus (HBV; a DNA virus) infection is serologically first noted by the appearance of HBV surface antigen (HBsAg). This is followed by HBV e antigen (HBeAg) and then HBV IgM core antibody (HBc IgM antibody). During recovery, the HBV surface and e antigens disappear from the circulation, HBc IgM antibody converts to negative, and HBc total antibody appears, followed by HBe antibody (HBeAb), and then HBs antibody (HBsAb).

In cases of chronic HBV infection, HBsAg remains positive. HBeAg positivity is variable, and its presence indicates increased infectivity. HBe antibody positivity is also highly variable. Immunization results in positivity for HBsAb, but not HBcAb, as the immunogen used for immunization is recombinant DNA HBsAg.

Hepatitis C virus (HCV; an RNA virus) is the most common viral cause of chronic hepatitis with 40% to 80% of acute infections leading to chronic hepatitis (e.g., hepatic disease exceeding 6 months duration). A positive HCV antibody test does not distinguish acute from chronic

Hepatitis serologic tests are used to diagnose viral hepatitis or recognize past exposure or immunization to a virus that can cause hepatitis.

infection, and it does not distinguish patients with active infection from those who have recovered. HCV antibody positivity can be confirmed by the recombinant immunoblot assay (RIBA). However, RIBA testing has the same diagnostic limitations as the HCV antibody testing. Evidence of active HCV infection is provided by elevations in transaminases, liver biopsy, or detection of HCV RNA by nucleic acid testing (e.g., RT-PCR, bDNA, or transcription-mediated amplification testing). Normal levels of AST and ALT do not exclude chronic HCV infection. A thorough discussion of viral nucleic acid testing is beyond the scope of this chapter.

Hepatitis D virus (HDV; a DNA virus) is a defective virus that requires coinfection of the host with HBV for the expression of HDV hepatitis. HBV and HDV infection can occur concurrently or HDV infection can be superimposed on chronic HBV infection. IgM antibody to HDV indicates acute infection. HDV total antibody has the same diagnostic limitations as HCV antibody, notably, active infection is not differentiated from recovery, and acute and chronic infections are not distinguished.

SELECTED LIVER DISEASES AND LABORATORY TESTS USED IN THE EVALUATION OF LIVER FUNCTION

Alpha-1 Antitrypsin Deficiency

In individuals with unexplained and/or early onset emphysema or liver disease, alpha-1 antitrypsin deficiency should be considered. Alpha-1 antitrypsin is an antiprotease that protects the lungs from endogenous elastases, collagenases, and proteases. Deficiency from alpha-1 antitrypsin can produce early onset panlobular emphysema. The liver disease results an inability to release a mutated alpha-1 antitrypsin protein.

Mutations in the *Pi* (protease inhibitor) gene *SERPINA1* result in alpha-1 antitrypsin deficiency. The normal allele is denoted as "M." A common abnormal allele is "Z." Homozygosity for Z (e.g., Z/Z) causes alpha-1 antitrypsin deficiency.

Glycogen Storage Diseases

GSDs are disorders of glycogen production (GSD type 0) or glycogen breakdown. GSDs are a group of heterogenous disorders affecting the liver, skeletal muscle, and/or myocardium. GSD types I, III, and VI can produce fasting hypoglycemia. GSD type I (von Gierke disease) results from a deficiency of glucose-6-phosphatase (type 1a). However, variants exist as type Ib: T1 transporter defects; type 1aSP: glucose-6-phosphatase stabilizing protein deficiency; type 1c: T2 beta transporter deficiency; and type 1d: GLUT7 glucose transporter deficiency. GSD type III (Cori or Forbes disease) is a deficiency of amylo-1,6 glucosidase. GSD type VI (Hers disease) results from a deficiency of liver phosphorylase or phosphorylase b kinase.

Hemochromatosis

Iron overload in the absence of chronic transfusion therapy most commonly results from hemochromatosis type 1 (HH1) that is inherited as an autosomal recessive disorder. HH1 results from mutations in the HFE gene that is encoded within the major histocompatibility complex located on the short arm of chromosome 6. Two possible genotypes cause HH1: C282Y/C282Y or C282Y/H63D. Homozygosity for H63D (H63D/H63D) does not cause clinical disease. HFE mutations lead to deficient hepatic secretion of hepcidin. In turn, hepcidin deficiency permits excessive expression of ferroportin with consequent hyperabsorption of iron from the GI tract.

Increased transferrin saturation is the earliest biochemical marker of hemochromatosis. Elevations in ferritin follow. Percent transferrin saturation is the recommended screening test. Elevated ferritin is not specific for iron overload. Ferritin is elevated as an acute phase reactant, and ferritin is released from the liver with disease or injury.

HH1 has a population frequency of ~1 in 300, with a 5:1 to 7:1 excess of affected males over females. The onset of symptoms is typically between 40 and 50 years of age. Iron deposition occurs in the heart (potentially causing cardiac failure), liver (producing liver disease including cirrhosis), endocrine organs (causing diabetes, hypopituitarism, hypothyroidism, and/or hypogonadism), and skin. Arthropathy is another feature of HH1.

Iron overload in the absence of chronic transfusion therapy most commonly results from hemochromatosis type 1 (HH1) that is inherited as an autosomal recessive disorder.

There are several other types of hemochromatosis in addition to HH1. HH2a results from hemojuvelin mutations, while HH2b is caused by primary hepcidin deficiency. HH2a and HH2b present in childhood. Mutations in the transferrin receptor 2 (TfR2) cause HH3. HH4 causes greater iron deposition in the reticuloendothelial system than in the solid organs and liver. HH4a is a consequence of ferroportin mutations. Aceruloplasminemia causes HH4b. Hemochromatosis can be differentiated from transfusion-related iron overload by noting whether the patient has a history of repeated transfusions. Iron overload from transfusion and hemochromatosis rarely coexist.

Wilson Disease

Wilson disease is a rare autosomal recessive disorder estimated to affect 1 in 200,000 persons. Mutations in *ATP7B* result in copper overload with consequent copper deposition in the brain, liver, kidneys, and cornea (the Kayser–Fleischer ring). *ATP7B* is the product of the copper-transporting ATPase gene on chromosome 13q. *ATP7B* moves copper into the bile. In >90% of patients with Wilson disease, the ceruloplasmin level is decreased. Copper excretion is increased in the urine, and therefore urinary copper is a highly useful noninvasive test in the investigation of possible Wilson disease. Liver biopsy can provide a quantitative measure of the degree of copper overload, as elevated hepatic copper is highly supportive of the diagnosis of Wilson disease. The most common presentation of Wilson disease is chronic liver disease (including cirrhosis) but it can present as acute, fulminant hepatitis that may require liver transplantation for survival.

Hepatocellular Carcinoma and Alpha-fetoprotein (AFP)

AFP is the major plasma protein produced by the fetal liver early in gestation. In adults, in contrast, AFP concentrations are normally very low. AFP may be elevated in many circumstances. It may be transiently increased with acute liver disease or persistently increased in chronic liver disease and cirrhosis. In patients with chronic liver disease or cirrhosis, an elevated AFP should trigger evaluation of the patient for hepatocellular carcinoma. For this cancer, elevated AFP levels serve as a tumor marker with a 40% to 80% sensitivity.

Hepatic Encephalopathy and Ammonia

Ammonia is an endproduct that results from amino acid deamination. The urea cycle captures ammonia (and thus nitrogen) for excretion by the kidney in the form of urea. Significant impairments in liver function produce hyperammonemia. In turn, hyperammonemia is associated with hepatic encephalopathy. A characteristic physical finding in patients with a toxic or metabolic encephalopathy is asterixis (unintended jerking movements particularly of the hands when they are dorsi-flexed).

Acute (fulminant) hepatic failure can result from a wide variety of insults but the most common causes are acute viral hepatitis, toxins (e.g., *Amanita phalloides* mushrooms), and poisonings (e.g., acetaminophen).

Cholestasis of Pregnancy and Serum Bile Acid

Serum bile acid concentrations reflect the ability of the liver to remove bile acids from the circulation and excrete them into the bile as part of the normal bile enterohepatic recirculation. Impaired hepatocyte uptake or secretion of bile acids, and portosystemic shunting, can elevate serum bile acid levels. Serum bile acids are often measured in women with cholestasis of pregnancy; otherwise, serum bile acids are rarely measured as they add little valuable information to the standard tests of hepatic function thus far discussed. Many argue that the diagnosis of cholestasis of pregnancy can be readily established without the measurement of serum bile acids.

Acute (Fulminant) Hepatic Failure

Acute (fulminant) hepatic failure can result from a wide variety of insults but the most common causes are acute viral hepatitis (e.g., HBV and less commonly HAV), toxins (e.g., *Amanita phalloides* mushrooms), and poisonings (e.g., acetaminophen). Other causes of acute hepatic failure include adenovirus infection, varicella-zoster virus (VZV) infection, acute fatty liver of pregnancy, Wilson disease, Reye syndrome, and portal vein thrombosis.

TABLE 16–9   **Commonly Observed Laboratory Findings in Hepatic Failure**

	Comment(s)
Elevated conjugated and unconjugated bilirubin	Defects in conjugation and excretion of bilirubin
Hypoalbuminemia	Decreased albumin synthesis
Elevated ALT and AST	Elevations of ~100-fold with acute liver failure; rapid decline to normal can indicate permanent loss of hepatocytes; in chronic liver disease, ALT and AST can be normal
Hyperammonemia	Impaired urea cycle
Hypoglycemia	Impaired gluconeogenesis in the fasting state after glycogenolysis has exhausted liver glycogen stores
Prolonged PT	Decreased production of clotting factors, malabsorption of vitamin K, and decreased clearance of fibrin-split products
Thrombocytopenia	As a result of DIC or thrombopoietin deficiency
Anemia	Bone marrow suppression leads to chronic anemia; blood loss from esophageal varices
Elevated creatinine and BUN	Decreased urine output; the hepatorenal syndrome may be present; elevated BUN and a normal creatinine can indicate a GI bleed

DIC, disseminated intravascular coagulation; GI, gastrointestinal; PT, prothrombin time.

In acute liver failure, the clinical course is rapid. Unless spontaneous recovery takes place or liver transplantation is performed, the outcome is fatal. Acute and chronic liver failure share many potential characteristics (**Table 16–9**): profound hyperbilirubinemia, coagulopathy (e.g., bleeding with a prolonged PT and thrombocytopenia), hypoproteinemia (e.g., hypoalbuminemia with edema), hypoglycemia, hyperammonemia with encephalopathy, and oliguric renal failure (the hepatorenal syndrome). Chronic liver failure is also associated with intrapulmonary shunting leading to hypoxia and clubbing of the digits. Liver failure that occurs after 6 months of recognized liver disease is chronic liver failure.

Cirrhosis

Cirrhosis is the outcome of any chronic disorder of the liver parenchyma or intrahepatic biliary tract that causes continuous or repeated episodes of cellular necrosis and inflammation, followed by subsequent episodes of repair. At some point, recurrent injury to the liver can destroy the connective tissue that is the reticular structure of the liver. This results in scarring with the deposition of increasing amounts of collagen. Bridging fibrosis can disturb intrahepatic blood flow, leading to portal hypertension, with the consequent development of ascites and esophageal varices. The liver becomes small and firm from fibrosis, yet on physical examination the abdomen is distended because of ascites. In some patients, reopening of the umbilical vein occurs and produces periumbilical varices termed "caput medusa" (after the mythical Greek character Medusa). Cirrhosis can predispose to hepatocellular carcinoma. Histologically, proliferating hepatocytes appear as regenerating nodules among the fibrotic bands. Nodules can be small (<3 mm—micronodular) or large (>3 mm—macronodular).

Ethanol abuse is the most common cause of cirrhosis in Westernized countries, accounting for 60% to 70% of cases. Other causes include chronic viral hepatitis (~10%), biliary tract diseases (~5% to 10%), and hereditary hemochromatosis (~5%). NAFL is increasingly being recognized as a cause of cryptogenic cirrhosis, that is, cirrhosis of otherwise unknown origin.

Patients with cirrhosis can experience severe functional liver impairment, also called "end-stage liver disease." Such patients have a mixed unconjugated and conjugated hyperbilirubinemia, profound hypoalbuminemia, hypoglycemia, coagulopathy (from decreased clotting factor production, decreased clearance of fibrin-split products, and thrombocytopenia), and hyperammonemia.

Ethanol abuse is the most common cause of cirrhosis in Westernized countries, accounting for 60% to 70% of cases.

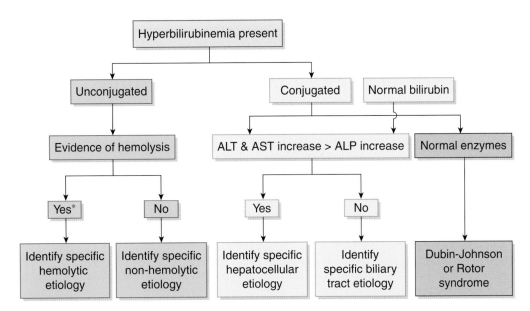

FIGURE 16-1 **One approach to the evaluation of liver function. (*) Increased LD, decreased haptoglobin; with or without an abnormal peripheral smear.**

Laboratory data can indicate the degree of liver dysfunction. However, cirrhosis remains a clinical diagnosis until definitive diagnosis is established by the results of a liver biopsy.

Primary Biliary Cirrhosis

Primary biliary cirrhosis (PBC) affects the interlobular bile ducts and is a chronic autoimmune biliary tract disease with obstructive jaundice. Thus, patients with PBC show a conjugated hyperbilirubinemia and relative elevations in ALP exceeding the ALT and AST elevations. ALT and AST can be normal.

Approximately 95% of patients with PBC are positive for AMA. Portal inflammation and progressive scarring can progress to liver failure requiring liver transplantation. The condition most often affects women between the ages of 40 and 50 years.

Primary biliary cirrhosis (PBC) affects the interlobular bile ducts and is a chronic autoimmune biliary tract disease with obstructive jaundice.

Primary Sclerosing Cholangitis

PSC affects the larger bile ducts. Men are more commonly affected than women (70:30 ratio), with a mean age at onset near 40 years. Tests for AMA are negative in patients with PSC. Inflammatory bowel disease, such as Crohn disease or ulcerative colitis, is identified in about 75% of patients with PSC. The definitive diagnosis of PSC is made by liver biopsy.

APPROACH TO THE PATIENT WITH LIVER DISEASE

One reasonable approach to the evaluation of liver function is to first consider the bilirubin concentration (**Figure 16-1** and **Tables 16-3** to **16-6**). If there is an unconjugated hyperbilirubinemia, possible hemolysis should be investigated. If this is absent, other causes of an unconjugated hyperbilirubinemia need to be considered, such as neonatal jaundice, Gilbert syndrome, and Crigler–Najjar syndrome.

If there is a conjugated hyperbilirubinemia, the liver enzymes can be used to separate hepatocellular disease (e.g., predominant elevations in ALT and AST) and biliary tract disease (e.g., predominant elevations in ALP, or if measured, GGT and 5′-NT). Disorders are then investigated based on their relative frequency and whether the disease is acute or chronic. Not noted in **Figure 16–1** is end-stage liver disease in which there can be significant elevations in both the conjugated and unconjugated fractions. In the absence of hyperbilirubinemia, the focus on liver dysfunction becomes the pattern of enzyme elevation.

REFERENCES

Dufour DR, et al. Diagnosis and monitoring of hepatic injury. I. Performance characteristics of laboratory tests. *Clin Chem.* 2000;46(December):2027–2049.

Dufour DR, et al. Diagnosis and monitoring of hepatic injury. II. Recommendations for use of laboratory tests in screening, diagnosis, and monitoring. *Clin Chem.* 2000;46(December):2050–2068.

Dufour DR, et al. *The National Academy of Clinical Biochemistry, laboratory medicine practice guidelines, laboratory guidelines for screening, diagnosis and monitoring of hepatic injury.* http://www.aacc.org/members/nacb/Archive/LMPG/HepaticInjury/Pages/HepaticInjuryPDF.aspx. Accessed 28 May, 2009.

Fix OK, Kowdley KV. Hereditary hemochromatosis. *Minerva Med.* 2008;99(December):605–617.

Hogarth DK, Rachelefsky G. Screening and familial testing of patients for alpha 1-antitrypsin deficiency. *Chest.* 2008;133(April):981–988.

Langner C, Denk H. Wilson disease. *Virchows Arch.* 2004;445(August):111–118.

Limdi JK, Hyde GM. Evaluation of abnormal liver function tests. *Postgrad Med J.* 2003;79(June):307–312.

Mallory MA, et al. Abnormal liver test results on routine screening. How to evaluate, when to refer for a biopsy. *Postgrad Med.* 2004;115(March):53–56, 59–62, 66.

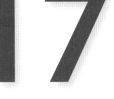

Pancreatic Disorders

Fritz F. Parl and Michael Laposata

LEARNING OBJECTIVES

1. Understand the differences between acute and chronic pancreatitis and the laboratory test results used to establish the diagnosis of each.

2. Learn the clinical, laboratory, and radiographic abnormalities in patients with cancer of the pancreas.

3. Learn the clinical and laboratory criteria for the diagnosis of diabetes mellitus, gestational diabetes mellitus, and hypoglycemia.

4. Identify the different islet cell tumors and learn their associated laboratory test results.

CHAPTER OUTLINE

INTRODUCTION

Disorders involving the pancreas are generally divided into 2 categories. One group includes diseases of the exocrine portion of the pancreas, which secretes digestive enzymes into the gastrointestinal tract. The other category includes the disorders of the endocrine portion of the pancreas, which contains beta cells for secretion of insulin, alpha cells for secretion of glucagon, and delta cells for secretion of somatostatin. The cells that secrete hormones are arranged in islets within the exocrine pancreas. The most frequently encountered disorders of the exocrine pancreas are pancreatitis and pancreatic tumors. Pancreatitis may be acute or chronic with recurrent bouts of acute pancreatitis. Pancreatic tumors of the exocrine pancreas almost always originate in the pancreatic ductal epithelium. The major disease of the endocrine pancreas is diabetes mellitus (DM). Other relatively rare disorders of the endocrine pancreas include the islet cell tumors.

ACUTE PANCREATITIS

Description

Acute pancreatitis is a potentially lethal disorder associated with intracellular activation of digestive enzymes in the pancreas. This results in autodigestion of the pancreatic tissue by the powerful enzymes normally secreted into the gastrointestinal tract to degrade ingested foods. The damage to the pancreas can produce inflammation, edema, necrosis, hemorrhage, and liquefaction, and may obstruct the pancreatic duct and block the flow of pancreatic enzymes into the gastrointestinal tract. The obstruction further enhances the progression of acute pancreatitis.

TABLE 17–1   Laboratory Evaluation for Acute and Chronic Pancreatitis and Pancreatic Carcinoma

Disorder	Test	Expected Result
Acute pancreatitis	Serum amylase	Increased
	Serum lipase	Increased
	Amylase/creatinine clearance	Increased
Chronic pancreatitis	Serum amylase	Increased, normal, or decreased
	Serum lipase	Increased, normal, or decreased
	Amylase/creatinine clearance	Increased, normal, or decreased[a]
	Fecal elastase	Decreased
	Bentiromide test	Positive
	Serum trypsinogen	Decreased
Pancreatic carcinoma	CA 19-9	Increased

[a]In chronic pancreatitis, the amylase/creatinine clearance ratio can be increased even when the serum amylase is normal or only slightly elevated. The amylase/creatinine clearance ratio is: [urine amylase (U/L) × serum creatinine (mg/L)]/[serum amylase (U/L) × urine creatinine (mg/L)] × 100.

Clinically, a bout of acute pancreatitis is characterized by mid-epigastric pain frequently radiating to the back, nausea, and vomiting.

The cause of acute pancreatitis in the majority of the cases is either alcohol abuse or gallstones. There are, however, other causes, such as hypertriglyceridemia, hypercalcemia, selected infections, obstructing pancreatic tumors, and trauma to the pancreas. Hereditary forms of acute pancreatitis have also been described due to mutations in the trypsinogen gene or the trypsin inhibitor gene. In addition, many medications have been associated with the development of acute pancreatitis. Selected examples are asparaginase, azathioprine, estrogens, furosemide, sulfonamides, tetracycline, and thiazide diuretics. The mechanism of pancreatic injury following ingestion of these medications may be related to hypersensitivity to the drug or accumulation of a toxic drug metabolite in the pancreas. In about 20% of cases of acute pancreatitis, a specific cause cannot be identified. This is known as idiopathic acute pancreatitis.

Diagnosis

In acute pancreatitis, the laboratory findings vary with the severity of the disease and other factors. There are typically elevations in serum amylase, serum lipase, urine amylase, and the amylase/creatinine clearance ratio (described below) (**Table 17–1**). Not all patients with acute pancreatitis exhibit hyperamylasemia, and in addition, amylase may be elevated in a number of other disorders. Additional nonspecific laboratory findings of acute pancreatitis may include a mild to moderate leukocytosis with a shift toward immature forms, hyperglycemia, mild hyperbilirubinemia, and a decreased serum calcium level. Serum aminotransferases and alkaline phosphatase may also be elevated.

Amylase is the most commonly used laboratory test in the evaluation of acute pancreatitis. However, an elevated lipase is more specific. Amylase activity measures the collective contribution of amylase isoenzymes, 1 of which is alpha-amylase (see below). This isoenzyme is derived mostly from the pancreas, with a small serum fraction originating from the salivary glands. Serum amylase levels typically become elevated 2 to 12 hours after the onset of acute pancreatitis, and are above the upper limit of normal in 85% to 90% of patients by 24 hours. In most cases, the serum amylase level reaches its peak concentration by 24 hours and returns to normal within 48 to 72 hours of the onset of acute pancreatitis. However, if there is continuing destruction of exocrine cells in the pancreas, the serum amylase level will remain elevated beyond 72 hours.

Many pancreatic and nonpancreatic conditions other than pancreatitis have been associated with an elevated serum amylase level. These include trauma to the pancreas, pancreatic injury from drugs such as opiates and heroin, biliary tract diseases including cholecystitis and biliary tract lithiasis, and pancreatic neoplasms. Other intraabdominal diseases, such as perforated or nonperforated peptic ulcer, peritonitis, intestinal obstruction, intestinal infarct, and recent

> Amylase is the most commonly used laboratory test in the evaluation of acute pancreatitis. However, an elevated lipase is more specific. Many pancreatic and nonpancreatic conditions other than pancreatitis have been associated with an elevated serum amylase level.

abdominal surgery, can also increase serum amylase activity. Hyperamylasemia can occur from nonpancreatic release of amylase, such as during acute salivary gland disease, and in some cases because of the presence of macroamylase (see below).

Macroamylasemia is an established cause for an elevated serum amylase value. Macroamylase is a complex of alpha-amylase and other molecules, which may be proteins or carbohydrates. Because of its large molecular size, macroamylase is not filtered by the glomerulus in the kidney. Consequently, it accumulates in the serum, and produces a chronically elevated serum amylase level. The presence of macroamylase has been shown to account for an elevated serum amylase level in 1% to 3% of patients. Because macroamylase does not enter the urine, the urine amylase level is normal or low, unlike the situation in acute and chronic pancreatitis in which the urine amylase level is usually elevated along with the serum activity. Thus, patients with macroamylasemia have a combination of elevated serum amylase levels and normal or low urine amylase levels.

Alpha-amylase can be pancreatic or salivary, and both pancreatic and salivary amylase have more than 1 isoenzyme. Amylase can be separated into its component isoenzymes by selective enzymatic or chemical inhibition and by electrophoresis. In acute pancreatitis, there is an increase in pancreas-derived isoenzymes in almost all patients, but isoenzyme analysis is rarely required for diagnosis.

A urine amylase determination may be helpful in diagnosing pancreatic disorders, especially when the serum amylase level is normal or slightly elevated. As a general rule, urine amylase rises within 24 hours after an increase in serum amylase level, and remains abnormal for 7 to 10 days after the serum level returns to normal. Renal excretion of amylase depends on the glomerular filtration rate and, consequently, the urine amylase correlates with the creatinine clearance. In acute pancreatitis, the clearance of amylase into the urine may be increased compared with creatinine, resulting in an increased (amylase/creatinine clearance [A/CC]) ratio. The A/CC ratio is determined using the following formula:

$$\frac{\text{Urine amylase (U/L)} \times \text{Serum creatinine (mg/L)}}{\text{Serum amylase (U/L)} \times \text{Urine creatinine (mg/L)}} \times 100$$

Determination of the A/CC ratio involves simultaneous collection of serum and urine specimens but does not require a timed or complete 24-hour urine collection. The A/CC ratio becomes abnormal 1 to 2 days after an elevation of the serum amylase, and typically remains abnormal for as long as the urine amylase is high. As noted earlier, this typically occurs 7 to 10 days after the serum amylase level returns to normal.

> In acute pancreatitis, the clearance of amylase into the urine may be increased compared with creatinine, resulting in an increased (amylase/creatinine clearance [A/CC]) ratio.

Serum lipase is considered a more specific marker for damage to the pancreas than is serum amylase. Following the onset of acute pancreatitis, the serum lipase level rises slightly after the amylase. The initial rise is typically 3 to 6 hours after the onset of the disease, with a peak concentration around 24 hours. Lipase remains elevated slightly longer than amylase, but it also returns to the reference range in 7 to 10 days in most cases.

Renal failure is the most common extrapancreatic condition associated with an elevated serum lipase level. About 80% of patients with renal failure have lipase levels 2 to 3 times the upper limit of the reference range, and about 5% have an elevation more than 5 times the upper limit of normal. Other conditions associated with serum lipase elevation include acute cholangitis, intestinal infarction, and obstruction of the small intestine.

A number of laboratory tests and computed tomography may be useful to assess prognosis in patients with acute pancreatitis. One system to assign prognosis in acute pancreatitis is the simplified Glasgow criteria. Features associated with a worse prognosis include age >55 years, white blood cell count >15,000/μL, LDH >600 U/L, glucose >180 mg/dL, albumin <3.2 g/dL, calcium <8 mg/dL, arterial PO_2 <60 mmHg, and BUN >45 mg/dL.

CHRONIC PANCREATITIS

Description

Following an attack of acute pancreatitis, the patient may experience a complete recovery, have an additional recurrence without permanent damage to the pancreas, or suffer multiple recurrences leading to chronic pancreatitis and significant damage to the organ. In chronic pancreatitis, the cells that generate the digestive enzymes are destroyed and replaced with scar tissue, and the pancreatic ducts become dilated and filled with precipitated protein. Chronic pancreatitis can be divided into chronic calcifying pancreatitis and obstructive pancreas. Since chronic disease follows from recurrence of acute pancreatitis, chronic pancreatitis has various causes in adults. In the United States, the majority of cases of chronic pancreatitis are due to prolonged excessive alcohol consumption. Malnutrition-induced pancreatitis is more common in underdeveloped areas of the world. In children, the most common cause of chronic pancreatitis is cystic fibrosis (see Chapter 7).

Diagnosis

The diagnosis of chronic pancreatitis may be challenging because the disease can evolve subclinically over an extended period. The patient with chronic pancreatitis often has impaired glucose tolerance or, in severe cases, DM. Additional manifestations include abdominal pain, weight loss, pancreatic calcifications on X-ray, and steatorrhea. The sensitivity of laboratory tests to diagnose chronic pancreatitis depends on the extent of pancreatic tissue destruction and the length of time over which the damage has occurred (**Table 17–1**).

An elevated serum amylase level is an important finding in the diagnosis of chronic pancreatitis, but it is much less informative than it is in the diagnosis of acute pancreatitis. In about one half of the patients with chronic pancreatitis, the serum amylase level remains within the normal range. In other patients with the disorder, the values may be borderline or only slightly elevated, raising the possibility of a nonpancreatic cause for the elevated amylase. In chronic pancreatitis, the urine amylase level may be elevated when the serum amylase is within the normal range or only slightly elevated. Measurement of a 72-hour fecal fat provides an index of pancreatic exocrine function. It is increased in severe chronic pancreatitis. However, the test is neither sensitive nor specific. More recently, measurement of fecal elastase (decreased in chronic pancreatitis) and serum levels of trypsinogen (decreased in chronic pancreatitis) have been used as additional tests of pancreatic function.

The bentiromide test is a noninvasive test for assessing pancreatic function in patients suspected to have chronic pancreatitis. The test is based on the hydrolysis by chymotrypsin of a synthetic tripeptide, *N*-benzoyl-L-tyrosyl-*p*-aminobenzoic acid. The tripeptide, variously called bentiromide, NBT-PBA, or BTP, is administered orally, along with a test meal to stimulate pancreatic secretion. Chymotrypsin cleaves the *p*-aminobenzoic acid (PABA) molecule from the bentiromide in the duodenum. The PABA moiety is absorbed into the portal circulation, conjugated in the liver, and excreted by the kidneys as an arylamine. In the bentiromide test, the arylamines are quantitated in a 6-hour urine specimen, with the time started after the oral intake of bentiromide and the test meal. Decreased excretion (<50% of the test dose) suggests decreased absorption from the duodenum, which can occur with deficient activity of pancreatic chymotrypsin. The sensitivity of the test for diagnosis of chronic pancreatitis depends on the severity of the disease, with greater sensitivity of the test correlating with greater disease severity. Many nonpancreatic conditions, especially diseases of the kidney, are associated with a false-positive test result by decreasing the conjugation and/or excretion of the PABA metabolite in the urine. Conversely, a number of drugs (acetaminophen, lidocaine, procainamide, sunscreens containing PABA, and pancreatic enzyme supplements, as examples) may produce a falsely normal result in patients with chronic pancreatitis, because these products can increase the amount of arylamine in the urine.

Imaging studies including abdominal plain films may demonstrate calcifications. Ultrasound and computed tomography scans are relatively sensitive and specific. Duodenal intubation using endoscopic retrograde cholangiopancreatography (ERCP) with injection of X-ray contrast medium into the common bile duct and pancreatic ducts is the most sensitive test, but the test itself may induce pancreatitis and should therefore be reserved for selected cases. More recently endoscopic ultrasound has gained favor, and it is equally sensitive and specific for chronic pancreatitis as ERCP.

PANCREATIC CARCINOMA

Description

Masses within the pancreas can be either non-neoplastic or neoplastic. The non-neoplastic masses are almost always cystic. However, both benign and malignant pancreatic tumors may be cystic. A cyst can be congenital from abnormal development, but more often, it is a collection of

---

An elevated serum amylase level is an important finding in the diagnosis of chronic pancreatitis, but in about one half of the patients with chronic pancreatitis, the serum amylase level remains within the normal range.

pancreatic secretions and tissue debris following bouts of pancreatitis, and is known as a pseudocyst. In contrast to true cysts, pseudocysts lack an epithelial lining. Pancreatic cancer affects more than 30,000 adults in the United States annually and is usually rapidly fatal. The great majority of these tumors are ductal adenocarcinomas.

Diagnosis

CA 19-9 is the most widely used pancreatic tumor marker. CA 19-9 antigen is present in the normal adult and fetal pancreas, and it is also found in the esophagus, stomach, small intestine, gallbladder, bile duct, and salivary glands. Measuring the level of the CA 19-9 may be useful in patients with pancreatic cancer. In patients with early stage tumors, the CA 19-9 level is often normal. Therefore, the marker is of little value as a screening test. In patients with more advanced tumors, the CA 19-9 level is often elevated, and this finding may be helpful in suggesting a diagnosis of pancreatic cancer. CA 19-9 is most useful as an aid to monitor the patient response to therapy. However, CA 19-9 is not specific to pancreatic cancer and may be elevated in other types of gastrointestinal cancers and in some non-neoplastic disorders as well.

DIABETES MELLITUS

Description

Almost 13% of Americans have DM, of which 40% are unaware of their disorder. A significant fraction will already have some degree of nephropathy, neuropathy, and/or retinopathy when they are first diagnosed with DM. Importantly, many of the complications of diabetes can be avoided through early diagnosis and aggressive management.

The American Diabetes Association (ADA) sponsored the formation of an Expert Committee on the Classification and Diagnosis of Diabetes Mellitus to establish guidelines. The World Health Organization (WHO) adopted these guidelines, and further refined the diagnostic criteria for gestational diabetes.

DM represents a heterogenous group of disorders with the common feature of hyperglycemia due to defects in insulin secretion, insulin action, or a combination of these 2 factors. Central to the ADA guidelines are etiology based rather than treatment based definitions for type 1 and type 2 DM and other disorders of glucose regulation (**Table 17–2**). The treatment can vary with the disease course. For instance, patients termed "noninsulin-dependent" diabetics may eventually require insulin to control their hyperglycemia. The categories type 1 and type 2 diabetes are now designated by Arabic, rather than Roman, numerals. The majority of patients (90% to 95%) have type 2 diabetes.

> Almost 13% of Americans have DM, of which 40% are unaware of their disorder. A significant fraction will already have some degree of nephropathy, neuropathy, and/or retinopathy when they are first diagnosed with DM.

TABLE 17–2   1997 American Diabetes Association Classification of Diabetes Mellitus

Classification	Pathogenesis
Type 1 diabetes	Absolute deficiency of insulin secretion, usually due to immune-mediated beta-cell destruction
Type 2 diabetes	Varying degrees of insulin resistance; even if there is increased plasma insulin, it is insufficient to compensate for the resistance
Other specific types of diabetes	Heterogenous causes, subclassified as: genetic defects of beta-cell function, genetic defects in insulin receptors, exocrine pancreatic disease, drugs or chemicals toxic to islet cells or that antagonize insulin, infectious destruction of islet cells, uncommon forms of immune-mediated diabetes, or other endocrine diseases that impair glucose regulation
Gestational diabetes	Various causes, including unrecognized type 1 diabetes and subclinical incipient type 2 diabetes

TABLE 17–3   Summary of Diagnostic Criteria for Diabetes Mellitus and Impaired Fasting Glucose or Impaired Glucose Tolerance

State	Fasting Plasma Glucose (mg/dL)	Standard Oral Glucose Tolerance Test Plasma Glucose Values (mg/dL) at 2 Hours after 75 g Glucose Bolus
Normal	<100	<140
Impaired fasting glucose (IFG) or impaired glucose tolerance (IGT)	100–125 (IFG)	140–199 (IGT)
Diabetes mellitus	≥126 after a fast ≥8 hours or ≥126 and/or ≥200 and symptoms consistent with diabetes	≥200

To confirm a diagnosis of diabetes mellitus, the patient must satisfy any of the above criteria on a subsequent day.

Diagnosis

The following laboratory criteria are used to diagnose DM in the nonpregnant patient:

(a) symptoms of DM and any random plasma glucose ≥200 mg/dL, or

(b) fasting plasma glucose (FPG) >125 mg/dL after a fast of ≥8 hours, or

(c) plasma glucose ≥200 mg/dL 2 hours after the start of a 75 g oral glucose tolerance test (OGTT).

To confirm a diagnosis of DM using the above criteria, the patient must also satisfy any 1 of the above criteria on a subsequent day (**Table 17–3**).

In 2009, the International Expert Committee on the role of hemoglobin A1C in the diagnosis of diabetes concluded that the hemoglobin A1C assay may be a better means of diagnosing diabetes than the measurement of blood glucose. They suggest that the diagnosis of diabetes should be made if the hemoglobin A1C level is ≥6.5% (see below). However, they recommend that the diagnosis of diabetes should be confirmed with a repeat hemoglobin A1C test if the first one is greater than 6.5%, unless the patient already has clinical symptoms of diabetes or a blood glucose level greater than 200 mg/dL, in which case a single value greater than 6.5% is adequate to establish the diagnosis.

The most commonly used laboratory test for diagnosis of diabetes is the FPG, measured after at least 8 to 16 hours of fasting. The patient can drink water while fasting, but should abstain from eating, smoking, or taking medications. Acute illness, surgery, and hospitalization within the previous 8 weeks are relative contraindications to testing, as false-positive results can arise in these situations. The threshold of 125 mg/dL for the FPG test is lower than that used previously (140 mg/dL). The 125 mg/dL threshold corresponds to an epidemiological breakpoint, above which the risk for retinopathy and nephropathy increases dramatically. Patients with impaired fasting glucose (IFG) have a FPG ranging from 110 to 125 mg/dL. This group is considered at risk for subsequent development of DM, as well as for cardiovascular disease.

If the clinical picture merits further testing for diabetes in a patient with a FPG ≤125 mg/dL, an OGTT is indicated. The patient should have a regular diet during the preceding 3 days, with a carbohydrate intake of at least 100 g per day. The patient's activity should be unrestricted, and only severe illness or hospitalization represents relative contraindications. Minor illnesses with gastrointestinal manifestations are not significant. The glucose bolus for nonpregnant adults is 75 g of anhydrous glucose dissolved in 10 to 12 oz of water or a preformulated flavored drink containing 75 g of glucose, such as glucola. For children, 1.75 g of glucose per kilogram weight is administered, up to a maximum of 75 g. The bolus should be consumed over 5 minutes. The testing protocol has been simplified from previous versions to include only 2 specimens: a fasting specimen and one 2 hours after the bolus. A 2-hour postbolus plasma glucose level of ≥200 mg/dL is diagnostic of DM. A 2-hour postbolus plasma glucose level of ≥140 mg/dL but <200 mg/dL is found in patients with impaired glucose tolerance. Patients in this group, like those with IFG, are considered at risk for subsequent development of DM as well as cardiovascular disease.

The most commonly used laboratory test for diagnosis of diabetes is the fasting plasma glucose, measured after at least 8 to 16 hours of fasting.

TABLE 17–4   **High-Risk Individuals for Whom Diabetes Mellitus Screening Is Recommended by the American Diabetes Association**

Individuals of the following ancestry: African, Asian, Hispanic, Native American, and Pacific Islander
Mothers with newborns >9 lb or history of gestational diabetes mellitus
Individuals with hypertension ≥140/90, HDL cholesterol ≤35 mg/dL, or triglycerides ≥250 mg/dL
Individuals with a history of impaired fasting glucose or impaired glucose tolerance
Obese individuals weighing ≥120% of ideal body weight
Individuals with first-degree relatives with diabetes mellitus

HDL, high-density lipoprotein.

A random plasma glucose level of ≥200 mg/dL, combined with symptoms of DM (polyuria, polydipsia, and unexplained weight loss), also can be used to establish a diagnosis of DM. These criteria do not depend on the time since the last meal, but the test should not be done when the patient is acutely ill.

Although not meeting criteria for diabetes, an intermediate group of subjects exist whose glucose levels are too high to be considered normal. This group has FPG with fasting glucose levels ≥100 mg/dL but <126 mg/dL (these patients have IFG), or 2-hour values in the OGTT of ≥140 mg/dL but <200 mg/dL (these patients have impaired glucose tolerance or IGT) (**Table 17–3**).

Patients with IFG and/or IGT have a prediabetic condition, indicating a high risk for development of DM. In the absence of pregnancy, IFG and IGT are not clinical entities in their own right, but instead identify patients at risk for DM and its cardiovascular complications. Loss of 5% to 10% of body weight, exercise, and treatment with appropriate medications are measures taken to prevent or delay the development of DM in patients with "prediabetes."

As mentioned before, about half of all Americans with type 2 DM go undiagnosed and suffer from preventable complications of the disease. Therefore, the ADA has advocated screening everyone over 45 years old with a FPG test, with a repeat test every 3 years if the results are negative. Screening of groups with high risk has been proposed for individuals <45 years old (**Table 17–4**).

Blood specimens for all these tests should be collected in gray-top tubes, as the sodium fluoride anticoagulant will inhibit glycolysis. Without sodium fluoride, the metabolism of glucose by the white blood cells in a specimen can lower the plasma glucose levels by 5% to 7% per hour. Serum levels are comparable to plasma levels if the serum is separated from the cells within 1 hour and testing is performed within 8 hours. Capillary blood glucose levels are approximately 10 mg/dL lower than plasma levels when fasting, but are equal to or higher than plasma levels after a glucose load. For the diagnosis of DM from a circulating glucose concentration, a plasma sample is the preferred specimen.

The measurement of glycohemoglobin, specifically hemoglobin A1c (HbA1c), is essential for monitoring the success of therapy for patients with DM. HbA1c is formed by the nonenzymatic linkage of glucose to hemoglobin. Glucose enters the red blood cell, and it becomes bound to hemoglobin. An aldimine is first formed that then undergoes an Amadori rearrangement to form a stable ketoamine, which persists for the lifespan of the red blood cell (typically 120 days). The HbA1c concentration does not exhibit the wide diurnal fluctuations that occur with blood glucose. The blood glucose concentration varies substantially with exercise, food ingestion, and many other factors. The rate of formation of HbA1c is directly proportional to the glucose concentration in the blood. Because of this, the HbA1c concentration is a reflection of the glucose values over the preceding 8 to 12 weeks. HbA1c is primarily used for monitoring long-term glycemic status and to determine whether a diabetic patient has achieved adequate metabolic control.

In diabetic patients, the retinopathy incidence increases substantially at hemoglobin A1c values between 6.0% and 7.0%. There is a low prevalence of retinopathy at hemoglobin A1c levels less than 6.5%. A HbA1c value of <7% is widely recommended. The ADA recommends measurement of HbA1c at least twice per year in all persons with DM. As noted above, a report from the

The measurement of glycohemoglobin, specifically hemoglobin A1c (HbA1c), is essential for monitoring the success of therapy for patients with diabetes. HbA1c is formed by the nonenzymatic linkage of glucose to hemoglobin.

TABLE 17–5   **Laboratory Evaluation for Selected Other Causes of Diabetes Mellitus**

Etiology	Test(s) for Evaluation
Exocrine pancreatic disease	Amylase, lipase
Cushing syndrome	24-Hour urine-free cortisol
Glucagonoma	Plasma glucagon
Hyperthyroidism	Thyroid-stimulating hormone (TSH)
Hemochromatosis	Iron, ferritin, total iron-binding capacity

International Expert Committee in 2009 on the role of hemoglobin HbA1c concludes that large volumes of data from diverse populations provide strong justification for assigning a reproducible HbA1c level of >6.5% as adequate for the diagnosis of diabetes.

Considerable attention is now focused on the detection of autoantibodies as a screening tool for asymptomatic individuals with a strong family history of type 1 DM. The presence of autoantibodies to 2 or more of the following—glutamic acid decarboxylase (GAD65), islet tyrosine phosphatase (ICA512), or insulin—is a strong predictor of progression to type 1 DM (greater than 50%). It remains to be shown, however, whether early intervention can slow or prevent the subsequent onset of disease. Therefore, the ADA does not currently advocate screening for diabetes with these tests.

An important aspect of the ADA classification system is the prognostic value of the etiology of DM in a given patient. DM from certain causes, such as drug use or endocrine tumors, may be completely reversible. DM from other causes such as insulin receptor defects are not reversible, and are often difficult to manage. DM may be the initial manifestation of a disease affecting multiple organs. DM categorized as "other specific types of diabetes" in **Table 17–2** are much rarer than type 1 or type 2 DM. These types deserve some consideration whenever a new diagnosis of DM is made, as shown in **Table 17–5**.

The treatment goals for patients with DM include the prevention of disease progression and complications. Tight glycemic control in type 1 diabetics, defined by an HbA1c value of <6.5%, lowers the risk for the development and progression of microvascular disease. Currently, some laboratories are reporting HbA1c values with an average glucose value estimate, calculated using a formula. This approach permits the HbA1c result to be interpreted using the same units used for daily glucose monitoring. Fructosamine, also known as glycosylated albumin, is used in some institutions as a measure of glycemic control, because it reflects control over a shorter time frame than the HbA1c level. Monitoring and managing dyslipidemia, using total cholesterol, low- and high-density lipoprotein, and triglycerides as indicators, probably lowers the risk of developing macrovascular disease for both type 1 and type 2 diabetics. Trace excretion of urinary albumin, termed "microalbuminuria," is routinely measured in patients with DM as an early marker of nephropathy. This test is not usually a part of routine urinalysis, and must therefore be ordered as a microalbumin test, along with a creatinine level, on a random urine specimen (see Chapter 18).

GESTATIONAL DIABETES MELLITUS

Description

Gestational DM represents any level of glucose intolerance initially recognized during pregnancy, even if it may have been present but unrecognized before the pregnancy. When hyperglycemia occurs for the first time during pregnancy, it usually develops late in the second or in the third trimester. Most women will be normoglycemic after pregnancy. Among the complications of untreated gestational DM are macrosomia (birth weight >4,000 g or 8.82 lbs), intrauterine fetal demise, and pulmonary immaturity. Congenital malformations are increased only in women who have preexisting diabetes, which may or may not have been clinically appreciated. Approximately 1 in 25 pregnancies in the United States is complicated by gestational DM, with a higher incidence in some ethnic groups (up to 1 in 7 in Native Americans).

Gestational diabetes represents any level of glucose intolerance initially recognized during pregnancy, even if it may have been present but unrecognized before the pregnancy.

TABLE 17–6 **Laboratory Evaluation for Gestational Diabetes Mellitus (GDM)**

Test	Interpretation
1. Screening OGTT: 50 g glucose bolus • Patient need not fast	PG (1 hour postbolus): • ≥140 mg/dL is abnormal • <140 mg/dL is normal
2. Confirmatory OGTT: 100 g glucose • Patient must fast • Only for patients with abnormal screening OGTT	Abnormal if at least 2 of the following 4 are met: • PG (prior to bolus): ≥95 mg/dL • PG (1 hour postbolus): ≥180 mg/dL • PG (2 hours postbolus): ≥155 mg/dL • PG (3 hours postbolus): ≥140 mg/dL
3. Follow-up postpartum: fasting PG only • Only for patients who have had GDM; to be performed at 6 months and every 3 years postpartum	Use criteria for nonpregnant adults in **Table 17–3**

GDM; gestational diabetes mellitus; OGTT, oral glucose tolerance test; PG, plasma glucose.

Diagnosis

Screening for gestational DM was previously recommended for all pregnant women. Now it is argued that screening of women at low risk for gestational DM is not cost-effective, although some practitioners still advocate testing all pregnant women. These low-risk women are of Caucasian or Middle-Eastern ancestry, less than 25 years old, of normal weight, have no first-degree relatives with DM, and no history of abnormal glucose metabolism. Women with a high risk for gestational DM should be evaluated as soon as feasible. All other women should be screened between 24 and 28 weeks gestation, with the exception of women with clinical symptoms consistent with gestational DM before 24 weeks, who should be tested when symptoms appear.

The ADA criteria for screening are shown in **Table 17–6**. Patients with an abnormal finding with the screening OGTT (with 50 g glucose) must also have an abnormal confirmatory finding with the OGTT (with 100 g glucose) to warrant the diagnosis of gestational DM. If a patient has only 1 abnormal value during a confirmatory OGTT performed at 24 to 28 weeks of gestation, some authorities recommend repeating the test at 32 weeks. The WHO currently advocates a screening OGTT for gestational DM using a 75 g glucose bolus, which has been shown to be more sensitive at detecting women at risk than the test using 50 g. However, the ADA chose not to adopt this modification because of the wide use of the 50 g bolus.

Six weeks after the end of a pregnancy complicated by gestational DM, the woman should be retested. Normoglycemic women with a history of gestational DM should be rescreened at 3-year intervals, and women with IFG or impaired glucose tolerance should be screened more frequently.

HYPOGLYCEMIA

Description

Hypoglycemia is a low plasma glucose state. Symptoms result from activation of the autonomic pathways and from inadequate glucose delivery to the central nervous system. This explains the clinical features of hypoglycemia which are, in the acute form, intermittent episodes of sweating, tachycardia, anxiety, dizziness, slurred speech, double vision, and confusion, with complete recovery on restoration of plasma glucose to normal levels.

The plasma glucose level in hypoglycemic patients decreases well below the reference range, often to less than 40 mg/dL. Hypoglycemia can be divided into reactive postprandial hypoglycemia and fasting hypoglycemia. Overall, hypoglycemia is most commonly observed in patients being treated for diabetes.

The plasma glucose level in hypoglycemic patients decreases well below the reference range, often to less than 40 mg/dL. Hypoglycemia is most commonly observed in patients being treated for diabetes.

- *Reactive hypoglycemia*: Reactive hypoglycemia may occur in patients who have had gastric surgery, in children with inborn errors in enzymes leading to fructose intolerance, or following ethanol consumption. Normally, the ingestion of a high carbohydrate meal increases the plasma glucose level and stimulates the release of an appropriate amount of insulin. In reactive hypoglycemia, the peak concentration of insulin is inappropriately high and causes the plasma glucose level to decrease below the reference range. Reactive hypoglycemia is diagnosed if there are hypoglycemic symptoms, and a plasma glucose level below 50 mg/dL following a high carbohydrate meal, with resolution of symptoms after administration of glucose.

- *Fasting hypoglycemia*: Fasting hypoglycemia may result from a variety of causes including drugs (ethanol, sulfonamides, salicylate, and pentamidine), insulinoma and other islet cell tumors, autoantibodies to insulin or its receptor, malignancy (such as sarcoma and hematopoietic tumors), various inborn errors of metabolism, critical illness, and selected endocrine disorders, among other causes. In general, fasting hypoglycemia can be classified into hyperinsulinemic and nonhyperinsulinemic types. Patients who become hypoglycemic as a result of excess insulin secretion from an insulinoma will have a decreased plasma glucose level and/or an abnormal insulin to glucose ratio. Elevated blood insulin levels independent of high carbohydrate meals are found in patients with insulinomas. In addition, patients with insulinomas have a high serum level of C-peptide, which is formed during the conversion of pro-insulin to insulin within the beta cells of the pancreas. C-peptide appears in the blood in an approximately equimolar concentration with insulin and, thereby, provides a reliable indication of insulin synthesis by the beta cells of the pancreas.
- *Surreptitious insulin injection*: Patients who inject themselves with insulin to produce a hypoglycemic state will have the same hypoglycemic symptoms as patients with hypoglycemia from other causes. However, these patients can be differentiated from patients with insulinomas because, even though they have a high level of plasma insulin, they have decreased levels of C-peptide. In insulin used for injection, the C-peptide moiety is removed. The C-peptide is not present in patients with surreptitious insulin injection because the insulin found in their blood is not synthesized from pro-insulin in their pancreas.
- *Excess administration of sulfonylureas*: As with insulin, patients who have purposely taken sulfonylureas (an oral antidiabetic medication) in greater than prescribed doses suffer from hypoglycemia. Because oral antidiabetic medications are not naturally occurring compounds, a high serum concentration of these medications can reveal excess intake.
- *Impaired liver function*: Hypoglycemia can also occur in the presence of liver disease, often when it is associated with excess alcohol intake or ingestion of certain medications.

Diagnosis

To diagnose hypoglycemia, the following 3 criteria (known as Whipple's triad) must be met:

- characteristic signs and symptoms of hypoglycemia;
- blood glucose level below 45 to 50 mg/dL coincident with symptoms;
- symptom reversal within 15 to 45 minutes of the administration of glucose, in the absence of cerebral edema.

ISLET CELL TUMORS

Description and Diagnosis

Islet cell tumors, which may occur as a single mass or multiple masses, may be associated with hyperfunction of specific hormone-secreting cells within the islets of Langerhans of the pancreas. Some islet cell tumors are nonfunctional, and therefore may present only with symptoms of a mass lesion. Radiographic studies to identify the tumor and permit surgical removal are an important part of the evaluation of the patient for an islet cell tumor.

- Beta cell tumors are also known as *insulinomas* and are clinically significant when they produce enough insulin to induce hypoglycemia. The laboratory studies used in the detection of insulinoma include plasma glucose, C-peptide, insulin, and the insulin to glucose ratio.

Beta cell tumors are also known as *insulinomas* and are clinically significant when they produce enough insulin to induce hypoglycemia.

- Tumors of the pancreatic islets that secrete gastrin are known as *gastrinomas*. However, the most common site of gastrinomas is the duodenum. An elevated serum gastrin level from a gastrin-secreting tumor is associated with the development of peptic ulcer disease because gastrin stimulates acid secretion as well as watery diarrhea and malabsorption. This constellation of clinical and laboratory findings constitutes Zollinger–Ellison syndrome. Patients with peptic ulcer disease who do not have a *Helicobacter pylori* infection or a history of nonsteroidal anti-inflammatory drug use may have Zollinger–Ellison syndrome and should be evaluated for a gastrinoma. Patients with Zollinger–Ellison syndrome may also have multiple endocrine neoplasia I, with islet cell tumors that produce a variety of hormones. The secreted hormones found, in descending order of frequency, are: gastrin, insulin, serotonin, and vasoactive intestinal polypeptide (VIP) that is associated with watery diarrhea. The diagnosis of gastrinomas is based on the finding of an elevation in serum gastrin while fasting in association with increased gastric acid secretion.
- Tumors of the alpha cells of the pancreatic islets, also known as *glucagonomas*, are associated with elevated serum levels of glucagon. These tumors are associated with a characteristic migratory erythema, as well as glucose intolerance, weight loss, deep vein thrombosis, and depression.
- Tumors of the delta cells of the endocrine pancreas are known as *somatostatinomas*. These tumors are typically associated with diabetes-related symptoms, diarrhea, steatorrhea, cholelithiasis, and weight loss. These tumors are most often located in the duodenum or jejunum, rather than in the pancreas.
- Some islet cell tumors produce vasoactive intestinal peptide (VIP). These tumors, known as a *VIPomas*, induce a syndrome of watery diarrhea, hypokalemia, hypochlorhydria, and acidosis (WDHHA syndrome). Serum VIP levels are elevated in patients with VIPomas.

A portion of this chapter appeared previously in Clinical Laboratory Reviews (a publication for the Massachusetts General Hospital physicians) 2000;8:2 and 1999;7:4. It has been included with permission.

REFERENCES

American Diabetes Association. Diagnosis and classification of diabetes mellitus. *Diab Care.* 2008; 31:S55–S60.

Apple F, et al. Lipase and pancreatic amylase activities in tissues and in patients with hyperamylasemia. *Am J Clin Pathol.* 1991;96:610.

Blamey SL, Imrie CW, O'Neil J, et al. Prognostic factors in acute pancreatitis. *Gut.* 1984;25:1340–1346.

Brown CM, Valori RM. Non-radiological investigation of pancreatic disease. *Br J Hosp Med.* 1995;54:400.

Comi RJ. Approach to acute hypoglycemia. *Endocrinol Metab Clin North Am.* 1993;22:247.

Cowie CC. Full accounting of diabetes and pre-diabetes in the U.S. population in 1988–1994 and 2005–2006. *Diab Care.* 2009;33:S287–S294.

Diabetes Control and Complications Trial Research Group. The effect of intensive treatment of diabetes on the development and progression of long-term complications in insulin-dependent diabetes mellitus. *N Engl J Med.* 1993;329:977.

Fore WW. Noninsulin-dependent diabetes mellitus: the prevention of complications. *Med Clin North Am.* 1995;79:287.

Gottlieb PA, Eisenbarth GS. Diagnosis and treatment of pre-insulin dependent diabetes. *Annu Rev Med.* 1998;49:391.

Haffner SM. Management of dyslipidemia in adults with diabetes. *Diab Care.* 1998;21:160.

Hirsch IB. Insulin analogues. *N Engl J Med.* 2005;352:174–183.

Kazmierczak SC. Enzymatic diagnosis of acute pancreatitis. *Clin Lab Sci.* 1990;3:91.

Kazmierczak SC, et al. Diagnostic accuracy of pancreatic enzymes evaluated by use of multivariate data analysis. *Clin Chem.* 1993;39:1960.

Kemppainen EA, et al. Advances in the laboratory diagnostics of acute pancreatitis. *Ann Med.* 1998;30:169.

Li H, et al. Laboratory tests useful in the diagnosis of pancreatitis and pancreatic carcinoma. *Clin Lab Rev.* 2000;8:2.

Malesci A, et al. Clinical utility of CA 19-9 test for diagnosing pancreatic carcinoma in patients: a prospective study. *Pancreas.* 1992;7:497.

Marks V, Teale JD. Investigation of hypoglycemia. *Clin Endocrinol.* 1996;44:133.

Meko JB, Norton JA. Management of patients with Zollinger–Ellison syndrome. *Annu Rev Med.* 1995;46:395.

Metzger BE. Summary and recommendations of the fifth international workshop-conference on gestational diabetes mellitus. *Diab Care.* 2007;30:S251–S260.

Nathan DM, et al. Translating the A1C assay into estimated average glucose values. *Diab Care.* 2008;31:S1473–S1478.

Niederau C, Grendell JH. Diagnosis of pancreatic carcinoma. *Pancreas.* 1992;7:234.

Ohkubo Y, et al. Intensive insulin therapy prevents the progression of diabetic microvascular complications in Japanese patients with non-insulin-dependent diabetes mellitus: a randomized prospective 6-year study. *Diab Res Clin Pract.* 1995;28:103.

Palmer-Toy DE, Godine J. The role of the laboratory in the diagnosis of diabetes mellitus. *Clin Lab Rev.* 1999;7:4.

Parker SL, et al. Cancer statistics. *CA Cancer J Clin.* 1997;47:5.

Posner MR, Mayer RJ. The use of serologic tumor markers in gastrointestinal malignancies. *Hematol Oncol Clin North Am.* 1994;8:533.

Ritts RF, Pitt HA. CA 19-9 in pancreatic cancer. *Surg Oncol Clin North Am.* 1998;7:93.

Shepherd PR, Kahn BB. Glucose transporters and insulin action. *N Engl J Med.* 1999;341:248–257.

The International Expert Committee. International Expert Committee report on the role of the A1C assay in the diagnosis of diabetes. *Diab Care.* 2008;32:1–8.

Tietz NW. Lipase in serum—the elusive enzyme: an overview. *Clin Chem.* 1993;39:746.

UK Prospective Diabetes Study Group. Intensive blood-glucose control with sulphonylureas or insulin compared with conventional treatment and risk of complications in patients with type 2 diabetes (UKPDS 33). *Lancet.* 1998;352:837.

Weber HC, et al. Diagnosis and management of Zollinger–Ellison syndrome. *Semin Gastrointest Dis.* 1995;6:79.

Whitcomb DC. Acute pancreatitis. *N Engl J Med.* 2006; 354:2142–2150.

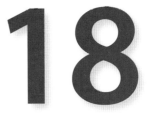

The Kidney

William E. Winter

CHAPTER OUTLINE

OVERVIEW OF RENAL DISEASE

The roles of the kidney include maintenance and regulation of fluid balance, acid/base and electrolyte balance (e.g., sodium, potassium, chloride, bicarbonate, calcium, phosphate, and magnesium), conservation of glucose, amino acids and proteins, the excretion of wastes, and the production of hormones such as erythropoietin and 1,25-dihydroxy vitamin D. The renal blood vessels provide blood to the glomerulus and the tubules for the generation of urine. The glomerulus filters blood to create a plasma ultrafiltrate by retaining cells and proteins, whereas the tubules "process" the plasma ultrafiltrate to urine, thereby concentrating wastes such as urea, creatinine, nitrogenous wastes, and hydrogen ions.

Renal disease is suggested by any of the following findings:

(1) Nonspecific symptoms of malaise, headache, visual disturbances, nausea, or vomiting (e.g., many of these findings suggest uremia or hypertension [see below]).
(2) Flank pain (from pyelonephritis, e.g.), pain that radiates to the groin (from ureteral colic as a result of nephrolithiasis, e.g.), or simple dysuria (from a lower urinary tract infection, e.g.).
(3) A reduction in the volume of urine output. In adults, oliguria, a pathologically reduced urine output, is defined as less than 500 mL of urine produced per day. Anuria, which is essentially absent urine production, is defined in adults as less than 100 mL of urine produced per day. In infants, oliguria can be defined as urine output of less than 1 mL/kg/hour, and in children older than infants, oliguria is defined as urine output of less than 0.5 mL/kg/hour.
(4) Hematuria.

TABLE 18–1 **Selected Consequences of Untreated Renal Failure**

Pathophysiology	Immediate Consequences	Later Possible Consequences
Salt and water retention	Hypertension	Heart failure, pulmonary edema
Potassium retention	Hyperkalemia	Cardiac arrhythmias
Phosphate retention	Hypocalcemia Hyperphosphatemia	Hyperparathyroidism with renal osteodystrophy
Decreased synthesis of 1,25-dihydroxy vitamin D	Hypocalcemia	Hyperparathyroidism with renal osteodystrophy
Decreased production of erythropoietin	Anemia	Heart failure
Decreased waste excretion	Azotemia, acidosis	Uremia
Decreased waste excretion	Platelet dysfunction	Bleeding tendency

(5) Discolored or malodorous urine (e.g., from a urinary tract infection).
(6) Elevations in the concentrations of creatinine or blood urea nitrogen (BUN) or an abnormal urinalysis.
(7) Malar rash (e.g., from systemic lupus erythematosus).
(8) Hypertension.
(9) Otherwise unexplained hypo- or hyperkalemia, hypocalcemia, hypo- or hyperphosphatemia, pathologic fractures, hypomagnesemia, acidosis, anemia, edema, or bleeding.

Renal function should be evaluated when patients are taking drugs that can damage the kidney (e.g., gentamicin) or drugs whose metabolism and/or excretion is dependent on the kidney (e.g., low-molecular-weight heparin).

Nitrogen retention, as shown by an elevated BUN concentration, is termed "azotemia." Azotemia can be classified as prerenal, renal, or postrenal. Prerenal azotemia refers to conditions with reduced blood flow to the kidney, and thereby reducing urine output and causing the retention of waste products. Examples of prerenal causes of azotemia are congestive heart failure, GI hemorrhage, renal artery stenosis, and severe dehydration.

Renal azotemia indicates that the kidney itself is dysfunctional. Renal azotemia results from diseases of the renal blood vessels, glomerulus, tubules, or renal interstitium.

Renal azotemia indicates that the kidney itself is dysfunctional. The number of individual causes of intrinsic renal disease is large. In the broad view, however, renal azotemia results from diseases of the renal blood vessels, glomerulus, tubules, or renal interstitium. Glomerulonephritides may be a result of a primary process in the kidney or a secondary disorder leading to glomerulonephritis. A biopsy is necessary to identify the type of glomerulonephritis. The histopathologic characteristics of the different glomerulonephridities are described in textbooks of anatomic pathology. Acute tubular necrosis can cause renal failure. This may occur as a result of exposure to a toxin or as a result of ischemic damage to the tubules.

Postrenal azotemia results from an anatomic obstruction to urine flow out of the kidney. The ureter, bladder outlet, or urethra may be obstructed by a stone (e.g., nephrolithiasis), congenital anomaly, inflammatory lesion, or neoplasm.

Among prerenal, intrinsic renal, and postrenal-induced renal failure, the dominant etiology is prerenal.

Uremia, unlike azotemia, is a clinical term that describes the patient's signs and symptoms when symptomatic end-stage renal failure is present. Findings in uremia include fatigue, headache, restlessness, depression, altered sensorium, nausea, vomiting, diarrhea, hiccups, bleeding, edema, shortness of breath, and pulmonary edema. Left untreated, uremia progresses to coma and death. Renal failure produces a wide variety of adverse clinical and metabolic consequences (**Table 18–1**).

Chronic renal failure is a deterioration in renal function that persists for more than 3 months. It occurs with progressive renal damage, and is independent of the cause of kidney disease. Chronic renal failure is an ultimate consequence of the loss of functioning nephrons. The dominant etiologies of chronic renal failure in adults are multifactorial, as in patients with diabetes, hypertension, glomeru-lonephritis, pyelonephritis/interstitial nephritis, cystic kidney disease, and toxicity from drugs. A significant percentage of patients with chronic renal failure have no known etiology for their disease.

Renal function can be assessed using a variety of clinical laboratory analyses. Acid/base and electrolyte balance is initially assessed by ordering a profile of tests that includes sodium, potassium, chloride, total serum CO_2, BUN, creatinine, calcium, and glucose.

A more detailed analysis of acid/base balance would also include a measurement of arterial blood gases (pH, pCO_2, pO_2, and calculated bicarbonate) and urine pH. The effect of erythropoietin is assessed by measuring the patient's hemoglobin, hematocrit, and red blood cell indices. The kidney's role in producing active vitamin D, that is, 1,25-dihydroxy vitamin D, and controlling phosphate excretion is evaluated, in part, through measurements of serum calcium or ionized calcium and albumin, phosphate, and parathyroid hormone (PTH). Measurements of 25-hydroxy vitamin D assess vitamin D stores. 1,25-dihydroxy vitamin D levels reflect the most active form of vitamin D in the body. However, measurements of 1,25-dihydroxy vitamin D are rarely required.

Urinary tract infections are especially common in females. Discussion of pathogenic organisms resulting in bacterial infections of the kidney appears in Chapter 5.

CLINICAL LABORATORY PARAMETERS

Creatinine

Creatinine is a breakdown product of creatine and phosphocreatine, also known as creatine phosphate. Creatine is produced in skeletal muscle, the kidney, and the pancreas and is then transported to the tissues, especially the skeletal muscle and brain, via the blood stream. Within cells, creatine is phosphorylated to phosphocreatine via the enzymatic action of creatine kinase (CK). Phosphocreatine provides a ready, rapid source of energy. For example, phosphocreatine is used as a short-term energy source as required during a sprint.

With an approximate 1% to 2% daily turnover rate, creatine and phosphocreatine are metabolized to creatinine at a fairly constant rate. Therefore, the plasma concentration of creatinine is usually stable day to day. Creatinine can be measured in the clinical laboratory by its ability to form an orange-red colored product in a chemical reaction with alkaline picric acid. This is the classic Jaffe reaction. Creatinine can also be measured enzymatically using creatininase. Modern alkaline picric acid methods have been improved to minimize interferences by other substances. Nonetheless, at this time creatinine measurements using the picric acid method can be falsely elevated by a number of substances including ketones, glucose, and various drugs, such as cephalosporins and sulfonamides. Using creatininase to measure creatinine, interferences are uncommon.

Creatinine is freely filtered. However, 10% of the total excreted creatinine is secreted by the tubules. Negligible amounts of creatinine are reabsorbed. The alkaline picric acid method overestimates serum creatinine by at least 10% because of endogenous positive interferences. Creatininase methods are calibrated to report a creatinine concentration comparable to creatinine measured by the alkaline picric acid method. Therefore, the creatininase methods to measure serum or plasma creatinine also display a positive bias. Standardization of creatinine measurements among analyzers has become an important goal for laboratory medicine.

The creatinine concentration in blood is inversely related to glomerular filtration rate (GFR; see below). If the GFR declines by 50%, the plasma creatinine approximately doubles. The creatinine concentration is directly related to skeletal muscle mass. Creatinine is higher in males than females, and increases with protein intake and with creatine intake. Creatine is sometimes used as a "nutritional" supplement by body builders or athletes. The clearance of creatinine by the kidney is a suitable estimate of GFR that is universally used by physicians.

> The glomerulus is investigated by determining the GFR. GFR is the number of milliliters of body fluid cleared by the kidneys per unit time reported in mL/minute.

The Glomerular Filtration Rate and Creatinine Clearance

Laboratory evaluation of the kidney as discussed in this chapter centers on assessments of glomerular and tubular function. The glomerulus is investigated by determining the GFR. GFR is the number of milliliters of body fluid cleared by the kidneys per unit time reported in mL/minute.

Ideally, GFR is measured using a substance that is produced by the body at a constant rate that is freely filtered by the glomerulus and is neither secreted nor reabsorbed by the tubules. As GFR is reduced, waste retention occurs. Measurable waste products excreted by the kidney include creatinine, urea, and uric acid. With a decline in the GFR, these waste products are retained and their circulating concentrations rise. Measurement of the GFR is a very important assessment of renal function. A steady decline in GFR can serve as a harbinger of eventual end-stage renal disease.

GFR measurements are most commonly based on the clearance of creatinine by the kidney. This entails a serum creatinine measurement and a concurrent timed urine collection for the measurement of excreted urinary creatinine and urine volume. In individuals aged 18 years and above, an estimate of the GFR (eGFR) can be calculated solely from the serum creatinine and various patient parameters such as age, sex, and ethnicity.

A complete urine collection is essential for an accurate determination of the creatinine clearance because the equation contains a measurement of urine volume. The blood sample for serum creatinine is collected at the beginning of the timed urine collection. The clearance is expressed in terms of volume of fluid cleared per unit time (e.g., mL/minute).

The basic formula for creatinine clearance is as follows (serum creatinine and plasma creatinine are used interchangeably in the formulae):

$$\frac{\text{Urine creatinine}}{\text{Serum creatinine}} \times \frac{\text{Urine volume (mL)}}{\text{Collection time (minute)}}$$

> GFR measurements are most commonly based on the clearance of creatinine by the kidney. This entails a serum creatinine measurement and a concurrent timed urine collection for the measurement of excreted urinary creatinine and urine volume.

The clearance can be corrected for the patient's body surface area to be compared to a standard body surface area of 1.73 M^2.

When corrected for body surface area, the formula for creatinine clearance is as follows:

$$\frac{\text{Urine creatinine}}{\text{Serum creatinine}} \times \frac{\text{Urine volume (mL)}}{\text{Collection time (minute)}} \times \frac{1.73}{\text{Body surface area (m}^2)}$$

For creatinine clearance (see the above formula), a 12- or 24-hour urine specimen is collected.

The GFR in persons aged 18 years and above can be reliably estimated (also known as the eGFR) solely from the patient's serum creatinine, age, gender, and ethnicity (e.g., African American or non-African American). The use of the modification of diet in renal disease (MDRD) equation, which is:

$$\text{eGFR} = 186(S_{Cr})^{-1.154} \times (\text{Age})^{-0.203} \times F$$

where $F = 0.742$ for females and 1.210 for African Americans, provides GFR estimates comparable to measured creatinine clearance when the GFR is less than 60 mL/minute/1.73 M^2. Because of difficulties in obtaining a complete timed urine collection, the National Kidney Foundation (NKF) advises that eGFR be used in place of creatinine clearance measurements when the GFR is between 15 and 60 mL/minute/1.73 M^2. It is not presently advised that eGFR be calculated in children because pediatric equations are not as well validated, unlike the MDRD equation that has been well validated in adults.

The MDRD equation provides eGFR determinations that are reliable between 15 and 60 mL/minute/1.73 M^2. However, below 15 mL/minute/1.73 M^2 and above 60 mL/minute/1.73 M^2, GFR should be estimated using the traditional creatinine clearance measurement. The lower limit of the reference range for GFR is 90 mL/minute/1.73 M^2. However, the upper limit of the reportable eGFR is 60 mL/minute/1.73 M^2. Therefore, there is a "gray" zone between the upper limit of the reportable eGFR and the lower limit of the reference interval (90 mL/minute/1.73 M^2). Therefore, it is practical to report eGFR values greater than 60 mL/minute/1.73 M^2 as simply "greater than 60 mL/minute/1.73 M^2" with a comment that "the lower limit of the reference interval is 90 mL/minute/1.73 M^2."

Many pathologic renal and systemic conditions can reduce the GFR. As GFR declines, creatinine clearance can, however, begin to overestimate GFR. This is because the fraction of the creatinine that is secreted by the tubules becomes a proportionately higher percentage of the urine creatinine excreted as GFR declines. However, since clinical practice is almost always based on

TABLE 18–2   **National Kidney Foundation Definitions of Kidney Damage Relative to the Glomerular Filtration Rate (GFR)**

Stage	GFR	Comment
0	≥90	Normal kidney function and no proteinuria
1	≥90	Kidney damage despite a normal or increased GFR
2	60–89	Mildly decreased GFR with evidence of kidney damage
3	30–59	Moderately decreased GFR
4	15–29	Severely decreased GFR
5	<15	Renal failure and dialysis or transplant needed

GFR is reported in mL/minute/1.73 M^2.

assessment of the creatinine clearance, the difference between the "true" GFR and the creatinine clearance as a reflection of the GFR is usually not problematic when making clinical judgments.

The development of renal impairment is frequently unrecognized until late in its course, when intervention is less likely to be successful. Screening for reductions in GFR has recently been championed by the NKF. The NKF provides guidelines for the interpretation of the GFR result (**Table 18–2**). It defines kidney damage as any pathologic kidney abnormality reflected by a marker of damage, as shown in a blood, urine, or imaging study. Kidney damage that is present for more than 3 months is termed "chronic" kidney damage.

The NKF stresses that the creatinine clearance (unlike the eGFR) does provide useful information in estimating the GFR in individuals who have exceptional dietary intakes (such as those on vegetarian diets or those taking creatine supplements) or muscle mass changes (such as people with amputations, malnutrition, or wasting conditions). Creatinine clearance measurements are also valuable when deciding on the initiation of dialysis. This decision is made when the GFR is <15 mL/minute/1.73 M^2; the eGFR is not reliable in this setting.

Urea and the Blood Urea Nitrogen

Urea is produced by the liver to create a metabolite of ammonia that can be excreted in the urine. The nitrogen in ammonia is derived from the deamination of amino acids.

The initially developed laboratory measurements of urea depended on liberating nitrogen from urea in whole blood. Therefore, the term "BUN" was created. However, modern laboratory methods actually measure urea in serum or plasma (and not whole blood) and back-calculate the nitrogen content, but the term "BUN" has persisted.

Urea is freely filtered by the glomerulus. However, because ~50% of urea is reabsorbed by the tubules, urea clearance greatly underestimates GFR and, therefore, urea clearance is not usually determined. Furthermore, while creatinine production by the body occurs at a fairly constant rate, providing stable serum creatinine concentrations over time (assuming there is no acute disease affecting the kidneys such as acute tubular necrosis), BUN levels can vary considerably. BUN is affected by the patient's state of hydration, protein intake, and the presence of large amounts of blood in the gastrointestinal tract. If a large gastrointestinal hemorrhage occurs, the metabolism of this additional protein originating from blood cells in the gastrointestinal tract leads to Urea production. With a decline in the GFR, BUN rises. Lastly, BUN can decline if there is liver failure, leading to decreased urea production or when there is malnutrition and amino acids are "conserved" for protein synthesis.

The 24-hour urea excretion in the urine can be used as an assessment of nutritional replacement in malnourished patients. If sufficient nitrogen is present in the diet and utilized by the body, normal levels of urea are excreted in the urine.

Modern laboratory methods actually measure urea in serum or plasma (and not whole blood) and back-calculate the nitrogen content, but the term "BUN" has persisted.

TABLE 18–3   Clinical Use of the BUN/Creatinine (Cr) Ratio

	Action
BUN and creatinine both within the reference range	Do not calculate the BUN/Cr ratio
BUN and/or creatinine above the reference range	Calculate the BUN/Cr ratio (reference range: 10:1–20:1) • ≥20:1 suggests prerenal azotemia or early postrenal azotemia • ≤10:1 suggests renal azotemia or late postrenal azotemia

The Blood Urea Nitrogen/Creatinine Ratio

If either the creatinine or BUN concentrations are above the upper limit of the reference interval, it is advised that the BUN to creatinine ratio (BUN/Cr) be calculated (**Table 18–3**). The normal BUN/Cr ratio is between 10:1 and 20:1. The ratio is helpful in determining the cause of renal impairment.

If the BUN/Cr ratio is 20:1 or higher, prerenal azotemia is likely to be present. Prerenal azotemia results from a reduction in the GFR while the kidney tubules are functioning.

The explanation why the BUN rises to a greater extent than creatinine involves 2 observations: 1) renal tubular secretion of creatinine persists even as GFR declines, opposing what would otherwise be a rise in serum creatinine, and 2) with decreased renal blood flow, the rate of capillary blood flow around the renal tubules is reduced, providing more time for the reabsorption of urea out of the urine in the tubules and back into the circulation, raising the serum BUN concentration.

When the BUN/Cr ratio is near 10:1, renal azotemia is likely, assuming that chronic urinary tract obstruction has been excluded. In cases of renal azotemia, the BUN and creatinine rise proportionate to one another because, in part, tubular dysfunction will not maintain the tubular secretion of creatinine.

In the early phase of postrenal obstruction, the BUN/Cr ratio is ~20:1 because urea is reabsorbed from urine that is "stagnant" in the excretory system because of the anatomic obstruction. Therefore, if the BUN/Cr ratio is elevated at the time of patient presentation, the treating physician is obligated to consider the possibility of an anatomic obstruction to urine flow, as well as prerenal azotemia. If there is persistent urinary tract obstruction, postrenal azotemia can evolve into renal azotemia from pressure damage to the kidneys. If renal impairment then supervenes, the BUN/Cr ratio would be 10:1, similar to other conditions associated with intrinsic renal disease.

Urine Protein Quantitation

The general health of the kidney is assessed in part by the measurement of urinary protein excretion. In normal adults, 24-hour urinary protein excretion does not exceed 150 mg. If one assumes that a normal adult urine output is 1,500 mL per day and a maximum of 150 mg of protein is excreted per day, the urine protein concentration should not exceed 10 mg/dL. Elevated concentrations of protein in the urine can result from glomerular disease, tubular disease, overflow from elevated concentrations of plasma proteins, such as immunoglobulins or immunoglobulin light chains in patients with myeloma, urinary tract inflammation, as found in interstitial nephritis or urinary tract infection, trauma, or neoplasia.

In adults, proteinuria greater than 1 g per day is considered to be very significant clinically. Levels of protein excretion of 3.5 g per day or greater are consistent with nephrosis. Nephrosis is the clinical syndrome of massive proteinuria, hypoalbuminemia, edema, and hyperlipidemia.

In children, an elevated level of urinary protein excretion is >4 mg/M²/hour. Nephrotic range proteinuria in children can be defined as >40 mg/M²/hour.

The most cost-effective way to initially screen for proteinuria is urine protein dipstick testing. In this semiquantitative system, proteinuria is reported as negative, trace (10 to 20 mg/dL), 1+ (30 mg/dL), 2+ (100 mg/dL), 3+ (300 mg/dL), and 4+ (1,000 to 2,000 mg/dL). Urine dipsticks for protein measurements are relatively insensitive to immunoglobulin light chains and, thus,

In adults, proteinuria greater than 1 g per day is considered to be very significant clinically. Levels of protein excretion of 3.5 g per day or greater are consistent with nephrosis.

TABLE 18–4   Interpretation of Albumin Excretion in the Urine

	Units	Normal	Microalbuminuria	Clinical Albuminuria
Spot collection	μg/mg Cr	<30	30–300	>300
Timed urine	μg/minute	<20	20–200	>200
24-Hour urine	mg/24 hour	<30	30–300	>300

Cr, creatinine.

TABLE 18–5   Laboratory and Blood Pressure Findings in Diabetic Nephropathy

Stage	GFR	UAE	Dipstick Proteinuria	Blood Pressure
1	Increased	Normal	Transient	Normal
2	Normal	Normal	Negative	Normal
3	Normal	Positive	Negative	± Increased
4	Decreased	Positive	Positive	Increased
5	Severely decreased	Positive	Positive	Severely increased

GFR, glomerular filtration rate; UAE, urinary albumin excretion.

a negative dipstick does not exclude Bence Jones (monoclonal light chain) proteinuria. A more accurate measure of proteinuria can be made using a 24-hour urine sample. The urine protein concentration in milligrams per deciliter is multiplied by the urine volume in milliliters per 24 hours yielding milligrams of protein excreted per 24 hours.

Minimal but persistent amounts of albumin in the urine are associated with diabetic nephropathy and with hypertensive renal damage. For this reason, people with diabetes are screened for minimal albumin excretion, also known as microalbuminuria. The albumin measurement is carried out using an immunoassay to provide analytical sensitivity, accuracy, and reproducibility. Microalbuminuria can be reported as the albumin to creatinine ratio obtained on a random urine sample, the albumin excretion in milligrams per minute on a timed urine sample collection (e.g., a 4-, 6-, or 12-hour collection), or the albumin excretion per 24 hours when a 24-hour urine sample is collected. **Table 18–4** provides an interpretation of microalbumin results.

It is recommended that all patients with type 2 diabetes mellitus be tested yearly for microalbuminuria from the time of diagnosis. For type 1 diabetes mellitus patients, testing is recommended to be performed annually beginning 5 years after the diagnosis of diabetes. Screening can begin with protein dipstick testing. If the dipstick is positive, microalbumin testing can be bypassed and testing should proceed to a 24-hour urine collection for the measurement of urine protein excretion. For patients with a negative dipstick result for proteinuria, microalbuminuria testing can be performed. If microalbuminuria is detected, a second sample should be obtained within 3 months. If the second sample does not display microalbuminuria, a third, tie-breaker sample is obtained. Thus, microalbuminuria must be present in 2 of 2 or 2 of 3 samples to classify the patient as having microalbuminuria.

With persistent microalbuminuria, the diabetic patient is diagnosed with stage 3 (e.g., incipient) diabetic nephropathy (**Table 18–5**). Stage 1 nephropathy immediately follows the diagnosis of type 1 diabetes mellitus and is characterized by renal hypertrophy and hyperfiltration. These patients have an elevated GFR from the expanded plasma volume induced by hyperosmolality caused by hyperglycemia. With the initiation of insulin treatment, stage 1 resolves but clinically silent histologic changes subsequently occur in the glomerulus with mesangial hypertrophy and thickening of the glomerular basement membrane. This is stage 2. With the recognition of incipient nephropathy (stage 3) and intervention with improved glycemic control and the administration of antihypertensive drugs, further progression to frank diabetic nephropathy can

Minimal but persistent amounts of albumin in the urine are associated with diabetic nephropathy and with hypertensive renal damage. For this reason, people with diabetes are screened for minimal albumin excretion, also known as microalbuminuria.

TABLE 18–6   **Approximate Molecular Weights of Selected Plasma Proteins**

Location on Serum Protein Electrophoresis Gel	Approximate Molecular Weight (kDa)
Prealbumin zone	
Retinol-binding protein	21
Transthyretin	54
Albumin zone	
Albumin	69
Alpha-1 globulin zone	
Alpha-1 antitrypsin	54
High-density lipoprotein	200–400
Thyroxine-binding globulin	54
Alpha-1-acid glycoprotein	40
Prothrombin	72
Alpha fetoprotein	69
Alpha-2 globulin zone	
Alpha-2 macroglobulin	800
Haptoglobin	86
Ceruloplasmin	160
Antithrombin	58
Erythropoietin	38
Beta globulin zone	
Transferrin	77
C-reactive protein	115–140
Complement component 3	185
Beta$_2$-microglobulin	12
IgA	170
Gamma globulin zone	
IgM	900
IgG	160

Also see serum protein electrophoresis in Chapter 2 on laboratory methods and Chapter 3 on autoimmune disorders.

be averted or at least delayed. Such patients show proteinuria by dipstick and have persistent hypertension (stage 4). Stage 5 nephropathy is characterized by the development of end-stage renal failure requiring either dialysis or transplantation.

Patterns of Proteinuria

When proteinuria is diagnosed, the subsequent diagnostic issues are the cause of the proteinuria and the structural part of the kidney that is functionally impaired. The glomerulus normally retains all plasma proteins with a molecular weight of greater than ~100,000 Da (**Table 18–6**). Variable amounts of plasma proteins with molecular weights between ~10,000 and ~100,000 Da are excreted into the urine. This includes albumin with a molecular weight of ~69,000 Da and free immunoglobulin light chains with a molecular weight of ~25,000 Da. Plasma proteins below ~10,000 Da, such as insulin, are essentially freely filtered by the kidney.

Urine protein electrophoresis can identify the following patterns of protein loss: glomerular, tubular, overflow, and nonselective proteinuria. Glomerular proteinuria is characterized by albuminuria and the excretion of beta globulins, notably transferrin. Tubular proteinuria is recognized in urine protein electrophoresis by an alpha-2 doublet in addition to increased albumin excretion.

Overflow proteinuria can result from a monoclonal immunoglobulin in high concentration in the plasma that "spills over" into the urine. Free monoclonal antibody light chains are detected by urine protein electrophoresis as an "M-spike," a band of restricted mobility, and confirmed to be present by immunofixation electrophoresis (IFE). The light chain loss occurs because the ability of the tubules to reabsorb filtered protein is exceeded. With extensive renal injury, intact monoclonal immunoglobulins can be lost. Persistent glomerular proteinuria can injure the tubule, resulting in a combined glomerular and tubular proteinuria. The excretion of multiple low-molecular-weight proteins that arise as part of the inflammatory acute phase response can also produce overflow proteinuria. Nonselective proteinuria, which can occur with severe renal dysfunction, is identified when the urine protein electrophoresis pattern is similar to that of serum.

The Fractional Excretion of Sodium as an Indicator of Tubular Function

Tubular dysfunction can result in many abnormalities: glycosuria, amino aciduria, renal tubular acidosis (bicarbonate wasting or failure to generate new bicarbonate), electrolyte wasting (e.g., hyponatremia, hypokalemia, and hypophosphatemia), and tubular proteinuria (see above). A readily available test of the resorptive function of the tubules is the "fractional excretion of sodium (FENa)."

FENa is calculated using creatinine and sodium measurements in serum or plasma and a simultaneously collected spot urine. The equation for the FENa is given as follows:

$$\text{FENa} = \frac{[U_{Na^+}]\ [S_{Cr}]}{[S_{Na^+}]\ [U_{Cr}]} \times 100$$

The unit is percent sodium excreted (%). Normally the FENa is less than 1%. If there is tubular disease or injury, such as acute tubular necrosis, sodium wasting will occur and the FENa exceeds 1%. Tubular reabsorption of sodium is 100% minus the FENa. FENa calculations are not valid when patients are treated with diuretics because the diuretic will induce urinary sodium loss.

Urinalysis

Examination of the physical, chemical, and microscopic contents of urine constitutes urinalysis testing. The physical characteristics of the urine include its color, clarity, and specific gravity. Chemical analyses of urine include pH and detection of glucose, protein, blood, ketones, bilirubin, urobilinogen, nitrite, and leukocyte esterase. The microscopic examination is an assessment for cells, bacteria, crystals, casts, lipids, and contaminants.

If the urine dipstick is completely normal, some laboratories will not perform the microscopic examination. A urinalysis should complement BUN and creatinine testing in any patient undergoing a renal evaluation.

The clinical significance of positive findings in urinalysis studies is briefly detailed below.

The color of normal urine is produced largely by pigments present in the diet, such as the pigments in vegetables, as well as metabolites of bile. Patients with elevated urine bilirubin or urobilinogen can have urine that is darkly colored, or some patients produce green urine because of the oxidation of bilirubin to biliverdin.

Hematuria refers to blood in the urine and usually both blood and hemoglobin are present. Hemoglobinuria is the presence of free hemoglobin in the urine, usually from hemolysis

Examination of the physical, chemical, and microscopic contents of urine constitutes urinalysis testing. A urinalysis should complement BUN and creatinine testing in any patient undergoing a renal evaluation.

of erythrocytes within the circulation. Hematuria occurs when at least 4 to 8 red blood cells are found per high-powered microscopic field. A positive dipstick test, which detects heme, establishes the presence of hemoglobin in the urine. To detect intact red blood cells, a microscopic examination of the urine sediment is required. If there is intravascular hemolysis, the dipstick test will be positive because it detects heme, and heme is present even if red blood cells are not intact and therefore not found microscopically. Diseases of the glomeruli are most often associated with red blood cell casts that are formed within the renal tubules. The casts are fragile and therefore they are most likely to be found in a fresh early morning urine specimen. Bleeding at any site in the urinary tract can produce hematuria without casts.

Proteinuria is thoroughly described earlier in this chapter.

Pyuria refers to increased white blood cells in the microscopic urine sediment. This is often considered to be at least 5 white blood cells per high-powered field. A test for leukocyte esterase enzyme activity, found in neutrophils, is on most urinalysis strips and can detect this activity whether the neutrophil is intact or disrupted. White blood cell casts originate in the tubules similar to red blood cell casts.

Urinary casts are formed in the kidney tubules and are indicators of renal disease. Cellular casts can be formed by red blood cells or white blood cells. Granular casts, which do not contain intact cells, and waxy casts can also be found in patients with chronic kidney disease.

Bacteriuria may be detected by a nitrite test on a urinalysis reagent strip, which is sensitive to the presence of clinically significant urinary bacteria concentrations. Bacteriuria is often asymptomatic but may reflect bacterial infection. It is frequently accompanied by pyuria.

Urine glucose is not useful to monitor patients with diabetes. There is only an approximate association between the level of plasma glucose and urinary glucose, as the renal threshold for glucose varies considerably among different individuals.

Urine pH can be altered by conditions associated with metabolic acidosis or alkalosis. Freshly collected urine specimens should have a pH between 5.0 and 6.5. A urine pH greater than 8.0 suggests delayed analysis or contamination.

Urine-specific gravity provides an assessment of the capacity of renal tubules to concentrate or to dilute urine. The specific gravity of urine should range between 1.003 and 1.035.

Bilirubin should not be present in the urine, and when it is detected, it is indicative of liver dysfunction or biliary obstruction.

Urinary urobilinogen is derived from bilirubin that is degraded by bacteria in the gastrointestinal tract. Conditions in which there is an elevated urinary urobilinogen include liver disease, because of failure to remove the urobilinogen from the blood, and hemolytic anemia in which bilirubin production increases the generation of urobilinogen.

Ketones most commonly appear in the urine of patients who have poorly controlled diabetes although they can also appear in hospitalized patients who do not have diabetes and in fasting patients.

Stones and Crystals Found in Urine

The process of kidney stone formation is known as nephrolithiasis or urolithiasis. The presence of a kidney stone is often associated with severe pain radiating from the back into the groin. Although most stones pass spontaneously, some do not. The size of the stone, among other factors, determines whether the stone will be passed or retained. Stones can form when there is increased excretion of the components found in stones or the urinary volume is decreased, leading to elevated concentrations of urinary components. Calcium, phosphate, and oxalate are the most commonly found chemical constituents in renal stones, and less commonly identified are urate and cystine.

If there is a sufficient amount of stone material for analysis, the composition of the stone can be determined. The value of knowing the composition of the stone is that information may be derived about the contributing factors to its formation. This can lead to treatment, sometimes involving dietary modification.

An elevated concentration of calcium in the urine can lead to the generation of calcium oxalate and calcium phosphate stones. An increased concentration of oxalate in the urine can occur in patients who have an excess absorption of dietary oxalate. Cystine can accumulate in the urine when there is defective transport of cystine out of the urine by the proximal tubules, allowing

If there is a sufficient amount of stone material for analysis, the composition of the stone can be determined. The value of knowing the composition of the stone is that information may be derived about the contributing factors to its formation.

cystine to reach a concentration at which it becomes insoluble in the urine. High concentrations of urinary uric acid are found in patients with gout, and such patients are predisposed to form urate stones, particularly when the urine has a pH below 5.4. Stones consisting of calcium carbonate and struvite ($MgNH_4PO_4$) can occur in patients with urinary tract infections, particularly those caused by *Proteus*. Many patients presenting with a kidney stone have no identifiable underlying cause for its formation.

Crystals are frequently observed in a microscopic urine examination, and the majority are normal urinary components. However, in patients predisposed to forming kidney stones, the crystals may provide information that suggests the composition of the stone.

Selected Additional Tests to Evaluate Renal Function

Cystatin C

Cystatin C is a low-molecular-weight protein of ~13,000 Da that is produced by the body at a constant rate. Because cystatin C appears to be cleared solely by the kidney, elevated cystatin C levels are inversely proportional to the GFR. Epidemiologic data demonstrate that increased cystatin C levels are positively correlated with mortality. Because creatinine measurements are readily available (and inexpensive) cystatin C is unlikely to replace creatinine clearance measurements in the near term.

Uric Acid

While it is true that uric acid concentrations rise as the GFR declines, uric acid is not a very helpful indicator of GFR. This is because serum uric acid levels vary widely according to diet. High-protein diets elevate uric acid, as does high cellular turnover. Neoplasias with high cellular turnover rates elevate uric acid as does cell death from chemotherapy. Uric acid levels are markedly affected by variation in the rates of production and reabsorption of uric acid, as found in patients with gout.

Calcium, Phosphate, and Parathyroid Hormone

Calcium, phosphate, and bone metabolism is impaired in patients with renal failure. PTH stimulates a net decrease in calcium excretion in the urine, as it stimulates calcium reabsorption in the distal tubule. PTH increases phosphate excretion into the urine, as it decreases the loss of calcium into urine. See Chapter 22 for additional information on this topic.

> Many patients presenting with a kidney stone have no identifiable underlying cause for its formation.

REFERENCES

Connolly JO, Woolfson RG. A critique of clinical guidelines for detection of individuals with chronic kidney disease. *Nephron Clin Pract.* 2009;111:c69–c73.

Eknoyan G, et al. *KDOQI Clinical Practice Guidelines for Chronic Kidney Disease: Evaluation, Classification, and Stratification.* http://www.kidney.org/professionals/KDOQI/guidelines_ckd/toc.htm. Accessed 28 May, 2009.

Kraut JA, Kurtz I. Metabolic acidosis of CKD: diagnosis, clinical characteristics, and treatment. *Am J Kidney Dis.* 2005;45(June):978–993.

Miller WG. Reporting estimated GFR: a laboratory perspective. *Am J Kidney Dis.* 2008;52 (October):645–648.

Myers GL, et al. National Kidney Disease Education Program Laboratory Working Group. Recommendations for improving serum creatinine measurement: a report from the Laboratory Working Group of the National Kidney Disease Education. *Clin Chem.* 2006;52(1):5–18.

Polkinghorne KR. Detection and measurement of urinary protein. *Curr Opin Nephrol Hypertens.* 2006;15(November):625–630.

Prigent A. Monitoring renal function and limitations of renal function tests. *Semin Nucl Med.* 2008;38 (January):32–46.

Thomas L, Huber AR. Renal function—estimation of glomerular filtration rate. *Clin Chem Lab Med.* 2006;44:1295–1302.

Vassalotti JA, et al. Testing for chronic kidney disease: a position statement from the National Kidney Foundation. *Am J Kidney Dis.* 2007;50(2):169–180.

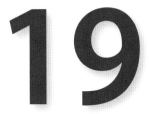

Male Genital Tract

D. Robert Dufour

LEARNING OBJECTIVES

1. Understand how prostate-specific antigen (PSA) is used in the diagnosis and monitoring of prostate cancer.

2. Learn how β-human chorionic gonadotropin (β-hCG), alpha-fetoprotein (AFP), and lactate dehydrogenase isoenzyme 1 (LDH-1) levels are used in the management of patients with certain germ cell testicular tumors.

3. Learn how tests of androgen metabolism and regulation can be used in diagnosis of male gonadal dysfunction.

CHAPTER OUTLINE

INTRODUCTION

The penis, the testes, the epididymis, and the prostate comprise the male genital tract. Circulating markers have been identified for prostate cancer and testicular cancer. For that reason, a discussion of these tumors and their serum markers is presented in this chapter (**Table 19–1**). Also, laboratory tests are often used in evaluating men with gonadal dysfunction. A summary of these tests and their usage is also provided. The male genital tract is the site of many infectious diseases, a significant proportion of which are sexually transmitted. These are discussed in Chapter 5.

PROSTATE CANCER

Description

Prostate cancer is a common malignancy of men that increases in incidence with age. It is the second most common cause of cancer death in males, behind only lung cancer. However, many cases are slowly progressive and do not cause major morbidity or lead to death. The unresolved challenge at this time is differentiating the rapidly progressive and fatal form of prostate cancer from the indolent forms that do not cause death. Mortality associated with the disease has been decreasing. This has been attributed by some to early detection, although a systematic review of published studies has shown no difference in prostate cancer mortality between those who have and those who have not been screened for the disease. Transrectal ultrasound instruments for tumor imaging and spring-loaded devices for biopsy collection have increased early detection. The use of laboratory assays to measure the serum prostate-specific antigen (PSA) concentration, however, has had the greatest impact on increased detection of this cancer.

TABLE 19-1   Clinical Utility of Serum Tumor Markers for Prostate Cancer and Testicular Cancer

Cancer Purpose	Prostate Cancer: Prostate-specific Antigen (PSA)	Testicular Germ Cell Tumors (LDH, AFP, HCG)
Screening	Controversial for men older than 50 years	Not useful
Establishing a diagnosis	Not useful	Can suggest histologic type(s) present, especially for small clusters of 1 tumor type that may be missed by histology
Indicator of disease extent	If PSA <20 ng/mL, bone metastasis unlikely	Of use in identifying clinically undetectable metastatic disease
Monitoring response to treatment	Useful to monitor success of treatment	Useful; markers should fall to undetectable with successful treatment
Monitoring for recurrence	Useful	Useful

Prostate-specific Antigen

PSA is an enzyme (part of the kallikrein family, also called human kallikrein 3) synthesized almost exclusively by the prostate and secreted into the seminal fluid. A small amount is also found in the blood. In the blood, PSA is largely bound to enzyme inhibitors such as alpha$_1$-antichymotrypsin and alpha$_2$-macroglobulin. A small fraction of circulating PSA is free.

PSA levels in blood are related to the size of the prostate. The larger the gland, the higher the PSA value. PSA may also increase transiently after a vigorous rectal examination, and after prostate biopsy or surgery. Inflammation and infarction of the prostate can also cause increased PSA, which returns to normal gradually. It is therefore recommended that PSA levels should be confirmed to be elevated by repeat measurement (at least 2 to 3 months apart) before any other action is taken, to exclude 1 of these insignificant causes of high PSA.

Prostate disease is common in men after the age of 50 years, and by age 70 years the majority of men have prostate disease. The 2 major diseases of the aging prostate are prostate carcinoma and benign prostatic hyperplasia (BPH). A number of factors have been evaluated to try to distinguish these causes of increased prostate size and/or increased PSA levels. In most laboratories, normal values for PSA are generally considered <4 ng/mL. In general, PSA is increased to a greater extent in prostate cancer than in BPH; PSA is rarely >20 ng/mL in BPH, and in only about 10% of cases is it >10 ng/mL, so higher values suggest cancer. A high PSA in a man with a small prostate gland on rectal examination is more worrisome for cancer than a similar PSA value in a person with a very large gland. The ratio of free PSA/total PSA may be a better diagnostic marker for prostate cancer than total PSA; in general, a lower proportion of free PSA is found in patients with prostate cancer, but there is a wide overlap in values.

PSA has been used for several purposes related to prostate cancer: screening (testing in persons without symptoms or signs of disease), prediction of course of disease, prediction of stage of disease, and follow-up after treatment. The most controversial use of PSA measurements is in screening. While several professional organizations recommend screening for prostate cancer, others do not or they suggest discussion between patients and doctors on a case-by-case basis. In 2008, the United States Preventive Services Task Force concluded that, in men over age 70 years, screening for prostate cancer actually caused more harm than good. The reason for this disagreement is that, to date, no evidence exists from controlled trials that persons identified with cancer by PSA screening have a lower likelihood of dying from prostate cancer. In a systematic review of screening programs, only 2 studies were found that evaluated screening in this way, and in those there was no difference in cancer mortality between those detected by screening and those not screened. Currently, 3 large prospective studies are underway to evaluate the benefits of screening, but the results will not be available till after 2010 at the earliest. It should be noted that PSA is not highly sensitive for detecting cancer. It is estimated that only about 50% to 60% of those with localized, and potentially curable, cancer have increased PSA,

PSA has been used for several purposes related to prostate cancer: screening (testing in persons without symptoms or signs of disease), prediction of course of disease, prediction of stage of disease, and follow-up after treatment. The most controversial use of PSA measurements is in screening.

and recent studies have found that many patients with less well-differentiated cancers actually have PSA values as low as 1 ng/mL.

Limited evidence suggests that the rate of rise in PSA can predict more aggressive cancers. A review of published studies found that persons with more rapid rises in PSA (a rise >0.35 ng/mL/ year 10 years before definitive diagnosis, or a rise >2 ng/mL in the year before definitive diagnosis) were far more likely to have recurrence after surgery and to die from cancer than those with more slowly rising PSA. In men who have decided to not have surgery, the rate of rise of PSA was also found to be predictive; if the PSA doubling time was less than 3 years, the likelihood of locally progressive disease was high, while it was very low for those whose PSA increased less than 2-fold over 10 years. More studies will be needed to confirm these findings and to determine whether this information can be useful in determining treatment.

PSA measurement is of some use in the initial staging of a patient with prostate cancer. In general, the higher the PSA, the less likely that cancer is localized to the prostate and the more likely that it has spread. Distant metastases are rare in persons with PSA <20 ng/mL, so performance of imaging studies of bone (the most common site of metastasis) for preoperative staging of cancer has little benefit in those with lower PSA values.

The most widely accepted use of PSA is to monitor patients after treatment. Since about 99% of prostate cancers produce PSA, and since PSA is made almost solely in the prostate, successful surgical removal of the gland (and cancer) should result in the loss of detectable PSA from the blood by 3 months after surgery. Failure of PSA to become undetectable indicates residual cancer that was not removed by surgery. With recurrence of cancer, PSA levels increase up to a year and a half before clinical evidence of recurrent cancer, allowing treatment of persons with rising PSA before their clinical condition deteriorates. With radiation therapy, PSA typically will fall to normal (usually to <1 ng/mL by 1 year after completion of radiation) with successful treatment, but will usually not be undetectable. Because prostate cancer responds to androgens, removal of the testes and the use of drugs that block androgen production are widely used to treat metastatic prostate cancer. The production of PSA is also androgen dependent. Rarely, PSA levels will fall dramatically with androgen deprivation even though there is little or no change in the amount of tumor. In most cases, though, PSA is a reliable marker of tumor response to androgen deprivation as a treatment for prostate cancer.

TESTICULAR CANCER

Description

Germ cell tumors and sex cord or stromal tumors are the 2 major categories of testicular tumors. Seminomas and nonseminomatous germ cell tumors (NSGCT) are the major groups of germ cell tumors, and more than 90% of testicular cancers arise from them. Most persons with germ cell tumors have a mixture of histologic varieties. Testicular germ cell tumors have a peak incidence in 15- to 34-year-old males, and are the most common type of tumor found in men of that age group. Testicular cancer is most commonly identified by finding an enlarged testicle during a routine physical or by a man on self-examination. If an ultrasound examination confirms the presence of an intratesticular mass, surgery is usually performed quickly to remove the testicle, its adnexa, and a long segment of the spermatic cord (radical orchiectomy). The diagnosis of testicular cancer, like most other cancers, is thus made by histopathologic examination of the testicle.

More than 90% of testicular cancers arise from germ cell tumors. Germ cell tumors often produce substances that can be used as tumor markers to evaluate the patient for complete removal of the tumor, detect recurrent cancer, and monitor treatment for any residual or recurrent tumor.

Diagnosis

Germ cell tumors often produce substances that can be used as tumor markers to evaluate the patient for complete removal of the tumor, detect recurrent cancer, and monitor treatment for any residual or recurrent tumor. Seminoma is associated with increased levels of the enzyme lactate dehydrogenase (LDH), particularly LDH isoenzyme 1 (LDH-1), in about 50% of cases, and also with the production of human chorionic gonadotropin (hCG). Of the NSGCT, several additional tumor markers may be useful. Yolk sac tumors produce alpha-fetoprotein (AFP), a normal product of the fetal liver and yolk sac, in about 90% of cases. Choriocarcinoma, a malignant tumor resembling the placental cells, produces hCG in close to 100% of cases. Because of the mixture of elements present in a given tumor, overall about 90% of patients with germ cell tumors have increases in hCG, AFP, LDH, or in all 3. As is generally true for circulating tumor markers, they are most useful for monitoring recurrence of disease or as a measure of response to therapy. Neither hCG nor AFP is useful in screening patients for testicular tumors, and they also have a limited role in establishing the diagnosis. Higher levels of hCG and LDH-1 at the time of diagnosis are associated with more aggressive cancers and, overall, a less favorable outcome.

hCG, LDH, and AFP are significantly affected by diseases in other organs. LDH is found in all cells. Therefore, damage to any cell can cause increased LDH. Since red blood cells contain LDH, a sample collected for LDH measurement in which there is red blood cell hemolysis will show an elevated LDH, with much of the LDH originating from red blood cells. This is also particularly problematic in the setting of chemotherapy, where transient increases occur from the cell damage expected from chemotherapy treatment. AFP is also produced by hepatocytes, as discussed in Chapter 16. Injury to the liver, as occurs with acute or chronic hepatitis, also commonly causes mild to moderate increases in AFP that can lead to suspicion of recurrent testicular carcinoma.

MALE GONADAL DYSFUNCTION

Description

While complete gonadal failure in men is rare (and is discussed more fully in Chapter 22), partial androgen deficiency is common with advancing age in men. This has also sometimes been referred to as andropause, and considered by some to be analogous to menopause, the age-related gonadal failure in women. There are a number of differences between age-related declines in gonadal function in men and women, however. While gonadal failure is inevitable in women, not all men develop low levels of testosterone. While menopause typically occurs between the mid-40s and mid-50s, partial androgen deficiency develops over a much broader age range in men. Estrogen and progesterone levels fall to extremely low levels in women and are accompanied by high gonadotropin (FSH and LH) levels. However, partial androgen deficiency in men is associated with mildly decreased testosterone levels and is usually not associated with abnormally high gonadotropin levels. According to the Endocrine Society consensus guidelines, only 7% of men in their 40s have low androgen levels. However, the figure rises to 30% of men in their 50s, almost half of those in their 60s, and to 90% of men in their 80s. As in women, routine use of hormone replacement in men is controversial. Androgens increase muscle and bone mass, and may protect against falls and bone fractures. Androgen deficiency can cause mood changes and sexual dysfunction, both of which may respond to androgen treatment. On the negative side, however, androgens are involved in the pathogenesis of both BPH and prostate cancer, and cause undesirable changes in blood lipids, which may increase the risk of myocardial infarction and stroke. Limited data on safety and effectiveness of androgen replacement are available, but a small placebo-controlled study published in 2006 found no clear benefit of androgen replacement.

7% of men in their 40s have low androgen levels. However, the figure rises to 30% of men in their 50s, almost half of those in their 60s, and to 90% of men in their 80s.

Diagnosis

Laboratory testing for partial androgen deficiency generally begins with measurement of serum testosterone. Normal levels are often stated to be greater than 250 to 350 ng/dL. Androgen deficiency is unlikely to be present if the total testosterone is >400 ng/dL. A problem with evaluation of total testosterone levels is that changes in the level of testosterone-binding proteins are common. Free testosterone, not bound to proteins, contributes significantly more to the biological effects of testosterone than does protein-bound testosterone. However, it is widely believed that testosterone bound to albumin (about 40% of total) may contribute partially to the biological effects of testosterone. The major testosterone-binding protein, sex hormone-binding globulin (SHBG), is increased by androgen deficiency, but decreased by obesity, both common problems in older men. Ideally, free testosterone is quantitated, but some assays for measurement of free testosterone are unreliable. This has led to the use of tests to determine "bioavailable testosterone," which are most helpful in those with testosterone levels between 200 and 400 ng/dL.

Transient decreases in testosterone and gonadotropin levels are commonly seen in persons who are acutely ill. Testing of gonadal function should be avoided in hospitalized individuals for that reason. Certain medications, as well as opiates and ethanol, can cause transient decreases as well.

In those with low testosterone, guidelines suggest measurement of LH. Generally, FSH follows LH and does not add additional information. It is expected that LH levels usually fall within the reference limits in age-related partial androgen deficiency. Very low levels of LH suggest a pituitary or hypothalamic problem, and require further evaluation of pituitary function, while high levels of LH suggest other causes of a low androgen level.

REFERENCES

Prostate Cancer

Amling CL. Prostate specific antigen and detection of prostate cancer: what have we learned and what should we recommend for screening? *Curr Treat Options Oncol.* 2006;7:337–345.

Carter HB, et al. Detection of life-threatening prostate cancer with prostate-specific antigen velocity during a window of curability. *J Natl Cancer Inst.* 2005;98:1521–1527.

D'Amico AV, et al. Preoperative PSA velocity and the risk of death from prostate cancer after radical prostatectomy. *N Engl J Med.* 2004;351:125–135.

Ilic D, et al. Screening for prostate cancer. *Cochrane Database Syst Rev. 3,* 2006.

Lin K, et al. U.S. Preventive Services Task Force: benefits and harms of prostate-specific antigen screening for prostate cancer: an evidence update for the U.S. Preventive Services Task Force. *Ann Intern Med.* 2008;149:192–199.

Nelson WG, et al. Mechanisms of disease: prostate cancer. *N Engl J Med.* 2003;349:366–381.

Oesterling JE, et al. The use of prostate specific antigen in staging patients with newly diagnosed prostate cancer. *JAMA.* 1993;269:57.

Thompson IM, et al. Prevalence of prostate cancer among men with a prostate-specific antigen level ≤4 ng per milliliter. *N Engl J Med.* 2004;350:2239–2246.

van den Bergh RC, et al. Prostate-specific antigen kinetics in clinical decision-making during active surveillance for early prostate cancer—a review. *Eur Urol.* 2008;54:505–516.

Testicular Cancer

Stenman UH Testicular cancer: the perfect paradigm for marker combinations. *Scand J Clin Lab Invest.* 2005;65:181–188.

Sturgeon CM, et al. National Academy of Clinical Biochemistry laboratory medicine practice guidelines for use of tumor markers in testicular, prostate, colorectal, breast, and ovarian cancers. *Clin Chem.* 2008;54(12):e11–e79.

von Eyben FE. Laboratory markers and germ cell tumors. *Crit Rev Clin Lab Sci.* 2003;40:377–427.

Male Sexual Dysfunction

AACE Male Sexual Dysfunction Task Force. American Association of Clinical Endocrinologists medical guidelines for clinical practice for the evaluation and treatment of male sexual dysfunction: a couple's problem—2003 update. *Endocr Pract.* 2003;91:77–95.

Allan CA, McLachlan RI. Age-related changes in testosterone and the role of replacement therapy in older men. *Clin Endocrinol (Oxf).* 2004;60:653–670.

Isidori AM, et al. Androgen deficiency and hormone-replacement therapy. *BJU Int.* 2005;96:212–216.

Nair KS, et al. DHEA in elderly women and DHEA or testosterone in elderly men. *N Engl J Med.* 2005;355:1647–1669.

Female Genital System

Stacy E.F. Melanson

INTRODUCTION

There are many conditions affecting the female genital system that involve clinical laboratory testing. These are reviewed in this chapter. The female genital tract is a common site for infections, which may be sexually transmitted, and it is a common site for tumors. The infections are presented in Chapter 5, and tumor descriptions are found in textbooks of anatomic pathology.

NORMAL PREGNANCY

Description

Normal pregnancy lasts approximately 40 weeks, as dated from the first day of the previous menstrual period, and is typically divided into three intervals or trimesters each lasting approximately 13 weeks. Five days after fertilization, a blastocyst implants in the uterus. Trophoblast cells of the blastocyst invade the endometrium with chorionic villi leading to a placenta and forming the embryo surrounded by amniotic fluid. The placenta nourishes the embryo and produces hormones vital to pregnancy such as human chorionic gonadotropin (hCG), progesterone, estradiol, estriol, and estrone. The amniotic fluid protects the embryo and changes composition as the pregnancy progresses. Lipids are a major component of the amniotic fluid and may reflect fetal lung maturity as discussed in Chapter 14. The embryo undergoes rapid cell division, differentiation, and growth in the first trimester (0 to 13 weeks). By 10 weeks, most major structures are

TABLE 20–1   Routine Testing in Normal Pregnancy

Test	Result in Pregnancy	Comments
Chemistry		
hCG	>10 IU/L	Should double every 2 days for the first 8 weeks
1st-trimester screen (free beta hCG, PAPP-A)	Dependent on multiple factors	To assess for trisomy 21
2nd-trimester "quad" screen (hCG, AFP, estriol, inhibin A)	Dependent on multiple factors	To assess for trisomy 21, neural tube defects, and other fetal anomalies
1-Hour glucose loading test	60 minutes: <140 mg/dL	To assess for gestational diabetes mellitus
Hematology		
Hematocrit	36%–48%	To assess for anemia
Blood bank		
Blood type	A, B, AB, O	Type and screen includes blood type, Rh typing, and antibody screen to assess for and/or help prevent HDN
Rh typing	Rh-positive/Rh-negative	
Antibody detection	Negative	
Microbiology		
Rubella screen, IgG	Positive/immune	All microbiology tests are performed to screen for immunity and to prevent adverse fetal outcome
Toxoplasma IgG	Negative	
Treponema pallidum IgG	Negative	To assess for syphilis
Hepatitis B surface antibody	Positive/immune	To assess for exposure to vaccine
Hepatitis B surface antigen	Negative	To assess for active hepatitis B
HIV antibody	Negative	To assess for exposure to HIV
Cervical culture for *gonorrhoeae* and *Chlamydia*	Negative	
Group B strep (GBS)	No group B beta hemolytic streptococci isolated	

Note: Results/reference values are laboratory dependent. hCG, human chorionic gonadotropin; PAPP-A, pregnancy-associated plasma protein-A; AFP, alpha-fetoprotein; HDN, hemolytic disease of the newborn.

Pregnancy has an effect on many laboratory tests, and these alterations should be considered when interpreting laboratory tests on pregnant women.

formed resulting in a fetus. The second trimester (13 to 26 weeks) is associated with rapid fetal growth. Completion of maturation occurs in the third trimester (26 to 40 weeks) resulting in a term pregnancy between 37 and 42 weeks.

Diagnosis

Ideally women should consult a physician prior to conception for a full medical examination. Once pregnancy has been achieved, many laboratory tests are routinely performed to help ensure an optimal maternal and fetal outcome (**Table 20–1**). Laboratory testing in complicated or abnormal pregnancies will be discussed later in the chapter. Most testing in pregnancy is performed on maternal serum because it is easy to obtain and provides minimal risk to the pregnancy, but maternal urine and amniotic fluid specimens may also be necessary. Pregnancy has an effect on many laboratory tests, and these alterations should be considered when interpreting laboratory tests on pregnant women (**Table 20–2**).

TABLE 20-2 **Effects of Pregnancy on Select Laboratory Tests**

Test	Result in Pregnancy	Comments
Hematocrit	Decreased	Due to an increased plasma volume
Coagulation factors	Several factors increase; some do not change; Factor XI decreases	The overall effect is an increased thrombotic risk
Lipids (triglycerides, cholesterol)	Increased	
Thyroxine-binding globulin, total T3 and T4	Increased	Patient remains euthyroid
Alkaline phosphatase activity	Increased	Due to production of placental, heat-stable, alkaline phosphatase
BUN, creatinine	Slightly decreased	Due to increased glomerular filtration rate
1,25-Dihydroxy vitamin D	Increased	Due to increased calcium and transfer of calcium to fetus
Parathyroid hormone	Increased	Ionized calcium remains normal

hCG is heterodimer composed of two nonidentical nonconvalently bound glycoprotein subunits, alpha and beta, that is synthesized by the syncytiotrophoblasts of the placenta. Only the intact molecule is biologically active. A single gene for the alpha subunit of all four glycoprotein hormones (thyroid-stimulating hormone [TSH], luteinizing hormone [LH], follicle-stimulating hormone [FSH], and hCG) is found on chromosome 6. hCG stimulates the LH receptor on the corpus luteum to produce progesterone and prevent pregnancy loss.

Detectable amounts of hCG (approximately 5 IU/L) are present in serum 8 to 11 days after conception, and hCG levels can be measured either qualitatively or quantitatively to diagnosis pregnancy (**Table 20-1**). Qualitative tests in urine or serum are usually sufficient for diagnosis, but the detection limits of qualitative tests range from 20 to 50 IU/L, limiting their use to the time following a missed menstrual period or greater than 11 days after conception. Home testing for hCG is available, and provides a qualitative measurement of urine hCG. First morning urine specimens are generally recommended for either qualitative laboratory or home-testing kits as they are concentrated and contain the most abundant hCG. As opposed to qualitative testing, quantitative testing offers a sensitivity as low as 2 to 5 IU/L and may be helpful to reveal problems in a pregnancy or predict prognosis in patients with a pregnancy complication, as will be discussed later in this chapter. In normal pregnancies, hCG doubles every 2 days for the first 8 weeks and peaks around 100,000 to 500,000 IU/L.

The serum contains many forms of hCG, including free subunits, hyperglycosylated and nicked forms, but the urine contains primarily free beta hCG. In addition, the hCG carbohydrate composition changes as the pregnancy progresses. Available hCG immunoassays for the diagnosis of pregnancy typically measure total hCG levels using antibodies either to both the alpha and beta subunits or to the intact molecule. False-negative results can be seen in early or abnormal pregnancies, in samples exposed to temperature or pH extremes, and in samples showing gross hemolysis, lipemia, or turbidity. False-positive results can be seen in gestational trophoblastic disease or in patient samples with heterophilic antibodies or interfering substances. In the first trimester, false-positives can be differentiated from normal pregnancies by the lack of doubling every 2 days.

Additional routine testing in pregnancy is performed to screen for common and/or treatable pregnancy complications such as anemia, hemolytic disease of the newborn (HDN), gestational diabetes mellitus (GDM), and infection (**Tables 20-1** and **20-2**). Maternal serum screening for conditions such as anemia is discussed below. HDN is a fetal hemolytic disorder caused by maternal antibodies directed against antigens on fetal erythrocytes, and maternal antibodies destroy fetal erythrocytes. Sensitization of women to fetal antigens usually occurs after a prior pregnancy or a previous blood transfusion. HDN is most common in D antigen-negative women who form antibodies due to the presence of the D antigen on fetal red blood cells. Severe forms lead to

Qualitative tests in urine or serum are usually sufficient for diagnosis, but the detection limits of qualitative tests range from 20 to 50 IU/L, limiting their use to the time following a missed menstrual period or greater than 14 days after conception.

hydrops fetalis and fetal demise. The severity of the erythrocyte destruction can be monitored by measuring the level of bilirubin in the amniotic fluid and/or the antibody titer. See Chapters 7 and 12 for more information on HDN. A positive screen on the glucose loading test is usually followed by a longer glucose challenge to confirm the diagnosis of GDM. Chapter 17 has a discussion of GDM. Infections during pregnancy or peripartum can contribute to fetal morbidity and mortality if left untreated. Additional discussions of infectious diseases are found in Chapter 5.

MATERNAL SERUM SCREENING

Description

Maternal serum screening can be performed to predict the risk of fetal anomalies, most commonly open neural tube defects (NTD), trisomy 21/Down syndrome, and trisomy 18. NTD result from failure of fusion of the neural plate and complete covering by the 27th day postconception. The extent and location of neural tissue exposed indicates the severity of the defect (i.e., anencephaly, meningomyelocele, and encephalocele). The result of a NTD is a direct communication of the amniotic fluid with fetal plasma proteins, and release of alpha-fetoprotein (AFP) into amniotic fluid and maternal serum. Rates of NTDs have decreased due to the addition of folic acid to grain as well as initiation of campaigns to recommend folic acid supplementation prior to conception. Trisomy 21 or Down syndrome is caused by an extra copy of chromosome 21 and is the most frequent chromosomal disorder among live-born children (1/600 to 1/800 live births). Risk factors for Down syndrome include advanced maternal age, the birth of a previously affected child, and balanced parental structural rearrangement of chromosome 21. Affected children suffer from mental retardation, hypotonia, congenital heart defects, and a flat facial profile. The main phenotypic features of trisomy 18 include hypertonia, prominent occiput, small mouth, micrognathia, short sternum, and horseshoe kidney.

> Maternal serum screening can be performed to predict the risk of fetal anomalies, most commonly open neural tube defects (NTD), trisomy 21/Down syndrome, and trisomy 18.

Diagnosis

The goal of maternal serum screening is to identify individuals who need further diagnostic evaluation for fetal anomalies such as NTD, trisomy 21, or trisomy 18 (**Table 20–3**). The first-trimester screen includes free beta hCG, pregnancy-associated plasma protein-A (PAPP-A), and nuchal

TABLE 20–3   First- and Second-Trimester Maternal Serum Screening

Maternal Serum Screen	Abnormal Results (<0.5 MoM or >2.0 MoM)	Indication
1st trimester (10–14 weeks) Free beta hCG PAPP-A Nuchal translucency		
	Increased free beta hCG Decreased PAPP-A Increased nuchal translucency	Risk of trisomy 21
2nd trimester (15–22 weeks) Total hCG AFP Estriol Inhibin A		
	Decreased AFP Increased hCG Decreased estriol Increased Inhibin A	Risk of trisomy 21
	Decreased AFP Decreased hCG Decreased estriol	Risk of trisomy 18
	Increased AFP	Risk of neural tube defect

hCG, human chorionic gonadotropin; PAPP-A, pregnancy-associated plasma protein-A; AFP, alpha-fetoprotein.

translucency (NT). The second-trimester "triple screen" (AFP, hCG, and estriol) has been available for many years and has recently been enhanced to create a second-trimester "quad screen" (AFP, hCG, estriol, and inhibin A). The quad screen and the first-trimester screen demonstrate increased sensitivity for Down syndrome detection and offer the potential for earlier diagnosis and management of fetal anomalies. First-trimester screening should be performed between 10 and 13 weeks, although 11 weeks appears to be the optimal time. Second-trimester screening is usually performed between 15 and 22 weeks.

First-trimester screening between 10 and 14 weeks is primarily performed to screen for trisomy 21 (**Table 20–3**). Free beta hCG is more accurate than intact hCG in the first trimester and is used instead of intact hCG for the first-trimester screen. PAPP-A is a protein produced by the placenta, and low levels have been associated with a risk of trisomy 21. NT is detected by ultrasound, not in the clinical laboratory. If an abnormal first-trimester screen is obtained, chorionic villus sampling, as opposed to amniocentesis, can be performed to obtain a sample for karotyping.

With regard to the individual markers in the second-trimester screening, AFP is the most abundant serum protein in the fetal circulation. It enters amniotic fluid through micturition and then diffuses to the placenta and into the maternal circulation. Maternal serum AFP is detectable at 10 weeks and peaks at 15 to 20 weeks. hCG function and measurement has been discussed previously. Estriol is the predominant estrogen of pregnancy and also the most difficult to measure because of low concentration and limited stability. Inhibin A, secreted by the ovaries and placenta, is a glycoprotein that inhibits FSH. Importantly, "normal" levels of AFP, hCG, estriol, and inhibin A are dependent on and are adjusted for gestational age, maternal weight, number of fetuses, and presence or absence of diabetes mellitus. Typically the laboratory provides absolute numbers to the genetic counselor caring for the patient. The genetic counselor ensures that the patient's history is accurate, adjusts the results according to the above-mentioned factors, and expresses the results in multiples of the median (MoM). Levels less than 0.5 MoM or greater than 2.0 MoM are generally considered abnormal. **Table 20–3** lists the results commonly associated with the risk of fetal anomalies. The most frequent causes of abnormal results include incorrect dating, the presence of twins, and fetal demise. For this reason, an ultrasound confirming the patient's history is the first line of testing in a patient with abnormal levels of any of the screening markers. Elevated amniotic fluid levels of AFP and acetylcholinesterase can predict the presence of NTDs more accurately than the second-trimester screen and should be performed if elevated serum levels of AFP are confirmed. Fetal karotyping is necessary to confirm chromosomal abnormalities.

ECTOPIC PREGNANCY

Description

Ectopic pregnancies arise if the fertilized egg implants in a location other than the body of the uterus, primarily in the fallopian tube. Of all reported pregnancies, 1.3% to 2% are extrauterine. The nonuterine location of implantation prevents normal development. Despite increased awareness and improved diagnostic modalities, such as serial hCG and transvaginal ultrasound, ectopic pregnancies remain a leading cause of maternal morbidity and occasionally mortality. Risk factors for ectopic pregnancy include tubal damage from either infection or disease, smoking, infertility, and previous miscarriage.

Diagnosis

Three classic symptoms of an ectopic pregnancy include lower abdominal pain, vaginal bleeding, and an adnexal mass. However, only 25% of women with ectopic pregnancy have these symptoms at the time of presentation, making laboratory testing and transvaginal ultrasound examination essential for diagnosis and management. In ectopic pregnancies, abnormal concentrations of hCG are present (**Table 20–4**). hCG concentrations in ectopic pregnancy range from undetectable to 200,000 IU/L, depending on the size and viability of the trophoblastic tissue. Levels typically are found to be in the range of 1,000 IU/L. Serial testing also reveals rates of hCG increase as slow as 35% over 2 days in ectopic pregnancy. Medical therapy with methotrexate or surgical management is available to women diagnosed with an ectopic pregnancy.

Three classic symptoms of an ectopic pregnancy include lower abdominal pain, vaginal bleeding, and an adnexal mass. However, only 25% of women with ectopic pregnancy have these symptoms at the time of presentation, making laboratory testing and transvaginal ultrasound examination essential for diagnosis and management.

TABLE 20-4   **Abnormal Pregnancy Conditions**

Condition	Laboratory Diagnosis
Ectopic pregnancy	Abnormal concentration and slow rate of increase in hCG
Gestational trophoblastic disease	Rise in serum hCG beyond that expected for gestational age
Pre-eclampsia	Modest increase in AST and ALT (4–10× upper limit) >0.3 g/L protein in 24-hour urine >1.0 g/L protein in random specimen
HELLP syndrome	Decreased platelets (<100,000 µL^{-1}) Elevated LDH (>600 IU/L) Elevated ALT and AST (200–700 IU/L)
Fatty liver of pregnancy	Mild increase in AST and ALT (AST > ALT) Serum bilirubin >6 mg/dL Hypoglycemia Increased uric acid Prolonged PT and PTT Low fibrinogen

hCG, human chorionic gonadotropin; PT, prothrombin time; PTT, partial thromboplastin time.

SPONTANEOUS ABORTION (MISCARRIAGE) AND RECURRENT ABORTION

Description

Spontaneous abortion or miscarriage refers to a pregnancy that ends spontaneously before the fetus has reached a viable gestational age. The most common complication of early pregnancy is spontaneous abortion, and it occurs in approximately 10% to 20% of all recognized pregnancies under 20 weeks gestation. The percentage increases if unrecognized or subclinical pregnancies are included. Risk factors include advancing maternal age, previous miscarriage, smoking, and alcohol or drug consumption. Chromosomal abnormalities account for approximately 50% of all miscarriages.

Recurrent spontaneous abortion is defined as three or more consecutive intrauterine pregnancy losses prior to the 20 to 24 weeks of gestation. It affects up to 1% to 5% of fertile couples. Primary aborters have had no live births, while secondary aborters were able to achieve at least one successful pregnancy. Assisted reproduction technologies are much less effective in women with recurrent fetal losses compared to those with infertility.

> The most common complication of early pregnancy is spontaneous abortion, and it occurs in approximately 10% to 20% of all recognized pregnancies under 20 weeks gestation.

Diagnosis

Women experiencing a miscarriage may present with a history of amenorrhea, vaginal bleeding, and lower abdominal pain. Serial measurements of hCG concentration in conjunction with physical examination and ultrasonography can be helpful in the diagnosis of spontaneous abortion. Decreasing hCG concentrations are consistent with a spontaneous abortion or nonviable pregnancy. Patients with a confirmed miscarriage can be managed expectantly, medically with misoprostol, or surgically. Following treatment, hCG levels can be monitored until the concentration is undetectable to confirm complete expulsion of products of conception. It may take 30 to 60 days before serum hCG levels are undetectable. The etiology of recurrent loss is often unclear, but can include genetic, anatomic, hormonal, thrombotic, placental, infectious, environmental, or psychological causes. Immunological factors may also play a role. Following a detailed history, physical examination, and radiological studies, certain laboratory tests may be helpful in determining the cause of the recurrent loss (**Table 20–5**). Of all the etiologic factors, only parental genetics has been shown to be a definitive cause of recurrent loss. Although uterine abnormalities, antiphospholipid antibodies, the Factor V Leiden mutation, and other thrombotic risk factors are definitely associated with recurrent loss, there is not sufficient proof of a causative role.

TABLE 20–5 Laboratory Evaluation of Recurrent Spontaneous Abortion

Analysis	Purpose
Parental and fetal tissue karotype	Tests for chromosomal abnormalities
LH, FSH, thyroid-stimulating hormone, prolactin	Tests for endocrine abnormalities
Thrombotic risk factors including protein C, protein S, antithrombin, Factor V Leiden and prothrombin gene 20210 mutations, Lupus anticoagulant, anticardiolipin antibodies	Tests for thrombophilic disorders
Antithyroid antibodies	Tests for autoimmune factors
Endometrial biopsy	Tests for luteal phase defect or inadequate endometrial maturation

GESTATIONAL TROPHOBLASTIC DISEASE

Description

Gestational trophoblastic diseases are a spectrum of disease processes originating from the placenta that include hydatidiform mole, invasive mole, and choriocarcinoma. Malignant gestational trophoblastic diseases have the potential for local invasion and metastasis.

Hydatidiform moles are the most common and occur in 1 of 600 therapeutic abortions and 1 of 1,100 pregnancies. Approximately 20% of patients will be treated for malignant sequelae after evacuation of a hydatidiform mole. Gestational choriocarcinoma occurs in approximately 1 in 30,000 pregnancies.

Diagnosis

Gestational trophoblastic diseases are usually diagnosed early in pregnancy. Patients present with abnormal bleeding and vague complaints. Ultrasound and serum hCG testing are used to make the diagnosis of gestational trophoblastic diseases. Ultrasound findings include the absence of a fetal heartbeat. hCG testing reveals hCG levels elevated beyond those expected for gestational age (**Table 20–4**). In addition, the free beta hCG/total hCG is higher in gestational trophoblastic disease than in normal pregnancies. Dilation and evacuation (D&E) procedures are performed to treat patients. Serial hCG measurements should be performed to ensure complete removal of tumor and monitoring of disease for recurrence. Chemotherapy may be necessary in cases of malignant transformation.

PRE-ECLAMPSIA AND ECLAMPSIA

Description

Pre-eclampsia is a multisystem disorder of unknown etiology, and it is a major cause of morbidity and mortality in pregnancy. Patients develop elevated blood pressure and proteinuria. In addition, coagulopathies, impaired liver function, renal failure, and cerebral ischemia may occur. Pre-eclampsia occurs in 2% to 8% of pregnancies. Eclampsia, in which women with pre-eclampsia have accompanying seizures, occurs less frequently. Eclampsia is more serious and carries a higher morbidity and mortality rate. Treatment includes controlling symptoms until delivery.

> Pre-eclampsia is a multisystem disorder of unknown etiology, and it is a major cause of morbidity and mortality in pregnancy. Pre-eclampsia is diagnosed by the occurrence of new hypertension and proteinuria in the second half of pregnancy.

Diagnosis

Pre-eclampsia is diagnosed by the occurrence of new hypertension and proteinuria in the second half of pregnancy. Hypertension in pregnancy is defined as a persistent systolic blood pressure ≥140 mmHg and/or a diastolic blood pressure ≥90 mmHg. Proteinuria is >300 mg/L protein in a 24-hour urine specimen or >1 g/L protein in a single urine specimen (**Table 20–4**). It should be demonstrated that seizures associated with eclampsia are not explained by a neurological disorder such as epilepsy.

HELLP SYNDROME

Description

The HELLP syndrome involves **h**emolysis, **e**levated **l**iver enzymes, and a **l**ow **p**latelet count. The syndrome can occur during pregnancy, typically between weeks 27 and 36, or in association with pre-eclampsia; it can also occur postpartum.

Diagnosis

The HELLP syndrome and pre-eclampsia have similar clinical presentations. A low platelet count and abnormal liver enzymes are important to make a diagnosis of the HELLP syndrome. The hemolysis in the HELLP syndrome is microangiopathic, and this results in schistocytes on the peripheral blood smear, an elevated indirect bilirubin, and an increased lactate dehydrogenase (LDH) activity.

FATTY LIVER OF PREGNANCY

Description

Approximately 1 in 13,000 pregnancies is affected by fatty liver of pregnancy. First pregnancies and multiple gestation pregnancies are at a higher risk. Symptoms, which are nonspecific and include nausea and vomiting, right upper quadrant pain, and lethargy, typically begin around the 36th week of gestation. Liver biopsies show accumulation of microvesicular fat, which may be caused by a defect in mitochondrial beta oxidation of fatty acids or a long-chain 3-hydroxyacyl CoA dehydrogenase deficiency. Treatment involves immediate delivery to prevent fulminant hepatic failure and liver transplant. Recurrence in subsequent pregnancies is rare.

Diagnosis

The diagnosis is made using both clinical symptoms and laboratory results. Although liver biopsy is virtually diagnostic in the setting of pregnancy, it is rarely necessary. The laboratory-test abnormalities include mild elevations in liver enzymes (AST > ALT), increased bilirubin, hypoglycemia, and hyperuricemia (**Table 20–4**). Abnormal coagulation test results, as indicated by a prolonged prothrombin time, a prolonged partial thromboplastin time, and a low fibrinogen, are found in acute fatty liver of pregnancy but not HELLP syndrome, and this helps differentiate the two conditions.

MALE AND FEMALE INFERTILITY

Description

Infertility is defined as the inability to achieve a successful pregnancy following 1 year of unprotected intercourse. It is estimated that 25% of couples will experience an episode of infertility. Couples with primary infertility have had no previous successful pregnancies. Couples with secondary infertility had prior pregnancies, but are currently unable to conceive. Both primary and secondary infertility have common causes, most often problems with the hypothalamic–pituitary–gonadal axis.

Diagnosis

Although male infertility is thought to cause 30% to 50% of cases of infertility, it may simply cause delayed conception in normal female partners. In many cases, the cause of infertility cannot be determined. Factors contributing to male infertility include endocrine (discussed in Chapter 22), anatomic, and psychosocial causes, abnormal spermatogenesis, and abnormal sperm motility. Following a detailed history and physical examination, laboratory evaluation of male infertility begins with a semen analysis (**Table 20–6**). Semen analysis should be performed after 2 to 3 days of sexual abstinence, and the specimen must be delivered to the laboratory within 1 hour of the time of collection and kept warm during transport. Some laboratories provide areas for specimen collection adjacent to the laboratory. The basic evaluation of semen includes semen volume,

Infertility is defined as the inability to achieve a successful pregnancy following 1 year of unprotected intercourse. It is estimated that 25% of couples will experience an episode of infertility.

TABLE 20-6   Laboratory Evaluation of Male and Female Infertility

Analysis	Purpose
Male	
Semen analysis	Tests for sperm inadequacy
Female	
Midluteal progesterone	Helps predict ovulation and formation of corpus luteum
Basal body temperature	Helps predict ovulation and formation of corpus luteum
LH surge	Helps predict ovulation and formation of corpus luteum
Day 3 FSH, estradiol, prolactin, thyroid-stimulating hormone	Tests for ovarian reserve and endocrine dysfunction

sperm concentration, forward motility, and morphologic analysis of the sperm. If the results of the semen analysis are abnormal, further endocrine, biochemical, or immunological testing can be performed in an attempt to identify the cause.

Factors contributing to female infertility include ovarian or hormonal, tubal, cervical, uterine, psychosocial, iatrogenic, and immunological factors. Ovulatory disorders such as hypergonadotropic hypogonadism and hypogonadotropic hypogonadism are the most common and are described in more detail in Chapter 22. Other disorders such as polycystic ovarian disease, obesity, thyroid dysfunction, androgen excess, and liver dysfunction can also contribute. Following a detailed history and physical examination, laboratory evaluation of female infertility is performed as outlined in **Table 20-6**. In addition to laboratory testing, a hysterosalpingogram can detect tubal or pelvic pathology. Midluteal progesterone concentrations greater than 10 ng/mL indicate normal ovulation while concentrations less than 10 ng/mL suggest anovulation, inadequate luteal phase progesterone production, or inappropriate timing of sample collection. Basal body temperature (rise in temperature by 0.5°F at the time of ovulation) and progesterone analysis help confirm that ovulation occurred. However, measuring the LH surge is more clinically valuable as it can predict ovulation 24 to 36 hours prior to ovulation and guide the timing of intercourse. Home kits employing two-site double monoclonal immunoassays can be purchased to monitor for urine LH and predict the LH surge. Serum levels of FSH and estradiol can be measured on day 3 of the menstrual cycle to indicate ovarian reserve. TSH and prolactin (PRL) can be used to assess for thyroid or pituitary dysfunction.

The LH surge can predict ovulation 24 to 36 hours prior to ovulation and guide the timing of intercourse. Home kits employing two-site double monoclonal immunoassays can be purchased to monitor for urine LH and predict the LH surge.

REFERENCES

Aitken RJ. Sperm function tests and fertility. *Int J Androl*. 2006;29:69.

Altman AD, et al. Maternal age-related rates of gestational trophoblastic disease. *Obstet Gynecol*. 2008;112:244.

Ashwood ER, Knight GJ. Clinical chemistry of pregnancy. In: Burtis CA, Ashwood ER, Bruns DE, eds. *Tietz Textbook of Clinical Chemistry and Molecular Diagnostics*. 4th ed. St. Louis, MO: Elsevier Saunders; 2006: 2153.

Baek KH, et al. Recurrent pregnancy loss: the key potential mechanisms. *Trends Mol Med*. 2007;13:310.

Barton JR, Sibai BM. Prediction and prevention of recurrent preeclampsia. *Obstet Gynecol*. 2008;112:359.

Borrelli PTA, et al. Human chorionic gonadotropin isoforms in the diagnosis of ectopic pregnancy. *Clin Chem*. 2003;49:2045.

Brassard M, et al. Basic infertility including polycystic ovary syndrome. *Med Clin North Am*. 2008;92:1163.

Christiansen OB, et al. Evidence-based investigations and treatments of recurrent pregnancy loss. *Fertil Steril*. 2005;83:821.

Duley L. Pre-eclampsia and the hypertensive disorders of pregnancy. *Brit Med Bull*. 2003;67:161.

Farquhar C. Ectopic pregnancy. *Lancet*. 2005;366:583.

Frey KA, Patel KS. Initial evaluation and management of infertility by the primary care physician. *Mayo Clin Proc.* 2004;79:1439.

Guntupalli SR, Steingrub J. Hepatic disease and pregnancy: an overview of diagnosis and management. *Crit Care Med.* 2005;33(suppl):S332.

Haymond S, Gronowski AM. Reproductive related disorders. In: Burtis CA, Ashwood ER, Bruns DE, eds. *Tietz Textbook of Clinical Chemistry and Molecular Diagnostics.* 4th ed. St. Louis, MO: Elsevier Saunders; 2006:2097.

Knox TA, Olans LB. Liver disease in pregnancy. *N Engl J Med.* 1996;335:569.

Makar RS, Toth TL. The evaluation of infertility. *Am J Clin Pathol.* 2002;117(suppl):S95.

Mihu D, et al. HELLP syndrome—a multisystemic disorder. *J Gastrointest Liver Dis.* 2007;16:419.

Pandey MK, et al. An update in recurrent spontaneous abortion. *Arch Gynecol Obstet.* 2005;272:95.

Papanna R, et al. Protein/creatinine ratio in preeclampsia. *Obstet Gynecol.* 2008;112:135.

Rai R, Regan L. Recurrent miscarriage. *Lancet.* 2006;368:601.

Rajasri AG, et al. Acute fatty liver of pregnancy (AFLP)—an overview. *J Obstet Gynaecol.* 2007;27:237.

Reddy UM, Mennuti MT. Incorporating first-trimester Down syndrome studies into prenatal screening. *Obstet Gynecol.* 2006;107:167.

Reddy UM, et al. Infertility, assisted reproductive technology, and adverse pregnancy outcomes. *Obstet Gynecol.* 2007;109:967.

Seeber BE, et al. Application of redefined human chorionic gonadotropin curves for the diagnosis of women at risk for ectopic pregnancy. *Fertil Steril.* 2006;86:454.

Seki K, et al. Advances in the clinical laboratory detection of gestational trophoblastic disease. *Clin Chim Acta.* 2004;349:1.

Shaw SW, et al. First- and second-trimester Down syndrome screening: current strategies and clinical guidelines. *Taiwan J Obstet Gynecol.* 2008;47:157.

Sibai BM. Diagnosis and management of gestational hypertension and preeclampsia. *Obstet Gynecol.* 2003;102:181.

Sibai BM. Diagnosis, controversies, and management of the syndrome of hemolysis, elevated liver enzymes, and low platelet count. *Obstet Gynecol.* 2004;103:981.

Smith GCS. Circulating angiogenic factors in early pregnancy and the risk of preeclampsia, intrauterine growth restriction, spontaneous preterm birth, and stillbirth. *Obstet Gynecol.* 2007;109:1316.

Soper JT. Gestational trophoblastic disease. *Obstet Gynecol.* 2006:108:176.

Su GL. Pregnancy and liver disease. *Curr Gastroenterol Rep.* 2008:10:15.

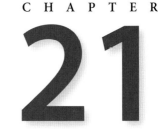

Breast

Karin E. Finberg

CHAPTER OUTLINE

INTRODUCTION

This chapter focuses on laboratory testing relevant to breast cancer. Infections of the breast are included in Chapter 5.

BREAST CANCER

Description

Cancers of the breast constitute a major cause of mortality in women of Western countries. In the United States, the lifetime probability that a woman will develop breast cancer is 1 in 8. Breast cancer accounts for 26% of new cancer cases and 15% of cancer deaths in American women. About 1% of breast cancers occur in males. The risk of developing breast cancer is influenced by several factors. These factors include increased age, family history of breast cancer (especially in a first-degree relative), hormonal factors (early age at menarche, older age of menopause, older age at first full-term pregnancy, fewer number of pregnancies, and use of hormone replacement therapy), clinical factors (high breast tissue density and benign breast diseases associated with atypical hyperplasia), obesity, and alcohol consumption. Since 1990, the mortality rate associated with female breast cancer has decreased in the United States, a decline that has been attributed to both therapeutic advances and early detection.

For localized breast cancer, primary treatment typically consists of either breast-conserving surgery and radiation or mastectomy. Most patients with invasive breast cancer subsequently receive systemic adjuvant chemotherapy and/or hormone therapy, both of which have been shown to reduce systemic recurrence and breast cancer-related mortality. However, the fact that some patients who lack lymph node involvement are cured by the combination of surgery and radiotherapy suggests that adjuvant treatment may not be necessary in all cases. Therefore, to rationally administer adjuvant therapy to patients with local disease, several prognostic factors are considered to assess the risk for recurrence. These prognostic factors include tumor size, axillary node involvement, histological type, cytological grade, lymphatic and vascular invasion, and certain biomarkers associated with breast cancer.

While adjuvant therapy improves patient outcomes, 25% to 30% of women with lymph node-negative and at least 50% to 60% of women with node-positive disease develop recurrent or metastatic disease. Metastatic breast cancer is currently regarded as incurable. Therapeutic options for metastatic disease include chemotherapy, hormone therapy, and molecularly targeted therapies. In the context of metastatic disease, information gained from serial monitoring of tumor markers detected in the serum may contribute to decisions to continue or terminate a particular treatment.

LABORATORY TESTING

Tissue-based Biomarkers in Breast Cancer

Assessment of biomarkers in tissue obtained from the patient's breast tumor is routinely performed to obtain prognostic information and to guide therapy.

Estrogen Receptor (ER) and Progesterone Receptor (PR)

ER and PR are intracellular receptors that bind to lipid-soluble steroid hormones that diffuse into target cells. Following ligand binding, 2 receptor subunits dimerize to form a single, functional DNA-binding unit that binds to specific DNA target sequences to induce transcription of target genes. There are 2 different forms of the ER, termed ER-α and ER-β, which are encoded by separate genes. Clinical assays assess ER-α, the classical form of the receptor. PR has 2 isoforms that differ in molecular weight but are encoded by a single gene.

> Assessment of biomarkers in tissue obtained from the patient's breast tumor is routinely performed to obtain prognostic information and to guide therapy.

Measurement of the ER and PR status of the tumor is recommended in all patients with breast cancer. ER expression is present in approximately 70% of breast cancers, is associated with a favorable prognosis, and suggests that the growth of the tumor may be estrogen-dependent. The primary purpose of determining ER and PR status in breast cancers is to identify those patients, in both the adjuvant and metastatic settings, who are likely to respond to endocrine treatments. These treatments act by either preventing the formation of estrogen from its precursors or blocking estrogen from binding to its receptors. Endocrine treatments include tamoxifen, ovarian ablation (surgical or chemical), aromatase inhibitors (anastrazole, letrozole, and exemestane), and irreversible ER inhibitors (e.g., fulvestrant). In patients with ER-positive tumors, 5 years of adjuvant treatment with tamoxifen significantly reduces annual death rates from breast cancer, while in patients with ER-negative tumors, tamoxifen shows little effect on recurrence or death, and it does not significantly modify the effects of polychemotherapy.

ER/PR status is routinely assessed by immunohistochemistry (IHC) in the clinical setting. IHC evaluates the percentage of cells with nuclear ER/PR staining and may also assess the staining intensity. The use of validated antibodies is required, and a positive control (i.e., a control tissue with tumor cells known to express the respective receptor) must be examined in parallel. For ER, normal breast epithelial cells in adjacent tissue can provide an internal positive control. To avoid false-negative results, at least 6 to 8 hours of formalin fixation is recommended to preserve ER and PR epitope recognition.

HER-2

HER2 (also known as *ERBB2* and *NEU*) is a proto-oncogene located at chromosome 17q11 that is a member of the epidermal growth factor receptor (EGFR) family. Like other EGFR family members, HER2 is a transmembrane receptor with cytoplasmic tyrosine kinase activity. Dimerization of the receptor leads to phosphorylation of a variety of substrates, resulting in the activation of intracellular signaling pathways important for cell proliferation and survival.

While normal cells contain 2 copies of the *HER2* gene (1 copy on each chromosome 17), in approximately 25% of breast cancers *HER2* gene copy number is increased at least 2-fold relative to the number of copies of chromosome 17, a phenomenon termed gene amplification. Gene amplification results in overexpression of the HER2 protein at the cell surface, which in turn promotes tumor cell proliferation and survival. Tumors that overexpress *HER2* behave more aggressively than those lacking overexpression, and they are associated with poorer clinical outcomes.

Assessment of *HER2* status of the tumor is recommended in all patients with invasive breast cancer. The primary purpose of *HER2* testing is to identify those patients with early or advanced breast cancer who are eligible for treatment with trastuzumab, a recombinant monoclonal antibody that recognizes HER2. Although its exact mechanism of action remains to be fully elucidated, trastuzumab has been shown in both in vitro assays and animal studies to inhibit proliferation of human tumor cells that overexpress HER2. In patients with *HER2*-positive early stage breast cancer, the addition of trastuzumab to adjuvant chemotherapy significantly improves disease-free and overall survival. Additionally, in patients with *HER2*-positive metastatic breast cancer, the addition of trastuzumab to adjuvant chemotherapy significantly increases the time until disease progression. Because a small percentage of patients treated with trastuzumab develop cardiotoxicity, the elimination of false-positive *HER2* results is important so that patients are not exposed to this risk unnecessarily.

HER2 status is routinely assessed in formalin-fixed tissues by either fluorescence in situ hybridization (FISH) or IHC. FISH assesses *HER2* status at the DNA level. A fluorescent-labeled nucleic acid probe that recognizes the *HER2* gene on chromosome 17 is hybridized on tissue sections, and the average number of *HER2* signals per nucleus is determined in areas of invasive tumor. In some assay systems, an additional probe that recognizes the centromeric region of chromosome 17 (CEP17) (and which is labeled with a different fluorophore) is included to allow the ratio of the average number of copies of *HER2*:CEP17 (the "FISH ratio") to be calculated. Tumors with >6 *HER2* gene copies per nucleus or with a FISH ratio >2.2 are scored as positive for gene amplification. Tumors with <4 *HER2* gene copies per nucleus or a FISH ratio <1.8 are scored as negative for gene amplification. Tumors with intermediate results are considered equivocal for gene amplification; in these cases, IHC for HER2 protein may be performed to resolve *HER2* status.

In contrast to the FISH assay, IHC assesses HER2 status at the protein level. The level of HER2 protein expression is scored on a semi-quantitative scale that ranges from "0" (no immunostaining) to "3+" (uniform intense membrane staining of greater than 30% of the invasive tumor cells). Tumors with 3+ protein expression are scored as positive for HER2 protein expression, while tumors with 0 or 1+ protein expression are scored as negative. Tumors with intermediate staining patterns (e.g., cases showing complete membrane staining that is weak in intensity) are considered equivocal; in these cases, FISH may be performed to resolve *HER2* status.

Serum-based Biomarkers in Breast Cancer

Serum-based tumor markers may be useful in the identification and management of patients with breast cancer. The ideal breast cancer marker would be both specific for breast cancer and sufficiently sensitive for screening purposes. Unfortunately, no marker identified to date meets these criteria. However, some markers may have utility in evaluating the progression of disease after initial therapy and for monitoring subsequent treatment.

When considering the use of serum tumor markers, several points should be kept in mind: 1) none of the currently available markers is elevated in all patients with breast cancer, even in the setting of advanced disease, so that a normal tumor marker level does not exclude a malignancy; 2) these markers are most sensitive for detecting metastatic disease and have little value in the diagnosis of local or regional recurrences; 3) the magnitude of change in marker levels that correlates with disease progression or regression has not been firmly established; 4) tumor marker levels may paradoxically rise after initiation of chemotherapy, a phenomenon attributed to therapy-mediated apoptosis or necrosis of tumor cells; 5) tumor marker levels may be increased in the setting of certain benign diseases.

CA 15-3 and CA 27.29

CA 15-3 and CA 27.29 represent different but overlapping epitopes of the MUC1 protein, a large, complex glycoprotein expressed at the luminal surface of glandular epithelial cells. In malignant cells, MUC1 may be overexpressed, and increased amounts of MUC1 may be shed into the circulation. MUC1 levels in serum may be assessed by immunoassays employing distinct monoclonal antibodies that recognize either the CA 15-3 or CA 27.29 epitopes. Results obtained from assays assessing CA 15-3 and CA 27.29 are highly correlated. Importantly, CA 15-3 elevations have been shown to occur in other malignancies and, to a lesser extent, in non-neoplastic disease. These pathologic conditions include adenocarcinomas of the colon, lung, ovary, and pancreas, as well as chronic hepatitis, cirrhosis, sarcoidosis, tuberculosis, and systemic lupus erythematosus.

In early stage breast cancer, elevated CA 15-3 levels are associated with a worse prognosis. However, because CA 15-3 and CA 27.29 show fairly low sensitivity for detection of early disease, the role of these markers in the management of early stage breast cancer remains unclear. Measurement of either CA 15-3 or CA 27.29 is therefore not recommended for screening, diagnosis, or staging of breast cancer. After primary and/or adjuvant therapy, increases in CA 15-3 or CA 27.29 can predict recurrence several months before other testing modalities or the development of symptoms. However, because prospective, randomized clinical trials have yet to demonstrate if such early detection of occult or asymptomatic metastases impacts disease-free or overall survival, the routine use of CA 15-3 and CA 27.29 for this application is not currently recommended. In patients with metastatic disease who are undergoing active therapy, CA 15-3 or CA 27.29 testing may be used in conjunction with history, physical exam, and diagnostic imaging to monitor the response to treatment. While the use of CA 15-3 or CA 27.29 alone to monitor response to treatment is not recommended, in the absence of readily measurable disease, an increasing CA 15-3 or CA 27.29 may be used nonetheless to identify treatment failure. In most clinical trials to date, a significant alteration in CA 15-3 has been defined as a concentration change of at least 25%.

Carcinoembryonic Antigen (CEA)

CEA is a cell-surface glycoprotein involved in cell adhesion that is normally expressed in the developing fetus. CEA levels in the blood decrease to very low levels after birth, though levels may be elevated slightly in smokers. CEA expression may be elevated in several types of cancer, including cancers of the breast, colon, pancreas, lung, and ovary, because of antigen shedding into the circulation. CEA may also be elevated in non-neoplastic diseases, including inflammatory bowel disease, pancreatitis, and liver disease. CEA is detected by immunoassay.

In early stage breast cancer, elevated CEA levels are associated with a worse prognosis. CEA is not recommended for screening, diagnosis, staging, or routine surveillance of breast cancer patients after primary therapy. Like CA 15-3 and CA 27.29, CEA testing may be used in conjunction with history, physical exam, and diagnostic imaging to monitor the response to treatment in patients with metastatic disease who are undergoing active therapy. However, CEA should not be used alone for this purpose. Compared to CA 15-3, CEA is generally a less sensitive marker for breast cancer. However, in some patients with breast cancer, elevations of CEA may occur in the setting of normal CA 15-3 or CA 27.29 levels.

HEREDITARY BREAST AND OVARIAN CANCER SYNDROME

Description

While most cases of breast cancer are caused by acquired somatic mutations, approximately 5% to 10% of breast cancer cases are attributed to a germline mutation in a highly penetrant cancer predisposition gene. A large proportion of these hereditary cases are associated with mutations in 2 genes, *BRCA1* and *BRCA2*. Mutations in *BRCA1* and *BRCA2* cause the hereditary breast and ovarian cancer syndrome, an autosomal dominant disorder in which the risk of both breast and ovarian cancer is significantly increased compared to the general population. *BRCA1* and *BRCA2*, which are located at chromosome 17q21 and 13q12, respectively, are tumor suppressor genes that play essential roles in the repair of double-stranded DNA breaks and thus in the maintenance of genome stability. Accordingly, in tumors from individuals with hereditary breast and ovarian cancer syndrome, the wild-type *BRCA1* or *BRCA2* allele is deleted, consistent with a tumor suppressor function for *BRCA1* and *BRCA2*.

A woman's risk for harboring either a *BRCA1* or *BRCA2* mutation is increased by certain factors related to her personal and family medical history. Personal factors include: 1) early onset breast cancer (i.e., diagnosis before 50 years of age); 2) bilateral or multifocal breast cancers; and 3) a history of both breast and ovarian cancer. Factors from the family history include: 1) breast cancer or breast and ovarian cancer in a pattern consistent with autosomal dominant transmission; and 2) breast cancer in a male relative.

> Approximately 5% to 10% of breast cancer cases are attributed to a germline mutation in a highly penetrant cancer predisposition gene. A large proportion of these hereditary cases are associated with mutations in 2 genes, *BRCA1* and *BRCA2*.

Hereditary breast and ovarian cancer syndrome shows incomplete penetrance. Among women with either a *BRCA1* or *BRCA2* mutation, the lifetime risk of developing breast cancer is 60% to 80%. The lifetime risk of developing ovarian cancer is 15% to 60% for women with *BRCA1* mutations and 10% to 27% for women with *BRCA2* mutations. Mutations in *BRCA1* and *BRCA2* also increase the risk of male breast cancer. Individuals with hereditary breast and ovarian cancer syndrome are also at risk for other tumors, including melanoma and cancers of the prostate (in males) and pancreas.

Determination of *BRCA1* and *BRCA2* mutation status is an important clinical assessment, as the identification of a deleterious mutation may alter clinical management. Interventions available to *BRCA1* and *BRCA2* mutation carriers include intensive screening, chemoprevention, prophylactic mastectomy, and prophylactic oophorectomy. Prophylactic oophorectomy, which reduces the risk of breast cancer as well as ovarian cancer, is recommended for all mutation carriers at the completion of childbearing.

Determination of *BRCA1* and *BRCA2* Mutations

Genetic testing for *BRCA1* and *BRCA2* mutations should be offered to individuals with a personal or family history suspicious for hereditary breast and ovarian cancer syndrome, and to women at risk because of a family member known to harbor a deleterious mutation in 1 of these genes. It is critical that testing be offered in the setting of appropriate genetic counseling, so that individuals are provided appropriate information regarding the risks, benefits, and limitations of genetic testing. Such counseling should also include consideration of how the results of such testing might affect other family members.

Study of kindreds with hereditary breast and ovarian cancer syndrome has identified hundreds of different deleterious mutations in the *BRCA1* and *BRCA2* genes. Most consist of frameshift or nonsense mutations, which are predicted to result in a loss of function of the encoded gene product. Due to the large number of different mutations described, genetic testing to assess for most of these involves examination of the DNA sequence of the entire coding region of each gene. Additional molecular testing may also be employed to assess for certain large genomic rearrangements that cannot be detected by routine DNA sequencing. In cases where a known deleterious mutation has already been identified in a family member, targeted mutation analysis is performed to specifically assess for the familial mutation.

When possible, genetic testing should be performed on an individual who has been diagnosed with breast or ovarian cancer because this strategy provides the most information for other members of the family. Genetic testing can lead to 4 possible outcomes: a true-positive result, a true-negative result, an uninformative result, and a variant of uncertain significance. A true-positive result occurs when a deleterious mutation known to be associated with increased cancer risk is identified; such a result confirms the diagnosis of hereditary breast and ovarian cancer syndrome. A true-negative result occurs only when the tested individual is found to lack a specific deleterious mutation already known to run in the family; a true-negative result thus reduces the tested individual's risk of developing breast and/or ovarian cancer to that of general population. An uninformative result occurs when a mutation is not identified in an individual from a family in which a deleterious mutation has not yet been identified; an uninformative result does not exclude the possibility of a *BRCA1* or *BRCA2* mutation that cannot be detected by current testing methodologies, nor does it exclude the possibility of a mutation in another cancer susceptibility gene. Genetic variants of uncertain significance are typically missense variants of unknown functional significance or intronic variants not predicted to disrupt mRNA processing; individuals harboring variants of unknown significance may still be at increased risk for cancer, and their medical management should be based on the known family history. In all cases, post-test genetic counseling should be performed to ensure that individuals fully comprehend the implications of their testing results.

Genetic testing for *BRCA1* and *BRCA2* mutations should be offered to individuals with a personal or family history suspicious for hereditary breast and ovarian cancer syndrome, and to women at risk because of a family member known to harbor a deleterious mutation in 1 of these genes

REFERENCES

Allain DC. Genetic counseling and testing for common hereditary breast cancer syndromes: a paper from the 2007 William Beaumont hospital symposium on molecular pathology. *J Mol Diagn.* 2008;10(5):383–395.

American Cancer Society. *Breast Cancer Facts & Figures* 2007–2008.

Atlanta: American Cancer Society, Inc.; 2007. http://www.cancer.org/docroot/STT/content/ STT_1x_Breast_Cancer_Facts__Figures_2007-2008.asp; Accessed 01.03.09.

Brooks M. Breast cancer screening and biomarkers. *Methods Mol Biol.* 2009;472:307–321.

Clarke M, et al. Adjuvant chemotherapy in oestrogen-receptor-poor breast cancer: patient-level meta-analysis of randomised trials. *Lancet.* 2008;371(9606):29–40.

Duffy MJ. Serum tumor markers in breast cancer: are they of clinical value? *Clin Chem.* 2006;52(3):345–351.

Duffy MJ. Estrogen receptors: role in breast cancer. *Crit Rev Clin Lab Sci.* 2006;43(4):325–347.

Early Breast Cancer Trialists' Collaborative Group. Effects of chemotherapy and hormonal therapy for early breast cancer on recurrence and 15-year survival: an overview of the randomised trials. *Lancet.* 2005;365(9472):1687–1717.

Gown AM. Current issues in ER and HER2 testing by IHC in breast cancer. *Mod Pathol.* 2008;21 (suppl 2):S8–S15.

Gulati AP, Domchek SM. The clinical management of BRCA1 and BRCA2 mutation carriers. *Curr Oncol Rep.* 2008;10(1):47–53.

Harris L, et al. American Society of Clinical Oncology 2007 update of recommendations for the use of tumor markers in breast cancer. *J Clin Oncol.* 2007;25(33):5287–5312.

Hicks DG, Kulkarni S. HER2+ breast cancer: review of biologic relevance and optimal use of diagnostic tools. *Am J Clin Pathol.* 2008;129(2):263–273.

Jemal A, et al. Cancer statistics, 2008. *CA Cancer J Clin.* 2008;58(2):71–96.

Sauter G, et al. Guidelines for human epidermal growth factor receptor 2 testing: biologic and methodologic considerations. *J Clin Oncol.* 2009;27(8):1323–33.

Sturgeon CM, et al. National Academy of Clinical Biochemistry laboratory medicine practice guidelines for use of tumor markers in testicular, prostate, colorectal, breast, and ovarian cancers. *Clin Chem.* 2008;54(12):e11–e79.

Tan DS, et al. Hereditary breast cancer: from molecular pathology to tailored therapies. *J Clin Pathol.* 2008;61(10):1073–1082.

U.S. Preventive Services Task Force. Genetic risk assessment and BRCA mutation testing for breast and ovarian cancer susceptibility: recommendation statement. *Ann Intern Med.* 2005;143(5):355–361.

Wolff AC, et al. American Society of Clinical Oncology/College of American Pathologists guideline recommendations for human epidermal growth factor receptor 2 testing in breast cancer. *Arch Pathol Lab Med.* 2007;131(1):18.

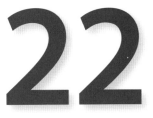

The Endocrine System

Michael Laposata, Samir L. Aleryani,
and Alison Woodworth

LEARNING OBJECTIVES

1. Learn the physiology and biochemistry of the relevant hormones and other important mediators.

2. Understand the laboratory tests used in the diagnosis of the more commonly encountered disorders.

3. Identify the clinical disorders associated with each of the endocrine glands and the role of specific laboratory tests in their diagnosis.

CHAPTER OUTLINE

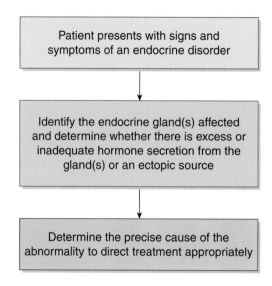

FIGURE 22–1 **An approach to the patient with an endocrinologic disorder.**

INTRODUCTION

This chapter on endocrine disorders is divided into separate discussions of each of the endocrine glands. Each section begins with an overview of the physiology and biochemistry of the relevant hormones. In addition, because of the large number of (often complex) laboratory tests in endocrinology, each section has a brief description of the laboratory tests most frequently used to diagnose the disorders in that disease group. Tests for which either serum or plasma is an acceptable specimen for analysis are noted as serum tests. Tests specifically requiring plasma are indicated by inclusion of the word "plasma" before the test name. As with all other chapters, each disorder is presented with a description of the disease and information useful in establishing a diagnosis. **Figure 22–1** shows a general approach to the patient with endocrine disease.

THYROID

Physiology and Biochemistry

Production of thyroid hormones is regulated by the hypothalamic–pituitary–thyroid axis (**Figure 22–2**). Thyrotropin-releasing hormone (TRH) is produced in the hypothalamus and induces thyrotropin-stimulating hormone (TSH) production in the anterior pituitary. TSH, in turn, stimulates thyroid hormone production and release by the thyroid gland. TSH production is inversely related to plasma thyroxine (T_4) and triiodothyronine (T_3) concentrations. The 2 primary hormones synthesized and secreted by the thyroid gland are T_4 and, in lesser quantities, T_3 (**Figure 22–3**). They are transported by plasma proteins—notably T_4-binding globulin, transthyretin, and albumin—to various tissue sites where T_4 is deiodinated to T_3 and the inactive form of T_3, known as reverse T_3 (rT_3). Thyroid hormones act through nuclear receptors that are transcription factors for numerous genes. These genes regulate a number of critical physiologic functions in development and metabolism.

Laboratory Tests

TSH

A "generational" classification has been applied for TSH assays based on the assay sensitivity. Third-generation assays can accurately measure TSH as low as 0.01 mU/L. This allows the physician to distinguish mildly subnormal TSH values (often seen in euthyroid hospitalized patients with nonthyroidal illness) from the low values of hyperthyroid patients. The third-generation

A "generational" classification has been applied for TSH assays based on the assay sensitivity. Third-generation assays can accurately measure TSH as low as 0.01 mU/L.

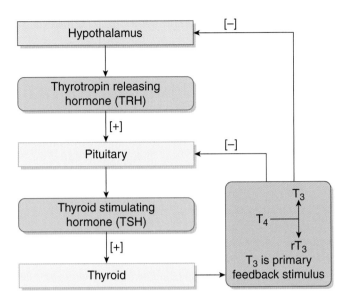

FIGURE 22–2 **Hypothalamic–pituitary–thyroid interactions. [+] Stimulation; [–] Inhibition.**

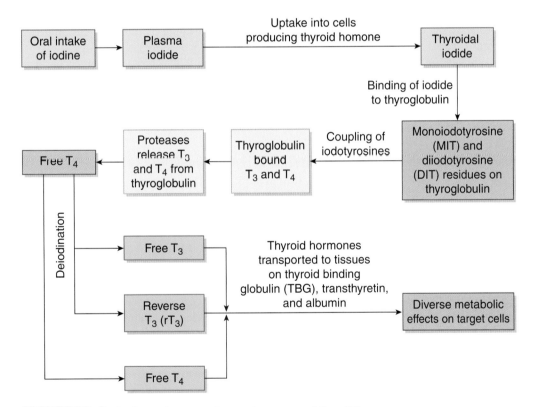

FIGURE 22–3 **The formation, secretion, and transport of thyroid hormones.**

tests are also useful for evaluating the effectiveness of the thyroid hormone replacement in hypo-thyroid patients. Third-generation assays are essential for monitoring TSH suppression therapy in patients with a TSH-responsive thyroid tumor.

The relationship between TSH and the thyroid hormones, particularly free T_4, is an inverse log-linear. Therefore, very small changes in free T_4 result in large changes in TSH. Thus, TSH is the most sensitive first-line screening test for suspected thyroid abnormalities. If the TSH is within the reference range (0.5 to 5.0 mU/L), no further testing is performed. If the TSH is outside of the reference range, a free T_4 is obtained.

Total Thyroid Hormone Measurements

Assays are available for both total T_4 and total T_3 measurements. These assays are quite specific and suffer little interference. However, a rise or fall in serum thyroid hormone carrier proteins will usually affect the total T_4 level and total T_3 level. Therefore, an assessment for free T_4 (see below) is usually more helpful in evaluating thyroid function. The concentration of T_4 in the blood is usually 100 to 200 times greater than the T_3 level. In hyperthyroidism, total T_3 concentrations correlate with total T_4 levels in all but a small subset of patients who have an elevation only in T_3. For that reason, T_3 should be measured in the serum of patients clinically suspected to be hyperthyroid and who have normal concentrations of serum T_4. Levels of T_3 are not useful in the assessment of hypothyroidism. Total T_3 is also decreased in euthyroid sick syndrome (ETS).

Free Thyroid Hormones and Thyroid Hormone-binding Capacity

"Direct" free thyroid hormone assays, without the need for a preliminary step to separate free hormones from hormones bound to protein carriers, have become available for measurement of free T_4 and free T_3. Only a small fraction of T_4 (<0.1%) circulates unbound to proteins, and this has made the accurate quantitation of free T_4 analytically difficult. Free T_4 is a better indicator of thyroid status than total T_4 because, as noted above, the total T_4 is altered by changes in the amounts of thyroid-binding globulin (TBG), albumin, and other thyroid hormone-binding proteins. About 0.3% of T_3 circulates as free T_3. In general, free T_3 concentrations correlate well with total T_3, but as with T_4, the concentrations of thyroid hormone-binding proteins influence the total T_3 level.

Although the free T_4 index offers an approximation of free T_4, this measure is largely obsolete due to improvements in the free hormone assays. The free T_4 index is calculated by multiplying the total T_4 by the measure of available hormone-binding sites on TBG in an assay known as the percent T_3-uptake. Because of the dependence on the amount of TBG, the free T_4 index and the T_3-uptake are affected by changes in the amount of thyroid-binding proteins induced by a variety of stimuli.

Reverse Triiodothyronine

Under acute stress or in illness, there is a shift in the T_4 deiodination in favor of the inactive rT_3 form rather than the active T_3. Numerous immunoassays are available for the measurement of rT_3 using antisera that do not cross-react significantly with T_3 or T_4. rT_3 is markedly increased in ETS syndrome (see below), but its measurement is rarely required for this diagnosis because its increase is proportional to the decrease in T_3.

Antithyroid Antibodies

> Antithyroid antibodies are present in approximately 15% of the general population and are the most common cause of thyroid disease.

Antithyroid antibodies are present in approximately 15% of the general population and are the most common cause of thyroid disease. They are also present in selected autoimmune diseases not usually associated with thyroid dysfunction. Descriptions of 3 types of antithyroid antibodies follow:

- *Antimicrosomal/antithyroid peroxidase antibodies (anti-TPO)*—These antibodies are directed against a protein component of thyroid microsomes, the enzyme TPO. They are present in almost all patients with Hashimoto thyroiditis, in about 85% of patients with Graves' disease (both discussed below), and in some patients with type 1 insulin-dependent diabetes mellitus, celiac disease, and Addison disease. An elevated anti-TPO antibody test in the context of symptoms of thyroid dysfunction is diagnostic for autoimmune thyroid disease. The presence of TPO antibodies before or during pregnancy is a good predictor of those women who will develop postpartum thyroid disease (discussed below). Normal concentrations are not well established because the antibodies may be found in healthy people (up to 12% of the population), and the reference range depends on the method used to perform the test.
- *Antithyroglobulin antibodies*—These are also called colloidal antibodies. They are present in more than 85% of patients with Hashimoto thyroiditis and in more than 30% of patients

with Graves' disease. Like anti-TPO, antithyroglobulin antibodies also may be found in other autoimmune diseases. In iodine-sufficient areas, antithyroglobulin antibody test is used less often, in favor of anti-TPO. However, in patients with suspected iodine deficiency, antithyroglobulin antibody is a better indicator of autoimmune thyroid disease.

- *TSH receptor antibodies*—These are a diverse group of immunoglobulins that bind to TSH receptors and influence receptor action. They are found in most patients with Graves' disease and in patients with selected other autoimmune disorders involving the thyroid. The biological functions of these antibodies vary from thyroid stimulation to thyroid inhibition (by blocking stimulation induced by TSH). Antibodies referred to as thyroid-stimulating immunoglobulins are present in 95% of patients with untreated Graves' disease. In vitro bioassays can assess the ability of stimulatory antibodies to induce functional responses in cultured cells by measuring cyclic adenosine monophosphate increases or adenylate cyclase activity. Assays are available that measure the capability of the inhibitory antibodies, called thyrotropin-binding inhibitory immunoglobulins, to block the binding of labeled TSH to its receptors.

Radioactive Iodine Uptake and Thyroid Scans

The radioactive iodine uptake and thyroid scan measurements involve the in vivo administration of radioactive iodine. Accumulated radioactivity in the thyroid is measured at intervals within 24 hours using a gamma scintillation counter. A nuclear imaging scan that examines the anatomic distribution of radioactive iodine uptake within the thyroid gland also may be obtained. This information may be useful in differentiating between possible causes of hyperthyroidism.

Thyroglobulin

Thyroglobulin is stored in the follicular colloid of the thyroid as a prohormone. Thyroglobulin measurements are used to monitor treatment in thyroid cancer. Persistent serum thyroglobulin after thyroidectomy is evidence of incomplete ablation or metastatic thyroid cancer. Thyroglobulin concentrations should always be assessed in the context of an antithyroglobulin antibody test because these autoantibodies can cause false-positive or -negative thyroglobulin results.

Fine Needle Aspiration (FNA) Cytology

FNA is the procedure of choice to collect a specimen for microscopic review to distinguish benign from malignant nodules. The sensitivity of thyroid FNA for detection of thyroid cancer and other disorders varies from 70% to 97%. It depends greatly on the quality of the specimens and the experience of the cytopathologist. Thyroglobulin can also be measured in FNA aspirates to diagnose and monitor thyroid cancer.

Hyperthyroidism Overview and Associated Disorders

Description and Diagnosis

Hyperthyroidism, also known as thyrotoxicosis, is a collection of disorders associated with excess thyroid hormone (**Table 22–1**). It can be caused by conditions associated with hyperfunction of the thyroid, such as Graves' disease or toxic multinodular goiter. It also may be caused by diseases associated with thyroid damage and increased release of thyroid hormones after cell injury. Rare causes of hyperthyroidism are ectopic thyroid tissue that produces thyroid hormones and intentional thyroid hormone overingestion in factitious hyperthyroidism. Patients with hyperthyroidism demonstrate a spectrum of hypermetabolic features, including nervousness, palpitations, muscle weakness, increased appetite, diarrhea, heat intolerance, warm skin, and perspiration. Affected patients also may have exophthalmos, emotional changes, menstrual changes, and a fine tremor of the hands. In the presence of a clinical history and physical examination consistent with hyperthyroidism, a diagnosis of hyperthyroidism (but not necessarily its cause) can be established by the demonstration of a low TSH level and a high free T_4. In uncommon situations, only the total T_3 level is elevated and the serum free T_4 is normal (T_3 thyrotoxicosis). To determine the etiology

In the presence of a clinical history and physical examination consistent with hyperthyroidism, a diagnosis of hyperthyroidism (but not necessarily its cause) can be established by the demonstration of a low TSH level and a high free T_4.

TABLE 22–1   Laboratory Evaluation of Patients for Thyroid Disease

Disorder	Laboratory Test Results Suggestive of Diagnosis in the Appropriate Clinical Setting
Hyperthyroidism	
Graves disease	TSH low; T_4 high; in some cases, T_3 is elevated and T_4 is normal; TSI elevated
Toxic multinodular goiter	TSH low; T_4 and T_3 high; suggestive radioactive iodine uptake and thyroid scan for toxic multinodular goiter
Toxic adenoma	TSH low; T_4 and T_3 high; suggestive radioactive iodine uptake and thyroid scan for toxic adenoma
Subacute thyroiditis	TSH low; T_4 and T_3 high; erythrocyte sedimentation rate increased; decreased radioactive iodine uptake
Chronic thyroiditis	TSH low; T_4 and T_3 high; erythrocyte sedimentation rate normal; decreased radioactive iodine uptake
Hypothyroidism	
Hashimoto thyroiditis	TSH high; T_4 normal and then low, preceding a decline in T_3; antithyroid peroxidase and antithyroglobulin positive
Ablative hypothyroidism	TSH high; T_4 and T_3 low following procedure that ablates thyroid
Infantile hypothyroidism	TSH high; T_4 and T_3 low in a newborn or infant
Euthyroid sick syndrome	*Moderately ill patients*: T_4 normal, T_3 low, rT_3 high; TSH low *Severely ill patients*: T_4 low, T_3 low, rT_3 high; TSH normal

rT_3, reverse triiodothyronine; T_3, triiodothyronine; T_4, thyroxine; TSH, thyrotropin-stimulating hormone; TSI, thyroid-stimulating immunoglobulins.

of the hyperthyroidism, additional testing is usually necessary. Graves' disease, toxic multinodular goiter, and toxic adenoma account for the vast majority (>95%) of cases of hyperthyroidism. It should be noted that diffuse or focal enlargement of the thyroid gland, also known as goiter, can be associated with hyperfunction, normal function, and hypofunction of the gland.

Thyroid Storm

Thyroid storm is a relatively uncommon, but life-threatening manifestation of hyperthyroidism caused by excess circulation of thyroid hormones. Symptoms of thyroid storm are similar, but much more severe than traditional hyperthyroidism, including a markedly high fever of 105°F to 106°F, tachycardia, hypertension, neurological, and gastrointestinal abnormalities. Thyroid storm is precipitated by acute illnesses such as sepsis, diabetic ketoacidosis, and preeclampsia, as well as surgical or other diagnostic or therapeutic action such as radioactive iodine use, anesthesia, excessive thyroid hormone ingestion, or thyroid palpitation. Thyroid storm is fatal in nearly all cases unless detected early. The diagnosis is based on the presence of clinical signs and symptoms of severe hyperthyroidism in the context of a precipitating cause. In addition, marked elevations in free and total T_4 are common in thyroid storm. Total T_3 is unreliable in this setting because concomitant non-thyroidal illness may cause T_3 to decrease significantly.

Graves' Disease

Graves' disease is a relatively common hyperthyroid disorder occurring more frequently in women. It has a familial predisposition. It is an autoimmune disease caused by thyroid-stimulating immunoglobulins that bind to TSH receptors. While many patients have the classic signs and symptoms of thyrotoxicosis, in elderly patients with Graves' disease, apathy, muscle weakness, and cardiovascular abnormalities occur more often than hypermetabolic symptoms.

Laboratory tests show undetectable TSH and increased free T_4. In some cases, the T_3 is elevated and the T_4 is normal. The differential diagnosis includes toxic multinodular goiter, toxic adenoma, subacute thyroiditis, ectopic thyroid tissue, and anxiety states (see below for descriptions). Radioactive iodine uptake and nuclear thyroid scans are helpful in distinguishing among these possibilities, as these entities can have different appearances on thyroid scans.

Graves' disease is a relatively common hyperthyroid disorder occurring more frequently in women. It is an autoimmune disease caused by thyroid-stimulating immunoglobulins that bind to TSH receptors.

Toxic Multinodular Goiter

The cause of hyperthyroidism in patients with toxic multinodular goiter is an apparent functional autonomy of certain areas within the thyroid gland. The disorder is seen more commonly in elderly patients. The degree of hyperthyroidism is generally less severe than that found in Graves' disease. Cardiovascular symptoms are prominent, such as arrhythmias, atrial fibrillation, or congestive heart failure, with weakness and wasting.

Laboratory tests usually show elevated free T_4 and T_3 concentrations, undetectable TSH, and no evidence of thyroid autoantibodies. As noted above, a radioactive iodine uptake study and a thyroid scan can be helpful in differentiating toxic multinodular goiter from other causes of hyperthyroidism.

Toxic Adenoma

Thyroid adenomas that secrete thyroid hormones and cause hyperthyroidism are known as toxic adenomas. Thyroid hormone synthesis by a toxic adenoma is usually independent of TSH regulation, and it results in suppression of the serum TSH level. These tumors can usually be distinguished from toxic multinodular goiter and Graves' disease by a radioactive iodine uptake study and thyroid scan.

Thyroiditis

Subacute Thyroiditis. Subacute thyroiditis is produced by a viral infection that alters thyroid function. This disease usually lasts for months, with thyroid function eventually returning to normal. The patient often has an associated upper respiratory infection and local pain mimicking a sore throat or an earache.

Patients in the early stage of this disease may have hyperthyroidism, with elevated T_4 and T_3 levels and a low TSH level. Laboratory findings also often include a high erythrocyte sedimentation rate and a decreased radioactive iodine uptake. If the disease progresses and the thyroid hormones are depleted, the patient develops hypothyroidism with low T_3 and T_4 levels and an elevated TSH.

Postpartum Thyroiditis. Postpartum thyroid disease is a transient autoimmune disease that has an onset of 1 to 6 months postpartum. Although the etiology is unclear, it is thought to be caused by a rebound in the immune system in response to the general state of immunosuppression that occurs during pregnancy. This disease can present as either hyperthyroidism or hypothyroidism. The typical disease course begins with a period of hyperthyroidism with elevated free T_4 followed by a period of hypothyroidism associated with reduced concentrations of free T_4 that completely resolve after 1 year. Approximately 20% of women with postpartum hypothyroidism develop permanent disease, requiring lifelong treatment and monitoring. The presence of anti-TPO antibodies prior to and during pregnancy is associated with an increased risk for postpartum thyroiditis.

Chronic (Painless) Thyroiditis. Patients with chronic thyroiditis have a transient thyrotoxicosis, but recurrences are common. The thyroid is firm, slightly enlarged, and not tender. The etiology of this disorder is unclear. Episodes of thyrotoxicosis usually fade within a few months.

Typically the T_4 and T_3 levels are elevated with a low TSH level. The patient will also have a markedly depressed radioactive iodine uptake. Chronic thyroiditis can be distinguished clinically from subacute thyroiditis because an elevated erythrocyte sedimentation rate and local pain in the region of the thyroid are more consistent with subacute thyroiditis. A definitive diagnosis can be made by microscopic review of cells obtained by aspiration or biopsy. Thyroglobulin measurements can differentiate among patients with chronic thyroiditis from those with thyrotoxicosis caused by surreptitious thyroid hormone intake.

Hypothyroidism Overview and Associated Disorders

Description and Diagnosis

When hypothyroidism occurs during development and in infancy, it results in a condition known as cretinism, which is marked by retardation of physical and intellectual growth. When hypothyroidism first appears in older children and adults, the collection of signs and symptoms is known as myxedema. In 95% of cases, hypothyroidism originates in the thyroid gland itself. If a patient has an increased serum TSH and a decreased free T_4—together with appropriate

When hypothyroidism occurs during development and in infancy, it results in a condition known as cretinism, which is marked by retardation of physical and intellectual growth. When hypothyroidism first appears in older children and adults, the collection of signs and symptoms is known as myxedema.

clinical symptoms—a diagnosis of hypothyroidism is confirmed (**Table 22–1**). If the increased TSH is accompanied by a normal or low-normal T_4, it may be indicative of an early stage of primary hypothyroidism. High titers of anti-TPO antibodies suggest Hashimoto thyroiditis (see below) or postpartum thyroid dysfunction in a postpartum woman.

Hypothyroidism also may be a result of inadequate stimulation of the thyroid by TSH. This is known as secondary hypothyroidism. A subnormal free T_4 with a decreased TSH is suggestive of secondary hypothyroidism from decreased TSH production or production of a biologically inactive form of TSH in the pituitary. It is usually accompanied by other pituitary hormone deficiencies, and it is much less common than primary hypothyroidism.

Clinical pictures of hypothyroidism differ, depending on the age. Congenital hypothyroidism is characterized by low production of thyroid hormones and can result in growth and intellectual delay if untreated. In the United States, all states screen for congenital hypothyroidism by testing for elevated TSH or a combination of elevated TSH and decreased fT_4. Significant changes in thyroid function occur in the neonatal period and throughout childhood. Therefore, TSH and free T_4 concentrations should be assessed using age-specific reference intervals. In particular, T_4 is typically elevated in newborns. In adults, hypothyroidism can have an insidious onset, especially in the elderly. Symptoms are usually nonspecific in the early stage and then progress to more definitive characteristics of hypothyroidism with dry hair, dry skin, periorbital puffiness, dull expression, large tongue, and enlarged heart. If untreated, myxedema coma with respiratory failure may occur. Treatment involves hormone replacement. The optimal dose is determined by clinical signs and symptoms and the serum TSH level.

Hashimoto Thyroiditis

Hashimoto thyroiditis is a common chronic inflammatory disease of the thyroid that accounts for as many as 90% of all cases of hypothyroidism. Autoimmune factors are thought to be the cause, as Hashimoto thyroiditis is often associated with other autoimmune diseases such as Sjögren syndrome and pernicious anemia.

Patients with Hashimoto thyroiditis carry anti-TPO and antithyroglobulin antibodies. Firm thyroid enlargement is characteristic, but atrophy is also seen. Patients typically have an increased TSH level and may have a normal free T_4 and an elevated radioactive iodine uptake in the early stage of the disease. Over time, serum T_4 declines first, followed by a decline in T_3 as hypothyroid symptoms become predominant.

Postablative Hypothyroidism

Postablative hypothyroidism is a relatively common cause of hypothyroidism in adults. Thyroid ablation occurs with total or subtotal thyroidectomy, or following treatment with radioactive iodine for hyperthyroidism.

A history of ablative therapy along with an elevated TSH and a low free T_4 concentration indicates that ablation has produced a hypothyroid state.

Infantile Hypothyroidism

Severe hypothyroidism in infancy is known as cretinism and, as previously noted, is characterized by irreversible mental retardation and growth impairment unless treated promptly. The appearance of symptoms depends on the severity of the disorder. However, even severe hypothyroidism is not usually apparent at birth. Early diagnosis and treatment with thyroid hormone prevents the manifestations of the disease. Elevated TSH and a low T_4 in a newborn or young infant are indicative of infantile hypothyroidism.

Pregnancy-related Thyroid Disease

Normal pregnancy is associated with a number of physiologic changes in thyroid function resulting in differences in "normal" laboratory values for thyroid function tests. The increase in estrogen stimulates hepatic synthesis of TBG, resulting in a net increase in total T_3 and total T_4 by about 1.5-fold. Significant homology exists between HCG, the pregnancy-associated glycoprotein hormone (see Chapter 20), and TSH. Because of this, HCG can directly stimulate the thyroid to produce thyroid hormone. Excess production of thyroid hormone signals a down-regulation

Hashimoto thyroiditis is a common chronic inflammatory disease of the thyroid that accounts for as many as 90% of all cases of hypothyroidism. Patients with Hashimoto thyroiditis carry anti-TPO and antithyroglobulin antibodies.

of TSH secretion. In the first trimester of pregnancy, increasing HCG concentrations are directly mirrored by decreasing TSH concentrations, which return to low normal in the second and third trimesters. Thus, TSH measurements in pregnancy should be considered in the context of gestational age and a reduced upper limit of normal.

Thyroid dysfunction during pregnancy can result in increased risks for the mother and fetus. Hypothyroidism during pregnancy is associated with an increased risk of miscarriage or preterm delivery and impaired neurological development in the fetus. Although controversial, it is recommended to screen all high-risk and symptomatic pregnant women for hypothyroidism by measuring TSH. Hyperthyroidism in pregnancy is associated with an increased risk of spontaneous abortion, preterm delivery, preeclampsia, and thyroid anomalies in the newborn. A subnormal TSH test result should be followed with free T_4 testing. An elevated free T_4 with the presence of autoantibodies confirms the diagnosis of hyperthyroidism in pregnancy. In mothers with confirmed thyroid disease, fetal thyroid function can be evaluated with ultrasound and amniotic fluid testing for TSH, free T_4, and total T_4. Normal reference intervals are instrument-specific for amniotic fluid thyroid function tests.

Euthyroid Sick Syndrome (ETS)

Description

It is estimated that 40% of emergency department patients have ETS at presentation. Stress, trauma, and illness can alter thyroid hormone production, transport, and metabolism, and thereby TSH levels, because of disruption of the normal feedback relationship between TSH and T_3 and T_4. This condition with altered thyroid hormone levels and no intrinsic disorder of the thyroid gland is called Euthyroid sick syndrome (ETS) or nonthyroidal illness (NTI), of which there are several variants.

The condition with altered thyroid hormone levels and no intrinsic disorder of the thyroid gland is called Euthyroid sick syndrome (ETS) or nonthyroidal illness (NTI), of which there are several variants.

Diagnosis

There is no consensus in the literature regarding the diagnosis and also therapy of ETS. The cause of ETS is different from patient to patient and is dependent on the history and any endocrinologic diagnosis. In moderately ill patients with ETS, serum T_4 levels are within the reference range, while serum T_3 is decreased and rT_3 is increased. Serum TSH levels are normal (except for a transient increase that may occur during recovery), and the normal TSH level is useful in distinguishing ETS in moderately ill patients from primary hypothyroidism. A second form of ETS occurs in more seriously ill patients. In these individuals, the T_4 and T_3 levels are usually below normal, as is the serum TSH concentration. In primary hypothyroid patients with severe illness, the TSH level remains elevated, unlike severely ill patients with ETS (who do not have primary hypothyroidism) with a low TSH level. Serum rT_3 is increased because of slow thyroid hormone clearance and greater than normal conversion of T_4 to rT_3 rather than to T_3. An elevated rT_3 in the appropriate clinical setting, with appropriately suggestive laboratory test results, points to ETS syndrome.

Thyroid Tumors

Description

Masses or "nodules" in the thyroid may be associated with normal function, hyperfunction, or hypofunction, and for that reason, they are considered apart from hyperthyroidism and hypothyroidism. Most solitary masses detected with physical examination are either the dominant nodule in a multinodular goiter, a cyst, or an asymmetric enlargement of the gland. Benign thyroid adenomas account for most of the neoplastic nodules. Adenomas are usually hyperfunctioning and appear as "hot nodules" by nuclear scan because they take up radioactive iodine while uptake is suppressed in the remainder of the gland. Less commonly, benign adenomas can appear "cold" by nuclear scan, usually when infarction has converted a formerly hyperfunctioning adenoma to a hypofunctioning nodule. Malignant tumors of the thyroid are nearly always hypofunctioning ("cold" by scan) and are only rarely associated with hyperfunction. The morphologic variants of thyroid cancer, diagnosed with histopathologic review of a biopsy specimen or aspirate (in order of frequency), are papillary carcinoma, follicular carcinoma, medullary thyroid carcinoma, and anaplastic carcinoma.

Diagnosis

The diagnosis is established by histopathologic review of a specimen obtained with FNA or biopsy. The accuracy of the diagnosis is increased with the use of guided ultrasound examination for sample collection.

ADRENAL CORTEX

Physiology and Biochemistry

The adrenal cortex secretes many steroid hormones that have a wide variety of physiologic effects. The hormones can be grouped into 3 major categories: glucocorticoids, mineralocorticoids, and sex steroids that include androgens, progestogens, and estrogens. The glucocorticoids and mineralocorticoids are collectively known as corticosteroids. Steroid hormones are synthesized from cholesterol in the adrenal glands and in the gonads. Steroid hormones are transported in the blood bound to carrier proteins, such as albumin and hormone-binding globulins, or as free hormone. Steroids may be modified with glucuronate or sulfate to increase their water solubility and permit excretion via the kidneys or the gastrointestinal tract. The percentage of steroid hormone that is bound to protein varies with the hormone affinity for carrier proteins and ranges from 60% to nearly 100%. Quantitatively, the glucocorticoids and mineralocorticoids are the most important group of hormones produced by the adrenal cortex. The major corticosteroids are cortisol (a glucocorticoid) and aldosterone (a mineralocorticoid). The synthesis and metabolism of the steroid hormones are illustrated in **Figure 22–4**. The liver is the main site for conjugation of steroid hormones, and the kidney excretes approximately 90% of the conjugated steroids. Glucocorticoids alter carbohydrate

> The adrenal cortex secretes hormones that can be grouped into 3 major categories: glucocorticoids, mineralocorticoids, and sex steroids that include androgens, progestogens, and estrogens.

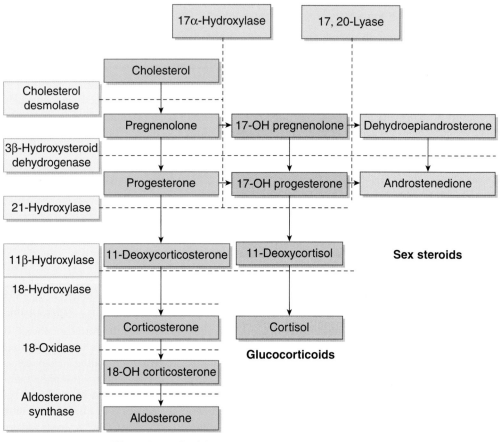

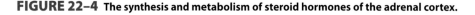

FIGURE 22–4 **The synthesis and metabolism of steroid hormones of the adrenal cortex.**

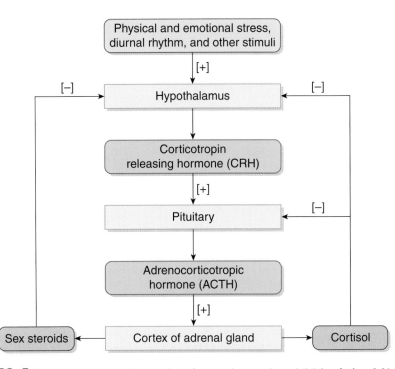

FIGURE 22–5 **Hypothalamic–pituitary–adrenal cortex interactions. [+] Stimulation; [–] Inhibition.**

metabolism by increasing gluconeogenesis and decreasing glucose utilization. Additional effects include the inhibition of amino acid uptake and protein synthesis in peripheral tissues. Mineralo- corticoids promote sodium conservation and potassium loss and thereby considerably influence the retention or loss of fluid. Among the naturally occurring mineralocorticoids, aldosterone has the highest mineralocorticoid activity followed by deoxycorticosterone and corticosterone.

Secretion of adrenal glucocorticoids and adrenal androgens is regulated by corticotropin (ACTH) that is secreted by the pituitary gland (**Figure 22–5**). Aldosterone and mineralocorticoid production are controlled by a different pathway known as the renin–angiotensin system. The hypothalamic– pituitary–adrenal (HPA) axis begins with the episodic release of corticotropin-releasing hormone (CRH) from the hypothalamus. CRH stimulates the episodic release of ACTH from the pituitary. ACTH then stimulates the adrenal cortex to produce cortisol in a diurnal or circadian manner. Cortisol concentrations are highest in the early morning between 4 and 8 AM and about 25% lower in the late evening. Physical and mental stress can elevate cortisol concentrations and blunt the circadian rhythm. ACTH release is under negative feedback control from the cortisol fraction not bound to proteins. Two adrenal sex steroids—dehydroepiandrosterone (DHEA) and androstenedione—are secreted in parallel with cortisol. Adrenal androgen production reaches a peak in the second decade, with a rise during late childhood. It gradually decreases and reaches a low level in the elderly.

As shown in **Figure 22–6**, aldosterone secretion is controlled by the renin–angiotensin sys- tem. Renin is an enzyme synthesized and stored in cells of the juxtaglomerular afferent arterioles of the renal glomeruli. The circulating renin hydrolyzes angiotensinogen to produce angiotensin I, which is rapidly converted to angiotensin II by angiotensin-converting enzyme. Angiotensin II then stimulates the cells of the adrenal cortex to produce aldosterone. Angiotensin II is also a po- tent vasoconstrictor. The primary stimuli for renin release are decreased perfusion of the kidney and a negative sodium balance.

> Cortisol concentrations are highest in the early morning between 4 and 8 AM and about 25% lower in the late evening. Physical and mental stress can elevate cortisol concentrations and blunt the circadian rhythm.

Laboratory Tests

The functional status of the adrenal cortex can be evaluated by measuring the circulating levels of the components of the HPA axis and the renin–angiotensin system. In addition to measurement of the plasma, serum, or urinary concentrations of these compounds, dynamic stimulation and suppression tests are valuable in identifying certain abnormalities.

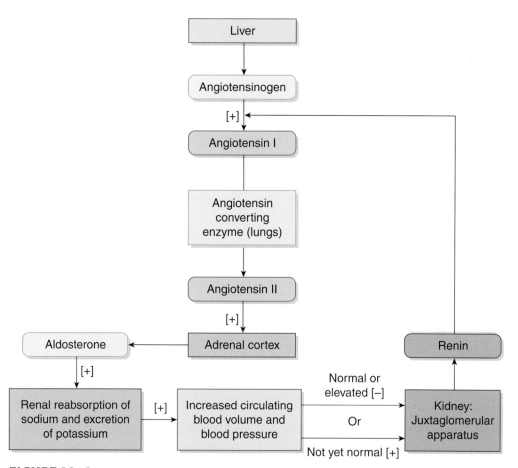

FIGURE 22–6 The renal and adrenal interactions in the renin–angiotensin system.

Cortisol

Because the secretion of cortisol is pulsatile, a single, random serum cortisol measurement is not usually diagnostic for adrenal dysfunction. The 24-hour urinary excretion of cortisol, an index of plasma-free cortisol during that 24-hour time frame, is a reliable gauge of excess cortisol secretion by the adrenal cortex. This is because urine cortisol is not influenced by the normal circadian variation found in the serum cortisol level. Salivary cortisol is another assay that is gaining acceptance. Salivary cortisol has not yet come into wide use and challenges in specimen collection and handling contribute to this limited use.

Low-dose Dexamethasone Suppression Tests

Dexamethasone is a substitute for endogenous cortisol and suppresses ACTH and CRH secretion. It can be administered as 1 mg at midnight in an overnight dexamethasone suppression test, or in a 2-day low-dose dexamethasone suppression test (LDST) by giving the patient 0.5 mg every 6 hours for 8 doses. If the dexamethasone is effective, it will suppress ACTH secretion and, thereby, suppress cortisol production. An abnormal response to the low-dose dexamethasone test will result in an abnormal production of cortisol, which is measured using a serum or a 24-hour urine sample.

High-dose Dexamethasone Suppression Test

In the high-dose dexamethasone suppression test, 2 mg of dexamethasone is administered every 6 hours for 8 doses over 2 days. The effect of dexamethasone is assessed by measuring the suppression of cortisol production in serum.

Metyrapone Test

The metyrapone test is a sensitive assessment of pituitary ACTH secretory reserve. The conversion of 11-deoxycortisol to cortisol is inhibited by metyrapone. Since 11-deoxycortisol does not inhibit ACTH secretion, when the plasma cortisol concentration declines following oral metyrapone administration, ACTH secretion increases and adrenal steroid synthesis is stimulated. The standard metyrapone test is 3 days from start to finish and involves metyrapone ingestion every 4 hours in six 750-mg doses. An alternative to the standard 3-day test is the overnight single dose (adjusted for weight) metyrapone test. Plasma ACTH, cortisol, and 11-deoxycortisol are measured in both assays. The metyrapone test is not widely used as the standard test is cumbersome. However, this test has a comparable specificity and sensitivity to the high-dose dexamethasone test.

ACTH

The optimum time of day for determination of plasma ACTH concentration is between midnight and 2 AM when the plasma-circulating levels of ACTH and cortisol are at their lowest point. At this time, the ability to detect an abnormality in ACTH secretion is the greatest.

CRH Stimulation Test

CRH can be administered intravenously to determine the response of the pituitary to stimulation by hypothalamic hormone. Stimulation of ACTH secretion by CRH is a means to measure a patient response to ACTH. The plasma ACTH and cortisol concentrations are measured in this stimulation test, which is useful in determining the etiology of adrenal insufficiency.

Aldosterone

The most important assay to establish a diagnosis of hyperaldosteronism or hypoaldosteronism is the serum aldosterone level. Aldosterone can be measured in the serum as the unmodified hormone, and in the urine as the 18-glucuronide conjugated metabolite of aldosterone. Screening for primary aldosteronism can include the determination of the ratio of plasma aldosterone concentration (PAC)/plasma renin activity (PRA).

Renin

Plasma renin activity is assayed by measuring its ability to convert angiotensinogen to angiotensin I, which is then quantitated by an immunoassay. When primary aldosteronism is present, often because of either resistant or severe hypertension, the PAC/PRA ratio will be elevated.

Steroid Measurements to Identify Enzyme Deficiencies in Congenital Adrenal Hyperplasia

Congenital adrenal hyperplasia (CAH) represents a spectrum of diseases resulting from enzyme deficiencies that impair normal hormone synthesis in the adrenal cortex. The decrease in cortisol production in most forms of CAH leads to an overproduction of steroid precursors and a shunting of the steroid precursors into the androgen synthesis pathway. These disorders are described in the section "Alterations in the Synthesis of Glucocorticoids, Mineralocorticoids, and Sex Steroids: Congenital Adrenal Hyperplasia." The assays used to identify the specific enzyme deficiencies include measurement of 17-hydroxyprogesterone, either unstimulated or after ACTH stimulation, 17-hydroxypregnenolone after ACTH stimulation, deoxycorticosterone, 11-deoxycortisol, and several androgens (androstenedione, DHEA, and testosterone). DNA-based tests also can be used to identify certain gene mutations that result in enzyme deficiencies found in CAH.

Cushing syndrome is a disorder of excess cortisol production, which is more commonly ACTH-dependent than ACTH-independent.

Hyperfunction Involving Glucocorticoids With or Without Mineralocorticoids: Cushing Syndrome

Description

Cushing syndrome is a disorder of excess cortisol production, which is more commonly ACTH-dependent than ACTH-independent. The early clinical features of Cushing syndrome are hypertension and weight gain. Truncal obesity with a round face, often known as a "moon facies," and an accumulation of fat in the posterior neck and regions of the back close to the neck, known as a "buffalo hump," appear with progression of the disease. Decreased muscle mass and proximal limb weakness occur from atrophy of muscle fibers induced by the high level of cortisol, which inhibits protein synthesis and uptake of glucose by the cells. Patients with Cushing syndrome often have elevated blood glucose levels with glucosuria. Other clinical signs and symptoms include striae of the skin, osteoporosis, hirsutism, menstrual abnormalities in women, and mental status changes involving mood swings with depression.

Cushing syndrome is separated into 3 main disease entities, with excess production of cortisol by the adrenal cortex as the common theme. Independent of the 3 naturally occurring forms of Cushing syndrome, the administration of glucocorticoids as a medication is a common cause of Cushing syndrome. This should be evident from the medication history. The naturally occurring forms of Cushing syndrome are described as follows:

- *Cushing disease*—This is the most common form of Cushing syndrome and is 4- to 6-fold more prevalent in women. It is caused most often by small tumors in the pituitary (<1 cm in size) known as microadenomas. These adenomas can be detected with various radiographic techniques after appropriate hormone tests suggest a pituitary etiology. On rare occasions, the tumors are large and present as macroadenomas.
- *Adrenal Cushing syndrome*—This form of Cushing syndrome is most commonly associated with a benign or malignant tumor in the adrenal cortex. Adrenal adenomas synthesize cortisol efficiently, but adrenal carcinomas often synthesize cortisol inefficiently and overproduce sex steroids, resulting in virilization.
- *Cushing syndrome from ectopic ACTH production*—Small cell lung carcinoma and bronchial carcinoid patients account for most of the Cushing syndrome cases in this category. This form of Cushing syndrome is more common in men because of the higher incidence of lung cancer in men. In the absence of signs and symptoms specifically associated with the lung carcinoma or carcinoid, these patients are clinically indistinguishable from those with pituitary Cushing disease. Because the syndrome often appears in patients with significant clinical manifestations of cancer, the symptoms from ectopic ACTH production often go unrecognized. Another very rare cause of Cushing syndrome with an ectopic focus and high serum ACTH level is a tumor, most frequently a bronchial carcinoid tumor, which secretes CRH instead of ACTH.

The strategy for the diagnosis of Cushing syndrome, and the subsequent identification of 1 of the 3 forms of Cushing syndrome, involves tests for urine-free cortisol, as measured in a 24-hour urine collection, serum cortisol (less useful because of the episodic nature of cortisol secretion), and plasma ACTH.

Diagnosis

The diagnosis of Cushing syndrome, or Cushing disease, discussed below collectively as Cushing syndrome, requires evidence of increased cortisol production and loss of suppression of cortisol synthesis or loss of cortisol diurnal variation. Screening for Cushing syndrome is difficult because 1) its prevalence is low; 2) several common conditions can lead to high cortisol levels and not produce the clinical manifestations of Cushing syndrome; 3) the screening tests have a high rate of false-positive results; and 4) a variety of algorithms are present for the suggested evaluation of patients for Cushing syndrome.

The strategy for the diagnosis of Cushing syndrome, and the subsequent identification of 1 of the 3 forms of Cushing syndrome, involves tests for urine-free cortisol, as measured in a 24-hour urine collection, serum cortisol (less useful because of the episodic nature of cortisol secretion), and plasma ACTH. ACTH levels are low in patients with adrenal tumors, but normal or elevated with pituitary or ectopic ACTH-producing tumors. **Table 22–2** summarizes the laboratory evaluation for Cushing syndrome.

The following steps to diagnose and differentiate Cushing syndrome can be made using first-line and then second-line diagnostic tests respectively.

First-line Tests

1. A 24-hour urinary-free cortisol (UFC) or salivary cortisol is sensitive first-line test. If the UFC or salivary cortisol test is normal, 2 more specimens are collected and tested. If all 3 UFCs are normal, Cushing syndrome is ruled out. The patient can return after 6 months for re-screening if signs or symptoms worsen.
2. If cortisol measurements are elevated on 2 occasions, a diagnosis of Cushing syndrome is ruled in. The patient can then be evaluated for the cause of the syndrome.

TABLE 22–2 Laboratory Evaluation for Cushing Syndrome

Laboratory Test	Pituitary Cause	Adrenal Cause	Ectopic ACTH Secretion
24-Hour urine-free cortisol or salivary cortisol	Elevated	Elevated	Elevated
Low-dose dexamethasone suppression test—high dose if clinical suspicion after normal low-dose test	No ACTH suppression and therefore no cortisol suppression; elevated levels of 24-hour urine-free cortisol	No ACTH suppression and therefore no cortisol suppression; elevated levels of 24-hour urine-free cortisol	No ACTH suppression and therefore no cortisol suppression; elevated levels of 24-hour urine-free cortisol
Plasma ACTH	Elevated or occasionally normal	Low	For ectopic ACTH-secreting tumors, ACTH is elevated and often at higher levels than found in Cushing disease (pituitary cause)
Imaging study	Pituitary tumor may be demonstrated	Adrenal tumor may be demonstrated	A tumor outside the adrenal may be demonstrated

ACTH, adrenocorticotropic hormone (corticotropin).

3. Positive first-line testing is confirmed with a 1 mg LDST. If cortisol production is suppressed by a low dose of dexamethasone in an overnight test and the urine-free cortisol is normal, Cushing syndrome is ruled out. If the clinical suspicion for Cushing syndrome is still high in the presence of a non-suggestive result for Cushing syndrome, a high-dose dexamethasone suppression test can be performed. If there is a lack of suppression by high-dose dexamethasone, further evaluation of the patient for Cushing syndrome is recommended. Taken together, failure of suppression by dexamethasone diverts the evaluation to differentiate between the 3 forms of Cushing syndrome beginning with a more definitive 2-day LDST.

4. There are many clinical conditions that can induce Cushing syndrome, and these must be considered. These include severe obesity, pregnancy, depression, diabetes mellitus, and glucocorticoid resistance.

Second-line Tests

Once Cushing syndrome is confirmed, a series of tests can then be performed to locate the cause of the hypercortisolism.

1. If an ACTH-secreting pituitary adenoma is suspected, MRI of the pituitary gland to identify a mass or petrosal sinus sampling to collect blood samples coming directly out of the pituitary after CRH stimulation are used as confirmation tests. A ratio of petrosal ACTH to serum ACTH above suggested cutoff values before and after CRH administration are consistent with a pituitary cause.

2. An imaging study is likely to be informative to identify an adrenal tumor and indicate an adrenal cause.

3. If an ectopic ACTH-secreting tumor is suspected, this can be challenging to locate, but imaging studies are often valuable. Chest, pancreas, colon, and gall bladder carcinomas have been shown to be sources of cortisol secretion.

"Pseudo-Cushing syndrome," which can be produced by alcohol abuse and other disorders, mimics both the clinical and biochemical features of the true syndrome.

Hypofunction Involving Glucocorticoids With or Without Mineralocorticoids: Adrenal Insufficiency

Description

Adrenal insufficiency can either be primary, from destruction of the adrenal cortex by a local disease process or a systemic disorder, or secondary from pituitary or hypothalamic disease that reduces stimulation of the adrenal gland. The most common cause of primary adrenal

Adrenal insufficiency can either be primary, from destruction of the adrenal cortex by a local disease process or a systemic disorder, or secondary from pituitary or hypothalamic disease that reduces stimulation of the adrenal gland.

insufficiency, in which all classes of adrenal cortical steroids are deficient, is autoimmune adrenalitis. In this particular disorder, the adrenal medulla and its catecholamine synthesis are spared. In other primary adrenal insufficiency disorders in which the adrenal gland is damaged, the adrenal medulla may be damaged along with the adrenal cortex. In secondary adrenal insufficiency, in which there is deficient stimulation of the adrenal gland because of pituitary or hypothalamic abnormalities, the adrenal medulla is not affected and, in addition, aldosterone deficiency is not usually present. Aldosterone secretion is more dependent on angiotensin II stimulation of the adrenal cortex than on stimulation of the adrenal cortex by ACTH (as discussed below).

- *Primary adrenal insufficiency*—There are many causes of primary adrenal insufficiency. Dysfunction in one or more sites in the HPA axis is the major cause of the primary adrenal insufficiency. Chronic primary adrenal insufficiency is known as Addison disease, which occurs mostly in adults. The most common cause was formerly tuberculous adrenalitis, and it is now autoimmune adrenalitis. Other causes of chronic primary adrenal insufficiency are systemic fungal infections, AIDS, and carcinomas metastatic to the adrenal gland. Primary adrenal insufficiency is characterized by hyperpigmentation of the skin and mucous membranes. The melanocytes are stimulated by the elevated levels of pituitary-derived ACTH that develop because there is little negative feedback from the adrenal gland to shut off ACTH production. Hyperkalemia is present if there is deficient aldosterone (see the sections on primary and secondary hypoaldosteronism). Primary adrenal insufficiency usually has a gradual onset but may occur abruptly, especially in critically ill patients. The rapid onset form of adrenal insufficiency is often the result of adrenal hemorrhage or thrombosis that impairs blood supply to the gland.
- *Secondary adrenal insufficiency*—A deficiency of ACTH secretion from any cause can lead to adrenal insufficiency. Long-term glucocorticoid therapy can result in prolonged suppression of CRH from the hypothalamus and cause transient secondary adrenal insufficiency. Patients with pituitary tumors who have pituitary gland surgery suffer from decreased ACTH production in the pituitary. Patients with space-occupying lesions in the pituitary, those who have received radiation therapy for pituitary or other central nervous system lesions, and patients with head trauma can develop decreased secretion of multiple pituitary hormones. Secondary adrenal insufficiency of abrupt onset from a pituitary-associated disorder can occur with postpartum pituitary necrosis, also known as Sheehan syndrome, in which bleeding occurs within the pituitary.

Acute primary adrenocortical failure (also called Addisonian crisis) can be triggered by a severe infection, sepsis, or abrupt withdrawal of steroids. It is a life-threatening emergency, characterized by abnormal electrolytes, hypotension, and hypoglycemia. Sudden death can occur if it is not treated promptly.

Diagnosis

The management of adrenal insufficiency first requires the determination if it is primary or secondary, followed by an identification of the specific cause for the adrenal insufficiency. The tests that are useful in the diagnosis of primary and secondary adrenal insufficiency are shown in **Table 22–3**. Adrenal insufficiency may involve a deficiency of glucocorticoids or both glucocorticoids and mineralocorticoids. On that basis, there will be low levels of serum cortisol and, if mineralocorticoid synthesis is also involved, low levels of serum aldosterone. The ACTH stimulation test, using CRH to stimulate ACTH production, is the most specific test to confirm a diagnosis of adrenal insufficiency and identify it as primary or secondary. Patients with primary adrenal insufficiency do not usually show cortisol secretion following ACTH stimulation because the defect is within the adrenal gland. Patients with mild or recent onset of secondary adrenal insufficiency (and a still viable adrenal cortex) respond to the ACTH because the defect is not within the adrenal gland. A chronic lack of stimulation of the adrenal cortex by ACTH in secondary adrenal insufficiency can result in cortical atrophy and limited cortisol production following ACTH stimulation by CRH. The CRH stimulation test can distinguish between secondary adrenal insufficiency caused by ACTH deficiency and that caused by CRH deficiency. Plasma ACTH and serum cortisol are measured after administration of CRH; increases are observed in hypothalamic

Adrenal insufficiency may involve a deficiency of glucocorticoids or both glucocorticoids and mineralocorticoids. On that basis, there will be low levels of serum cortisol and, if mineralocorticoid synthesis is also involved, low levels of serum aldosterone.

TABLE 22-3 Laboratory Evaluation for Adrenal Insufficiency

Laboratory Test	Primary Adrenal Insufficiency	Secondary Adrenal Insufficiency
ACTH stimulation test	Exogenous ACTH does not stimulate cortisol secretion because the dysfunctional adrenal cortex is already maximally stimulated by endogenous ACTH	If the secondary adrenal insufficiency is mild or of recent onset, there is an increase in cortisol secretion; there is a minimal increase, if any, in plasma cortisol after administration of ACTH in patients with long-standing disease because the adrenal cortex is atrophied in secondary adrenal insufficiency from a chronic lack of stimulation by ACTH
Serum cortisol measured between 8 and 9 AM	Low	Low
Plasma ACTH	Elevated, because feedback inhibition by the adrenal is absent	Low, because the origin of the disorder is in the hypothalamus or pituitary
Serum aldosterone	Low in cases in which the destruction of the adrenal gland impacts both cortisol production and aldosterone production	Often normal, although it may be depressed if there is significant atrophy of the adrenal glands as a result of chronic lack of stimulation by ACTH
CRH stimulation test	Not useful	This test can distinguish between ACTH deficiency (from the pituitary) and deficiency of CRH (from the hypothalamus); plasma ACTH and cortisol are measured after administration of CRH; if secondary adrenal insufficiency is the result of a hypothalamic disorder, the CRH will produce an increase in plasma ACTH and cortisol
Adrenal autoantibody tests	This is a test for detection of antibodies against the adrenal cortex and is performed by indirect immunofluorescence on sections of bovine or human adrenal cortex; autoimmune adrenalitis is a common cause of primary adrenal insufficiency	Not useful

ACTH, adrenocorticotropic hormone (corticotropin); CRH, corticotropin-releasing hormone.

disorders, but not in pituitary disorders. A serologic test for anti-adrenal antibodies is useful to determine if autoimmune adrenalitis is the cause of primary adrenal insufficiency.

Hyperfunction and Hypofunction Involving Mineralocorticoids: Hyperaldosteronism and Hypoaldosteronism

Description and Diagnosis

Aldosterone is a mineralocorticoid produced in the adrenal glands. It is largely responsible for sodium retention and water resorption, and thereby control of blood volume. It also promotes the excretion of potassium into the urine. Aldosterone concentration in the blood is regulated by the renin–angiotensin system (**Figure 22–6**). In response to decreased blood volume, the juxtaglomerular apparatus of the kidney secretes renin, which converts angiotensinogen to angiotensin I. Angiotensin I is converted to angiotensin II by angiotensin-converting enzyme in the lungs. Angiotensin II is a potent vasoconstrictor and also stimulates the adrenal glands to generate aldosterone, which then increases blood volume by promoting sodium retention in exchange for potassium that is lost into the urine.

Aldosterone levels in disease may be high (hyperaldosteronism) or low (hypoaldosteronism). An abnormal (high or low) level of serum aldosterone may be the result of a defect originating inside (primary disorder) or outside (secondary disorder) the adrenal gland (**Table 22–4**).

> Aldosterone is a mineralocorticoid produced in the adrenal glands. It is largely responsible for sodium retention and water resorption, and thereby control of blood volume. It also promotes the excretion of potassium into the urine.

Primary Hyperaldosteronism

In this disorder, there is excess secretion of aldosterone as a result of an abnormality within the adrenal gland. Most often, the high level of aldosterone is produced by bilateral hyperplasia of the adrenal glands or by an aldosterone-secreting adenoma, resulting in a disorder known as Conn syndrome. Less often, primary hyperaldosteronism is a result of primary (unilateral) adrenal

TABLE 22–4   **Laboratory Evaluation for Hyperaldosteronism and Hypoaldosteronism**

Laboratory Test	Primary Hyperaldosteronism	Secondary Hyperaldosteronism	Primary Hypoaldosteronism	Secondary Hypoaldosteronism
Serum potassium	Usually low, but a low-sodium diet may result in a normal value	Usually low, but a low-sodium diet may result in a normal value	Usually elevated	Usually elevated
Serum sodium	Mildly elevated in most cases	Normal or mildly elevated	Usually low	Low or low normal
Serum aldosterone	Elevated in samples collected from patients recumbent 1 hour and on an unrestricted sodium diet (>100 mmol/day) for at least 3 days	Elevated in samples collected on patients recumbent for 1 hour and on an unrestricted sodium diet (>100 mmol/day) for at least 3 days	Usually low	Usually low
Plasma renin activity	Low for most causes of hyperaldosteronism; the low value for plasma renin makes the ratio of serum aldosterone to plasma renin very elevated in primary hyperaldosteronism	Elevated when there is decreased perfusion of the kidneys, a common cause of secondary hyperaldosteronism	Normal or elevated	Hypoaldosteronism may be secondary to a variety of disorders associated with low renin production, and in these disorders the renin is low; with other causes of secondary hypoaldosteronism, the renin may be normal or elevated

hyperplasia or a cancerous tumor. In primary hyperaldosteronism, the plasma renin activity (PRA) is low because the high level of plasma aldosterone concentration (PAC) maintains an adequate or more than adequate blood volume. The ratio of the PAC/PRA is widely used as a screening test for primary aldosteronism in hypertensive patients. A ratio of greater than 25 is used to identify patients with this disorder.

Secondary Hyperaldosteronism

In this disorder, there is excess secretion of aldosterone as a result of an abnormality outside the adrenal gland. It is much more common than primary hyperaldosteronism. Decreased renal perfusion is the most common cause of secondary hyperaldosteronism. The decreased blood flow into the kidney results in an elevation of the PRA. The elevation in plasma renin level (as shown in **Figure 22–6**) produces the increase in aldosterone. Congestive heart failure, nephrotic syndrome, cirrhosis of the liver, and other hypoproteinemic conditions in which there is chronic depletion of plasma volume can produce an elevation in serum aldosterone.

The clinical and laboratory features common to both primary and secondary hyperaldosteronism include hypertension associated with hypervolemia and low or low-normal levels of serum potassium. The serum sodium also may be slightly elevated. Additional clinical features include nocturnal polyuria, polydipsia, and weakness from the low potassium levels.

Primary Hypoaldosteronism

This disorder is much less common than primary hyperaldosteronism. Primary hypoaldosteronism is most often a result of destruction of the adrenal gland from various causes (as noted in the section "Hypofunction Involving Glucocorticoids With or Without Mineralocorticoids: Adrenal Insufficiency"), including autoimmune adrenalitis, adrenal infection by tuberculosis, metastatic tumors to the adrenal, adrenalectomy, CAH associated with low aldosterone production (see the section "Alterations in the Synthesis of Glucocorticoids, Mineralocorticoids, and Sex Steroids: Congenital Adrenal Hyperplasia"), and hemorrhage into the adrenal gland. There is an additional disorder associated with primary hypoaldosteronism, known as pseudohypoaldosteronism, in which the tissues are resistant to the action of aldosterone. In this disorder, the serum aldosterone and plasma renin levels are very elevated.

The clinical and laboratory features common to both primary and secondary hyperaldosteronism include hypertension associated with hypervolemia and low or low-normal levels of serum potassium.

Secondary Hypoaldosteronism

In this disorder, aldosterone hyposecretion results from factors originating outside the adrenal gland. One cause is a deficiency of ACTH production in the pituitary, often accompanied by deficiencies of other pituitary hormones. As noted earlier, the adrenal cortex can become atrophied as a result of a chronic lack of stimulation by ACTH, decreasing aldosterone as well as cortisol production. Another cause is long-term glucocorticoid administration. A low level of ACTH can occur with prolonged glucocorticoid therapy because the glucocorticoids provide a negative feedback signal to the pituitary for ACTH production. Secondary hypoaldosteronism can also occur as a result of deficient renin production and from inhibition of angiotensin-converting enzyme by medications.

Clinical and laboratory features common to primary and secondary hypoaldosteronism include hypotension, which may be orthostatic, and high serum potassium levels. Slightly low serum sodium values also may be present. The clinical signs and symptoms vary significantly and depend on the specific defect leading to the hypoaldosteronism. Patients with pseudohypoaldosteronism have clinical features found in patients with true hypoaldosteronism because their tissues are unresponsive to aldosterone. However, these patients do not have the low aldosterone values found in true hypoaldosteronism, but instead have elevated levels.

Alterations in the Synthesis of Glucocorticoids, Mineralocorticoids, and Sex Steroids: Congenital Adrenal Hyperplasia

Description and Diagnosis

CAH is caused by any 1 of a group of enzyme deficiencies in the biosynthetic pathways for cortisol and aldosterone. Because cortisol production is decreased, and cortisol provides the inhibitory feedback to the pituitary for ACTH secretion, the lack of cortisol results in an increase in ACTH and excess stimulation of the adrenal gland (see **Figures 22–5** and **22–6** for the regulation of cortisol and aldosterone production). This results in greater flux through pathways around an existing enzymatic defect, producing elevations in adrenal hormones whose synthesis is not affected by the enzyme deficiency. Most of the known enzyme deficiencies in the synthetic pathways for aldosterone and cortisol result in an elevation in sex steroid synthesis, which has a virilizing effect on the patient. The most common of the enzymatic defects is a deficiency of 21-hydroxylase. This deficiency accounts for 90% to 95% of the cases of CAH. The clinical manifestations for 4 of the enzyme deficiencies producing CAH are noted below. **Figure 22–4** shows the intermediate compounds in the synthesis of aldosterone, cortisol, and androgens in the adrenal gland and the enzymes in the pathway, some of which may be deficient. **Table 22–5** presents the laboratory evaluation for CAH.

- *21-Hydroxylase deficiency*—This is the most common form of CAH. In female infants, this deficiency results in hypertrophy of the clitoris and pseudohermaphroditism as a result of disruption in the synthesis pathways for cortisol and aldosterone. In postpubertal females, it results in amenorrhea, infertility, and hirsutism. In males, the virilization results in enlargement of the external genitalia and precocious puberty. As seen in **Figure 22–4**, 21-hydroxylase deficiency will result in a decrease the generation of both cortisol and aldosterone.
- *11-Beta-hydroxylase deficiency*—This is the second most common enzyme deficiency. The clinical and laboratory features of patients with this abnormality are largely similar to those found in patients with 21-hydroxylase deficiency. In addition, the patients with this disorder develop mineralocorticoid-induced hypertension and hypokalemia from an elevation in deoxycorticosterone, an aldosterone precursor with significant mineralocorticoid activity.
- *17-Alpha-hydroxylase deficiency*—This deficiency is rare and accounts for approximately 1% of all CAH cases. In this deficiency, there is no inhibition of aldosterone synthesis, but there is a block in the synthesis of both cortisol and sex steroids. The elevation of aldosterone results in hyperaldosteronism that produces hypertension and hypokalemia. In females, the androgen deficiency results in a lack of development of secondary sex characteristics because the androgens are biochemical precursors of estrogens. In males, pseudohermaphroditism appears.

Most of the known enzyme deficiencies in the synthetic pathways for aldosterone and cortisol result in an elevation in sex steroid synthesis, which has a virilizing effect on the patient. The most common of the enzymatic defects is a deficiency of 21-hydroxylase.

TABLE 22–5   Laboratory Evaluation for Congenital Adrenal Hyperplasia

Enzyme Deficiency	Relevant Laboratory Findings (Focusing on Compounds Most Likely to Be Measured in an Evaluation)
21-Hydroxylase	Elevated: 17-hydroxyprogesterone, androstenedione, DHEA, and its sulfated metabolite (DHEA-S) testosterone; ACTH and plasma renin activity because of the deficiencies of cortisol and aldosterone
	Decreased: aldosterone, cortisol
11-Beta-hydroxylase	This defect results in a decrease in aldosterone production and cortisol synthesis and the elevations shown above for 21-hydroxylase deficiency. An assay for 11-deoxycortisol or deoxycorticosterone is necessary to differentiate the 21-hydroxylase deficiency from the 11-beta-hydroxylase deficiency. These steroids are elevated in 11-beta-hydroxylase deficiency and low in 21-hydroxylase deficiency
17-Alpha-hydroxylase	Elevated: aldosterone; deoxycorticosterone
	Decreased: androgens, cortisol
3-Beta-hydroxysteroid dehydrogenase	Elevated: DHEA; ACTH and plasma renin activity because of the deficiencies of cortisol and aldosterone
	Decreased: aldosterone, cortisol
	Assays for 17-hydroxypregnenolone and 17-hydroxyprogesterone, as well as assays for DHEA and androstenedione, are helpful in the differentiation of 3-beta-hydroxysteroid dehydrogenase deficiency from 21-hydroxylase deficiency and 11-beta-hydroxylase deficiency; the 17-hydroxypregnenolone to 17-hydroxyprogesterone ratio and the DHEA to androstenedione ratio in 3-beta-hydroxysteroid dehydrogenase deficiency are extremely high

ACTH, adrenocorticotropic hormone (corticotropin); DHEA, dehydroepiandrosterone.

- *3-Beta-hydroxysteroid dehydrogenase deficiency*—This is another rare CAH disorder. This enzymatic deficiency results in a metabolic block in the production of aldosterone and cortisol, with no inhibition of the synthesis of DHEA, an androgen. In its severe form, this enzyme deficiency manifests as early masculinization in males and amenorrhea and pseudohermaphroditism in females.

ADRENAL MEDULLA

Physiology and Biochemistry

The main sites of production of the catecholamines are the brain, the chromaffin cells of the adrenal medulla, and the sympathetic neurons. The catecholamines include dopamine, epinephrine, and norepinephrine as the most potent of the endogenously produced compounds. Of these, in the adrenal medulla, epinephrine production is quantitatively the greatest. The catecholamines have a wide variety of biological effects. They have a marked impact on the vascular system, and are therefore important in the regulation of blood pressure. Epinephrine influences many metabolic pathways, especially carbohydrate metabolism. In some tissues, epinephrine and norepinephrine produce opposite effects. Alpha-adrenergic receptors on cells interact effectively with both epinephrine and norepinephrine, and the beta-adrenergic receptors respond primarily to epinephrine with little activation by norepinephrine.

Catecholamine synthesis and metabolism in the adrenal medulla is illustrated in **Figure 22–7**. The pathway begins with an amino acid, tyrosine. This is metabolized to a catecholamine, dihydroxyphenylalanine (DOPA). DOPA is then converted to dopamine, which is transformed to norepinephrine, which is subsequently converted to epinephrine. Because of their great potency, the catecholamines must be rapidly inactivated through re-uptake into storage granules, conversion to metabolites, or excretion. Unlike the steroid hormones, catecholamines are not bound to proteins as they circulate. In plasma, they have a very short half-life of approximately 2 minutes. Urine catecholamines, on the

The catecholamines include dopamine, epinephrine, and norepinephrine as the most potent of the endogenously produced compounds. Of these, in the adrenal medulla, epinephrine production is quantitatively the greatest.

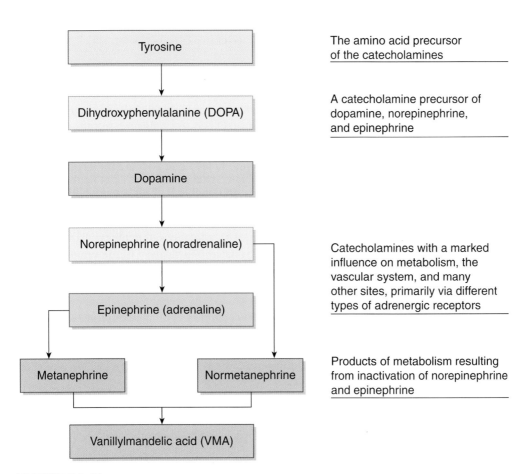

FIGURE 22–7 **Catecholamine synthesis and metabolism in the adrenal medulla.**

other hand, represent a pool of catecholamines delivered into urine in the preceding hours. There are a number of degradative products of epinephrine and norepinephrine. The compounds noted in **Figure 22–7**—metanephrine, normetanephrine, and vanillylmandelic acid—are the ones that are measured in clinical assays to assess catecholamine production and degradation.

Laboratory Tests

Epinephrine and Norepinephrine

Total or fractionated (epinephrine or norepinephrine) catecholamines can be measured in plasma or urine samples. The plasma concentration reflects the rate of synthesis and release of catecholamines by the adrenal medulla and their half-life in the circulation. Catecholamines are secreted into the urine as free hormones.

Metanephrines (Metanephrine and Normetanephrine)

Both metanephrine and normetanephrine undergo conjugation with sulfate or glucuronide. The metanephrines can be measured in a randomly collected single urine specimen. If the result is not definitive for a diagnosis, a 24-hour urine collection for quantitation of urinary metanephrines is often performed. Total and fractionated metanephrines can be measured in plasma samples.

Vanillylmandelic Acid

This compound is the major metabolite of both metanephrine and normetanephrine. It is measured in the urine and, although it is indicative of catecholamine synthesis and metabolism, it is inferior to urinary metanephrine quantitation for this purpose.

There are a number of degradative products of epinephrine and norepinephrine. Metanephrine, normetanephrine, and vanillylmandelic acid are the ones that are measured in clinical assays to assess catecholamine production and degradation.

Pheochromocytoma

Description

A pheochromocytoma, which may be benign or malignant, is a chromaffin cell tumor of the adrenal medulla or autonomic nervous system that secretes catecholamines. On this basis, it is a cause of hypertension. However, it is a rare cause of hypertension with approximately 5 pheochromocytomas per 100,000 hypertensive cases. Other catecholamine-secreting chromaffin cell tumors are paragangliomas and neuroblastomas. It is essential that a pheochromocytoma be rapidly and accurately identified in patients with hypertension because surgical resection of the tumor, with elimination of the hypertension and its complications, is successful in at least 90% of cases, and the disease may be otherwise fatal. The diagnosis is made most often in patients between the ages of 30 and 60 years. The clinical features of a patient with pheochromocytoma include, most importantly, the presence of sustained or paroxysmal hypertension. The attacks of hypertension occur abruptly and subside slowly, with a total duration of less than 1 hour in approximately 80% of patients. They may be precipitated by palpation of the tumor, postural changes, exertion, anxiety, trauma, pain, intake of foods or beverages containing tyramine (such as certain cheeses, beer, and wine), and the ingestion of certain medications. Headaches are common in patients with pheochromocytoma, and they are usually severe. Generalized sweating and palpitations with tachycardia occur frequently. Other common signs and symptoms are anxiety, chest pain, nausea, fatigue, and weight loss. Of all pheochromocytomas, approximately 10% are familial and coexist with a form of multiple endocrine neoplasia (MEN) (see later section), 10% are malignant, 10% are extra-adrenal in location and are called paragangliomas (and therefore 90% are in the adrenal), and 10% are bilateral.

> It is essential that a pheochromocytoma be rapidly and accurately identified in patients with hypertension because surgical resection of the tumor, with elimination of the hypertension and its complications, is successful in at least 90% of cases, and the disease may be otherwise fatal.

Diagnosis

As noted before, the most biologically significant catecholamines synthesized by a pheochromocytoma are epinephrine and norepinephrine. These compounds are metabolized into

TABLE 22-6   Laboratory Evaluation for Pheochromocytoma

Laboratory Test	Results/Comments
Plasma metanephrines	Measurement of fractionated, free plasma metanephrines is the preferred screening test to rule out pheochromocytoma; a low level of metanephrines reliably excludes the diagnosis of pheochromocytoma
Urinary metanephrines	More than 95% of patients with pheochromocytoma will have an elevated level of urinary metanephrines; the measurement of metanephrines per gram of creatinine can be made with a randomly collected single urine specimen, or if the result is not definitive, with a 24-hour urine collection; an elevated urinary metanephrine level in the presence of clinical signs and symptoms consistent with pheochromocytoma can establish the diagnosis
Plasma catecholamines	Concentrations of plasma catecholamines are elevated in pheochromocytoma; if hypertension is paroxysmal (epinephrine and norepinephrine) rather than sustained, blood must be obtained for catecholamine measurement during a spontaneous or provoked hypertensive episode to demonstrate an elevated plasma catecholamine level; because plasma catecholamines increase with stress, the sample for plasma catecholamine measurement must be collected with careful regard to minimize stress to the patient; blood is optimally obtained after at least 20 minutes of rest and drawn through a previously inserted venous cannula; the medications that the patient is ingesting at the time of or immediately prior to the test may also influence catecholamine levels
Urinary catecholamines	Urinary catecholamines may be used in the initial assessment of a possible pheochromocytoma; however, the test for urinary metanephrines has a higher sensitivity for detection of pheochromocytoma
Urinary vanillylmandelic acid	Urinary VMA is elevated in the majority of patients who have a pheochromocytoma, but it is less sensitive than the test for urinary metanephrines for diagnosis of the disorder; the urinary VMA level is not needed to establish the diagnosis; ingestion of tricyclic antidepressants and selected other medications may produce spurious results in this assay

metanephrine and normetanephrine, respectively (**Figure 22–7**), and both of these compounds can be metabolized to vanillylmandelic acid. Measurement of fractionated, free plasma metanephrines is the preferred screening test to rule out pheochromocytoma. Follow-up testing for patients with suspected pheochromocytoma and a positive plasma metanepherines screening test includes measurement of metanephrines in a random or 24-hour urine sample and then fractionated catecholamines in plasma or urine. The diagnosis of pheochromocytoma is based on the detection of increased levels of urinary or plasma metanephrines, and possibly plasma or urinary catecholamines, in the appropriate clinical setting of sustained or paroxysmal hypertension. A number of radiographic techniques can be used to localize a pheochromocytoma. In addition, blood sampling from an individual adrenal gland can be used to locate a tumor when all other localization methods fail. Laboratory tests used for diagnosis of pheochromocytoma are described in **Table 22–6**.

PARATHYROIDS

This section is focused on parathyroid hormone (PTH) and disorders associated with high or low levels of this hormone. Most parathyroid disorders alter calcium metabolism, and thereby have an effect on bone. However, there are also a number of disorders associated with hypercalcemia or hypocalcemia, or alterations in bone density, in which a change in the PTH level is not a major factor. Therefore, in addition to hyperparathyroidism and hypoparathyroidism, this chapter also briefly describes a few selected disorders associated with hypercalcemia, hypocalcemia, or altered bone density in which PTH does not play a major role.

Physiology and Biochemistry

PTH is a polypeptide secreted from the parathyroid glands. The primary function of PTH is the regulation of the concentration of ionized calcium in extracellular fluids. An increase in secretion of PTH produces a rise in serum ionized calcium and a decrease in the serum phosphorus concentration. A normal or an elevated blood calcium provides negative feedback to the parathyroid gland to reduce the secretion of PTH (see **Figure 22–8**).

The resorption of bone induced by PTH is mediated by increased activity of osteoclasts. PTH can also promote an increase in the renal tubular reabsorption of calcium.

Vitamin D is an intermediary in the action of PTH to elevate the serum calcium level. It is a fat-soluble hormone required for calcium absorption in the gut, bone metabolism, and development of cells and the immune system. Vitamin D also influences phosphorus metabolism. Vitamin D_2 is known as ergosterol, and vitamin D_3 is known as cholecalciferol.

Food can be fortified with either vitamin D_2 or D_3, both of which can be used as vitamin D supplements. Cholecalciferol is ingested in the diet, and it is also synthesized in the skin upon ultraviolet irradiation of 7-dehydrocholesterol. The cholecalciferol is transported to the liver where it is hydroxylated to produce 25-hydroxycholecalciferol [25-$(OH)D_3)$] The 25-(OH)D_3 has limited biological activity, but in the kidney it undergoes further hydroxylation to form dihydroxy metabolites, the most potent of which in calcium metabolism is 1,25-$(OH)_2D_3$. An increase in this vitamin D metabolite results in increased intestinal absorption of calcium and an elevation in plasma calcium levels. The production of this dihydroxy metabolite of vitamin D is regulated by the need for calcium in the circulation. Decreased blood calcium results in a stimulation of the parathyroid glands to secrete PTH that leads to the increased production of 1,25-$(OH)_2D_3$ in the renal proximal tubules. Thus, PTH is responsible for maintaining the necessary levels of calcium in the body by extracting sufficient calcium from the diet, resorbing it from bone, or preventing its excretion through the renal tubules. **Figure 22–8** shows the regulation of PTH secretion. Ingested Vitamin D_2 is hydroxylated into 25-$(OH)D_2$ and follows the same metabolism to 1,25-$(OH)_2D_2$.

Calcitonin has an opposing action to PTH, but in humans it appears to play a minor role in calcium homeostasis. As a drug, its pharmacologic action is more definitive. It inhibits osteoclastic bone resorption. It also decreases renal tubular reabsorption of calcium, and by these mechanisms opposes the action of PTH. Calcitonin synthesis occurs in the parafollicular cells of the thyroid gland.

An increase in secretion of PTH produces a rise in serum ionized calcium and a decrease in the serum phosphorus concentration. Calcitonin has an opposing action to PTH, but in humans it appears to play a minor role in calcium homeostasis.

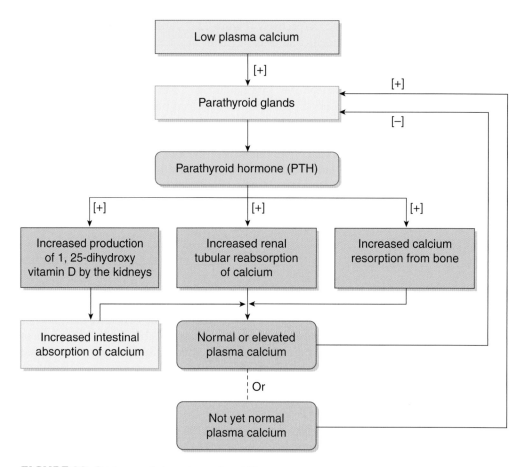

FIGURE 22–8 **The regulation of parathyroid hormone secretion. [+] Stimulation; [–] Inhibition.**

Only about 1% of the calcium in the bones is exchangeable with the extracellular fluid, and it is this pool that is most significantly affected by the level of PTH.

Approximately 98% of calcium is present in the body within the bones in the form of hydroxyapatite, a crystal lattice composed of calcium, phosphorus, and hydroxide. Of the calcium not within the bones, about half is present in extracellular fluid and the remainder is present in a variety of tissues, particularly skeletal muscle. Only about 1% of the calcium in the bones is exchangeable with the extracellular fluid, and it is this pool that is most significantly affected by the level of PTH. Calcium exists in the plasma in 3 distinct forms, 1 of which is free or ionized calcium. This is the physiologically active form of calcium and accounts for approximately 45% to 50% of the total calcium in the plasma. Another 40% to 45% of calcium in the plasma is bound to plasma proteins. The protein that binds most of this calcium is albumin, but calcium also binds to some globulins. The remaining 10% to 15% of the total calcium forms a complex with a variety of anions. The most commonly found complexes are calcium phosphate and calcium citrate. The distribution of the 3 forms of calcium changes with alterations in pH in the extracellular fluid and with changes in plasma protein concentration. In general, the serum ionized calcium increases in acidosis and decreases in alkalosis; an increase in the concentration of plasma proteins that bind calcium results in a corresponding increase in total calcium; and a decrease in the plasma proteins may result in a decrease in total calcium.

The metabolism of phosphorus is linked to the metabolism of calcium. About 85% of the phosphorus in an adult is present in the bone as part of hydroxyapatite. Most of the remaining phosphorus in the body is within phospholipids, proteins, carbohydrates, nucleotides, and other important biochemical compounds. Phosphorus is present in virtually all foods, and dietary deficiencies do not occur. The phosphorus in the extracellular fluid exists primarily as HPO_4^{2-} and $H_2PO_4^-$, which are collectively known as inorganic phosphorus. The relative amounts of these 2 phosphate anions are pH-dependent. Food ingestion can alter the serum inorganic phosphorus concentration significantly, with an increase in serum phosphorus concentration following the ingestion of phosphate-rich food.

Laboratory Tests

Calcium

Whole blood, serum, or plasma specimens can be used for measurement of total calcium levels. For accurate measurement of the ionized or free form of calcium, the specimen must be transported on ice and must not be exposed to air.

Inorganic Phosphorus

About 15% of the inorganic phosphorus, predominantly HPO_4^{2-} and $H_2PO_4^-$, in the plasma is protein-bound, and the remainder is free or complexed to another ion. Organic phosphorus (not measured in the assay for inorganic phosphorus) refers to the phosphorus within phospholipids, proteins, carbohydrates, nucleic acids, and other organic substances.

PTH

The most important test in the differential diagnosis of hypercalcemia is the assay for serum PTH. The biological activity of PTH resides in the first 34-amino terminal amino acids.

The intact hormone (iPTH) with 84 amino acids accounts for much of the circulating PTH, but there are many circulating PTH fragments. The assay for iPTH has largely superseded earlier tests for various PTH fragments.

Intraoperative PTH Assay

Primary hyperparathyroidism requiring parathyroidectomy is a challenge because of variability in the location and number of parathyroid glands. Of parathyroid adenomas, 15% to 20% are ectopic rather than adjacent to the thyroid gland, and approximately 5% of patients have 5 parathyroid glands rather than 4. The success of parathyroid surgery has been improved by intraoperative PTH measurement. The intraoperative PTH assay is used to detect decreases in plasma PTH levels on excision of parathyroid tumors in surgery. Use of this intraoperative test has resulted in a higher incidence of complete removal of hypersecreting parathyroid gland tissue, reduced the need for extensive exploration of the neck, and decreased the need for repeat surgery.

The success of parathyroid surgery has been improved by intraoperative PTH measurement. The intraoperative PTH assay is used to detect decreases in plasma PTH levels on excision of parathyroid tumors in surgery.

Vitamin D

The quantitation of selected vitamin D metabolites is useful in assessing vitamin D metabolism. Vitamin D metabolites of greatest relevance to calcium metabolism include $25\text{-}(OH)D_3$ (also known as 25-hydroxy vitamin D) and $1,25\text{-}(OH)_2D_3$ (also known as 1,25-dihydroxy vitamin D). Currently the most commonly ordered test is the total 25-(OH) vitamin D, which is a combination of the 25-(OH) vitamin D_2 and 25-(OH) vitamin D_3. Recently, tandem mass spectrometry has increased in use and allowed for measurement of vitamin D_2 and vitamin D_3 in either form [i.e., 25-(OH) or 1,25-(OH)]. 25-(OH) vitamin D is the most abundant metabolite of vitamin D, and it has a long half-life. It is the component measured in most immunoassays for vitamin D. In contrast, 1,25-(OH) vitamin D has a much lower serum concentration, and a shorter half-life (4 to 6 hours).

PTH-related Protein (PTHrP)

This protein, nearly twice the size of PTH, is equipotent with PTH in causing hypercalcemia. Like PTH, it stimulates renal proximal tubular reabsorption of calcium. The assay to measure PTHrP shows less than 1% cross-reactivity with PTH.

Bone Markers

Markers for bone turnover can be classified into 2 groups, markers of bone formation and resorption. Bone markers should not be used as definitive tests for the diagnosis of osteoporosis. Their primary utility is to monitor response to treatment for bone disease. The markers with the most clinical utility are described below.

Bone Formation Markers

Alkaline Phosphatase. This enzyme is present in a wide variety of tissues, one of which is the bone. Most laboratory assays for alkaline phosphatase (ALP) measure total ALP. The bone-derived fraction of ALP can be differentiated from its isoenzymes in serum by bone-specific ALP immunoassay or based on its instability. Bone ALP is denatured by heat and urea.

Osteocalcin. Serum osteocalcin is a moderately specific marker for bone formation. Serum concentrations are highest in adolescence, and in the newborn when bone growth is most active, and in renal failure due to clearance impairment. The serum osteocalcin concentration rises in women from the 4th to the 10th decade as the bone turnover increases. Menopause induces a marked increase in bone turnover, often with an increase in serum osteocalcin. Although not as sensitive as collagen markers, measurement of osteocalcin can help predict bone loss in postmenopausal women.

Procollagen Type I Intact N-Terminal Propeptide (PINP). PINP, which is formed during collagen synthesis, is the most sensitive marker of bone formation. Measurement of PINP by radioimmunoassay in serum is recommended for monitoring of therapy to bone disease. It should be measured prior to initiation of therapy and then subsequently 3 to 6 months later. PINP exhibits less intraindividual biovariability than other collagen markers.

Bone Resorption Markers

N- and C-Terminal Telopeptide of Type 1 Collagen (NTx and CTx). NTx and CTx are peptide fragments formed during bone resorption through proteolytic processing of the N- and C-terminal ends of type I collagen, respectively. These can be measured by immunoassay in both serum and urine to assess response to treatment of bone disease. Significant intraindividual variability exists in CTx concentrations because it is affected by diet, exercise, and time of day. NTx should be measured prior to initiation of therapy and then 3 to 6 months later to assess bone disease status.

Pyridinium Crosslinks. Pyridinium crosslinks, including deoxypyridinoline (DPD), are a group of products formed during bone resorption as a result of collagen breakdown. These can be measured by immunoassay and are useful in monitoring therapy. Urine pyridinium crosslink concentrations can determine efficacy of bone disease treatment after as little as 2 months of therapy.

Primary Hyperparathyroidism
Description

In primary hyperparathyroidism, there is excess secretion of PTH in the absence of an appropriate stimulus. The disease affects women about twice as frequently as it affects men, and the incidence increases with age. The majority of cases of primary hyperparathyroidism result from a single parathyroid adenoma, with hyperplasia of the parathyroids and parathyroid carcinoma being less common causes. The hypercalcemia in hyperparathyroidism occurs as a result of the direct action of PTH to increase resorption of bone calcium, PTH-induced renal tubular reabsorption of calcium, and synthesis of $1,25\text{-}(OH)_2D_3$ that promotes the intestinal absorption of calcium. Primary hyperparathyroidism is often identified in asymptomatic individuals who have an unexpected serum hypercalcemia. Symptomatic patients with primary hyperparathyroidism may present with kidney stones, chronic constipation, mental depression, neuromuscular dysfunction, recurrent pancreatitis, peptic ulcer, or an unexplained osteopenia.

The majority of cases of primary hyperparathyroidism result from a single parathyroid adenoma, with hyperplasia of the parathyroids and parathyroid carcinoma being less common causes. In the diagnosis of primary hyperparathyroidism, the total serum calcium is the initial test.

Diagnosis

In the diagnosis of primary hyperparathyroidism, the total serum calcium is the initial test. The ionized calcium also should be determined, especially in patients with abnormal serum concentrations of total protein or albumin. As noted earlier, the total serum calcium is 45% to 50% free and ionized, 40% to 45% protein-bound (mostly to albumin), and 10% to 15% complexed with small inorganic and organic ions. On demonstration of hypercalcemia, serum PTH and fasting serum phosphorus (because the phosphorus level in the serum is altered by diet) should be measured. Assays for PTH can measure the intact molecule, carboxy-terminal, or midregion segments. The use of the intact PTH assay is preferred, especially in patients with renal disease because PTH carboxy-terminal fragments can accumulate with decreased renal function. The diagnosis of hyperparathyroidism is made when persistent hypercalcemia and an elevated serum

TABLE 22–7 Laboratory Evaluation for Hyperparathyroidism and Hypoparathyroidism

Laboratory Test	Primary Hyperparathyroidism	Secondary Hyperparathyroidism	Hypoparathyroidism	Hypercalcemia of Malignancy
Serum total or ionized calcium	Elevated	Low or normal	Low	Elevated
Serum intact PTH	Elevated	Elevated	Low or undetectable	Low or normal
Serum PTH-related protein	Undetectable	Undetectable	Undetectable	Detectable in some cancers
Serum 1,25-dihydroxy vitamin D	May be elevated but not usually required for diagnosis	May be elevated, normal or low depending on the blood concentrations of calcium and phosphorus	Low	Low or normal
Serum phosphorus (inorganic)	Low or normal	Normal	Elevated	Low or normal

PTH, parathyroid hormone.

PTH level are both demonstrated. The serum inorganic phosphorus may be normal in patients with primary hyperparathyroidism. Patients with severe hyperparathyroidism can have bone pain, skeletal deformities, and even bone fractures (**Table 22–7**).

Secondary Hyperparathyroidism
Description
Secondary hyperparathyroidism occurs when there is chronic hypocalcemia and an excessive compensatory secretion of PTH. Chronic hypocalcemia is often a result of vitamin D deficiency or renal disease with calcium losses into the urine. Inadequate dietary intake of calcium is a rare cause of hypocalcemia. Renal failure with calcium loss, which leads to the elevation in PTH in secondary hyperparathyroidism, can, in turn, produce bone disease, because of the excessive resorption of calcium from the bone in secondary hyperparathyroidism.

Diagnosis
In secondary hyperparathyroidism, there is an elevation in the PTH, but unlike primary hyperparathyroidism, the total and ionized calcium in the serum is low or normal. Tests to identify causes of primary hyperparathyroidism, such as a parathyroid adenoma, should have negative results. Tests should be performed to identify the cause of the chronic hypocalcemia leading to secondary hyperparathyroidism, to establish a diagnosis. Vitamin D deficiency and renal disease, as noted previously, are the 2 most common causes of chronic hypocalcemia, and these may be diagnosed with the appropriate laboratory assays (**Table 22–7**).

Hypoparathyroidism
Description
Hypoparathyroidism occurs most frequently with unintentional removal of the parathyroids in the surgical excision of the thyroid gland. Other causes of hypoparathyroidism are much less common. Hypocalcemia resulting from the hypoparathyroidism produces characteristic signs and symptoms, including numbness and tingling, and for patients with very low serum calcium levels, convulsions and muscle spasms.

Diagnosis
In hypoparathyroidism, the total and ionized calcium levels in the serum are low, with a low or undetectable serum PTH concentration. There is an elevation in the serum inorganic phosphorus associated with the decrease in serum calcium (**Table 22–7**).

Hypoparathyroidism occurs most frequently with unintentional removal of the parathyroids in the surgical excision of the thyroid gland. In hypoparathyroidism, the total and ionized calcium levels in the serum are low, with a low or undetectable serum PTH concentration.

Pseudohypoparathyroidism

Description

As the name implies, patients with pseudohypoparathyroidism have signs and symptoms that are characteristic of hypoparathyroidism. This disorder results from a resistance of the tissues to the action of PTH and not a PTH deficiency, hence the use of the term "pseudo."

Diagnosis

Pseudohypoparathyroidism can be distinguished from true hypoparathyroidism by the high concentration of serum PTH, in the presence of a low serum calcium concentration, in patients with the signs and symptoms of hypoparathyroidism. In addition, patients with pseudohypoparathyroidism demonstrate a lack of metabolic response when infused with PTH.

Hypercalcemia of Malignancy

Description

The most common cause of severe hypercalcemia in an inpatient hospital population is malignancy. Tumors most often associated with hypercalcemia of malignancy include breast carcinoma, multiple myeloma, and lung carcinoma. The serum calcium level may be elevated as a result of osteolysis in the bone from metastases or humoral-induced hypercalcemia. In humoral-induced hypercalcemia, tumor production of PTHrP acts similarly to PTH to produce hypercalcemia. The assay for PTHrP is potentially useful when malignancy is suspected as a cause of hypercalcemia.

> The most common cause of severe hypercalcemia in an inpatient hospital population is malignancy. Tumors most often associated with hypercalcemia of malignancy include breast carcinoma, multiple myeloma, and lung carcinoma.

Diagnosis

Hypercalcemia of malignancy must be differentiated from hyperparathyroidism. Patients with hypercalcemia of malignancy will have an elevated total and ionized serum calcium, in the presence of a low PTH value. The low PTH value is the differentiating feature of hypercalcemia of malignancy from primary and secondary hyperparathyroidism, which are associated with high concentrations of serum PTH (**Table 22–7**). For patients in whom humorally induced hypercalcemia is suspected, the most specific confirmatory test is the assay for PTHrP.

Osteoporosis

Description

Osteoporosis is the most common metabolic disease of the bone associated with decreased bone mass. The causes of osteoporosis are many and varied. Osteoporosis may be primary or secondary. It can occur in association with hyperparathyroidism as described before, as well as with Cushing syndrome, acromegaly, prolonged use of heparin, excess vitamin D intake, and immobilization, among other conditions and disorders.

Bone mineral density (BMD) studies are preferred for diagnosis of primary osteoporosis. BMD estimates obtained by imaging studies are compared to BMD in normal populations to generate a T-score. The WHO defines osteoporosis as a T-score ≤ -2.5. T-scores between -1.0 and -2.4 confirm osteopenia. Laboratory testing is preferred for the evaluation of secondary disease. Bone turnover markers can be used to monitor treatment.

Diagnosis

Osteoporosis as a primary disorder is inferred by the absence of another disease known to induce osteoporosis. Primary osteoporosis is generally idiopathic, postmenopausal, or senile. Secondary osteoporosis is established by demonstrating an underlying process or treatment that leads to osteoporosis.

Osteomalacia

Description

Osteomalacia is deficient mineralization of bone that results from disturbances in calcium and phosphorus metabolism. It can result from a nutritional deficiency of vitamin D, defects in vitamin D metabolism or action, defects in mineral metabolism, or disturbances of the bone cells in the bone matrix. When osteomalacia occurs before the cessation of growth, it is known as rickets. Skeletal deformities appear in rickets because of the compensatory overgrowth of epiphyseal cartilage.

Diagnosis

Radiographic studies can demonstrate the disorder, and the specific cause for osteomalacia, if it is identified, is generally established with laboratory testing. There are many disorders associated with the decreased mineralization of the bone.

Osteitis Deformans (Also Known As Paget Disease of Bone)
Description

Osteitis deformans is associated with osteoclastic resorption of bone and extensive production of abnormal, poorly mineralized osteoid. This results in a bone that is structurally weak and prone to deformity and fracture. The disorder may involve 1 bone or may be more generalized.

Diagnosis

In osteitis deformans, there is a greatly elevated level of serum ALP, which reflects osteoblastic proliferation in the deformed bone. The serum calcium and inorganic phosphorus levels are usually normal, but may be increased in some patients.

TESTES AND OVARIES

Male Physiology and Biochemistry

The male testes serve 2 important functions (**Figure 22–9**). One is the production of sperm, and the other is the synthesis and secretion of androgens. Sertoli cells within the testes secrete inhibin, and this glycoprotein inhibits the pituitary secretion of follicle-stimulating hormone (FSH). FSH acts on the Sertoli cells to stimulate sperm production and the synthesis of inhibin. Leydig cells in the testes are responsible for the production of androgens. The Leydig cells in the testes receive stimulation by luteinizing hormone (LH) to promote the conversion of cholesterol, through many intermediates, to testosterone. Testosterone, 1 of the androgens, is important for both the maturation of sperm and providing negative feedback to the anterior pituitary and hypothalamus to reduce the stimulation of the male testes. The hormone secreted by the hypothalamus in the hypothalamic–pituitary–gonadal axis is gonadotropin-releasing hormone (GnRH). GnRH stimulates the release of both LH and FSH from the pituitary in pulsatile patterns. Higher values for LH and FSH are found in the early morning hours.

The androgens are a collection of 19 carbon steroids that produce masculinization and male secondary sex characteristics. The main androgen secreted by the Leydig cells of the testes is testosterone. Other androgens secreted by the testes include androstenedione and DHEA. These compounds can be metabolized to testosterone and dihydrotestosterone (DHT) in target tissues. Circulating testosterone is a precursor to DHT. As previously noted, a number of androgens are secreted by the adrenal glands, including DHEA, DHEA-sulfate (DHEA-S), androstenedione, and androstenediol. Women also produce testosterone, but only 5% to 10% as much as men. Testosterone, as well as androstenedione, can be converted to estrogens. Approximately 6% to 8% of the testosterone is converted to DHT, but only about 0.3% to estradiol. Most of the testosterone and DHT in the plasma is bound to plasma proteins. Only approximately 3% is free. The 2 major proteins that bind testosterone and DHT are sex hormone-binding globulin (SHBG) and albumin. In men, approximately 45% to 65% of protein-bound testosterone is associated with SHBG and 35% to 50% is bound to albumin. Protein-bound testosterone in women is distributed approximately two thirds on SHBG and one third on albumin. The bioavailable testosterone includes the small fraction which is free and that protein-bound fraction that is bound to albumin. Testosterone is weakly bound to albumin, and therefore available for tissue uptake when associated with albumin. The main excretory metabolites of testosterone, androstenedione, and DHEA are collectively known as 17-ketosteroids that can be quantitated in the urine.

The androgens are a collection of 19 carbon steroids that produce masculinization and male secondary sex characteristics. The main androgen secreted by the Leydig cells of the testes is testosterone. Other androgens secreted by the testes include androstenedione and DHEA.

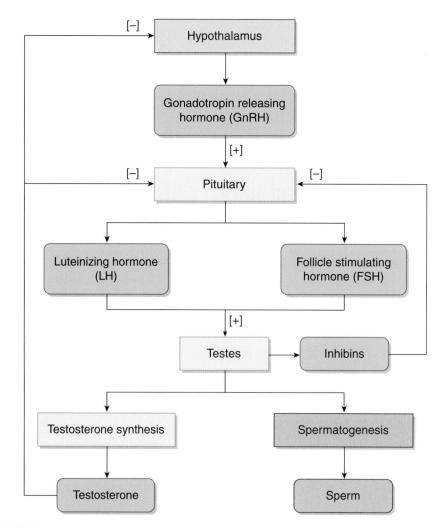

FIGURE 22–9 **The hypothalamic–pituitary–gonadal axis in males. [+] Stimulation; [–] Inhibition.**

Laboratory Tests

Total Testosterone
Total testosterone measured by immunoassay is a commonly used first-line test in evaluating a male or gonadal dysfunction. Total serum testosterone represents both protein-bound and non-protein-bound testosterone.

Free and Weakly Bound Testosterone
This is the bioavailable pool of circulating testosterone. In cases where total testosterone is abnormal, free testosterone can be assessed as a part of a panel that determines bioavailable testosterone and SHBG. Testosterone and SHBG are measured by immunoassay, and concentrations of free and bioavailable testosterone are derived from a mathematical equation based on the constants for the binding of testosterone to albumin and/or SHBG. This assay is not recommended for women and children because the testosterone concentrations are much lower. Therefore, for women and children, testosterone and SHBG are measured by tandem mass spectrometry, and again free and bioavailable testosterone are determined by the same mathematical equation.

SHBG can be measured by immunoassay separately, but the utility is largely in evaluating bioavailable testosterone in men with suspected hypogonadism.

Testosterone Precursors and Metabolites
Immunoassays are available for quantitation of DHT, androstenedione, DHEA, DHEA-S, and other related compounds.

Total testosterone measured by immunoassay is a commonly used first-line test in evaluating a male or gonadal dysfunction.

DHEA and DHEA-S

Serum levels of DHEA and DHEA-S provide an assessment of adrenal androgen production, which may be altered in patients with various conditions, including adrenal hyperplasia, adrenal tumors, delayed puberty, and hirsutism. DHEA is almost entirely derived from the adrenal glands, and DHEA-S in the circulation originates mostly from the adrenal glands, although in men some of it is derived from the testes. There is a circadian rhythm for the serum concentration of DHEA, but not for DHEA-S because it has a longer half-life.

Urinary 17-Ketosteroids

As noted above, the 17-ketosteroids in the urine are a collection of metabolites of androgenic steroids secreted by the testes, the adrenal glands, and in women, by the ovaries. The urine 17-ketosteroid test detects androsterone, DHEA, and several other steroids. However, it does not detect cortisol, estrogens, pregnanediol, testosterone, and DHT because they do not have a ketone functional group. In men, approximately 33% of the urinary 17-ketosteroids represent metabolites of testosterone secreted by the testes, and most of the remaining 17-ketosteroids are derived from steroids generated in the adrenal glands. In women, on the other hand, the 17-ketosteroids are derived almost exclusively from androgens generated in the adrenal glands. The main purpose of measuring these steroid metabolites is to assess androgen production by the adrenal gland. However, in men, a decrease in 17-ketosteroids in the urine may result also from decreased production of testosterone by the testes. Although the urine 17-ketosteroids are sometimes ordered to evaluate male androgenic status, this test does not detect the major androgens—testosterone and DHT. Therefore, if low androgens are suspected, serum testosterone is the preferred test, rather than 17-ketosteroids. Many clinicians now prefer the assessment of serum DHEA-S over urinary 17-ketosteroids for investigation of adrenal androgen production because a 24-hour urine collection is not required and many drugs interfere with the measurement of 17-ketosteroids.

Endocrinologic Disorders Affecting Male Reproduction

Description and Diagnosis

Hypogonadotropic Hypogonadism. Hypogonadotropic hypogonadism in males is associated with absent or decreased function of the testes. If this impairment is manifested early in life, sexual development is retarded. In hypogonadotropic hypogonadism, there is a defect in the hypothalamus or pituitary that reduces normal gonadal stimulation. There are many causes for this abnormality, including pan-hypopituitarism and GnRH deficiency. A deficiency of GnRH in the hypothalamus is responsible for the most common form of hypogonadotropic hypogonadism, and this disorder is known as Kallmann syndrome.

Patients with hypogonadotropic hypogonadism have below normal serum concentrations of LH, FSH, and testosterone. Because there are many causes for the disorder, there is much heterogeneity in the severity of these hormonal deficiencies. A clinical picture of sexual infantilism and low levels of LH, FSH, and testosterone in the serum are characteristic features of hypogonadotropic hypogonadism.

Hypergonadotropic Hypogonadism. This disorder results from a defect in the testes, which may be a result of injury to the testes. There is active stimulation of the testes, but they are unresponsive in this disorder. Apart from testicular injury, aging is among the commonly encountered causes of hypergonadotropic hypogonadism. The disorder can also result from testicular damage from radiation or chemotherapy.

Patients with hypergonadotropic hypogonadism have elevated concentrations of LH and FSH in the presence of decreased levels of testosterone.

Androgen Insensitivity Syndrome (Testicular Feminization Syndrome). Patients with androgen insensitivity syndrome (AIS), as it is now called, have a severe defect in androgen action, with resistance to the masculinizing effect of the androgenic hormones. This results in a female habitus, with breast tissue and a vagina that ends in a blind pouch, and undescended male testes.

The circulating concentration of testosterone in patients with AIS (**Table 22–8**) is normal or elevated for a male. An elevation in testosterone can result in estrogen formation in these individuals because testosterone is a precursor for estrogen. The serum concentration of LH is

Patients with androgen insensitivity syndrome (AIS), as it is now called, have a severe defect in androgen action, with resistance to the masculinizing effect of the androgenic hormones. This results in a female habitus, with breast tissue and a vagina that ends in a blind pouch, and undescended male testes.

TABLE 22–8   **Laboratory Evaluation for Males with Hypogonadism and Complete Androgen Insensitivity Syndrome (AIS)**

Disorder	Laboratory Test Results for LH, FSH, and Testosterone
Hypogonadotropic hypogonadism	Low serum concentrations of LH, FSH, and testosterone
Hypergonadotropic hypogonadism	Elevated serum concentrations of LH and FSH with a low serum concentration of testosterone
Testicular feminization syndrome	Elevated or occasionally normal serum testosterone for a male, with an elevated serum LH

FSH, follicle-stimulating hormone; LH, luteinizing hormone.

increased, presumably because of resistance to the negative feedback of testosterone within the pituitary and hypothalamus.

Impotence. There are many causes for the persistent inability to develop or maintain a penile erection sufficient for intercourse and ejaculation. Although psychogenic impotence is the most common (up to 50%), there are many endocrinologic and non-endocrinologic disorders that are associated with impotence. These include vascular disease, diabetes mellitus, hypertension, neoplasms, and adverse drug effects.

An endocrinologic study of the patient may be pursued by measuring the serum testosterone in the early morning, along with LH and FSH, to assess the hypothalamic–pituitary–male gonadal axis for testosterone production. Chapter 19 has additional discussion of this topic.

> There are many causes for the persistent inability to develop or maintain a penile erection sufficient for intercourse and ejaculation. Although psychogenic impotence is the most common (up to 50%), there are many endocrinologic and non-endocrinologic disorders that are associated with impotence.

Female Physiology and Biochemistry

The ovaries function to produce ova and secrete sex hormones, notably estrogens and progestins. Estrogens maintain the female secondary sex characteristics. They are also essential in the regulation of the menstrual cycle, and breast and uterine growth in the maintenance of pregnancy (see Chapter 20 for a discussion on pregnancy). The estrogens have a major impact on calcium metabolism, and the estrogen depletion associated with menopause results in a loss of bone mineral content. Most of the estrogens in the body are secreted by the ovarian follicles and the corpus luteum. During pregnancy, estrogen is also synthesized in the placenta. Only minute quantities are synthesized by the adrenals. The normal human ovary produces estrogens, progestins, and androgens, but the primary products are estradiol and progesterone. More than 20 different estrogens have been identified. Those with clinical importance are estradiol, also known as E_2; estrone, also denoted as E_1; and estriol that is E_3. Estradiol is derived almost exclusively from the ovaries, and for that reason the serum estradiol level is considered a reflection of ovarian function. In the nonpregnant state, most of the estrogen (microgram quantities) is derived from the ovaries. In pregnant women, the major source of estrogen is the placenta, which secretes estriol as the major product in milligram amounts. Like most other steroid hormones, the vast majority of the circulating estrogen is bound to plasma proteins. More than 95% of circulating estradiol is bound with high affinity to SHBG and, less avidly, to albumin.

Progesterone is a female sex hormone in the progestin family that plays a central role in female reproductive endocrinology. It is involved in regulation of the menstrual cycle and is produced during pregnancy by the placenta. In the nonpregnant state, progesterone is produced largely by the ovary. The adrenal cortex is only a minor source of progesterone production in both sexes, and progesterone is made in very small quantities in the testes in men. More than 90% of the progesterone is protein-bound in the circulation. Progesterone can be metabolized to 3 groups of metabolites, one of which is the pregnanediols. Urinary pregnanediol concentration can be used as an index of endogenous production of progesterone because it correlates with alterations in progesterone synthesis and metabolism.

There is a tightly coordinated feedback system among the hypothalamus, anterior pituitary, and ovaries in adolescent and adult women to regulate menstruation. Each menstrual cycle consists of a follicular and a luteal phase. Day 1 is the first day of menstrual bleeding. The follicular phase is associated with follicle growth and is the first part of the cycle. Ovulation occurs around day 14 of the menstrual cycle, and the luteal phase follows in the last half of the cycle.

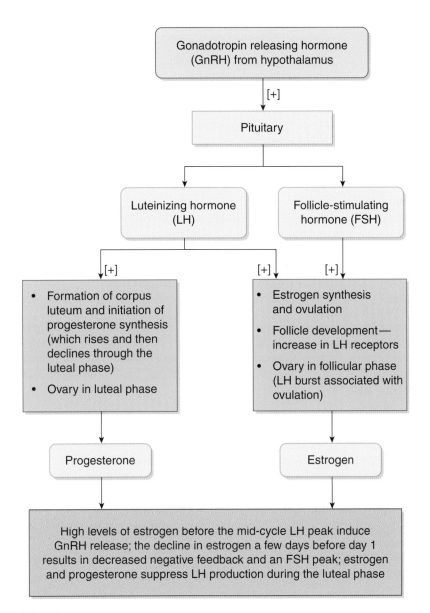

FIGURE 22–10 **The hypothalamic–pituitary–gonadal axis in menstruating females. [+] Stimulation.**

In general, follicular growth in the ovary is stimulated by FSH, and ovulation and progesterone secretion from the developing corpus luteum are driven by LH. During the menstrual cycle:

- FSH increases during the early part of the follicular phase and then declines until ovulation; there is a gradual decrease in FSH through the luteal phase.
- LH secretion increases around the middle of the follicular phase and just before ovulation; estrogen secretion in the follicular phase stimulates the pituitary to release LH in a surge, with the peak value for LH appearing 10 to 12 hours before ovulation.
- The estradiol level increases under the influence of FSH in the follicular phase and rises rapidly as the follicle matures. The estradiol concentration then falls abruptly after ovulation but rises again as the corpus luteum forms in the luteal phase.
- Progesterone is at very low levels during the follicular phase; with the midcycle surge of LH and ovulation, progesterone production begins to increase and reaches a maximum approximately 8 days after the midcycle LH surge. The progesterone then declines to baseline levels at the end of the luteal phase.

Figure 22–10 illustrates the complex relationships in the hypothalamic–pituitary–female gonadal axis.

In general, follicular growth in the ovary is stimulated by FSH, and ovulation and progesterone secretion from the developing corpus luteum are driven by LH.

Laboratory Tests

Estrogens

Serum estrogen levels are represented by the estradiol (E_2) concentration, because estriol (E_3) in a nonpregnant woman is derived almost exclusively from estradiol. In addition, blood estrone (E_1) levels typically parallel estradiol levels throughout the menstrual cycle, but at a lower concentration. Urinary estrogens can be quantitated as total estrogens or as fractionated estrogens with measurement of estradiol, estrone, and estriol. Since estradiol is derived primarily from the ovaries, the estradiol level in the urine can provide a more accurate reflection of ovarian function than total urinary estrogen.

Progesterone

The progesterone concentration in serum is a reflection of progesterone production. Assays for urinary progesterone metabolites are used much less frequently to assess progesterone synthesis than tests for serum progesterone.

Endocrinologic Disorders Affecting Female Reproduction

Description and Diagnosis

Healthy women display considerable variations in the length of the menstrual cycle, but most women have cycles between 25 and 30 days in length. The absence of menstrual bleeding is known as amenorrhea. Primary amenorrhea refers to women who have never menstruated, and secondary amenorrhea refers to women in their reproductive years in whom menstruation was present and then ceased after a variable period.

Primary Amenorrhea. Primary amenorrhea is established if spontaneous regular menstruation has not begun by the age of 16 years, whether or not secondary sex characteristics have developed. The list of causes of primary amenorrhea is lengthy. They include lower genitourinary tract defects such as imperforate hymen; uterine disorders such as endometritis; a host of ovarian disorders—approximately 40% of females with primary amenorrhea have Turner syndrome (45 X karyotype) or pure gonadal dysgenesis (either a 46 XX or XY karyotype); adrenal disorders such as CAH; thyroid disorders, notably hypothyroidism; pituitary–hypothalamic disorders such as hypopituitarism and Kallmann syndrome (which also affects men); and pregnancy.

Because of the long list of possible causes for primary amenorrhea, the diagnostic evaluation varies considerably. Depending on the clinical suspicion, the evaluation may include assays for FSH, LH, estrogen and progesterone, a karyotype to evaluate the patient for cytogenetic abnormalities, and measurements of other serum or urinary hormone concentrations (**Table 22–9**).

Secondary Amenorrhea. Secondary amenorrhea is more common than primary amenorrhea and is the absence of regular menstruation for at least 6 months in a woman who has previously had menses. Oligomenorrhea is present if a woman has less than 9 menstrual cycles per year. The causes of secondary amenorrhea include many of those for primary amenorrhea. However, there are a number of conditions associated with secondary amenorrhea that are independent of primary amenorrhea. Most notably, pregnancy is a common cause of amenorrhea and must be considered first in a patient who has stopped menses. An elevated prolactin concentration, which may be induced by a prolactin-secreting tumor, can produce oligomenorrhea or amenorrhea, presumably by inhibition of the release of LH and FSH by the prolactin. Patients with secondary amenorrhea can be divided into those with and without signs of hirsutism and androgen excess. Hirsutism is the excessive growth of terminal hair in women and in children, in a distribution similar to that which occurs in postpubertal men. Causes of hirsutism may be androgen-dependent, with abnormalities often originating in the ovary or the adrenal gland, or androgen-independent, sometimes from anti-epileptic medications. Adult women with hirsutism and androgen excess may carry a diagnosis of adult onset CAH, ACTH-dependent Cushing syndrome, or polycystic ovary syndrome, among other causes.

Because the list of disorders associated with secondary amenorrhea is even longer than the list associated with primary amenorrhea (**Table 22–9**), the initial evaluation is very broad

Primary amenorrhea refers to women who have never menstruated, and secondary amenorrhea refers to women in their reproductive years in whom menstruation was present and then ceased after a variable period.

TABLE 22–9   Laboratory Evaluation of Women With Amenorrhea

Disorder	Associated Disorders and Potentially Relevant Laboratory Tests
Primary amenorrhea	Turner syndrome and pure gonadal dysgenesis—karyotype analysis
	Congenital adrenal hyperplasia—adrenal hormone and enzyme activity measurements
	Hypothyroidism—selected thyroid hormone assays
	Hypopituitarism—pituitary hormone concentrations in serum
Secondary amenorrhea	Pregnancy—test for hCG
	Prolactin-secreting pituitary tumor—serum prolactin level
	Polycystic ovary syndrome—serum hormone levels and appropriate radiographic studies
	Cushing syndrome—see the section "Hyperfunction Involving Glucocorticoids With or Without Mineralocorticoids: Cushing Syndrome"
	Adult onset congenital adrenal hyperplasia—adrenal hormone and enzyme activity measurements as described in this chapter
	Hypothyroidism and hypopituitarism—as described above for primary amenorrhea

hCG, human chorionic gonadotropin.

until the differential diagnosis is narrowed by the results of physical examination, history, and initial radiographic and laboratory studies. In general, however, if the cause of amenorrhea is unclear, the estrogen status should be determined. The total or free testosterone and DHEA-S should be performed in women with hirsutism or virilization. An elevation of DHEA-S points to an adrenal origin as a cause for the hirsutism. An elevation in testosterone suggests either an adrenal or an ovarian source, or an androgen-secreting tumor outside the adrenal and ovaries.

Infertility and Pregnancy

These topics are presented in Chapter 20.

DISORDERS RELATED TO THE PITUITARY GLAND

Growth Hormone/Anterior Pituitary

Physiology and Biochemistry

Growth hormone (GH) is a major product of the pituitary gland. It is a single chain polypeptide that has structural similarities to prolactin and placental hormones, known as placental lactogens, with which it has overlapping biological activities. GH has secretory spikes, with a half-life of about 20 minutes, which typically occur several hours after meals and exercise. The secretion of GH also rises after the onset of sleep and reaches a peak in deepest sleep. Two hypothalamic factors control the release of GH from the pituitary. Growth hormone-releasing hormone (GHRH) stimulates GH release from the pituitary, and somatostatin (also known as growth hormone-inhibitory hormone or GHIH) inhibits GH release. The larger influence on the release of GH by the pituitary is the inhibitory action of somatostatin. To promote growth, GH in the circulation binds to target tissues, mostly cartilage, bone, and other soft tissues. GH exerts its effects directly, and also through insulin-like growth factors (IGFs) that are produced in the liver and other tissues under the influence of GH. GH has a number of effects on lipid, carbohydrate, and protein metabolism. IGFs, previously known as somatomedins, also have multiple effects on growth promotion and metabolism. There are a number of IGFs. Unlike most other

GH has secretory spikes, with a half-life of about 20 minutes, which typically occur several hours after meals and exercise. The secretion of GH also rises after the onset of sleep and reaches a peak in deepest sleep.

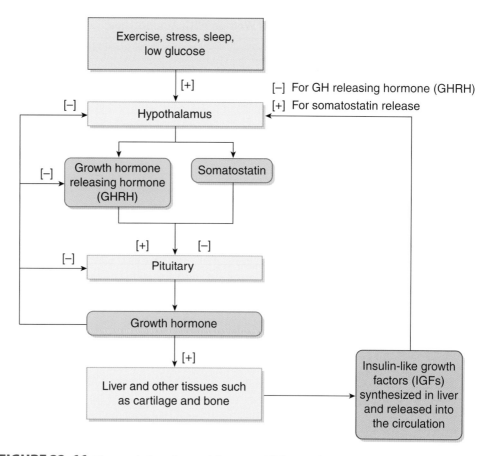

FIGURE 22–11 **The regulation of growth hormone (GH) secretion. [+] Stimulation; [–] Inhibition.**

peptide hormones, IGFs circulate in the blood in a complex with plasma-binding proteins. The hypothalamic–pituitary–GH axis is shown in **Figure 22–11**.

Laboratory Tests

Growth hormone
Most of the assays for GH are performed using serum, because the concentration of GH in urine is approximately 0.1% of that in serum. Human growth hormone exists in the pituitary gland and in the circulation as a heterogeneous mixture of isoforms. The presence of GH variants in serum can lead to discrepant results among the different assays for GH. Even if the assay problems did not exist, a single random level of GH is not usually clinically informative because of the episodic secretion of GH by the pituitary gland. Serum levels between pulses in healthy individuals are extremely low and may not even be detectable. As an alternative, GH secretion can be monitored using a continuous blood sample withdrawal pump or by collecting blood specimens for GH assay as often as every half hour over a 12-hour period. Because of the difficulties in assessment of the GH level created by pulsatile secretion of the hormone, provocative tests have been established to stimulate or suppress GH release as a better assessment of excess or deficient GH (**Table 22–10**). A commonly used stimulation test to assess the adequacy of GH secretion is the insulin tolerance test, which produces a transient hypoglycemia to provoke GH release. One GH suppression test involves the ingestion of an oral glucose load, which in healthy individuals suppresses the serum GH level.

Insulin-like Growth Factors
IGF-I is more GH-dependent and more potent in growth promotion than IGF-II. IGF-II has more insulin-like activity than IGF-I. The immunoassays for IGF-I (previously known as somatomedin C) have little cross-reactivity with IGF-II. IGF-I concentrations are elevated in GH excess and are

Because of the difficulties in assessment of the GH level created by pulsatile secretion of the hormone, provocative tests have been established to stimulate or suppress GH release as a better assessment of excess or deficient GH.

TABLE 22-10 Laboratory Evaluation for Growth Hormone Excess or Deficiency

Laboratory Test	Growth Hormone Excess	Growth Hormone Deficiency
Serum growth hormone (GH)	Single measurements of GH are not often reliable because GH secretion is episodic and other conditions can increase GH secretion; normal individuals have a markedly suppressed GH level in response to an oral glucose load, but patients with acromegaly/gigantism show an increase, no change, or slight decrease in GH level to the same challenge	Because GH may be low in both normal children and GH-deficient patients, it is necessary to show an inadequate rise of serum GH in response to 2 different provocative stimuli
Serum IGF-I	The specific form of IGF known as IGF-I is elevated in nearly all patients with acromegaly/gigantism	Low in most deficient patients, but low in many other clinical conditions as well
Radiology	Sellar enlargement in 90% of cases; if present, a pituitary tumor should be localized; radiographs of the hand show "arrowhead tufting" of distal phalanges and increased width of intra-articular cartilages; feet show similar changes	

GH, growth hormone; IGF, insulin-like growth factor.

low in states of GH deficiency. Therefore, measurement of IGF-I is valuable in assessing children with growth abnormalities for GH excess or deficiency. It is the assay of choice for the diagnosis of acromegaly because it has little variation in blood levels throughout the day, in contrast to GH that has a pulsatile pattern. There are marked differences in serum IGF-I concentration between adults and children, and because of this, it is very important to establish age-related reference ranges.

Growth Hormone Excess—Acromegaly and Gigantism

Description
The most common cause of excess GH production is a chromophobe adenoma of the pituitary gland. Molecular studies have shown that almost 50% of GH excess cases are due to a mutation in the receptor for GHRH. A prolonged excess of GH results in an overgrowth of the skeleton with acral enlargements, as well as overgrowth of the soft tissues, and these are found in 100% of the patients with this condition. In adults, this condition is known as acromegaly. Because GH has an action on the cartilaginous portion of the bone, GH excess in children before long bone growth is completed results in gigantism.

Diagnosis
The most important requirement for diagnosis of GH excess is a demonstration of inappropriate or excessive GH secretion. Because of the episodic secretion of GH, as many as 10% of patients with active acromegaly have a random serum GH level that falls within the normal reference interval. When patients with acromegaly are evaluated in a suppression test, with ingestion of a glucose load, they typically show either no change in the basal level of GH or an increase in the serum GH level; healthy individuals show marked suppression after oral ingestion of the glucose. Active acromegaly also may be detected by an elevated serum IGF-I level, and IGF-I concentrations correlate with the severity of the disease. The serum IGF-I level, even as a random test, correlates with the clinical severity of acromegaly better than the test for glucose-induced suppression of the GH level.

A prolonged excess of GH results in an overgrowth of the skeleton with acral enlargements. In adults, this condition is known as acromegaly. GH excess in children before long bone growth is completed results in gigantism.

Growth Hormone Deficiency

Description
A deficiency of GH may be congenital or acquired. Children who have inadequate GH production or action will not grow to full height. It should be noted that growth retardation is not

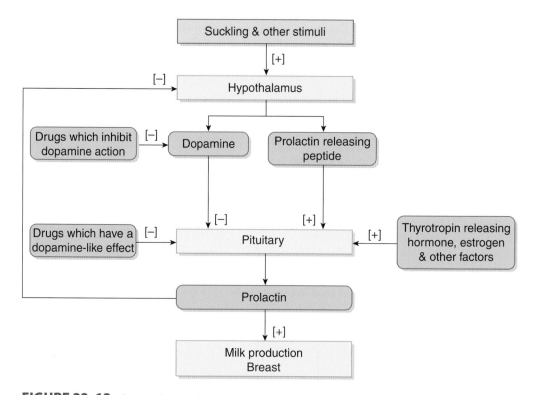

FIGURE 22–12 **The regulation of prolactin secretion. [+] Stimulation; [–] Inhibition.**

usually caused by GH deficiency, but by causes unrelated to GH. However, children with growth retardation with no obvious explanation should be evaluated for a GH deficiency. In children, causes of GH deficiency include anatomic damage to the pituitary or hypothalamus, isolated GH deficiency in the pituitary, and a combination of pituitary hormone deficiencies from a variety of causes. In adults, the most common causes of GH deficiency are pituitary irradiation and a pituitary adenoma that impairs GH secretion. Since adults are usually at full height, GH deficiency is not usually clinically significant.

Diagnosis
The diagnosis of GH deficiency as a cause of growth retardation requires the demonstration of a persistently low GH level in 2 different provocative stimulation tests (**Table 22–10**). The provocations for GH release that can be used include vigorous exercise, deep sleep, and treatment with glucagon, L-DOPA, insulin, arginine, or GHRH. Patients with GH deficiency and growth failure usually have low IGF-I levels. However, there are many other causes for a low IGF-I level besides GH deficiency.

Prolactin/Anterior Pituitary
Physiology and Biochemistry
Prolactin is secreted by the anterior lobe of the pituitary gland. It is a polypeptide with 199 amino acid residues that structurally resembles GH, and is also secreted by cells in the anterior pituitary. Prolactin production is regulated by stimuli from the hypothalamus, but unlike most other anterior pituitary hormones, its release is primarily controlled by inhibition rather than by stimulation (see **Figure 22–12** for the hypothalamic–pituitary–prolactin axis). The primary negative stimulus to the pituitary that limits prolactin secretion is provided by dopamine. There are various stimulatory factors for prolactin release, along with the inhibitory compounds. One stimulatory factor is TRH. Another mechanism to stimulate prolactin release from the pituitary is to decrease the inhibitory effect of dopamine. A number of medications inhibit dopamine action. Prolactin secretion, like that of several other anterior

Prolactin production is regulated by stimuli from the hypothalamus, but unlike most other anterior pituitary hormones, its release is primarily controlled by inhibition rather than by stimulation.

pituitary hormones, is episodic. The lowest levels of prolactin occur at midday, with the highest values shortly after the onset of sleep. The major physiologic stimulus for prolactin release is suckling of the breast. This results in a rise in maternal plasma prolactin levels within minutes to initiate breast feeding. Prolactin controls the initiation and maintenance of lactation only if the breast tissue is appropriately primed by estrogens and other hormones for ductal growth, development of the breast lobular and alveolar system, and the synthesis of specific milk proteins.

Laboratory Tests

Prolactin

As with GH, there is molecular heterogeneity in prolactin with multiple isoforms, which can lead to discrepant results among the immunoassays. The best serum specimen is one that is collected 3 to 4 hours after the subject has awakened. It is important to collect the specimen after an overnight fast, when the patient is still resting, because emotional stress, exercise, ambulation, and protein ingestion all elevate the baseline prolactin level. Multiple sampling may be necessary because of the episodic secretion of prolactin.

Hyperprolactinemia

Description. There are many causes for an elevated prolactin level, 1 of which is a pituitary adenoma. Pregnancy, chronic renal failure, chest wall trauma, primary hypothyroidism, and a host of medications can also elevate prolactin levels. Elevation of the serum prolactin concentration is associated with many different signs and symptoms. In women, these include anovulation, with or without menstrual irregularity, and amenorrhea. Men with prolactin-secreting pituitary adenomas often present with oligospermia, impotence, or both.

Diagnosis. A patient with a prolactin-secreting pituitary adenoma generally has a higher elevation of serum prolactin than someone with hyperprolactinemia from a different cause. Because so many medications can provoke prolactin release, and medications are the most common cause of an elevated serum prolactin level, a medication history is very important. Noteworthy medications that can elevate the serum prolactin level include estrogens, dopamine antagonists such as haloperidol, histamine receptor-blocking agents such as cimetidine, and tricyclic antidepressants.

Hypoprolactinemia

Description and Diagnosis. This condition is not detected unless a woman fails to lactate postpartum. A low prolactin level in a woman in this setting is consistent with hypoprolactinemia.

Antidiuretic Hormone (ADH)/Posterior Pituitary

Physiology and Biochemistry

The posterior pituitary secretes oxytocin and ADH, also known as arginine vasopressin. ADH is a small peptide with 9 amino acids. Oxytocin has a similar structure. Release of hormones from the posterior pituitary into the circulation occurs on stimulation of selected neurons. In the circulation, ADH and oxytocin are usually not bound to carrier proteins.

ADH secretion is regulated by the osmolality of the blood (**Figure 22–13**). Even a small increase in osmolality causes stimulation of ADH release to increase water retention and decrease the serum osmolality toward normal. ADH induces the reabsorption of water in the collecting tubules in the ascending limb of the loop of Henle in the kidney. ADH is also known as vasopressin because in adequate concentrations, it can induce vasoconstriction that increases the blood pressure. A change in blood volume can also alter ADH secretion, as can nonosmotic stimuli such as pain, stress, sleep, exercise, and a variety of pharmacologic compounds. Negative feedback for ADH release is provided by atrial natriuretic peptide. With an increased circulating blood volume or a decreased osmolality, atrial natriuretic peptide concentration increases to decrease ADH release. The osmolality of the plasma also impacts the thirst center to coordinate oral intake of water and conservation of water in the kidney.

Even a small increase in osmolality causes stimulation of ADH release to increase water retention and decrease the serum osmolality toward normal. ADH induces the reabsorption of water in the collecting tubules in the ascending limb of the loop of Henle in the kidney.

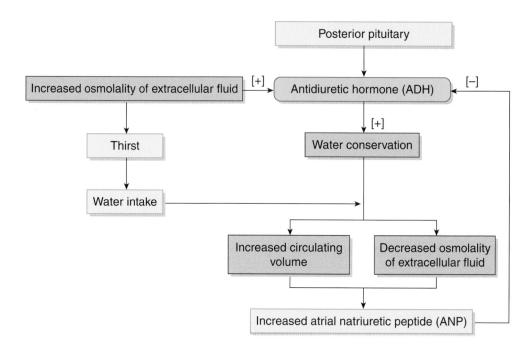

FIGURE 22–13 **The regulation of circulating fluid volume and osmolality. [+] Stimulation; [–] Inhibition.**

Laboratory Tests

Antidiuretic Hormone

ADH can be measured using an immunoassay. ADH is a temperature-sensitive peptide, and plasma testing should be performed within 24 hours after collection. Freezing the specimen stabilizes it for many months.

Serum and urine osmolality

Serum and urine osmolality are measured using a freezing point depression osmometer.

Polyuria

Description. A deficiency of ADH or resistance to the action of ADH results in the failure of the renal tubules to reabsorb water and, as a result, an increased amount of water is lost into the urine. Because urine output is dependent on fluid intake, a normal urine output cannot be defined. However, whenever there is more than 2.5 L of urine generated per day, an investigation for a cause of polyuria is usually indicated.

Polyuria can occur from 3 main causes. The first is deficient production of ADH, as occurs in hypothalamic diabetes insipidus. In this disorder, the pituitary gland fails to secrete normal amounts of ADH in response to stimuli. When the thirst mechanism is normal, increased fluid intake compensates for water lost into the urine and thereby prevents dehydration. Severe dehydration can occur if the thirst center is abnormal, and there is excess water loss into the urine. Neoplastic diseases, neurological surgery, head trauma, ischemia, and autoimmune disorders account for most of the cases of diabetes insipidus originating in the hypothalamus.

The second cause for polyuria is deficient ADH action in the kidney. This is known as nephrogenic diabetes insipidus and it occurs due to insensitivity of the kidneys to respond to ADH.

The third cause of a polyuric state is excessive water intake. This is known as psychogenic or primary polydipsia. In rare cases, hypothalamic disease can affect the thirst center and induce polydipsia. There are also many medications that can affect the thirst center and cause polydipsia.

Diagnosis. The differential diagnosis of a polyuric state is centered on measurements of plasma and urine osmolality and plasma ADH concentration. The first step is to document that polyuria

Polyuria can occur from 3 main causes. The first is deficient production of ADH, as occurs in hypothalamic diabetes insipidus. The second cause for polyuria is deficient ADH action in the kidney. The third cause of a polyuric state is excessive water intake.

TABLE 22–11 Laboratory Evaluation for Disorders of Water Uptake and Excretion

Baseline Disorder	Serum Sodium and Osmolality	Urine Sodium and Osmolality	Serum ADH
SIADH	Low	Normal-high	High
Hypothalamic diabetes insipidus	Normal-high	Low	Low
Nephrogenic diabetes insipidus	Normal-high	Low	Normal-high
Psychogenic polydipsia	Low-normal	Low	Low

SIADH, syndrome of inappropriate antidiuretic hormone secretion.

exists by establishing that the urine volume exceeds 2.5 L/day. Glycosuria must be excluded as a cause of the polyuria, as hyperglycemia with diabetes mellitus is a common cause of polyuria. Patients with hypothalamic diabetes insipidus have a low or inappropriately normal plasma ADH level because the hypothalamus is unable to secrete ADH. Patients with nephrogenic diabetes insipidus have a normal to high plasma level of ADH because the kidney is failing to respond, and the hypothalamus generates excess hormone in an attempt to compensate. Patients with primary polydipsia usually have a low serum ADH level (**Table 22–11**). An increase in urine osmolality of more than 10% in 1 hour following ADH administration indicates hypothalamic diabetes insipidus. The excess ADH promotes reabsorption of water by the kidney, resulting in a decreased urine volume and an increased urine osmolality. A failure to increase urine osmolality on ADH administration suggests nephrogenic diabetes insipidus because the defect in this disorder is a failure of the kidney to respond to ADH.

Syndrome of Inappropriate Antidiuretic Hormone Secretion (SIADH)

Description.
SIADH is an autonomous, sustained synthesis and release of ADH in the absence of stimuli. Thus, the ADH level in the plasma is inappropriately increased relative to the osmolality. There are a number of known causes of SIADH. One of them is production of ADH by a malignant tumor, especially a small cell carcinoma of the lung. In addition, there are a number of medications that stimulate the production of ADH. The patient's blood volume is modestly expanded, and the serum sodium level may be decreased along with plasma osmolality. SIADH is a commonly encountered cause of hyponatremia in hospitalized patients.

Diagnosis.
Patients with SIADH usually have a low serum osmolality, a urine osmolality greater than that of serum, and an elevated urine sodium concentration (**Table 22–11**). There are many causes for hyponatremia other than SIADH, including congestive heart failure, renal insufficiency, nephrotic syndrome, liver cirrhosis, and treatment with medications that stimulate ADH secretion. SIADH is not often assessed by measurement of plasma ADH because the ADH level is not usually necessary to make the diagnosis.

NEOPLASTIC DISORDERS

Multiple Endocrine Neoplasia
Description

MEN is a syndrome most often inherited as an autosomal dominant trait. The MEN syndromes are associated with hyperplasia or tumors in multiple endocrine glands at the same time. There have been many recent advances in the understanding of the genetic basis of the different types of MEN.

SIADH is an autonomous, sustained synthesis and release of ADH in the absence of stimuli. Thus, the ADH level in the plasma is inappropriately increased relative to the osmolality.

- *MEN 1 (Wermer syndrome)*—Multiple endocrine neoplasia type-1 (MEN 1) syndrome involves hyperplasia or neoplasms in 1 or more of the following: the parathyroid gland, the pancreatic islet cells, and the anterior pituitary. In the absence of a family history of the syndrome, however, at least 2 of these 3 sites must be involved for a diagnosis of MEN 1. The hormonal presentation of MEN 1 is highly variable because the pituitary and the pancreatic islet cells in neoplastic states can secrete many different hormones. Although the prevalence is reported to be 20 to 200 per million live births, it is likely to be greatly underestimated because the clinical expression of MEN 1 varies and often presents with mild symptoms. Patients with MEN 1 usually present in the fourth decade of life. MEN 1 has been linked to a gene mutation in the tumor suppressor gene MENIN on chromosome 11.
- *MEN 2 (Sipple syndrome)*—It is the multiple endocrine neoplasia type-2 (MEN 2). The most commonly found abnormality in the MEN 2 syndrome is medullary thyroid carcinoma that occurs in over 95% of patients with MEN 2. Pheochromocytoma develops in over 50% of patients with MEN 2, and parathyroid hyperplasia or adenoma produces hyperparathyroidism in 15% to 30% of patients with MEN 2. MEN 2 includes 3 major phenotypes. Over 90% of the cases of MEN 2 are MEN 2A that includes medullary thyroid carcinoma, pheochromocytoma, and hyperparathyroidism. The familial cases of MEN 2A are most often diagnosed in the third or fourth decade of life. In MEN 2B, parathyroid disease is rare and there are separate developmental abnormalities such as ganglioneuromatosis and marfanoid habitus, in addition to pheochromocytoma and medullary thyroid carcinoma. MEN 2B generally presents 10 years earlier than MEN 2A. It accounts for approximately 5% of all MEN 2 cases. MEN 2B is usually recognized early in life. The child with MEN 2B has a characteristic facial appearance with a failure to thrive, mucosal neuromas, and constipation or diarrhea due to the ganglioneuromatoses in the gut. The diagnosis can be made conclusively by demonstrating the presence of a mutation in the RET proto-oncogene. The RET proto-oncogene product is a receptor tyrosine kinase that transmits growth and differentiation signals. The third form of MEN 2 is familial medullary thyroid carcinoma. In this form of MEN 2, there is no pheochromocytoma and no hyperparathyroidism, only medullary thyroid carcinoma. This disorder has a later onset than MEN 2A or MEN 2B and usually has a good prognosis. The most common clinical presentation in the patient with medullary carcinoma is a mass in the neck. The diagnosis is most often made by histopathologic review of a specimen acquired by fine-needle biopsy.

Multiple endocrine neoplasia type-1 (MEN 1) syndrome involves hyperplasia or neoplasms in 1 or more of the following: the parathyroid gland, the pancreatic islet cells, and the anterior pituitary. The most commonly found abnormality in the MEN 2 syndrome is medullary thyroid carcinoma that occurs in over 95% of patients with MEN 2.

Diagnosis

Because there is such a variety of hormonal abnormalities in MEN 1, many different assays are needed to demonstrate hyperplasia or neoplasms of the parathyroid gland, pancreatic cells, and the anterior pituitary, all of which may be involved in MEN 1. Genetic mutations in the coding sequence of the RET proto-oncogene are found in the vast majority of patients with MEN 2 (both MEN 2A and MEN 2B) and those with isolated familial medullary thyroid carcinoma. Any first-degree relative of a patient carrying an MEN-associated mutation should also be evaluated.

Carcinoid Tumors
Description

Carcinoid tumors are the most common of the endocrine tumors. They are generally found in the wall of the gastrointestinal tract, but also can be found in the pancreas, rectum, ovary, and lung. Tumors originating from the primitive foregut include carcinoid of the bronchus, the stomach, the first portion of the duodenum, and the pancreas. These tumors often secrete 5-hydroxytryptophan, histamine, and other peptides. Carcinoid tumors originating from the primitive midgut are those found in the second portion of the duodenum, the jejunum, the ileum, and the ascending colon. These tumors secrete serotonin, also known as 5-hydroxytryptamine, and other peptides. They are associated with the development of carcinoid syndrome, which is characterized by cutaneous flushing, gastrointestinal hypermotility with diarrhea, heart disease, bronchospasm, myopathy, and increased skin pigmentation. Tumors originating from the primitive hindgut include those of the transverse colon, descending colon, and rectum. These tumors are typically silent because they are usually nonsecretory. Therefore, functioning carcinoid tumors are more likely to be detected if they secrete a compound that has biological activity. The serotonin-secreting carcinoid tumors arising from the primitive midgut or foregut are the ones most often detected. Silent carcinoid tumors are most often discovered incidentally at surgery for other disorders in the gastrointestinal tract. Patients with silent carcinoid tumors may have vague abdominal pain that is either undiagnosed or attributed to irritable bowel syndrome.

Diagnosis

Serotonin (5-hydroxytryptamine) is transported in the blood by platelets. It is metabolized to 5-hydroxyindoleacetic acid (5-HIAA). 5-HIAA is quantitatively the principal metabolite of serotonin, and the majority of it is excreted into the urine and thus used as an indicator of serotonin production. Patients with serotonin-secreting carcinoid tumors of midgut origin usually have markedly elevated levels of urinary 5-HIAA. If there is a borderline concentration of 5-HIAA in a random or 24-hour urine specimen, a repeat collection should be made with an avoidance of foods or medications that might elevate the 5-HIAA level. Only when the 5-HIAA is normal or borderline is the measurement of serotonin needed to document the diagnosis. Platelets contain almost all the serotonin found in the blood and for that reason, the serotonin is measured in whole blood (with platelets) or in platelet-rich plasma.

Functioning foregut tumors may also be detected by the urinary 5-HIAA assay, even though they secrete 5-hydroxytryptophan rather than serotonin. Urinary 5-HIAA is elevated because the 5-hydroxytryptophan released from these tumors is converted to serotonin in other tissues and is subsequently metabolized to 5-HIAA. In addition, urine histamine is generally elevated in patients with functioning foregut carcinoid tumors because these tumors (in contrast to midgut carcinoids) usually produce histamine.

> 5-HIAA is quantitatively the principal metabolite of serotonin, and the majority of it is excreted into the urine and thus used as an indicator of serotonin production. Platelets contain almost all the serotonin found in the blood and for that reason, the serotonin is measured in whole blood (with platelets) or in platelet-rich plasma.

REFERENCES

Ascoli P, Cavagnini F. Hypopituitarism. *Pituitary*. 2006;9:335.

Ayuk J, et al. Growth hormone and its disorders. *Postgrad Med J*. 2006;82:24.

Baylis PH. The syndrome of inappropriate antidiuretic hormone secretion. *Int J Biochem Cell Biol*. 2003;35:1495.

Bertino EM, et al. Pulmonary neuroendocrine/carcinoid tumors: a review article. *Cancer*. 2009;115:4434.

Bhagavath B, Layman LC. The genetics of hypogonadotropic hypogonadism. *Semin Reprod Med*. 2007;25:272.

Bhangoo A, Jacobson-Dickman E. The genetics of idiopathic hypogonadotropic hypogonadism: unraveling the biology of human sexual development. *Pediatr Endocrinol Rev*. 2009;6:395.

Blackwell J. Evaluation and treatment of hyperthyroidism and hypothyroidism. *J Am Acad Nurse Pract*. 2004;16:422.

Bloomfield D. Secondary amenorrhea. *Pediatr Rev*. 2006;27:113.

Boelaert K, Franklyn JA. Thyroid hormone in health and disease. *J Endocrinol*. 2005;187:1.

Bornstein SR. Predisposing factors for adrenal insufficiency. *N Engl J Med*. 2009;360:2328.

Bostwick JR, et al. Antipsychotic-induced hyperprolactinemia. *Pharmacotherapy*. 2009;29:64.

Bronstein MD. Prolactinomas and pregnancy. *Pituitary*. 2005;8:31.

Bryant J, et al. Pheochromocytoma: the expanding genetic differential diagnosis. *J Natl Cancer Inst*. 2003;95:1196.

Carling T. Multiple endocrine neoplasia syndrome: genetic basis for clinical management. *Curr Opin Oncol*. 2005;17:7.

Carrol T, et al. Late-night salivary cortisol for the diagnosis of Cushing's syndrome: a meta-analysis. *Endocr Pract*. 2009;6:1.

Dattani M, Preece M. Growth hormone deficiency and related disorders: insights into causation, diagnosis, and treatment. *Lancet*. 2004;363:1977.

Demers LM, et al. The thyroid: pathophysiology and thyroid function testing. In: Burtis CA, Ashwood ER, Burns DE, eds. *Tietz Textbook of Clinical Chemistry*. 4th ed. Philadelphia: WB Saunders; 2006:1967.

Demers LM, et al. The thyroid: pathophysiology and thyroid function testing. In: Burtis CA, Ashwood ER, Burns DE, eds. *Tietz Textbook of Clinical Chemistry*. 4th ed. Philadelphia: WB Saunders; 2006:2003.

Demers LM, et al. Pituitary function. In; Burtis CA, Ashwood ER, Burns DE, eds. *Tietz Textbook of Clinical Chemistry*. 4th ed. Philadelphia: WB Saunders; 2006:2053.

Doody KM, Carr BR. Amenorrhea. *Obstet Gynecol Clin North Am.* 1990;17:361.

Eastell R, et al. Diagnosis of asymptomatic primary hyperparathyroidism: proceedings of the third international workshop. *J Clin Endocrinol Metab.* 2009;94:340.

Eisenhofer G. Biochemical diagnosis of pheochromocytoma—is it time to switch to plasma-free metanephrines? *J Clin Endocrinol Metab.* 2003;88:550.

Eisenhofer G, et al. Biochemical diagnosis of pheochromocytoma: how to distinguish true- from false-positive test results. *J Clin Endocrinol Metab.* 2003;88:2656.

Fatourechi V. Subclinical hypothyroidism: an update for primary care physicians. *Mayo Clin Proc.* 2009;84:65.

Funder JW, et al. Case detection, diagnosis, and treatment of patients with primary aldosteronism: an Endocrine Society clinical practice guideline. *J Clin Endocrinol Metab.* 2008;93:3266.

Garber JR. *Harvard Medical School Thyroid Disease: Understanding Hypothyroidism and Hyperthyroidism.* Stamford, CT: Harvard Medical School-Consumer Health Publishing Group; 2007:1.

Garcia C, et al. The role of the clinical laboratory in the diagnosis of Cushing syndrome. *Am J Clin Pathol.* 2003;120:S38.

Genazzani AD, et al. Diagnostic and therapeutic approach to hypothalamic amenorrhea. *Ann N Y Acad Sci.* 2006;1092:103.

Gharib H, et al. American Association of Clinical Endocrinologists and Associazione Medici Endocrinologi medical guidelines for clinical practice for the diagnosis and management of thyroid nodules. *Endocr Pract.* 2006;12:63.

Giacchetti G, et al. Management of primary aldosteronism: its complications and their outcomes after treatment. *Curr Vasc Pharmacol.* 2009,7.244.

Giraldi PF. Recent challenges in the diagnosis of Cushing's syndrome. *Horm Res.* 2009;1:123.

Hindié E, et al. 2009 EANM parathyroid guidelines. *Eur J Nucl Med Mol Imaging.* 2009;36:1201.

Ilias I. A clinical overview of pheochromocytomas/paragangliomas and carcinoid tumors. *Nucl Med Biol.* 2008;1:S27.

Layman LC. Hypogonadotropic hypogonadism. *Endocrinol Metab Clin North Am.* 2007;36:283.

Lechan RM. The dilemma of the nonthyroidal illness syndrome. *Acta Biomed.* 2008;79:165.

Maeda SS, et al. Hypoparathyroidism and pseudohypoparathyroidism. *Arq Bras Endocrinol Metab.* 2006;50:664.

Majzoub JA, Srivatsa A. Diabetes insipidus: clinical and basic aspects. *Pediatr Endocrinol Rev.* 2006;1:60.

Marx SJ. Molecular genetics of multiple endocrine neoplasia types 1 and 2. *Nat Rev Cancer.* 2005;5:367.

Master-Hunter T, Heiman DL. Amenorrhea: evaluation and treatment. *Am Fam Physician.* 2006; 73:1374.

Minowada S. Hypogonadism [primary, secondary]. *Nippon Rinsho.* 2006;2:237.

Mulatero P, et al. Differential diagnosis of primary aldosteronism subtypes. *Curr Hypertens Rep.* 2009;11:217.

Mullis PE. Genetics of growth hormone deficiency. *Endocrinol Metab Clin North Am.* 2007; 36:17.

Nakamoto J. Laboratory diagnosis of multiple pituitary hormone deficiencies: issues with testing of the growth and thyroid axes. *Pediatr Endocrinol Rev.* 2009;6:291.

Neumann HP, et al. How many pathways to pheochromocytoma? *Semin Nephrol.* 2002;22:89.

Osamura RY, et al. Pathology of the human pituitary adenomas. *Histochem Cell Biol.* 2008;130:495.

Pecori GF, et al. The dexamethasone-suppressed corticotropin-releasing hormone stimulation test and the desmopressin test to distinguish Cushing's syndrome from pseudo-Cushing's states. *Clin Endocrinol.* 2007;66:251.

Pinchot SN, et al. Carcinoid tumors. *Oncologist.* 2008;13:1255.

Pivonello R, et al. Cushing's syndrome. *Endocrinol Metab Clin North Am.* 2008;37:135.

Practice Committee of American Society for Reproductive Medicine. Current evaluation of amenorrhea. *Fertil Steril.* 2008;90:S219.

Rodgers S, et al. Primary hyperparathyroidism. *Curr Opin Oncol.* 2008;20:52.

Rosano TG, et al. Pituitary function. In: Burtis CA, Ashwood ER, Burns DE, eds. *Tietz Textbook of Clinical Chemistry.* 4th ed. Philadelphia, PA: WB Saunders; 2006:1033.

Rossi GP, et al. Primary aldosteronism: an update on screening, diagnosis and treatment. *Hypertension.* 2008;26:613.

Savage MO, et al. Work-up and management of paediatric Cushing's syndrome. *Curr Opin Endocrinol Diabetes Obes.* 2008;15:346.

Sawka AM. A comparison of biochemical tests for pheochromocytoma; measurement of fractionated plasma metanephrines compared with the combination of 24-hour urinary metanephrines and catecholamines. *J Clin Endocrinol Metab.* 2003;88:553.

Schlechte JA. Clinical practice. Prolactinoma. *N Engl J Med.* 2003;349:2035.

Schmidt L. Diagnosis of adrenal insufficiency: evaluation of the corticotropin-releasing hormone test and basal serum cortisol in comparison to the insulin tolerance test in patients with hypothalamic–pituitary–adrenal disease. *J Clin Endocrinol Metab.* 2003;88:4193.

Silverberg SJ, et al. Presentation of asymptomatic primary hyperparathyroidism: proceedings of the third international workshop. *J Clin Endocrinol Metab*. 2009;94:351.

Sokol RZ. Endocrinology of male infertility: evaluation and treatment. *Semin Reprod Med*. 2009;27:149.

Sowers JR, et al. Narrative review: the emerging clinical implications of the role of aldosterone in the metabolic syndrome and resistant hypertension. *Ann Intern Med*. 2009;150:776.

Steiner BS. Hypogonadism in men. A review of diagnosis and treatment. *Adv Nurse Pract*. 2002;10:22.

Toumpanakis CG, Caplin ME. Molecular genetics of gastroenteropancreatic neuroendocrine tumors. *Am J Gastroenterol*. 2008;103:729.

Vaidya B, et al. Addison's disease. *BMJ*. 2009;339:b2385.

Young DS. *Effects of Drugs on Clinical Laboratory Tests*. 5th ed. Washington, DC: AACC Press; 1990:331.

Young WF. Primary aldosteronism: renaissance of a syndrome. *Clin Endocrinol*. 2007;6:6607.

Index

Page numbers in bold indicate figures and tables.